Textbook of
CHILD NEUROLOGY

JOHN H. MENKES, M.D.

Clinical Professor of Pediatrics, Neurology and Psychiatry
University of California at Los Angeles and
Chief of Neurology—Neurochemistry Laboratory
Brentwood V. A. Hospital

Textbook of

in consultation and with a contribution by

Marcel Kinsbourne, M.D., Ph.D.

Professor of Paediatrics (Neurology), University of Toronto School of Medicine,
Professor of Psychology, University of Toronto

and contributions by

Ulrich Batzdorf, M.D.

Associate Professor of Neurosurgery
University of California at Los Angeles

Ronald S. Gabriel, M.D.

Associate Clinical Professor of Neurology and Pediatrics
University of California at Los Angeles

and

Marvin L. Weil, M.D.

Associate Professor of Neurology and Pediatrics
University of California at Los Angeles
Harbor General Hospital, Torrance, California

CHILD NEUROLOGY

Lea & Febiger · Philadelphia

Reprinted, 1975

Library of Congress Cataloging in Publication Data

Menkes, John H
    Textbook of child neurology.

    1. Pediatric neurology. I. Title.
[DNLM: 1. Nervous system diseases—In infancy and childhood. WS340 M545t 1974]
RJ486.M45   618.9'28   73–20251
ISBN 0–8121–0408–0

Library of Congress Catalog Card Number 73–20251

Published in Great Britain by Henry Kimpton Publishers, London

PRINTED IN THE UNITED STATES OF AMERICA

To My Teachers:

B.G.B.

S.S.G.

A.S.N.

S.C.

D.B.C.

Preface

Even in a textbook, prefaces are written not to be read but rather to blunt inevitable criticisms. One must therefore first ask, why, in view of the existence of several first-rate pediatric neurology texts, was this book ever written. The main excuse for becoming involved in such an undertaking, and for imposing another book upon an already overwhelmed medical audience, is the hope of being able to offer a new viewpoint of the field. More than any other branch of clinical neurology, pediatric neurology has felt the impact of the many recent advances in the neurosciences. Their magnitude becomes evident when the neurologic literature of the last century is read. At that time clinical descriptions achieved a degree of clarity and conciseness, which has not been improved upon, and which at present is only rarely equalled. Yet the reader who finds the explanation of Tay-Sachs disease* offered during the last years of the nineteenth century must experience a sense of achievement at the great strides made during a relatively brief historical period. However, at the same time, one cannot but wonder how many of our "explanations," accepted and taught today, will make as little sense fifty years hence.

* Namely, "an inherited weakness of the central nervous system, especially of the ganglion cells, and a premature degeneration due to exhaustion caused by this."

It is the aim of this text to incorporate some of the knowledge derived from the basic neurologic sciences into the clinical evaluation and management of the child with neurologic disease. Obviously this can only be done to a limited extent. For some conditions the basic sciences have not yet offered any help, while for others, available experimental data only provide tangential information. Even when biochemical or physiologic information is pertinent to the conditions under discussion, their full presentation has been avoided, for to do so with any degree of completeness would require an extensive review of several scientific disciplines, which would go far beyond the intent of the text. The author and his colleagues have therefore chosen to review only aspects of the neurologic sciences with immediate clinical impact, and to refer the reader to the literature for some of the remaining information. They have also deemed it appropriate *not* to include a section on the neurologic examination of children. This subject is extremely well presented by R. S. Paine and T. E. Oppe, *The Neurological Examination of Children,** a work everyone seriously interested in pediatric neurology should read.

In covering the field, extensive use of literature references has been made. These, generally serve one or more of the following purposes:

(1) A classic or early description of the condition.

* London: Wm. Heinemann, 1966.

(2) Background information pertaining to the relevant neurologic sciences.

(3) A current review of the condition.

(4) In the case of some of the rarer clinical entities, the presentation of several key references was preferred to a brief and obviously inadequate summary.

It is hoped that this approach will serve to keep the text reasonably compact, yet allow it to be used as a guide for further reading.

The author is indebted to a number of colleagues for their critical manuscript reviews and suggestions:

Dr. John M. Adams, Department of Pediatrics, UCLA.

Dr. Barbara F. Crandall, Division of Genetics, UCLA.

Dr. Theodore L. Munsat, Department of Neurology, University of Southern California.

Dr. Robert C. Neerhout, Department of Pediatrics, UCLA.

Dr. Gerhard Nellhaus, Division of Pediatric Neurology, University of Colorado School of Medicine.

Dr. James B. Peter, Department of Medicine, UCLA.

Dr. Alvin D. Sidell, Barrows Neurological Institute, Phoenix, Arizona.

Dr. Richard E. Stiehm, Department of Pediatrics, UCLA.

The Brain Information Service, UCLA, provided valuable assistance in literature retrieval.

JOHN H. MENKES, M.D.
Los Angeles, California

Contents

Metabolic Diseases of the Nervous System

CHAPTER 1

While the diseases considered in this chapter are various in both their clinical and pathologic aspects, their genetic transmission implies that they are directly or indirectly the results of inborn enzymatic defects.

Over the past twenty years the number of disorders to which we are able to assign a known enzymatic lesion has increased strikingly. Even so, they are relatively uncommon, and their importance lies, in part, in the insight they offer into the normal development and function of the human nervous system. In some of the metabolic disorders such as sucrosuria,[1] cystathioninuria,[2] or hyperprolinemia,[3] the association of a neurologic disturbance may be fortuitous and merely the result of subjecting retarded children, a highly selected group, to biochemical examination. A survey of the normal adult population for the presence of inborn errors of metabolism is needed to determine which of these conditions represent harmless metabolic variants.

For practical purposes, the metabolic disorders are divided into five groups:

1. Disorders of amino acid metabolism associated with neurologic symptoms
2. Disorders in amino acid transport
3. Disorders of carbohydrate metabolism
4. Disorders of lipid metabolism
5. Other metabolic disorders

DISORDERS OF AMINO ACID METABOLISM

PHENYLKETONURIA

Phenylketonuria is an inborn error of metabolism manifested by the inability of the body to convert phenylalanine to tyrosine; it produces a clinical picture highlighted by mental retardation, seizures, and imperfect hair pigmentation.

Følling in 1934[4] first called attention to the condition in a report of 10 mental defectives who excreted large amounts of phenylpyruvic acid. The disease has been found in all parts of the world, although it is rare in Negroes or in Jews of European descent. Its frequency in the general population of the United States, as determined by screening programs, is approximately 1 in 14,000.[5] Among mentally defective individuals the frequency of the condition, as determined by surveys such as that of Jervis,[6] is approximately 1 in 200.

The genetics of phenylketonuria have been well-studied. Jervis[6] found that of 1094 siblings of phenylketonurics, 433 (40 percent) were affected. When statistically corrected for uncounted families of heterozygous parents with only normal children, the percentage of affected children of heterozygous parents becomes 27 percent, a close approximation to the 25 percent expected for an autosomal recessive condition.

Biochemical Pathology

Jervis,[7] Udenfriend and Bessman,[8] and Wallace et al.[9] have proved the metabolic defect responsible for phenylketonuria to be an inability to convert phenylalanine to tyrosine (Fig. 1–1).

In man phenylalanine is an essential dietary constituent and is necessary for protein synthesis. In mammals, the conversion of phenylalanine to tyrosine is irreversible, and the latter cannot replace phenylalanine in a minimal diet. Kaufman and Levenberg have found that phenylalanine hydroxylase, the enzyme mediating this step, can be fractionated into two protein components, differing in their heat lability.[10] Enzyme I, the heat labile fraction found in liver, kidney, and pancreas but not brain,[11] is deficient in the classic form of phenylketonuria. It has been found to exist in the form of two isozymes in human fetal liver, and as three isozymes in adult rat liver.[12] The heat stable enzyme II, dihydropteridine reductase, is present in normal amounts (Table 1–1). The hydroxylation of phenylalanine also requires reduced pyridine nucleotide (NADPH), reduced iron, oxygen, and a dihydrobiopterin.[13] The cofactor is converted to a tetrahydropteridine in the dihydro-

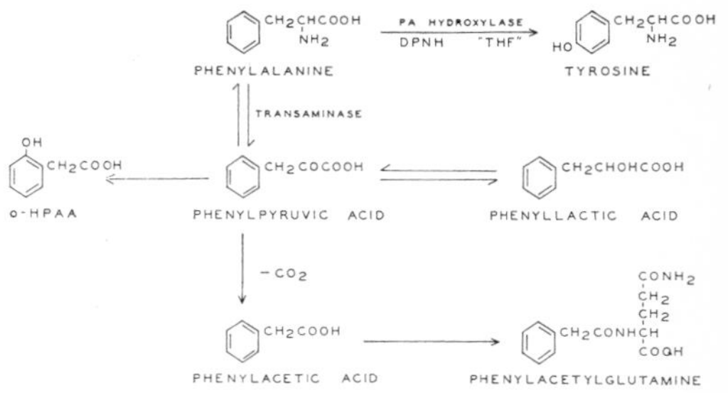

Fig. 1–1. Phenylalanine metabolism. The hydroxylation of phenylalanine to tyrosine is blocked in phenylketonuria. All the intermediary metabolites depicted above have been found in urine or blood.

pteridine reductase catalyzed reaction. Reduced tetrahydropteridine participates directly in the hydroxylation of phenylalanine,[14] and the addition of reduced pteridine, oxygen, and phenylalanine to the enzymes occurs sequentially.[15]

The reaction as proposed by Kaufman is set forth in Figure 1–2.[16] As expected from this mechanism, amethopterin or other folic acid antagonists inhibit the conversion of phenylalanine to tyrosine in both animals and humans.[17] Due to a partial deficiency of the cofactor and probably also of fraction II, phenylalanine hydroxylase activity in human fetal liver is less than in the adult.[18] The enzyme activity reaches adult levels by the third to twelfth day, but until then serum

TABLE 1-1.
THE ENZYMATIC DEFECT IN PHENYLKETONURIA*

Additions	Enzyme Activity ($\Delta\mu$mol of tyrosine/60 min)			
	Phenylketonurics		Normals	
	Case 1 (Age-3 yr)	Case 2 (Age-5 yr)	Case 1 (Age-8 yr)	Case 2 (Age-15 yr)
Liver homogenate	0.020	0.018	0.069	0.059
Liver homogenate + cofactor	0.022	0.026	0.165	0.177
Liver homogenate + enzyme I	0.310	0.078		
Liver homogenate + enzyme I + cofactor	0.618	0.480	0.661	0.560
Liver homogenate + enzyme II	0.020	0.020	0.070	0.068
Liver homogenate + enzyme II + cofactor	0.021	0.018	0.169	0.157
Enzyme I + enzyme II + cofactor	0.700	0.550	0.448	0.355

The liver homogenates from patients with phenylketonuria are compared with those from normal subjects with respect to the ability to hydroxylate phenylalanine to tyrosine.

* From Kaufman.[16]

phenylalanine levels are somewhat higher than those of older infants or adults (up to 7.5 mg% contrasted with a normal range of 1.0 to 2.5 mg%).[19] This transitory defect in phenylalanine hydroxylation is even more pronounced in premature infants.[20]

Phenylketonuric children are born with only slightly elevated phenylalanine blood levels, but due to the absence of phenylalanine hydroxylase activity, the amino acid derived from food proteins accumulates in serum and cerebrospinal fluid and is excreted in large quantities. In lieu of the normal degradative pathway, phenylalanine is converted to phenylpyruvic acid, phenylacetic acid, and phenylacetylglutamine (Fig. 1–1).

The transamination of phenylalanine to phenylpyruvic acid is sometimes deficient for the first few days of life, and the age when phenylpyruvic acid may be first detected varies from 2 to 34 days. From the first week of life on, o-hydroxyphenylacetic acid is also excreted in large amounts.[21] This derivative is formed in liver and kidney from phenylpyruvic acid, the conversion requiring ascorbic acid and an enzyme related to p-hydroxyphenylpyruvic acid oxidase.[22,23]

Liver contains sufficient phenylpyruvic acid hydroxylase to convert all of the phenylpyruvic acid formed by transamination of phenylalanine to o-hydroxyphenylacetic acid, and any phenylpyruvic acid in urine is probably formed in muscle, brain, or heart.[23a]

The abnormal concentration of metabolites in serum and urine is depicted in Table 1–2.[24,25,26]

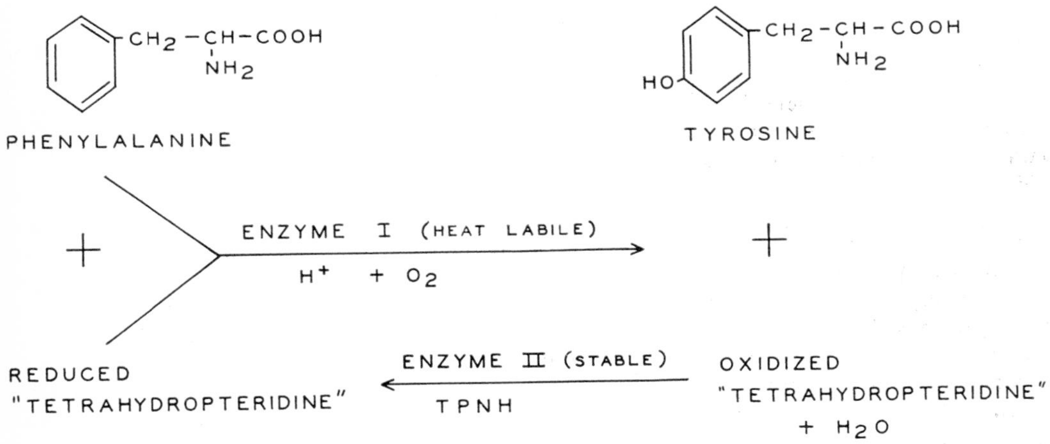

Fig. 1–2. Mechanism of phenylalanine hydroxylation. The thermolabile factor (enzyme I) is deficient in phenylketonuria. Enzyme II, dihydropteridine reductase, reconverts the quininoid or oxidized form of the pteridine to tetrahydropteridine.

TABLE 1-2.

CONCENTRATION OF PHENYLALANINE METABOLITES IN PHENYLKETONURICS*

	Phenylketonurics		Normals	
	Serum	Urine	Serum	Urine
Phenylalanine	15–100+ mg/100 ml	0.4 gm/24 hr	0.84–2.64 mg/100 ml	18 mg/24 hr
Phenylpyruvic acid	0.31–1.78 mg/100 ml	0.7–2.8 gm/24 hr	Appr 0	Appr 0
o-Hydroxyphenylacetic acid	—	0.1–0.4 gm/24 hr	—	<1 mg/24 hr

* Compiled from Jervis,[24] LaDu and Michael,[25] and Armstrong et al.[26]

In addition to the disruption of phenyl-alanine metabolism, tryptophan and tyrosine also are handled abnormally. Large amounts of indolyl-3-lactic acid, indolyl-3-acetic acid, indolyl-3-pyruvic acid, and indican have been found in the urine.[27,28,29] Conversely, the levels of 5-hydroxytryptamine (serotonin) in serum and of 5-hydroxyindolylacetic acid in urine are decreased.[30]

In vitro studies and work on phenylalanine loaded rats suggest that this alteration in 5-hydroxyindole production is the result of an inhibition of 5-hydroxytryptamine synthesis at as many as three different sites.[31]

Intestinal transport of L-tryptophan and tyrosine is impaired in phenylketonuria, and fecal tryptophan and tyrosine content is increased. These abnormalities are reversed following dietary correction of the plasma phenylalanine levels.[32]

Miyamoto and Fitzpatrick have suggested that a similar interference may occur in the oxidation of tyrosine to dihydroxyphenylal-anine (DOPA), a melanin precursor, and may be responsible for the deficiency of hair and skin pigment in phenylketonuric individuals.[33]

Pathologic Anatomy

The pathology of phenylketonuria has been incompletely defined on account of uncertainty as to which of the cerebral lesions are due to the basic disease and which are the outcome of anoxia accompanying seizures.

The alterations within the brain are non-specific, usually confined to white matter, and probably progress in severity with increasing age. They are of three types:

1. Interference with the normal maturation of the central nervous system. Impaired cortical layering, delayed outward migration of neuroblasts, and heterotopic gray matter may be observed.[34,35] These changes suggest a period of abnormal brain development during the last trimester of gestation (Fig. 1–3).

2. Defective myelination. This may be generalized or limited to those areas where one may expect postnatal myelin deposition. Except in some of the older patients, products of myelin degeneration are unusual[36] (Fig. 1–4).

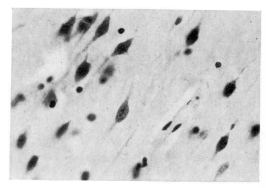

Fig. 1–3. Phenylketonuria. Cresyl violet stained section showing spindle-shaped immature neuron in the center of the field. These cytoarchitectural abnormalities are nonspecific. Together with the convolutional abnormalities they indicate a developmental arrest. × 350. (Courtesy of Dr. N. Malamud, Langley Porter Neuropsychiatric Institute, San Francisco, California.)

3. Cystic degeneration of gray and white matter. Lacking electron microscopic examination it is not known whether the cysts represent dilatation of the glial cells or of the myelin sheath.

In addition to the above, pigmentation of the substantia nigra and locus caeruleus is diminished or absent. As these areas are normally pigmented in albinos and as tyrosinase activity cannot be demonstrated in normal neurons within the substantia nigra,[37] this is not a result of tyrosinase inhibition by phenylalanine or its derivatives. Rather neuromelanogenesis in the phenylketonuric patient must be interrupted at some other metabolic point, such as the metal-catalysed pseudoperoxidation of dopamine derivatives probably responsible for the melanization of substantia nigra lipofuscin.[37]

The association of ulegyria or micro-polygyria with phenylketonuria has been considered to be coincidental, or the result of prolonged seizures.

Clinical Manifestations

Phenylketonuric infants appear normal at birth. During the first two months of life, vomiting—which may even be projectile—and irritability are frequent. By four to nine months delayed intellectual development becomes apparent.[38] In the classic case, men-

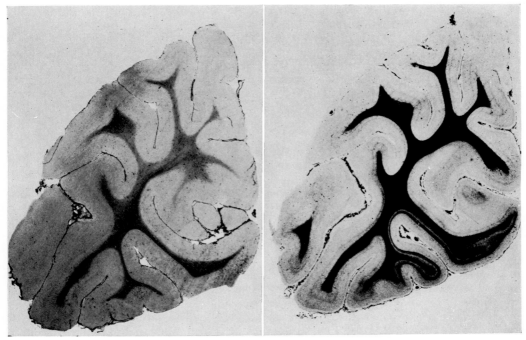

Fig. 1–4. Phenylketonuria. Myelin preparation to show relative reduction in volume of white matter in occipital lobe as compared to normal brain of corresponding age (right). In this brain there was no evidence of demyelination. × 2.5. (Courtesy of Dr. L. Crome, Queen Mary's Hospital for Children, Carshalton, Surrey, England.)

tal retardation may be severe, precluding speech and toilet training. Children in this category have an intelligence quotient below 50. Seizures are common in the more severely retarded. These usually start before 18 months of age and may cease spontaneously. During infancy they may take the form of infantile spasms, later changing into grand mal attacks.

The typical child is blond and blue-eyed, with normal and often pleasant features. The skin is rough and dry, and there may be eczema. A peculiar musty odor, attributable to phenylacetic acid, may suggest the diagnosis. Significant neurologic abnormalities are rare. Microcephaly may be present, as well as a mild increase in muscle tone, particularly in the lower extremities. The plantar response is often variable or extensor.

Older children are quite restless and hyperactive; they are prone to repetitive movements of body and hands. We have observed intellectual deterioration in several of our patients—the outcome of the institutional environment or a function of the natural history of the disease.

A variety of electroencephalographic abnormalities has been found, but hypsarrhythmic patterns, recorded even in the absence of seizures, and single and multiple foci of spike and polyspike discharges are the most common.[39,40]

Untreated phenylketonuria is not invariably accompanied by intellectual deficit. There are a number of individuals with intelligence quotients above 90 who have the classical biochemical picture of phenylketonuria.[41,42]

On theoretical grounds individuals heterozygous for phenylketonuria are considered to have a partial deficiency of phenylalanine hydroxylase. According to Perry[43] fasting phenylalanine levels and phenylalanine-tyrosine ratios determined spectrophotometrically tend to be higher in heterozygotes than in normal subjects. Criteria for diagnosing a heterozygote are a fasting serum phenyl-alanine level of 1.80 mg% or higher and a phenylalanine-tyrosine ratio greater than 1.60. While such criteria may serve to dis-tinguish a group of heterozygotes from a group of normal individuals, it is doubtful whether the genotype of a given subject can be ascer-tained by either fasting amino acid levels or the response to a phenylalanine load.

Heterozygous mothers may have abnormal plasma phenylalanine levels during the latter part of pregnancy and following delivery. In at least one instance, a plasma phenylalanine value of 13.0 mg% (upper limit of normal: 2.5 mg%) was recorded at 32 weeks' gesta-tion.[44]

Although the incidence of spontaneous abortions is high, a number of phenyl-ketonuric women have had children; most of the offspring, although heterozygotes, showed pre- and postnatal growth retardation, micro-cephaly, severe intellectual delay, and, in a few instances, major congenital malforma-tions. It seems likely that the high amino acid level in the pregnant phenylketonuric mother may damage the fetus.[41,45,46]

Since a diet restricted in phenylalanine may induce nutritional deficiencies as detri-mental to the fetus as phenylketonuria, it is best to advise phenylketonuric mothers against having children.

The pathogenesis for mental retardation in phenylketonuria is still unclear.[31] It is likely that no single factor is responsible, but rather that impairment of amino acid transport across the blood-brain barrier, defective proteolipid protein synthesis, impaired my-elination, and low levels of neurotransmitters such as serotonin are responsible to varying degrees.[47,47a]

Diagnosis

The diagnosis of phenylketonuria can be suspected from the clinical features of the disease and from the examination of the patient's urine by means of the ferric chloride test.[48]

Add three to five drops of 10 percent ferric chloride to 1 cc of urine without prior acidification. Note the color change which occurs immediately and over the subsequent three to four minutes. Phenylpyruvic acid turns the urine an emerald green, which fades in 20 to 40 minutes. The reaction probably involves the formation of an enol tautomer, which becomes conjugated with the ferric salt. An even more transient green is produced by urines containing p-hydroxy-phenylpyruvic acid. By contrast, the green-brown color seen in most urines from patients with histidinemia is permanent.[49] The urine in maple syrup disease sometimes yields a navy blue color with this reagent.

When there are ketones or salicylates in the urine, addition of ferric chloride yields a purple color. Phenothiazines, isoniazid, and high concentrations of epinephrine produce a green color.

In adequately preserved specimens, phenyl-pyruvic acid decomposes to benzaldehyde, and the ferric chloride test becomes negative. The addition of a dilute solution of 2,4-dinitro-phenylhydrazine produces a copious yellow precipitate in both fresh and old specimens. Initial confirmatory evidence may be ob-tained by finding an elevation of plasma phenylalanine levels or an abnormal phenyl-alanine tolerance curve. For routine screen-ing a simple stick test (Phenistix) is available for use both in urine and on wet diapers.

As mentioned previously, plasma phenyl-alanine levels are elevated in the cord blood of phenylketonurics and rise rapidly within a few hours of birth. Inasmuch as there may be a delay in the appearance of phenyl-pyruvic acid, the ferric chloride and 2,4-dinitrophenylhydrazine tests are inadequate during the neonatal period. A screening pro-gram involving microbiologic or spectro-fluorometric estimation of blood phenyl-alanine levels has therefore been suggested.[50,51]

Blood from a skin puncture is spotted on a piece of thick filter paper and mailed to a central laboratory where the phenylalanine content is measured by its effectiveness in overcoming growth inhibition of *Bacillus subtilis* (A.T.C.C. 6051) by 2-thienylalanine, or is determined spectrofluorometrically after the formation of a phenylalanine-ninhydrin-copper complex, the fluorescence of which is enhanced by L-leucyl-L-alanine.[51] While this method has wide applicability, false-positive results occur with a frequency of 1/2100.[52] Some of these are due to a delay in the induction of phenylalanine hydroxylase, while the rest are hyperphenylalaninemias to be discussed below.

False-negative tests may be expected in phenylketonuric infants tested prior to the institution of a normal caloric intake.

Hyperphenylalaninemia

The widespread use of screening programs to detect the newborn infant whose blood phenylalanine concentration is higher than normal has uncovered several other conditions characterized by elevated blood phenylalanine levels during the neonatal period.

TABLE 1-3.

CONDITIONS EXHIBITING ELEVATED BLOOD PHENYLALANINE

Conditions	Biochemical Findings
Phenylketonuria	Blood PA* 20 mg/100 ml or higher Urine positive for PPA,† o-HPAA‡ Tyrosine levels low normal
Phenylalaninemia (type II)	Blood PA variable, normal to above 20 mg/100 ml Excretion of PPA and o-HPAA inappropriately low for serum PA concentrations
Phenylalaninemia (type III)	Blood and urine findings identical to classic PKU. Defect becomes less marked with increasing age, but ability to handle phenylalanine is never normal
Phenylalaninemia (type IV) (atypical PKU)	Blood PA below 20 mg/100 ml on normal diet. PPA and o-HPAA excretions correlated with blood levels. Tyrosine levels normal
Phenylalaninemia of premature and immature infants	Tyrosine levels much higher than PA levels. FeCl₃ positive because of presence of p-hydroxyphenylpyruvic acid in urine Defect is transient

* PA   phenylalanine.
† PPA   phenylpyruvic acid.
‡ o-HPAA   o-hydroxyphenylacetic acid.

Their clinical and biochemical characteristics are summarized in Table 1-3.

Aside from phenylketonuria, phenylalaninemia—type IV (Table 1-3) appears to be the most common variant and has previously been termed "atypical phenylketonuria."[53,54] Patients have an impaired ability to convert phenylalanine to tyrosine, but on a normal protein intake their phenylalanine levels range between 7 mg/100 ml and 20 mg/100 ml. Fasting blood levels in parents have been normal, but tolerance tests have often been abnormal in one of the two parents. The gene distribution of this entity differs from that of phenylketonuria, with a relatively high prevalence among Jews of European descent. This is probably a different genetic disorder, transmitted as an autosomal dominant trait; or possibly these patients are homozygous for a third allele at the phenylalanine locus.[55,56] Hepatic phenylalanine hydroxylase activity ranges between 1/10 and one-half of control values in the presence of added tetrahydropteridine.[54]

Less commonly a defect in phenylalanine hydroxylation is coupled with a temporary or permanent abnormality of phenylalanine transamination (phenylalaninemia, type II, Table 1-3).[57] In these patients the excretion of phenylpyruvic and o-hydroxyphenylacetic acids is inappropriately low for the serum phenylalanine concentrations and the ferric chloride test is negative on a normal diet; it may become slightly positive during an acute phenylalanine load. In another variant (phenylalaninemia, type III) the phenylalanine tolerance improves gradually over the first few months of life, but while the ability to metabolize phenylalanine is greater than in phenylketonuria, it is never normal. No enzymatic studies have been performed on this variant.

In addition, elevated blood phenylalanine levels were observed in 25 percent of premature infants and in an occasional full term newborn. In all these patients tyrosine levels were increased to a much greater extent.[20] In view of the existence of several other entities associated with elevated blood phenylalanine, phenylketonuria can only be diagnosed if the following criteria are satisfied:[52]

1. Blood phenylalanine concentrations ex-

ceed 20 mg/100 ml within seven days following birth, but blood tyrosine levels remain normal or lower than normal (2.5 mg/100 ml).

2. In untreated infants, the urinary ferric chloride tests are positive by 2 to 36 days of age. Phenylpyruvic acid and o-hydroxyphenylacetic acid are excreted when the blood phenylalanine concentrations are above 10–15 mg/100 ml.

3. When the infant is temporarily returned to a normal diet between 4 and 9 months of age, the blood phenylalanine concentration rises to 20 mg/100 ml or higher and he begins to excrete phenylpyruvic and o-hydroxyphenylacetic acids.

4. After an acute phenylalanine load, the blood tyrosine concentration does not rise. The blood phenylalanine concentration increases and remains markedly elevated for one or more days.

The distinction between phenylketonuria and phenylalaninemia is more than academic. Children with phenylalaninemia do not fare well on dietary therapy. Phenylalanine levels tend to fall precipitously, and side reactions such as hypoglycemia and symptoms of protein deficiency are prone to develop. These have been known to induce intellectual retardation and other neurologic symptoms.[58]

Treatment

The generally accepted therapy for phenylketonuria restricts the dietary intake of phenylalanine. A commercially available casein hydrolysate from which phenylalanine has been removed by absorption on charcoal is the sole source of amino acids. Generally, patients tolerate this diet quite well, and within one to two weeks the concentration of phenylalanine in serum becomes normal. Various complications of dietary treatment, all due to insufficient intake of phenylalanine, include x-ray evidence of osteoporosis, cupping of the long bones, and spicule formation in the metaphyses, hypoglycemia,[59] megaloblastic anemia,[60] cutaneous lesions, and poor weight gain. There is some evidence that prolonged nutritional deprivation during infancy interferes with intellectual development.[61] To avoid these symptoms of amino acid deficiency, enough milk is added to the

diet to keep serum levels of the amino acid between 4 mg% and 15 mg%.[61] A recent retrospective study indicates that the critical level of phenylalanine may even be higher than 15 mg/100 ml and suggests that severe dietary restrictions may not be required.[58a] Samples of low phenylalanine menus are given by Centerwall.[62] Frequent serum phenylalanine determinations are essential to insure adequate regulation of diet. Since urinary phenylpyruvic acid becomes minimal at or below serum phenylalanine levels of 15 mg% to 20 mg%, both the ferric chloride and the 2,4-dinitrophenylhydrazine tests are quite unreliable for this purpose. As restriction of phenylalanine intake has definite inherent risks, the criteria for initiating treatment of infants with phenylalanine elevation now need reevaluation. Infants whose phenylalanine levels remain below 20 mg% on a normal protein intake (phenylalaninemia, type IV) do not become retarded [5,52,63,64] and there is no justification for their treatment.

At present we have insufficient evidence for or against the need of treating children whose phenylalanine blood level is higher than 20 mg%, but who do not excrete phenylpyruvate (phenylalaninemia, type II). Restriction of dietary phenylalanine is therefore indicated for these patients.

In addition, the author has made it a practice to reinstate briefly a normal protein intake during the latter part of the first year of life in all patients receiving a restricted phenylalanine diet. In a significant percentage of infants who initially had a blood phenylalanine concentration of 20 mg/100 ml or higher, amino acid levels did not rise when a normal diet was given for a 72-hour period three months following diagnosis.[63]

When the patient with classic phenylketonuria is maintained on a low phenylalanine diet, seizures disappear and the EEG tends to revert to normal. Abnormally blond hair regains its natural color.

The effects on mental ability are, unfortunately, less clear-cut. Studies prior to 1965 suggested that, as a group, infants whose treatment was started before six months achieved higher developmental quotients than those started at a later age.[65] However, about 30 percent of infants placed on a diet shortly after birth have phenylalaninemia type IV, which does not lead to mental retardation; therefore this represents a different population from those children who present for treatment at a later age with high phenylalanine levels and neurologic symptoms.[66,67] Fuller and Shuman[68] have found that treated phenylketonuric children fall into a tri-modal distribution with respect to their Binet intelligence quotient or Gesell language-adaptive quotient. In their experience neither the age at which therapy was initiated nor the degree of dietary control determined into which of the three groups a given child would fall. However, patients who were started on treatment prior to six months, some of whom may have had phenylalaninemia, were represented only in the two higher performance modes.

In most of the other studies some deficit in IQ has been found in infants treated at an early age, as compared to their parents and unaffected siblings. Even when the measured IQ is normal, neuropsychologic handicaps which result in poorer school progress than would be predicted from the IQ alone—are common.[69] Minor structural malformations of the central nervous system may well be responsible for this difference[34] (Fig. 1–3). In some instances, prenatal brain damage may lower the IQ, while in others normal intellectual development may be possible in the absence of any dietary management. Finally, in a third group dietary treatment may be beneficial when phenylalanine concentrations are maintained sufficiently high to allow normal protein synthesis. In a few instances treatment may even result in some clinical improvement when instituted later than infancy. However, it should be kept in mind that evaluation of the effectiveness of treatment for older children is complicated by the placebo effect of increased medical and parental interest in a child who previously has only been "mentally retarded." As yet we have no way of ascertaining into which of the three groups a given patient will fall.

The duration of treatment is also controversial, and various centers have advocated terminating dietary restrictions at 4, 9, or even 15 years of age.[69,70,70a] However, discontinuation of the low phenyl-

alanine diet is followed by a decrement in performance for those children who have been under strict dietary control (phenylalanine levels 2–9 mg%) prior to discontinuing treatment, and by no significant decrement for those who were under looser control (phenylalanine levels over 9 mg%).[71]

Frequent clinical and development follow-up examinations are advisable once patients are returned to a regular diet.[69]

The marked hyperactivity of phenylketonurics, which often presents a problem to both parents and institutions, may respond to very large doses of chlorpromazine (up to 10 to 20 mg/kg/day).

HEREDITARY TYROSINEMIA

This is an inherited disorder associated with a partial deficiency of several hepatic enzymes, including the methionine activating enzyme, cystathionine synthase, tyrosine transaminase, and p-hydroxyphenylpyruvic acid oxidase.[72] It leads to an elevation of serum tyrosine and methionine, renal rickets, hepatic cirrhosis, and severe growth retardation, but experience to date has indicated that the nervous system is usually spared.

MAPLE SYRUP URINE DISEASE

This condition is a familial cerebral degenerative disease due to a defect in branched-chain amino acid metabolism and characterized by the passage of urine possessing a sweet, maple-syrup-like odor. It was first described in 1954 by Menkes and others.[73] Since then, numerous other cases have been diagnosed throughout the world. The disease occurs in both Caucasian and Negro infants and is transmitted by an autosomal recessive gene.

Biochemical Pathology

The disease is characterized by the accumulation of three branched-chain keto acids: alpha-ketoisocaproic acid (KICA), alpha-ketoisovaleric acid (KIVA), and alpha-keto-beta-methylvaleric acid (KMA), the derivatives of leucine, valine, and isoleucine, respectively.[74] Their accumulation suggests a defect in oxidative decarboxylation of branched-chain ketoacids (Fig. 1–5).

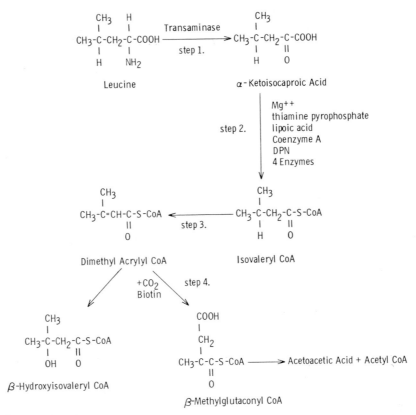

Fig. 1–5. Degradation of leucine in mammalian tissues. In maple syrup urine disease the metabolic block is located at step 2. In isovaleric acidemia the block is confined to step 3. A rare entity with a possible metabolic block at step 4 has also been reported.

In mammalian tissue at least two specific enzymes are required for the decarboxylation of the three branched-chain ketoacids.[75] The enzyme system for oxidative decarboxylation of KICA and KMA is found in hepatic mitochondria, and can also be demonstrated in human leukocytes.[76,77] Dehydrogenation of KIVA requires a second, biochemically distinct, enzyme. Fibroblasts from patients with maple syrup disease have a marked reduction in the ability to decarboxylate all three branched-chain amino acids.[77] The alpha-keto acid dehydrogenase complexes from mammalian sources have been reviewed by Reed.[78] In maple syrup disease a single gene defect affects more than one enzyme. The probability is small that in mammals two enzymes governing related biochemical reactions are located on one operon, for even in microorganisms operon linkage is restricted to sequential reactions within a metabolic pathway. A more likely explanation is that the two or three enzymes affected in maple syrup disease have a common polypeptide chain which is under the control of a single gene. As a consequence of the defect, the aforementioned keto acids accumulate in serum and cerebrospinal fluid and are excreted in large quantities in urine.[79] Plasma levels of the respective amino acids (viz., leucine, isoleucine, and valine) are elevated secondary to the rise in keto acid concentrations. Alloisoleucine, probably formed by transamination of KMA, has also been found in serum.[80] In some cases the branched-chain hydroxy acids, most prominently alpha-hydroxyisocaproic acid, are also excreted and a derivative of alpha-hydroxybutyric acid, the decarboxylation of which is impaired by accumulation of KMA, is responsible for the characteristic odor of the patient's urine and perspiration.[74]

Pathologic Anatomy

Structural alterations in the nervous system of infants who survive long enough are limited to cerebral white matter, and are similar to but more severe than those in phenylketonuria. The brain is soft and edematous. The cytoarchitecture of the cortex is generally immature, with fewer cortical layers and the persistence of ectopic foci of neuroblasts. The number of oligodendrocytes and the amount of myelin are less than would be seen in a normal brain of comparable age. There is marked astrocytosis and generalized cystic degeneration.[81] On chemical examination, the concentration of myelin lipids is markedly reduced, with cerebrosides, sulfatides, and proteolipid protein almost completely absent. These abnormalities are not found in infants dying of the disease within the first days of life, nor in patients treated by restriction of branched-chain amino acid intake.[82,83]

Clinical Manifestations

In the original four patients reported by Menkes[73] as well as in subsequent cases,[84] opisthotonus, intermittent increase in muscle tone, and respiratory irregularities appeared within the first week of life in babies apparently normal at birth. Subsequently, there was rapid deterioration of the nervous system and all but one died within one month. Other patients, spastic and intellectually retarded, have survived for several years.

About half develop severe hypoglycemia, perhaps in part due to glucose malabsorption. Leucine-induced hyperinsulinism or inhibition of gluconeogenesis may also play a role.[85] Intermittent keto-aciduria, accompanied by periods of ataxia, drowsiness, and behavior disturbance, has been noted. In this condition there is reduced ability to decarboxylate all three keto acids in both fibroblast cultures and peripheral leukocytes.[77,86,87] While in the classical form of maple syrup disease both parents have about half of the normal enzyme activities, in the intermittent form only one parent has decreased keto-acid

oxidase activity.[87] A third variant of maple syrup disease has been described in mildly to moderately retarded children devoid of severe neurologic manifestations. In this condition leukocytes possess a small fraction of normal decarboxylase activity for each of the three branched-chain keto-acids.[88,89] In a fourth variant, encountered in a retarded child, the serum levels of the branched-chain amino acids are lower, and the condition responds to thiamine (10 mg/day).[90]

The cause of rapid cerebral deterioration in infants with maple syrup disease is unknown. Since a reduced intake of branched-chain amino acids has prevented the evolution of the more severe neurologic symptoms, damage probably results from the accumulation of some metabolite. Interference with amino acid transport into brain and incorporation into cerebral proteins and neurotransmitters has some experimental support.[91]

Diagnosis

Maple syrup disease is diagnosed by the characteristic odor of the patient and a positive, 2,4-dinitrophenylhydrazine test on the urine. The ferric chloride test sometimes produces a navy blue color. Chromatography of the urine for keto-acids or of the serum for amino acids confirms the diagnosis. KICA decarboxylase has been demonstrated in cultivated amniotic fluid cells as early as 10 weeks' gestation, making antenatal diagnosis possible.

Treatment

As in phenylketonuria, a diet containing restricted amounts of leucine, isoleucine, and valine has been used in treatment. For optimal results it should be initiated during the first few days of life. A sample synthetic amino acid diet has been prepared by Snyderman.[92] The dietary management of these patients is extremely complex and requires frequent quantitative measurements of the serum amino acids. Prompt and vigorous treatment of even mild infections is mandatory and a number of children on this synthetic diet have succumbed to septicemia.[84] Peritoneal dialysis has been used to correct the initial acute neurologic symptoms.[94] At the present time a few children maintained on such a regimen are known to have achieved a fairly adequate intellectual development, with developmental quotients ranging from 55 to 100.[92,93] Pathologic examination on one treated patient indicates that myelination proceeds normally when the intake of branched-chain amino acids is restricted.[83,95]

DEFECTS IN UREA CYCLE METABOLISM

Five inborn errors in the urea cycle have been described with one defect at each of the five steps in the conversion of ammonia to urea (Fig. 1–6). These include argininosuccinic aciduria, citrullinuria, and two conditions termed hyperammonemia, the more common one due to a defect of ornithine transcarbamylase, the other probably the result of defective carbamyl phosphate synthetase. Congenital lysine intolerance is also associated with periodic ammonia intoxication, most likely due to interference by lysine with the enzyme arginase. These diseases have in common an autosomal recessive transmission, moderate to severe mental retardation, seizures, vomiting, and intermittent episodes of stupor or coma. In all conditions the enzyme defect is partial, for complete failure of urea formation would be incompatible with life. While urea synthesis is reduced, it proceeds at a nearly normal rate once the substrate-binding capacity of the mutant enzyme involved is overcome by the mass effect of increased substrate concentration.

Neurologic symptoms are believed to result from chronic hyperammonemia, but since the urea cycle is functional in brain, they could also be the result of an accumulation of urea cycle intermediates in the central nervous system.

Argininosuccinic Aciduria

This is probably the most common of the urea cycle disorders and is characterized by mental retardation, poorly formed hair, and accumulation of the dipeptide argininosuccinic acid in body fluids. It was first described in 1958 by Allan and others.[96]

Biochemical Pathology

Argininosuccinic acid is a normal intermediary metabolite in the synthesis of urea (Fig. 1–6). A deficiency in argininosuccinase has been demonstrated in liver, erythrocytes, and brain.[97,98,99] When the sensitivity of the assay method has permitted, traces of residual argininosuccinase activity have been found.

The synthesis of urea is only slightly depressed, but a large proportion of labelled ammonium lactate administered to affected individuals is converted to glutamine.[100] The manner in which children synthesize urea is not clear, although it appears likely that in

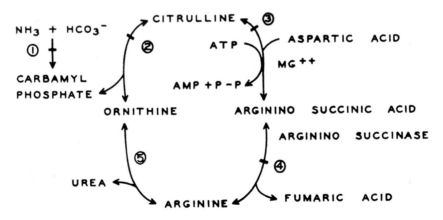

Fig. 1–6. Normal urea cycle. The cycle is completely reversible. In argininosuccinic aciduria the cycle is blocked at step 4. In citrullinuria the block occurs at step 3. In the two forms of hyperammonemia the blocks are at steps 1 and 2, respectively. In congenital lysine intolerance, lysine interferes with arginase, the enzyme converting arginine to ornithine.

argininosuccinic aciduria, as well as in the other defects of the urea cycle, substrate accumulates to a concentration at which the decreased substrate binding capacity of the mutant enzyme is overcome by a mass effect.

Pathologic Anatomy

The liver architecture is normal with increased fat deposition. The brain in one patient, who died at nine days of age, was edematous with poor demarcation of gray and white matter. The cortical layers were poorly developed and myelination was defective with vacuolated myelin sheaths and cystic degeneration of white matter.[101] In an older patient there were atypical astrocytes similar to the Alzheimer's cells seen in Wilson's disease and in severe chronic liver disease.[102]

Clinical Manifestations

The clinical picture is variable. Nearly all patients suffer from recurrent generalized convulsions, poorly pigmented, brittle hair (trichorrhexis nodosa), ataxia, hepatomegaly, and severe intellectual limitation.[103] However, some have been seizure-free and have presented with little more than learning difficulties.[104] In other patients the disease has followed an acute course, with neonatal seizures and death.[101]

Diagnosis

The large quantities of argininosuccinic acid excreted are readily detected on staining paper chromatograms for amino acids. In all instances in which it has been examined, the spinal fluid has been abnormal. In contrast to normal fluid in which glutamine is the predominant amino acid, argininosuccinic acid is the principal ninhydrin reactor in these patients. In the fasting state the blood ammonia level may be normal or only slightly elevated, but marked elevations occur after protein loading.[103]

Treatment

Most of the neurologic symptoms of argininosuccinic aciduria, as well as of the other urea cycle disorders, can be attributed to ammonia intoxication, and are therefore a function of the amount of protein ingested. Restriction of protein intake to 1–2 gm/kg/day usually lowers the blood ammonia to a level which allows the patient to be symptom-free. The quantity of protein intake which is adequate for growth, yet prevents hyperammonemia, must be adjusted on an individual basis. The reduction of blood ammonia in argininosuccinic aciduria has been accompanied by improved growth, reduction in liver size, and cessation of seizures. In some patients the brittle hair has returned to normal with treatment.

Citrullinemia

In 1963 McMurray and his associates reported a mentally retarded infant who had a metabolic block in the conversion of citrulline to argininosuccinic acid (Fig. 1–6, step 3).[105] A deficiency of argininosuccinic acid synthetase was demonstrated by liver biopsy in one patient and in cultured fibroblasts in another.[106,107] In tissue culture argininosuccinate synthetase has decreased affinity for its substrate, citrulline, and conversion of citrulline to argininosuccinic acid is only possible at high citrulline concentrations.[107]

As a result of the enzymatic defect the concentration of citrulline in urine, serum and cerebrospinal fluid is increased, and administration of a protein meal results in a dramatic rise of blood ammonia. Blood and urinary urea values are normal, indicating that urea production is not completely blocked. In one patient serum concentrations of homocitrulline, homoarginine, and lysine were elevated, suggesting the presence of an alternate mechanism for ammonia disposal and urea formation. This would involve a second urea cycle, which includes homocitrulline, homoargininosuccinic acid, homoarginine, and lysine.[107a]

Citrullinemia is a rare disease, and its characteristic clinical picture has not been established.[106,108] Citrullinuria in the absence of citrullinemia may be seen in patients with cystinuria.[106] In this instance citrulline is derived from arginine which is poorly absorbed from the intestine.[109]

Hyperammonemia with Ornithine Transcarbamylase Deficiency

Two defects in the urea cycle are characterized by a relatively normal amino acid excretion and chronic elevation of blood ammonia levels. The more common of these two entities was first reported in 1962 by Russell and coworkers[110] in two cousins with markedly depressed activity of hepatic ornithine transcarbamylase (Fig. 1–6, step 2). The activity of the other urea cycle enzymes is normal, with the exception of carbamylphosphate synthetase, which for as yet unknown reasons is reduced to 20 to 50 percent of normal.[111]

This condition is transmitted as a sex-linked disorder. In males the enzyme is completely absent, while in females the enzyme deficiency is partial.[111a] As a consequence of this enzyme defect blood ammonia levels are strikingly and consistently elevated (0.4 to 1.0 mg/100 ml, contrasted with normal values of less than 0.1 mg/100 ml). CSF ammonia is at least 10 times normal. Serum glutamine, and sometimes also serum glycine, and ornithine levels are elevated.

As in argininosuccinic aciduria, the neuropathologic picture is highlighted by the presence of Alzheimer's cells throughout the brain.[112]

In males, the clinical picture is marked by severe hyperammonemia, which is often fatal during the neonatal period.[111a] In females, the hyperammonemia is less striking, and the clinical picture is highlighted by a failure to thrive, and episodic attacks of headache and vomiting, followed by a period of lethargy or stupor. These attacks are often the consequence of protein ingestion and are accompanied by high blood ammonia levels. A number of subjects, including obligatory heterozygotes, have had intermittent migraine, associated with a mild elevation of blood ammonia.[112] An asymptomatic adult with this disorder has also been documented.

Restriction of protein intake to the lowest level compatible with growth has not been successful in preventing a postprandial rise in blood ammonia, and smaller, more frequent meals have been recommended, with the addition of citric acid (2 gm/day in four divided doses) to facilitate ammonia excretion.[113]

A variant of this type of hyperammonemia has also been reported. The patient, a male, had a milder clinical picture and his liver ornithine transcarbamylase activity was decreased to 25% of normal, compared with 5%–7% in the usual patient with this condition.[114]

Hyperammonemia with Carbamyl Phosphate Synthetase Deficiency

Another disorder of the urea cycle manifests itself by a reduction in hepatic carbamyl phosphate synthetase activity (Fig. 1–6, step 1). This condition was first reported by Freeman and associates,[115] and subsequently by Hommes and associates.[116] In the latter patient carbamyl phosphate synthetase activity was 50% of normal in liver but only 6% in brain. Blood and urinary glycine is elevated in this condition, and there is a cyclic neutropenia. On autopsy there is ulegyria of cerebral and cerebellar cortex, and hypomyelination of the centrum semiovale and the central part of the brain stem. In contrast to argininosuccinic aciduria, no Alzheimer cells are seen.[116a]

Congenital Lysine Intolerance

Patients affected with this condition experience episodes of vomiting, lethargy, and coma in association with a high protein intake. Attacks can be provoked by the ingestion of lysine and are characterized biochemically by marked elevations of blood ammonia, lysine, and arginine.[117] In one patient, studied in detail, there was a partial deficiency of hepatic lysine dehydrogenase.[118] The subsequent rise in tissue lysine can be expected to inhibit competitively the action of arginase, which converts arginine to ornithine (Fig. 1–6). It is, however, not clear why hyperlysinemia (see p. 19) does not induce hyperammonemia.

Other Genetic Causes of Hyperammonemia

Aside from the above diseases hyperammonemia is also seen in other genetic disorders the biochemical basis of which is still unclear. These include a syndrome of familial protein intolerance with a defect in the transport of basic amino acids,[119] and intermittent hyperammonemia with abnormally high levels of ornithine in the blood, and homocitrulline in the urine.[120] Patients with the latter condition, termed ornithinemia, present with psychomotor retardation, prolonged neonatal jaundice, infantile spasms, and intermittent ataxia. Ornithine transcarbamylase levels are normal (Fig. 1–6, step 2), but hepatic ornithine-keto acid aminotransferase activity is reduced.[121] It is not clear why this defect in the conversion of ornithine to glutamic semialdehyde should by itself cause hyperammonemia; if anything this might be expected to favor the conversion of ammonia to urea because of the increased availability of ornithine.

Hyperammonemia, associated with depressed function of all five enzymes of the urea cycle, is seen in ketotic hyperglycinemia.[122]

Ammonia intoxication has also been noted in a cerebral-atrophic syndrome described by Rett,[123] seen mainly in females, and characterized by spasticity, seizures, and marked mental retardation. The cause of the hyperammonemia is unknown.

HISTIDINEMIA

This condition, which may represent a harmless metabolic variant, has been described in several children who presented with a variety of minor neurologic disturbances, such as delayed speech,[124] apparently due to impaired auditory memory. The major catabolic pathway for histidine proceeds via urocanic acid, formiminoglutamic acid, and glutamic acid. Histidinemia is the result of an interruption in the first step of this pathway because of a defect in histidase.

This enzyme is absent from epidermis and liver of affected individuals. As expected from the location of the metabolic block, histidine levels in both serum and urine are elevated, plasma levels being usually above 8 mg%, and large amounts of imidazole lactic, imidazole acetic, and imidazole pyruvic acids are excreted.[125] Urocanic acid, found in normal sweat, is absent in histidinemic patients.[126]

For unknown reasons blood and urine alanine is elevated. Addition of ferric chloride to the urine results in the appearance of an olive green color. The diagnosis is confirmed by an elevation of histidine in blood, and by the absence of urocanic acid from the stratum corneum of skin.[127] The presence of large amounts of urinary histidine is insufficient for the diagnosis of histidinemia, as this type of urinary amino acid pattern is a not uncommon finding in the normal population.

On pathologic examination, a number of cerebral malformations and reduced myelination is evident.[128] The clinical picture in histidinemia is variable. Of 23 cases in the literature up to 1970, 17 had retarded speech, but of these 15 were mentally retarded and would be expected to have slowed speech development.[129] A few patients have had seizures and ataxia, while others have been neurologically and intellectually normal.[124]

While it is tempting to postulate that histidine has a specific deleterious effect on the language center, it is interesting to note that untreated phenylketonuric children perform more poorly in language than in motor and personal-social behavior.

Treatment of histidinemia with a low histidine diet has been proposed, but in view of the uncertainty of the natural course of the disease, we have no way of judging the effectiveness of treatment.[128]

A variant of histidinemia, in which blood histidine levels were elevated but skin histidase activity was normal, has been described.[130] In another variant, loss of histidase activity has been incomplete.[131]

Two other rare defects of histidine metabolism have been reported by Japanese workers. In urocanic aciduria, impaired hepatic urocanase deficiency results in an increased excretion of the acid. Blood histidine levels are normal. The initially reported patient presented with mental retardation and hemiplegia, the latter a sequel of tuberculous meningitis.[132]

Patients with formiminotransferase deficiency also present with mental and physical retardation. Because of an intermittently high output of 4-amino-5-imidazole carboxamide, the ferric chloride test may yield a permanent gray-green color.[133]

DEFECTS IN THE METABOLISM OF SULFUR AMINO ACIDS

Homocystinuria

Homocystinuria is an inborn error of methionine metabolism manifesting itself by multiple thromboembolic episodes, ectopia lentis, and mental retardation. Although discovered in only 1962 by Field and reported by Carson and associates,[134] its incidence is second to that of phenylketonuria among the errors of amino acid metabolism affecting the nervous system and accounts for about 0.02% of inmates of institutions for the retarded in the United States and 0.3% in Northern Ireland.[135]

Biochemical Pathology

In the most common form of homocystinuria the metabolic defect is one of cystathionine synthase, the enzyme catalyzing the formation of cystathionine from homocysteine and serine (Fig. 1–7).[136] As a result of the block, increased amounts of homocystine, the oxidized derivative of homocysteine and its precursor methionine, are found in urine and plasma. Administration of a methionine load to affected individuals produces a striking and prolonged rise in plasma methionine but very little altera-

tion in the homocystine levels. In part this reflects the low renal threshold for this amino acid.[137]

At least three other sulfur-containing amino acids, including S-adenosylmethionine, S-adenosylhomocysteine, and homolanthionine are also excreted.[138,139] Homolanthionine may be synthesized by a condensation of homocysteine and homoserine, catalyzed by a defective cystathionine synthase, whose binding site for serine is altered to accept homoserine as well. Serum folate is reduced, probably as the result of increased utilization of its metabolite, N^5-methyltetrahydrofolic acid, in the remethylation of homocysteine to methionine (Fig. 1–7).

As cysteine cannot be formed from methionine it becomes an essential amino acid for homocystinurics. Cystathionine, normally present in high concentration in human brain, is absent from homocystinuric tissue, suggesting that cerebral cystathionine synthase is also defective.[140]

On the basis of the response to therapeutic

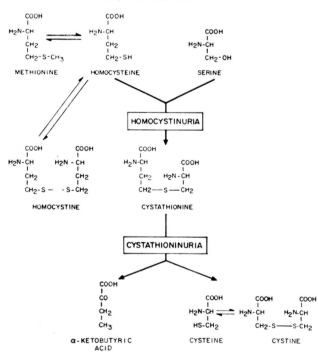

Fig. 1–7. Normal metabolism of sulfur amino acids. In the most common form of homocystinuria the defect is in the conversion of homocysteine to cystathionine. In cystathioninuria the block is located in the conversion of cystathionine to cysteine. A block in the conversion of homocysteine to methionine also produces homocystinuria, but serum methionine levels remain normal.

trials with pyridoxine, Vitamin B_{12}, and folic acid, several variants of homocystinuria can now be distinguished. In the most common form of homocystinuria administration of oral pyridoxine, the coenzyme for cystathionine synthase, does not alter homocystine excretion, while in one variant large doses of the vitamin (500 mg/day or higher) eliminate homocystine from plasma and urine. It would appear that biochemically unresponsive patients suffer from a deficiency of the enzyme, while the responsiveness of the other group of patients may result from stimulation of an enzyme having reduced affinity for its cofactor, or enhancement of alternative pathways of sulfur amino acid metabolism.[141]

Homocystinuria may also result from an impaired methylation of homocysteine to methionine (Fig. 1–7). When the metabolic block is at this point, plasma methionine concentrations are normal, rather than increased as is the case in the common form of homocystinuria. Methylation utilizes N^5-methyltetrahydrofolate as methyl donor and a B_{12} derivative as cofactor. Methylation may be impaired due to either lack of cofactor or enzyme. When synthesis of the B_{12} cofactor is defective the biochemical picture is characterized by increased excretion of methylmalonic acid and homocystine (vid. infr.). This abnormality is correctable with large doses of B_{12}. A defect in the methylation enzyme, methylenetetrahydrofolate reductase, has also been described. In this condition the biochemical abnormalities are corrected by folic acid.[142]

The clinical picture in patients with defective methylation of homocystine is protean. Some are retarded, others have recurrent episodes of vomiting and lethargy, or muscular weakness and seizures, while at least one subject has been physically and developmentally normal.[143]

Pathologic Anatomy

The primary structural alterations are noted in blood vessels of all calibers.[144] In most of these there is intimal thickening and fibrosis, while in the aorta and its major branches fraying of elastic fibers may be observed. Both arterial and venous thromboses are common in a number of organs.

Within the brain there are usually multiple infarcted areas of varying age. Dural sinus thromboses have been recorded.

The relationship between the metabolic defect and the propensity to vascular thromboses is unclear. Homocysteine in high concentrations may shorten clotting time in vitro, probably by activating the Hageman factor (Factor XII).[145] McCully has found that elevated concentrations of homocysteine alter the state of aggregation and fibrillar structure of proteoglycans, and in this manner produce the pathologic changes in the vasculature.[146] The ectopia lentis commonly seen in homocystinuria is due to a similar alteration in the normal fibrous structure of the zonular fibers.[147]

Clinical Manifestations

The condition is transmitted in an autosomal recessive manner. Homocystinuric infants appear normal at birth, and their early development is unremarkable until seizures, developmental slowing, or cerebrovascular accidents occur between 5 and 9 months of age. Ectopia lentis has been recognized by 18 months of age. The typical older homocystinuric child's hair is sparse, blond, and brittle, and there are multiple erythematous blotches over the skin, particularly across the maxillary areas and cheeks. The gait is shuffling, the extremities and digits long, and genu valgum is present in most instances. Ectopia lentis is invariable in older children, and secondary glaucoma and cataracts are common.[148]

In about half the patients reported, major thromboembolic episodes have occurred on one or more occasions. These include fatal thromboses of the pulmonary artery and of the renal artery and vein. Multiple major cerebrovascular accidents may result in hemiplegia and, ultimately, in a picture which closely resembles pseudobulbar palsy. It is likely that minor and unrecognized cerebral thrombi are the direct cause of the mental retardation which occurs in more than half the patients.[149] Routine laboratory studies are normal, but electromyographic examination suggests the presence of a myopathy in a high proportion of patients.[150] Radiographs show a delay in bone maturation, and an alteration in configuration resembling acromegalic gigantism.

Diagnosis

The diagnosis of homocystinuria suggested by the appearance of the patient may be confirmed by a positive urinary cyanide-nitroprusside reaction, by the increased urinary excretion of homocystine and by an elevated plasma methionine. The nitroprusside-cyanide screening test is performed as follows:[151]

To 5 ml of urine, add several drops of concentrated ammonium hydroxide and 2 ml of a 5 percent solution of sodium cyanide. After 5 to 10 minutes, a few drops of a 5 percent solution of sodium nitroprusside are added. A deep purple color indicates a positive reaction. The test is also positive in the presence of large amounts of cystine and acetone, and in the rare patient excreting glutathionine or beta-mercaptolactate-cysteine disulfide.[152]

While ectopia lentis, arachnodactyly, and cardiovascular symptoms are also seen in Marfan's syndrome, homocystinuria can be distinguished by its autosomal recessive transmission, the thromboembolic phenomena, and the peculiar facial appearance. The relatively long fingers of Marfan's syndrome are present at birth, and the skeletal disproportion remains constant. In homocystinuria the skeleton is normal for the first few years of life, but the limbs grow disproportionately long.

Cystathionine synthase has been found in cultivated amniotic fluid cells, and the condition can therefore be diagnosed prenatally.[153]

Treatment

Restriction of methionine intake lowers plasma methionine and eliminates the abnormally high urinary excretion of homocystine. A low methionine diet has been described which utilizes lentils, gelatin, and soya, protein sources low in this amino acid.[154]

Supplementation of this diet with folic acid has been suggested, on the supposition that the mental defect may be related to low serum folate levels.[63,155] Pyridoxine has also been used, and in large doses reduces homo-

cystine excretion of some patients. Although the biochemical picture can be improved by these means, or by administration of vitamin B_{12}, or folic acid in patients with homocystinuria due to defective methylation, there is no evidence of clinical benefit. Evaluation of long term treatment of patients placed on dietary restriction during infancy will have to take into account the variable clinical picture, particularly with respect to mental retardation.

Cystathioninuria

A grossly increased urinary excretion of the amino acid cystathionine has been observed in a small number of individuals.[156] The aminoaciduria is the result of a defect in cystathionase (Fig. 1–7),[157] an enzyme requiring pyridoxal phosphate as cofactor. As a result of the defect, brain cystathionine is markedly elevated. High doses of pyridoxine (B_6) induce a marked reduction in plasma and urinary cystathionine concentrations. Liver specimens from patients with the disease show a small amount of cystathionase activity, which can be enhanced considerably by the addition of pyridoxal phosphate. This phenomenon results from a structural alteration of the apoenzyme, which impairs coenzyme binding.[155,157] While some of the subjects encountered initially suffered from mental retardation or personality disturbances, it is now clear that cystathioninuria is a benign metabolic variant, and that the association with neurologic symptoms had been fortuitous.

Cystathioninuria is also seen in association with liver disease, pyridoxine deficiency, galactosemia, and neural crest tumors.[158]

Hypermethioninemia

A number of patients have presented with familial hepatic cirrhosis, renal tubular defects, rickets, hypoglycemia, and a peculiar body odor resembling that of boiled cabbage.[159] Even though serum methionine levels are often elevated, it appears likely that this entity is identical with tyrosinosis, a relatively common condition, in which neurologic symptoms are usually accompanied by severe hepatic or renal dysfunction.[160]

This condition differs from the methionine

malabsorption syndrome seen in a child presenting with mental deficiency, convulsions, diarrhea, attacks of hyperpnea, and a maple-syrup-like odor attributed to the presence of alpha-hydroxybutyric acid. Individuals affected by this condition have increased fecal methionine, and their diarrhea is exacerbated upon administration of a methionine load.[161] In contrast to the situation in maple syrup disease, this patient's amino acid excretion was normal.

Elevations of serum methionine are also seen in neonatal hepatitis, and in many infants, one to three months of age, receiving a high protein diet (at least 7 gm/kg/day).

Beta-mercaptolactate-cysteine disulfide has been isolated from the urine of a mentally retarded individual.[152] The metabolic defect responsible for its formation is still unknown.

OTHER RARE METABOLIC DEFECTS

Various studies have appeared in the literature describing a single case, or several cases with neurologic disturbances apparently associated with an abnormality in the amino acid pattern of serum or urine.

The Iminoacidurias

Several inborn metabolic errors are characterized by the increased excretion of proline and hydroxyproline, the two principal imino-acids. Normally the metabolism of proline proceeds via glutamic acid. Proline oxidase converts proline to Δ'-pyrroline-5-carboxylic acid (PC), which is then converted by PC dehydrogenase to glutamic acid. Analogous but distinct enzyme systems convert hydroxy-proline to Δ'-pyrroline-3-hydroxy-5-carboxylic acid (HPC), and this to γ-hydroxyglutamic acid.

Hyperprolinemia, Type I

This condition is characterized by increased proline in blood (8–11 mg%), and increased urinary excretion of proline, hydroxyproline, and glycine. Although often this metabolic error is associated with mental retardation, nerve deafness, photosensitive epilepsy, and congenital renal disease, some patients have had normal neurologic and renal function.[3,162] While the biochemical disturbance follows an autosomal recessive inheritance, the renal disease has behaved as a dominant trait and has been seen in individuals who lacked full expression of the biochemical disturbance. The biochemical basis involves a deficiency in proline oxidase which has been found to be absent from liver.[163] The increased serum proline results in a hyperaminoaciduria involving proline, hydroxyproline, and glycine. The output of the latter two amino acids reflects an overloading of their tubular transport system by the high concentrations of proline.[164]

Only a few postmortem studies are on hand: one showed a decrease in cortical neurons and a patchy loss of ganglion cells in the organ of Corti, while another showed vacuolization of white matter and delayed cerebral myelination.[165]

Hyperprolinemia, Type II

A second form of hyperprolinemia has been seen in asymptomatic children and in patients presenting with seizures and mental retardation. These individuals excreted both proline and Δ'-pyrroline-5-carboxylic acid. Serum proline levels run somewhat higher than in type I hyperprolinemia. The defect is one of Δ'-pyrroline-5-carboxylic acid dehydrogenase, the enzyme converting Δ'-pyrroline-5-carboxylic acid to glutamic acid.[166,167]

A mentally retarded individual with markedly increased concentrations of hydroxy-proline in blood and urine resulting from a deficiency of hydroxyproline oxidase has been described by Efron and others.[168]

Hyperlysinemia

At least three pathways are available for the degradation of lysine in mammalian tissues. The major one involves reversal of the synthetic steps and proceeds via saccharopine to alpha-amino-adipic-δ-semialdehyde (Fig. 1–8). The enzyme catalyzing the conversion of lysine to saccharopine (Fig. 1–8, step 1), lysine-α-ketoglutarate reductase, has been shown in human liver, and has reduced activity in patients with hyperlysinemia.[169]

At least six patients with hyperlysinemia have been identified. Four were retarded,

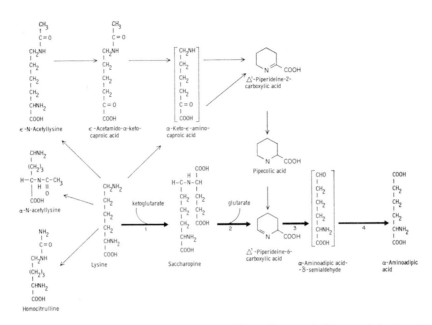

Fig. 1–8. Metabolic pathways of lysine in the human. The major metabolic route is indicated by heavy arrows. In hyperlysinemia the block is at step 1, and patients also excrete α-N-acetyllysine and homocitrulline. In saccharopinuria the block is at steps 2, 3, or 4. The metabolic block in pipecolatemia is still uncertain.

had seizures or electroencephalographic abnormalities and short stature and lax ligaments.[170]

The diagnosis of hyperlysinemia rests on the increased serum levels of lysine. High urinary excretion of lysine, usually accompanied by increased cystine excretion, but with normal blood levels of both amino acids, is seen in some heterozygotes for cystinuria.[171] Abnormally high excretion of the dibasic amino acids (lysine, arginine, and ornithine) in the face of normal plasma levels and a normal cystine excretion is characteristic of hyperdibasicaminoaciduria, a benign metabolic variant,[172] transmitted in a dominant manner. Increased output of lysine and arginine is encountered in a condition termed familial protein intolerance with dibasic aminoaciduria. This entity presents with retardation, recurrent vomiting and diarrhea, and hyperammonemia.[173] The underlying defect may be an impaired liberation of ammonia from glutamine.[174]

Another disorder of lysine metabolism is pipecolatemia.[175] This is a degenerative neurologic disease associated with a general-ized aminoaciduria, and elevated blood levels of pipecolic acid. Administration of lysine to such a patient did not increase pipecolic acid levels, suggesting that cyclization of lysine (Fig. 1–8) is a minor metabolic route.

In saccharopinuria, a condition presenting with mental retardation and progressive spastic diplegia,[176] the metabolic block may lie between saccharopine and alpha-amino-adipic-acid-δ-semialdehyde or at subsequent steps of lysine degradation (Fig. 1–8, steps 2, 3, 4).[176a]

A few other, extremely rare, defects of amino acid metabolism associated with neurologic symptoms are presented in Table 1–4. A number of other neurologic disorders that are accompanied by aminoaciduria are not included in this table. It has been the experience of a number of investigators, including our group, that when mentally retarded children are screened a few will exhibit a pathologic degree of aminoaciduria. Deficiency diseases, notably rickets, may account for some of these; the remainder are unexplained.

TABLE 1-4.
RARE DEFECTS OF AMINO ACID METABOLISM ASSOCIATED WITH NEUROLOGIC SYMPTOMS

Disease	Enzymatic Defect	Clinical Features	Diagnosis
Hypervalinemia[177]	Valine transaminase	Vomiting, failure to thrive, nystagmus, mental retardation	Increased blood and urine valine; no increase in keto acid excretion
Sarcosinemia[178,179]	Impaired sarcosine-glycine conversion	Mental retardation in some, normal intelligence in others	Increased blood and urine sarcosine, ethanolamine
Hyper-beta-alaninemia[180]	Beta-alanine-alpha-ketoglutarate transaminase	Seizures commencing at birth, somnolence	Plasma urine beta-alanine and beta-aminoisobutyric acid elevated; urinary gamma-aminobutyric acid elevated
Hyperalaninemia[181,182]	Pyruvate decarboxylase	Intermittent cerebellar ataxia and choreoathetosis	Increased serum alanine, lactate, and pyruvate
Carnosinemia[183,183a]	?Carnosinase	Grand mal and myoclonic seizures, mental retardation	Increased serum and urine carnosine; increased CSF homocarnosine
β-hydroxyisovaleric aciduria and beta-methyl crotonyl-glycinuria[184]	β-Methylcrotonyl-CoA carboxylase (step 4, Fig. 1–5)	Similar to infantile spinal muscular atrophy; urine smells like that of cat	Increased urine beta-hydroxyisovaleric acid, beta-methylcrotonylglycine
α-Methyl-β-hydroxy butyric aciduria[185]	Defective conversion of α-methylacetoacetate propionate	Recurrent severe acidosis	α-methyl acetoacetate and α-methyl-β-hydroxy butyric acid in urine
Cytosol tyrosine aminotransferase deficiency[186]	Soluble tyrosine amino transferase	Multiple congenital anomalies	p-hydroxyphenyl-pyruvic and p-hydroxyphenyl-lactic acid excretion increased

DISORDERS OF AMINO ACID TRANSPORT

Renal amino acid transport is handled by five specific systems that have nonoverlapping substrate preferences. The disorders that result from genetic defects in each of these systems are listed in Table 1–5.

HARTNUP'S DISEASE

This is a rare, familial condition characterized by photosensitive dermatitis, intermittent cerebellar ataxia, mental disturbances, and renal aminoaciduria. The name is that of the family in which it was first detected.[187]

Biochemical Pathology

The symptoms are the result of an extensive disturbance in the transport of neutral amino acids. There are four main biochemical abnormalities:[188]

Renal Aminoaciduria. The concentration of urinary amino acids is on the average about

TABLE 1-5.

DEFECTS IN AMINO ACID TRANSPORT

Transport System	Condition	Biochemical Features	Clinical Features
Basic amino acids	Cystinuria (3 types)	Impaired renal clearance and defective intestinal transport of lysine, arginine, ornithine, and cystine	Renal stones; no neurologic disease
	Lowe's syndrome	?Impaired intestinal transport of lysine and arginine; ?impaired tubular transport of lysine	Severe mental retardation, glaucoma, cataracts, myopathy; sex-linked transmission
Acidic amino acids	None known		
Neutral amino acids	Hartnup's disease	Defective intestinal and renal tubular transport of tryptophan and other neutral amino acids	Intermittent cerebellar ataxia; photosensitive rash
Proline, hydroxyproline, glycine	Iminoglycinuria	Impaired tubular transport of proline, hydroxyproline, and glycine	Harmless variant
Beta-amino acids	None known	Excretion of beta-aminoisobutyric acid and taurine in beta-alaninemia is increased due to competition at the tubular level	

10 times normal. That the outpouring of amino acids is due to a circumscribed defect in tubular function is proved by a normal renal clearance of proline, cystine, glycine, taurine, and the basic amino acids. In contrast, Jepson[189] has found that most neutral amino acids have higher clearances than normal, the maximum being 122 ml per minute for histidine. The latter value approaches the glomerular filtration rate of 140 ml per minute, indicating almost complete absence of histidine resorption.

Increased Excretion of Indican. Excretion of indoxyl sulfate is two to four times normal. Milne and his associates[188] believe this to be the result of impaired intestinal transport of tryptophan. They have shown that D-tryptophan is completely unabsorbed in patients with Hartnup's disease and that transport of D-tryptophan across the gut wall is greatly impaired. The unutilized amino acid remains in the gut where microorganisms convert it to indican. Neomycin, which sterilizes the intestinal tract, thereby abolishes indicanuria.

Increased Excretion of Indole-3-Acetic Acid, Indole-3-Acrylglycine, and Indole-3-Acetyl-L-Glutamine. The abnormally high output of these nonhydroxylated indole metabolites contrasts with the decreased excretion of such indole derivatives as kynurenine and 5-hydroxytryptamine (serotonin). This disturbance, like the increased output of indican, may in part be due to defective transport of D-tryptophan and L-tryptophan across the jejunal wall, with a subsequent increase in intestinal degradation of the amino acid by microorganisms. A similar impairment of cellular transport of L-tryptophan within the liver would result in less substrate being made available for oxidation by tryptophan peroxidase, an enzyme found in the soluble fraction of liver cells. The impaired formation of formylkynurenine from tryptophan could ultimately produce a deficiency of endogenous nicotinamide and cause pellagralike symptoms.

Increased Fecal Amino Acids. The impaired intestinal transport of neutral amino acids results in increased fecal amino acids showing a pattern resembling the urinary excretion of a typical Hartnup patient.[190]

Pathologic Anatomy

No pathologic studies have yet been reported.

Clinical Manifestations

The symptoms of Hartnup's disease are intermittent and variable, tending to improve with increasing age. Characteristically there is a red, scaly rash on the exposed areas of the face, neck, and extensor surfaces of the extremities. This resembles the dermatitis of pellagra and, like it, is aggravated by sunlight. Cerebral symptoms may precede the rash for several years. They include intermittent personality changes, psychoses, migrainelike headaches, photophobia, and bouts of cerebellar ataxia. Changes in hair texture have also been observed. The four children of the original Hartnup family underwent progressive mental retardation, but this is not invariable. For obscure reasons no typical cases of Hartnup's disease have been discovered in the United States. We have observed a patient with the clinical picture of Hartnup's disease, impaired intestinal absorption of neutral amino acids but no renal aminoaciduria. A somewhat similar case has been reported by Borrie and Lewis.[191]

Diagnosis

The diagnosis of Hartnup's disease should be considered in patients with intermittent cerebral symptoms even without skin involvement.

Other metabolic disorders that produce intermittent cerebellar ataxia include the intermittent variant of maple syrup disease,[87] hyperalaninemia,[181,182] and familial intermittent cerebellar ataxia.[192] Paper chromatography of urine for amino acids and indolic substances in the face of a normal serum pattern is diagnostic for Hartnup's disease. Another entity in which tryptophanuria is associated with elevated blood tryptophan has been encountered in Japan.[193]

Treatment

The similarity of Hartnup's disease to pellagra has prompted treatment with nicotinic acid. However, the tendency for symptoms to remit spontaneously and for general improvement to occur with advancing age makes such therapy difficult to evaluate.

LOWE'S SYNDROME (OCULOCEREBRORENAL SYNDROME)

This sex-linked recessive disorder is characterized by severe mental retardation, myopathy, congenital glaucoma or cataract, and biochemically by a generalized aminoaciduria of the Fanconi type, renal tubular acidosis, and rickets.[194]

Neuropathologic examination in two instances has disclosed rarefaction of the molecular layer of the cerebral cortex and parenchymal vacuolation.[195]

The fundamental biochemical defect is unknown but is now believed to be a defect in membrane transport.[196] The urinary levels of lysine are more elevated than those of the other amino acids, and defective uptake of lysine and arginine by the intestinal mucosa has been demonstrated in two patients.[196]

IMINOGLYCINURIA

Individuals homozygous for iminoglycinuria, very likely a harmless metabolic variant, have an increased urinary excretion of proline, hydroxyproline and glycine, and a defect in the renal tubular transport system common to these three amino acids. The heterozygote has an increased output of glycine only.[197]

Transient iminoglycinuria occurs normally during early infancy, and reflects a delay in the maturation of renal tubular function.[198] It is the single most common abnormal finding in mass screening of infants for amino acid disorders.[199]

Mental retardation is relatively commonly associated with renal aminoaciduria. This may be due to various congenital defects involving both brain and kidneys. It may also be secondary to the malnourished condition which frequently accompanies severe intellectual deficit. Finally, as has been pointed out by Berry,[200] Menkes and associates,[201] and Wright,[202] the wide normal variation in amino acid excretion must be taken into account before a "mild aminoaciduria" can be considered pathologic.

DISORDERS OF CARBOHYDRATE METABOLISM

GALACTOSEMIA

Hepatomegaly, splenomegaly, and failure to thrive associated with the excretion of galactose was first pointed out by Von Reuss in 1908.[203] Galactosemia is transmitted by an autosomal recessive gene. The prevalence of this condition varies widely. In Massachusetts it is seen with a frequency of 1:187,000; in Austria it is 1:40,000 to 1:46,000, while in England it is 1:72,000.[204]

Biochemical Pathology

In 1917 Göppert demonstrated that galactosemic children excreted the sugar following the ingestion of both lactose (milk) and galactose.[205] In 1956 Schwarz and his associates found that administration of galactose to affected children gave rise to an accumulation of galactose-1-phosphate.[206] This was confirmed by Kalckar and his group, who were able to demonstrate a deficiency in galactose-1-phosphate uridyl transferase, the enzyme that catalyzes the conversion of galactose-1-phosphate into galactose uridine diphosphate (UDP-galactose, Fig. 1–9).[207]

Transferase activity may normally be found in liver, erythrocytes, and to a lesser extent in brain. All other enzymes involved in galactose metabolism are found in adequate amounts in affected children, thus pinpointing the enzymatic lesion (Table 1–6).[208]

Immunologic studies have shown the presence of a protein in galactosemic erythrocytes which cross-reacts with normal transferase. This provides evidence for a point mutation resulting in a catalytically inactive transferase which retains its antigenic properties.[209] In parents of galactosemic infants, erythrocyte uridyl galactose-1-phosphate transferase activity is also decreased, averaging 64 percent of normal. Since this partial enzymatic defect is always found in both parents, the finding provides excellent biochemical support for the recessive transmission of the defect.[210]

Genetic surveys and electrophoretic examinations of galactose-1-phosphate uridyl transferase have revealed at least five forms of galactosemia:

1. "Classical" galactosemia. In this condition the enzymatic block, while severe, is not quite complete. In part this can be explained by assuming a structural modifica-

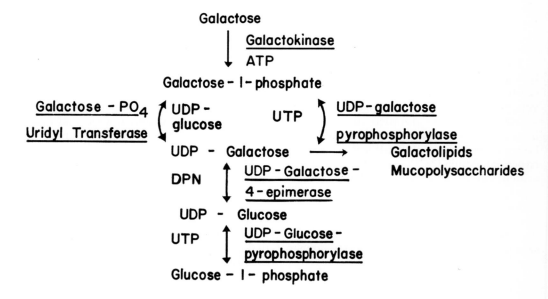

Fig. 1–9. Normal galactose metabolism. In galactosemia, galactose-1-phosphate uridyl transferase is defective.

TABLE 1-6.

ENZYMES OF GALACTOSE METABOLISM IN HUMAN RED CELL HEMOLYSATES

Condition of Subjects	Galactokinase		Gal-1-PO$_4$ Uridyl Transferase		Galactowaldenase		PP-uridyl Transferase	
	No. of Subjects	Activity	No. of Subjects	Activity	No. of Subjects	Activity	No. of Subjects	Activity
Normal	3	0.10	15	0.82	3	0.32	9	1.20
Galactosemic	3	0.08	10	0.02	3	0.35	8	1.85

Activity expressed in micromols substrate consumed per hour per milliliter packed cell hemolysate. From Isselbacher, et al.[208]

tion of the affected enzyme, rather than its complete absence. Fibroblast strains from galactosemic patients may show nearly normal levels of transferase activity under certain culture conditions, suggesting that the mutant enzyme is unstable under various physical conditions.[211] On the other hand the direct oxidation of galactose to galactonate contributes significantly to the ability of the galactosemic to convert small amounts of galactose to CO_2.[212,212a]

2. A subgroup is able to metabolize galactose to CO_2 at a normal rate despite the absence of transferase from red cells. In this variant, confined to Negroes, hepatic transferase activity is 10% of normal. Patients' white cells also lack transferase activity, but the parents' leukocytes have normal enzymatic activity, rather than the 50 percent reduction expected for heterozygotes.[213,214]

3. A number of asymptomatic individuals have erythrocyte transferase activity equal to that of heterozygotes for "classical" galactosemia but a different electrophoretic mobility. They are homozygous for a trait allelic with galactosemia, which is now termed the Duarte variant.[215] Its gene frequency is as high as five percent (Fig. 1–10).

4. In two siblings with the clinical picture of galactosemia, but with residual red cell transferase activity, starch gel electrophoresis revealed a transferase enzyme with a slower than normal mobility.[216] This condition has been termed "Rennes" galactosemia.

5. A deficiency of galactokinase (Fig. 1–9) has been discovered in patients with juvenile

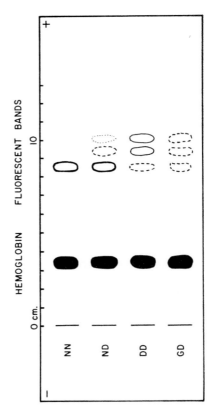

Fig. 1–10. Galactosemia variants. Starch gel electrophoresis showing the fluorescent bands of UDP-galactose-1-phosphate uridyl transferase. NN-normal individual; ND-heterozygote for Duarte variant; DD-homozygote for Duarte variant; GD-heterozygote for galactosemia and Duarte variant. (Courtesy of Dr. William R. Bergren, Children's Hospital, Los Angeles, California.)

cataracts, but neither hepatomegaly nor neurologic deficits are present.[217,218]

In children affected with "classical" galactosemia, lactose of human or cow's milk is hydrolyzed to galactose and glucose, the latter being handled in a normal manner. The metabolism of galactose, however, stops after the sugar is phosphorylated to galactose-1-phosphate. This phosphate ester accumulates in erythrocytes, lens, liver, and kidney.[219] While its presence may produce a variety of secondary metabolic disturbances, such as the inhibition of phosphoglucomutase,[220] it is not the sole toxic metabolite. Galactitol, the alcohol of galactose, is also found in the lens, brains, and urine of galactosemic individuals[221] and may be a major factor in the development of symptoms.

Administration of galactose to affected infants results in marked hypoglycemia. This has been explained by postulating increased insulin release, prompted by the large amounts of circulating reducing substance, or by assuming an interference on the part of galactose-1-phosphate with normal glycogen breakdown. It is probably the major cause of cerebral damage in galactosemic infants. The peripheral hypoglycemia is enhanced by competition between glucose and galactose at the level of the hexose transport across the blood-brain barrier. As a consequence the brain of galactosemic subjects is in a constant hypoglycemic environment. While actual brain glucose levels have not been assayed, the reduced cerebral concentrations of the alcohol derivative of glucose—myo-inositol—substantiate this argument.[222]

Intolerance to galactose decreases with increasing age. In part this may be due to the decreasing importance of milk as a food item, or it may reflect the finding that many of the older patients belong to the previously cited Negro variant of galactosemia and are able to increase their capacity to metabolize galactose as they get older. In subjects with classical galactosemia who have been tested on repeated occasions, no increase in erythrocyte transferase activity has been found.[223]

Pathologic Anatomy

The main pathologic lesions are found in the liver and brain. In the liver several stages are recognized. Initially one sees a severe, diffuse, fatty metamorphosis. The hepatic cells are filled with large, pale, fat-containing vacuoles (Fig. 1–11).[224] If the disease remains untreated, the liver cell cords become transformed into pseudoglandular structures. The final stage is pseudolobular cirrhosis. Cerebral alterations are nonspecific and are probably due to hypoglycemia. Edema, fibrous gliosis of white matter, and marked loss of cortical neurons and Purkinje cells are the most prominent findings.[225]

Chemical examination of the brain indicates a loss of phospholipids in both white matter and cortex.[226]

Clinical Manifestations

Infants with galactosemia appear normal at birth, although their cord blood may already contain abnormally high concentrations of galactose-1-phosphate. In severe cases, symptoms develop during the first week of life. These include vomiting, diarrhea, listlessness, and failure to gain weight. Many infants are markedly jaundiced. This may represent a persistence of neonatal jaundice, or the pigmentation may appear at three to five days of age. By two weeks hepatosplenomegaly and lenticular opacifications are easily detectable. The cataracts may be cortical or nuclear. The most frequently observed opacity is a central refractile ring.[227] The infants are hypotonic and often have lost their Moro reflex. Pseudotumor cerebri as a result of cerebral edema is not uncommon.[228] Usually the urine contains a reducing substance, although if food intake has been poor this may be present in a concentration of less than 100 mg% and thus fail to give a positive Benedict reduction test. There is a proteinuria and a marked aminoaciduria without an increase in serum amino acids. The liver function tests may be abnormal by one week of age. If untreated, growth failure becomes severe and the infant develops the usual signs of progressive hepatic cirrhosis: ascites, prothrombin deficiency, and esophageal varices. In some infants the disease may be less severe and may not manifest itself until three to six months of age when the patients present with delayed physical and

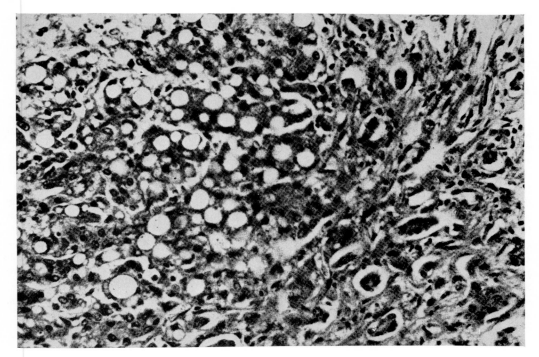

Fig. 1–11. Galactosemia, high-power view of liver. There is periportal fibrosis, a marked disruption of hepatic architecture, and an increase in the number of bile ducts. Considerable numbers of cells are distended with large, pale vacuoles. (Courtesy of Dr. G. N. Donnell, Children's Hospital, Los Angeles, California.)

mental development. By then cataracts may be well-established and the cirrhosis far advanced.

In another group of galactosemics the diagnosis is not made until the patients are several years old, often on evaluation for mental retardation. They may not have cataracts or albuminuria. Intellectual retardation is not consistent in galactosemics. When present, it is moderate; intelligence quotients range between 50 and 70. Asymptomatic homozygotes have also been detected.

Diagnosis

The urine often contains a reducing sugar, which unlike glucose gives a negative glucose oxidase reaction (Clinistix). Confirmation of the identity of the sugar is best accomplished by paper chromatography. The presence of galactose in urine does not in itself establish the diagnosis. Galactosuria, usually in combination with glucosuria or fructosuria, is seen in severe hepatic disorders of the neonatal period (e.g., neonatal hepatitis, tyrosinosis, or congenital atresia of the bile ducts). Families in whom several members are mentally defective and who have congenital cataracts without an abnormality in galactose metabolism have been described by Franceschetti and others.[229]

The enzyme defect is best documented by measuring the erythrocyte transferase activity. Currently, the most reliable technique for the enzyme assay is that of Beutler and Baluda.[230] In this assay, blood hemolysate is incubated at 37° C with UDP-glucose and galactose-1-phosphate. After the reaction is stopped, the amount of UDP-glucose consumed is determined following the addition of NAD and UDP-glucose dehydrogenase to the extract. Only 0.1 ml of blood is required for the analysis, which can be run on capillary blood obtained in the newborn nursery. Direct measurement of galactose-1-phosphate uridyl transferase activity in erythrocytes has been employed by Donnell and his group for the detection of heterozygotes.[231] The antenatal diagnosis of galactosemia can be made by enzymatic assay on cultured amniotic fluid cells.[232]

Treatment

When milk is withdrawn and lactose-free products such as Nutramigen and Mullsoy substituted, gastrointestinal symptoms are rapidly relieved and normal growth reinstituted. The progression of cirrhosis is arrested, and sometimes the cataracts disappear. In 85% of treated patients the IQ exceeds 90 but usually is still less than that of unaffected siblings.[233] The composition of a low galactose diet has been published by Cornblath and Schwarz.[234] Even though soybean powder contains galactose in the form of alpha-galactosides, these are not absorbed from the normal intestinal tract and no galactose uptake can be demonstrated on a soybean diet unless, in the presence of diarrhea, galactoside-splitting bacteria colonize the upper intestine.[235] Maintenance of the galactose-free diet and avoidance of milk and milk products is recommended until after puberty. Intermittent monitoring of erythrocyte galactose-1-phosphate levels have been suggested. In several children who returned to a milk-containing diet prior to puberty, cataracts flared up. There are also some who, even after that age, continue to be sensitive to milk products and prefer to avoid them.

Because infants have developed hypoglycemia when first placed on a galactose-free diet, it might be well to add excess of glucose to the formula.

GLYCOGEN STORAGE DISEASE (GLYCOGENOSES)

Of the nine types of glycogenoses only one form directly affects the central nervous system (Table 1–7). This condition, first described by Pompe[236] in 1932 and known as the generalized or cardiac form of glycogen storage disease (type II by Cori),[237] is a rare autosomal recessive disorder characterized by glycogen accumulation in skeletal muscles, heart, liver, and central nervous system.

Biochemical Pathology

Two groups of enzymes are involved in the degradation of glycogen. Phosphorylase initiates one set of breakdown reactions,

TABLE 1-7.

THE ENZYMATICALLY DEFINED GLYCOGENOSES

Type	Defect	Structure of Glycogen	Involvement	Neuromuscular Symptoms
—	UDPG-glycogen transferase	Normal	Liver, muscle	Hypoglycemic seizures
I	Glucose-6-phosphatase	Normal	Liver, kidney	Hypoglycemic seizures
II	Acid α-1,4-glucosidase	Normal	Generalized	Progressive weakness
III	Amylo-1,6-glucosidase and/or oligo-1,4→ 1,4-glucan-transferase	Limit dextrin	Generalized, liver, muscle	Hypoglycemic convulsions
IV	Amylo-1,4→ 1,6-transglucosylase	Amylopectin-like	Generalized	None
V	Muscle phosphorylase	Normal	Muscle	Muscular cramps, weakness, atrophy
VI	Liver phosphorylase	Normal	Liver, leukocytes	Hypoglycemia
VII	Phosphofructokinase	Normal	Muscle, erythrocytes	Muscular cramps, weakness
VIII	Phosphohexoseisomerase (inhibitor?)	Normal	Muscle	Muscular cramps, myoglobinuria
IX	Phosphorylase kinase	Normal	Liver	None

cleaving glycogen to limit dextrin, which then is acted upon by a debrancher enzyme (oligo-1, 4→1, 4-glucantransferase, and amylo-1, 6-glucosidase) to yield a straight-chain polyglucosan, which is cleaved to the individual glucose units by phosphorylase.

A second set of enzymes includes α-amylase which cleaves glycogen to a series of oligosaccharides, and two α-1, 4-glucosidases which cleave the α-1, 4 bonds of glycogen. There are two of these terminal glucosidases, one, located in the microsomal fraction, has a neutral pH optimum (neutral maltase); the other, found in lysosomes, has its maximum activity at an acid pH (3.5) (acid maltase).

The structure of glycogen in Pompe's disease is normal, and the activity of all other enzymes involved in carbohydrate metabolism is intact. In type II glycogenosis the latter enzyme (acid maltase) is deficient in lysosomes of liver, heart, and skeletal muscle,[238] and it has been postulated that acid maltase normally metabolizes the glycogen accumulating in lysosomes as a result of tissue turnover.

Pathology

Glycogen may be deposited in virtually every tissue. The heart is globular, the enlargement being symmetric and primarily ventricular. There is massive glycogen deposition within the muscle fibers. In cross section these appear with a central, clear area giving a "lacunate" appearance. Glycogen is also deposited in striated muscle, particularly the tongue, and in smooth muscle, kidney, and liver (Fig. 1–12). Ultrastructural studies of the liver show normal amounts of glycogen in cytoplasm, but increased concentrations within lysosomes.[239] In the central nervous system glycogen accumulates within neurons and in the extracellular substance. The anterior horn cells are predominantly affected, although deposits are seen in all parts of the neuraxis, including the cerebral cortex.[240] Chemical analysis indicates an excess of glycogen in both cerebral cortex and white matter and a deficiency in total phospholipid, cholesterol, and cerebroside. There is no evidence for primary demyelination.[240]

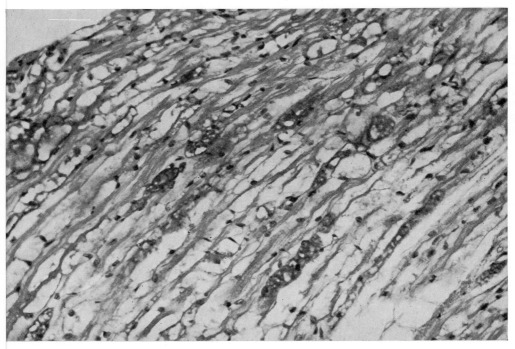

Fig. 1–12. Glycogen storage disease (type II-Cori). Muscle fibers showing vacuolated glycogen deposits. (Courtesy of Dr. J. B. Sidbury, Jr., Duke University Medical Center, Durham, North Carolina.)

Clinical Manifestations

The first symptoms usually appear during the second month of life or later. They include difficulty in feeding, with dyspnea and exhaustion interfering with sucking. Gradually muscular weakness and impaired cardiac function become apparent, although one or the other may predominate to such an extent that a division into cardiac and muscle types has been suggested.[241] In an occasional family, glycogen storage disease of the heart has been associated with Werdnig-Hoffmann disease in relatives.[242] Marked cardiac enlargement is present at an early age. The heart appears globular on radiographic examination; murmurs are usually absent but the heart tones have a poor quality and a gallop rhythm is often audible. The electrocardiogram is compatible with myocardial damage; the PR interval is markedly shortened, the R waves high and the T wave inverted. Affected infants have poor muscle tone and few spontaneous movements, although the deep tendon reflexes are often intact. Skeletal muscles may be enlarged and gradually acquire a peculiar rubbery consistency. Electromyography shows lower motor neuron degeneration. Convulsions, intellectual impairment, and coma have also been observed. The liver, while usually not enlarged, is abnormally firm and easily palpable. Splenomegaly is rare. Infants are prone to intercurrent infections, particularly pneumonia, and usually succumb to these or to bulbar paralysis by one year of age.

Acid maltase deficiency has also been seen in older children and adults. In these patients organomegaly is absent and muscle weakness is often slowly progressive or nonprogressive with maximum involvement of the proximal musculature of the lower extremities.[243] The biochemical difference between the two clinical forms of glycogen storage disease is unclear. It may involve the presence of a partially active but electrophoretically abnormal acid maltase in the milder form of the disease.[244,244a]

Diagnosis

When cardiac symptoms predominate, a differentiation from other causes of cardiomegaly and congestive failure in the absence of significant murmurs will be required. These include endocardial fibroelastosis, acute interstitial myocarditis, and aberrant coronary artery. When muscular weakness predominates, Werdnig-Hoffmann disease, muscular dystrophy, myasthenia gravis, and "atonic cerebral palsy" must be considered (see Chapter 12). Cardiac involvement is generally late in Werdnig-Hoffmann disease and muscular dystrophy. In contrast to glycogen storage disease, the intellectual deficit in atonic cerebral palsy is usually severe and early in onset. A muscle biopsy is usually required to confirm the diagnosis. Blood chemistries, including fasting blood sugars and glucose tolerance tests, are normal. The maltose-cleaving activity of leukocytes is markedly diminished, and a test for this reaction serves as an excellent diagnostic aid.[245] Acid maltase activity can also be shown in fibroblasts grown from normal amniotic cells; this method can be used for the antepartum diagnosis of Pompe's disease.[246]

Heterozygotes for this condition can be detected by observing the effect of phytohemagglutinins on lymphocyte enzymes. In the typical heterozygote phytohemagglutinin stimulation of a nonaffected enzyme will be greater than stimulation of acid maltase.[247]

Hug, Schubert, and Schwachman have described an infant with progressive ataxia, spasticity, and hepatomegaly, in whom glycogen storage was attributed to a deficiency in hepatic phosphorylase. In contrast to type VI glycogenesis, glucagon and epinephrine restored phosphorylase levels to normal.[248] The defect appeared to be the result of deranged control over the degree of activation of liver phosphorylase.

Treatment

Currently there is no effective treatment for Pompe's disease. Two approaches have been suggested. Intravenous administration of bacterial alpha-glucosidase has reduced hepatic glycogen content but induces a severe anaphylactic reaction. Hyperbaric oxygen therapy has also been proposed. This theoretically produces a transient leakage of glycogen from the lysosome into cytoplasm where it would be subject to the action of phosphorylase.

FRUCTOSE INTOLERANCE

Fructose intolerance, as distinguished from benign fructosuria, was first described by Chambers and Pratt in 1956.[249] It is relatively rare in the United States, but far more common in Europe, perhaps because of the tendency to supplement infant formulas with sucrose. The condition is usually transmitted by an autosomal recessive gene, and manifests itself by intestinal disturbances, poor weight gain, and attacks of hypoglycemia after fructose ingestion. Transient icterus with hepatic enlargement, fructosuria, albuminuria, and aminoaciduria follow intake of large quantities of fructose. Mild mental deficiency is frequent and there may be a flaccid quadriparesis.[250] The main pathologic abnormality is hepatic cirrhosis similar to that seen in galactosemia. The brain shows neuronal shrinkage, attributable to hypoglycemia, and retarded myelination.[251]

Biochemical Pathology

Finnish and French workers have demonstrated a deficiency of fructose-1-phosphate aldolase in liver, kidney, and mucosa of small intestine.[252,253] The activity of fructose-1, 6-diphosphate aldolase is lowered to a lesser extent (10–25% of normal in liver of affected infants). By electrophoresis it becomes evident that the principal hepatic aldolase, aldolase B, is inactive, while aldolase A, normally found in muscle and renal medulla, is normal.[254] This enzymatic pattern is similar to that seen in normal fetal tissue.

As a consequence of the metabolic defect ingested fructose, or sucrose, which is split into fructose and glucose, is converted to fructose-1-phosphate, which accumulates in tissues and is responsible for renal and hepatic damage. In the kidneys fructose-1-phosphate induces proximal tubular dysfunction within 30 minutes after its intake, while renal medullary function remains intact.[255] The cause of the fructose-induced hypoglycemia is unknown, but it is not related to excess insulin release, or to increased peripheral utilization of glucose. More likely, the conversion of hepatic glycogen to glucose is inhibited, possibly at the point of the cyclic AMP-induced activation of phosphorylase.[256]

Diagnosis

The diagnosis of hereditary fructose intolerance is made in part on the patient's clinical history, on the presence of a urinary reducing substance, and on the results of an intravenous fructose tolerance test (0.25 gm/kg). In most cases administration of this amount of fructose produces gastrointestinal symptoms, hypoglycemia, and a fall in the level of serum phosphorus. In the urine tyrosine, phenylalanine, proline, and phenolic acid excretion is increased. For confirmation a liver biopsy with determination of fructose-1-phosphate aldolase levels is necessary. Other causes for an increased excretion of fructose are fructosuria, an asymptomatic metabolic variant due to a deficiency of fructokinase, and impaired liver function.

Of the various forms of mellituria seen in infancy and childhood the most common are due to the increased excretion of a single sugar, predominantly glucose. Isolated lactosuria and fructosuria are also encountered. Lactosuria is usually explained on the basis of congenital lactose intolerance, or secondary lactose intolerance associated with enteritis, celiac disease, and cystic fibrosis. Essential pentosuria is due to the excretion of L-xylulose. Ribosuria occurs in muscular dystrophy, probably as the result of tissue breakdown. Sucrosuria has been reported in association with hiatus hernia and other intestinal disturbances.

A mixed sugar excretion can be seen in acute infections, liver disease, and gastroenteritis.[257]

Treatment

Treatment is relatively simple. It involves avoiding the intake of fruits and cane or beet sugar (sucrose). The composition of fructose-free diets has been published.[234]

MUCOPOLYSACCHARIDOSES (GARGOYLISM)

A syndrome consisting of mental and physical retardation, multiple skeletal deformities, hepatosplenomegaly, and clouding of the cornea was first described by Hunter in

TABLE 1-8.
A CLASSIFICATION OF THE MUCOPOLYSACCHARIDOSES

Type	Eponym	Clinical Features				Urinary MPS					Enzyme Defect
		Corneal Clouding	Dwarfism	Neurologic Signs	Cardiovascular Involvement	HS	DS	KS	C-4-S	C-6-S	
I	Hurler	Severe	Marked	Marked	Marked	+	+				α-L-iduronidase
II	Hunter	Absent (late?)	Marked	Mild to moderate	Late	+	+				?
III	Sanfilippo A, B	Absent (late?)	Moderate	None	Unknown	+					A. Heparan sulfate sulfatase B. α-acetylglucosaminidase
IV	Morquio	Late	Marked	None	Late			+			?
V	Scheie	Severe	Mild	Marked	Late	+	+			+	α-L-iduronidase (partial)
VI	Maroteaux-Lamy	Severe	Marked	Marked	Unknown	+	+				Sulfatase B
VII	Chondroitin-4 sulfate mucopolysaccharidosis	Mild	Marked	None (mild mental retardation)	None				+		?

Key to symbols: MPS = mucopolysaccharides; HS = heparan sulfate; DS = dermatan sulfate; C-4-S = chondroitin-4-sulfate; KS = keratan sulfate and C-6-S = chondroitin-6-sulfate

32

1917[258] and later by Hurler and Pfaundler in 1919 and 1920.[259] To Ellis and his associates in 1936 the "large head, inhuman facies, and deformed limbs" suggested the appearance of a gargoyle.[260] The syndrome actually represents seven or more entities, distinguishable by their genetic transmission, enzymatic defects, and urinary mucopolysaccharide pattern (Table 1–8).

Biochemical Pathology

The principal biochemical disturbance in the various mucopolysaccharidoses involves the metabolism of mucopolysaccharides (MPS).[261] These are polymers of high molecular weight in which uronic acids and amino sugars or their sulfate esters are the main structural units. Large amounts (75 to 100 mg per 24 hours) of fragmented chains of two sulfated mucopolysaccharides, chondroitin sulfate B (dermatan sulfate) and heparan sulfate are excreted by individuals affected with either of the two principal genetic entities, the autosomally transmitted type I (Hurler's type) and the rarer sex-linked type II (Hunter's type). This compares with a normal excretion of 5–25 mg per 24 hours for all MPS's. According to Varadi et al. this is distributed between chondroitin sulfate A (chondroitin-4-sulfate) (31%), chondroitin sulfate C (chondroitin-6-sulfate) (34%), chondroitin (25%), and heparan sulfate (8%).[263]

Another form of mucopolysaccharidosis has been included under the term Morquio or Morquio-Ullrich disease (type IV, Table 1–8). The urinary MPS excreted in this condition consists of almost 50% keratan sulfate and lesser amounts of chondroitin-6-sulfate.[264]

Yet another disorder, termed the Sanfilippo variant (type III, Table 1–8) and transmitted as an autosomal recessive trait, manifests itself by intellectual deterioration commencing at about three years of age. Hepatosplenomegaly and other physical stigmata are relatively unremarkable, and bony abnormalities are absent.[265] In this variant the principal urinary MPS is heparan sulfate.

Scheie first described an adult form which spares the nervous system and has been observed in individuals presenting with corneal dystrophy (type V, Table 1–8). Like Hurler's and Hunter's disease, these patients excrete dermatan sulfate and heparan sulfate.[266]

Two rarer mucopolysaccharidoses, the Maroteaux-Lamy syndrome,[267] and chondroitin-4-sulfate mucopolysaccharidosis[268] are outlined in Table 1–8. The former is associated with a deficiency of sulfatase B from liver, kidney, and spleen.[269]

The chemistry of mucopolysaccharides has been reviewed by Spranger.[270] MPS occurs as large polymers having a protein core, and multiple carbohydrate branches. Chondroitin-4-sulfate is found in cornea, bone, and cartilage. It consists of alternating units of D-glucuronic acid and sulfated N-acetyl galactosamine (Fig. 1–13).

Dermatan sulfate is a normal minor constituent of connective tissue, and a major component of skin. It differs structurally from chondroitin-4-sulfate in that L-iduronic acid takes the place of glucuronic acid in the alternating hexose moieties (Fig. 1–13).

Heparan sulfate consists of alternating units of D-glucuronic acid and N-acetylglucosamine, which is either sulfated in the 6-position or has an N-sulfate replacing the N-acetyl group. In some areas the N-acetylglucosamine may not be sulfated while in others it is doubly sulfated.[271] In both cases the mucopolysaccharide chains are linked to serine of the

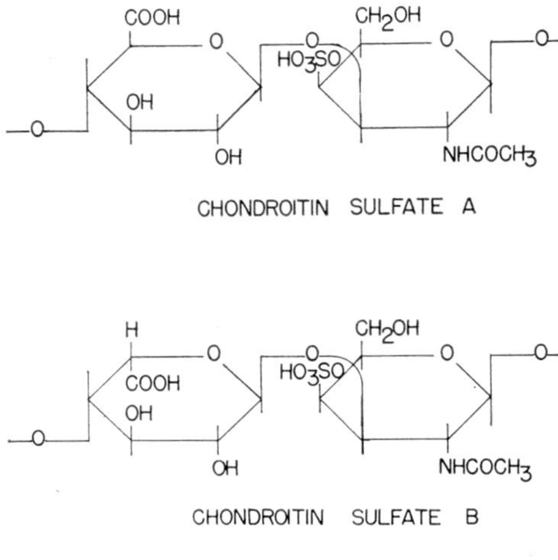

CHONDROITIN SULFATE A

CHONDROITIN SULFATE B

Fig. 1–13. Structure of chondroitin sulfate A (chondroitin-4-sulfate) and chondroitin sulfate B (dermatan sulfate).

protein core by means of a xylose-galactose-galactose-glucuronic acid-N-acetylhexosamine bridge.[272]

Over the last few years the pathways of MPS biosynthesis have been partly elucidated. Since MPS synthesis is puromycin-sensitive, the formation of a protein acceptor appears to be the primary reaction.[273] Hexosamine and hexuronic acid moieties are then attached to the protein, one sugar at a time, starting with xylose. The manner by which a chain of alternate groups of hexosamine and hexuronic acid are synthesized is still not clear. Sulfation occurs after the completion of polymerization. The sulfate groups are introduced through the intermediary of an active sulfate. This is a labile nucleotide, identified as adenosine-3'-phosphate-5'sulfatophosphate.[274] Desulfation and depolymerization may occur simultaneously, but the relevant steps are unknown. Connective tissue of patients with mucopolysaccharidoses contains normal amounts of dermatan sulfate and heparan sulfate. In tissues where there are pathologic amounts of MPS, such as in liver, spleen, and in the urine the protein core is completely lacking or only represented by a few amino acids.[275] Together with the finding of a decreased rate of MPS degradation by fibroblast cultures this suggests that the basic defect in the mucopolysaccharidoses is a malfunction of the degradative pathway.[276] The excessive accumulation of MPS in Hurler's fibroblasts is correctable by a protein isolated from normal fibroblasts or normal human urine which accelerates the degradation of the stored sulfated MPS and is identical with α-L-iduronidase.[277]

The material stored in brain of patients with Hurler's disease is of two types. Jervis found the ganglioside content of cerebral cortex, as determined from the fat-soluble neuraminic acid concentration, to be three to five times normal.[279] This increase is due to the presence of large amounts of two gangliosides, normally only present in trace quantities. One of these is the ganglioside stored in Tay-Sachs disease (G_{M2}), while the other is hexosamine-free and is identical with hematoside (G_{M3}).[280] The greater proportion of the material stored within affected neurons is in the form of MPS the exact structure of which is still uncertain.[281]

The enzymatic difference between Hurler's and Hunter's diseases is still unclear. While the MPS excretion pattern cannot be used to distinguish the two conditions, fibroblasts derived from patients with Hunter's disease will not prevent accumulation of MPS in Hurler's fibroblasts. The factor accelerating the degradation of dermatan sulfate in fibroblasts from patients with Hunter's disease has as yet not been shown to have any enzymatic activity.[281a] Similarly the metabolism of Hurler's cells is correctable by fibroblast strains derived from patients with Sanfilippo disease. However, fibroblasts from patients with Scheie's disease do not correct the accumulation of MPS in Hurler fibroblasts. This suggests that the enzymatic defect in these two conditions is identical, and that residual activity of α-L-iduronidase in Scheie's disease prevents its full phenotypic expression.[282]

Sanfilippo disease is biochemically heterogenous. On the basis of their enzymatic deficiencies, cultured fibroblasts of patients fall into two subgroups: type A in which heparan sulfate sulfatase is deficient, and type B with a defect in N-acetyl-α-D-glucosaminidase (Table 1–8).[282a,282b]

Pathologic Anatomy

The visceral alterations in Hurler's and Hunter's diseases are widespread and involve almost every organ.[283,284] Large vacuolated cells (gargoyle cells) containing acid MPS and believed to be derived from fibroblasts may be found in cartilage, tendons, periosteum, the endocardium, and the vascular walls, particularly the intima of the coronary arteries. By electron microscopy another cell type containing a glycolipid has been identified in the mitral valves.[285] There are abnormalities in the cartilage of the bronchial tree, and the alveoli are filled with lipid-laden cells. The bone marrow is replaced in part by connective tissue, which contains many vacuolated fibroblasts. The liver is unusually large, most parenchymal cells being about double or more their normal size. On electron microscopy MPS are noted to accumulate in the lysosomes of most hepatic parenchymatous cells.[286] The Kupffer cells are swollen and contain abnormal amounts of MPS. In the spleen the reticulum cells are larger than normal and contain the same storage material. In Hurler's and Sanfilippo disease there are widespread changes in the central nervous system. The neurons are swollen and vacuolated and their nuclei are peripherally displaced. Neuronal distention is most conspicuous in the cerebral cortex, but the cells in the thalamus, brain stem, and particularly in the anterior horns of the spinal cord are also involved. In the cerebellum, the Purkinje cells contain abnormal lipid material and demonstrate a fusiform swelling of their dendrites. In white matter, the perivascular spaces are often distended and filled with aggregates of fat-laden cells. Frequently, the leptomeninges are markedly fibrosed and contain a similar storage material. These alterations produce a partial obstruction of the subarachnoid spaces and are responsible for the hydrocephalus which is often observed.

Clinical Manifestations[270,287]

Children affected with Hurler's disease usually appear normal at birth and during the greater part of their first year. Slowness in development may be the first evidence of the disorder. Bony abnormalities of the upper extremities are observed by one to two years. According to Caffey, these changes are much more marked here than in the lower extremities, the most striking being swelling of the central portion of the humeral shaft[288] (Fig. 1–14), produced by a thickening of the cortex and dilatation of the medullary canal.

Typically, the patient is small with a large head and peculiar gross features (Fig. 1–15). The eyes are widely spaced. The bridge of the nose is flat and the lips are large. The mouth is open and there is an almost constant nasal obstruction or upper respiratory infection. Kyphosis is marked and appears early. The hands are wide, the fingers short and stubby. The abdomen protrudes, an umbilical hernia is often present, and there is gross hepatosplenomegaly. The hair is profuse and coarse. In older children a unique skin lesion is occasionally observed.[290]

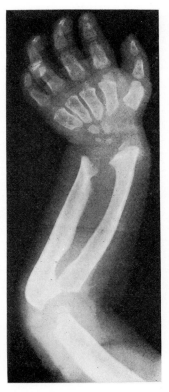

Fig. 1–14. Hurler's disease. Roentgenogram of upper extremity. The ulna and radius are short and wide, their epiphyseal ends irregular. The metacarpal bones and phalanges are also thickened and irregular.

It consists of an aggregation of white, nontender papules of varying size, found symmetrically around the thorax and upper extremities. Corneal opacities are frequent in Hurler's disease. In most cases there is progressive spasticity and mental deterioration. Deafness and optic atrophy may develop ultimately.

Generally, the course is downhill with the disease progressing more slowly in those children whose symptoms had a somewhat later onset. McKusick has pointed out that all patients who have survived for 20 years or longer have been male and probably have had Hunter's disease.[287]

Death is usually due to bronchopneumonia secondary to the previously described pulmonary and bronchial alterations. Conges-

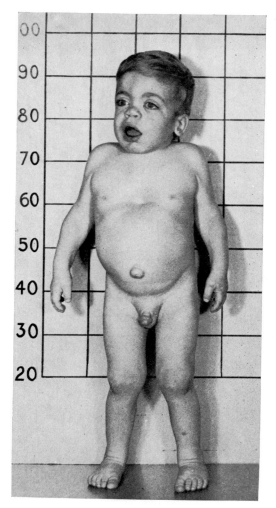

Fig. 1–15. Hurler's disease in a 4-year-old. The boy demonstrates the unusual, coarse facies, depressed bridge of nose, open mouth, and large tongue. The hands are spadelike, the abdomen protrudes, and there is an umbilical hernia. (Courtesy of Dr. V. A. McKusick, Johns Hopkins Hospital, Baltimore, Maryland.)

tive heart failure and coronary artery disease may also prove fatal, even as early as age seven.[291]

Hunter's disease is less severe than Hurler's disease. While the major clinical manifestations are similar, mental deterioration progresses at a slower rate, and corneal clouding is usually absent or minimal in the older patient. Retinitis pigmentosa has been ob-served and may progress to complete blindness. While Hurler's disease is transmitted as an autosomal recessive disorder, Hunter's disease has a sex-linked recessive inheritance with the female carrier being clinically unaffected. It is about one-fifth as frequent as Hurler's disease.

Sanfilippo disease, an autosomal recessive disease, is characterized by mental deterioration beginning at about the third year of life in the face of minor somatic signs. These include facial abnormalities, hepatosplenomegaly, and minor skeletal alterations, apparent radiologically.

The clinical manifestations of Morquio's disease include retarded growth and deformities of the vertebral bodies and epiphyseal zones of the long bones. Corneal opacities and mental retardation are occasionally present, and patients with these signs have, in the past, been designated as having Morquio-Ullrich disease. But the characteristically high urinary output of keratan sulfate is also present in patients who lack mental retardation.[292]

In Scheie's disease the major manifestation is corneal clouding. Intelligence is unaffected, and neurologic symptoms are limited to a high incidence of carpal tunnel syndrome (compression of the median nerve as it traverses the carpal tunnel of the wrist).

In Maroteaux-Lamy disease and in chondroitin-4-sulfate mucopolysaccharidosis intelligence is usually normal, and there are no neurologic symptoms.

Diagnosis

While classic gargoylism offers little in the way of diagnostic difficulty, children are frequently seen in whom some of the cardinal signs such as hepatosplenomegaly, mental deficiency, bony abnormalities, or a typical facial configuration, are minimal or completely lacking. A useful screening test for increased output of urinary MPS has been suggested by Renuart.[293]

To 1 ml of a 5 percent solution of cetyltrimethylammonium bromide (CAB) in a 1 molar citrate buffer, pH 6.0, 5 ml of previously filtered urine are added. The solutions are mixed and allowed to stand in an incubator or a water bath at 25° C for 30 minutes. A flocculent precipitate represents a positive test.

A small increase in the output of urinary MPS has been seen in Marfan's disease, celiac disease, idiopathic hypercalcemia, and in the various collagen vascular diseases. Small infants may also give falsely positive results with this test.

Further differentiation of the mucopolysaccharidoses rests on the electrophoretic patterns of of the urinary MPS (Table 1–8). The accumulation of metachromatic material in fibroblast cultures can also be used for diagnostic purposes, and is of particular assistance in making an antenatal diagnosis utilizing amniotic fluid cells.[261,262]

X-ray abnormalities in Hurler's syndrome are extensive and have been reviewed by Caffey[288] (Figs. 1–14 and 1–16). The cerebrospinal fluid is normal. When blood smears are studied carefully, 20–40 percent of lymphocytes will be seen to contain metachromatically staining cytoplasmic inclusions (Reilly granules) in Hurler's, Hunter's, and Sanfilippo diseases.[289]

In a number of conditions, the facial configuration seen in Hurler's disease, the bony abnormalities and hepatosplenomegaly are unaccompanied by an abnormal MPS ex-

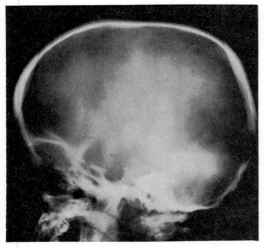

Fig. 1–16. Hurler's syndrome. Roentgenogram of skull. The skull bones are somewhat thickened and the sella turcica is enlarged and the posterior clinoid is hooked forward. (Courtesy of Dr. O. M. Gatewood, Johns Hopkins Hospital, Baltimore, Maryland.)

cretion. The best defined of these entities is generalized G_{M1} gangliosidosis, formerly known as pseudo-Hurler's disease. This condition is characterized by hepatosplenomegaly, mental retardation, and bony abnormalities, but a normal MPS output. The basic defect is one of ganglioside degradation, and the condition will be considered with the disorders of lipid metabolism. Patients presenting with dwarfism, early psychomotor retardation, unusual facies, but a clear or only faintly hazy cornea, and a normal MPS excretion[294] manifest a syndrome termed lipomucopolysaccharidosis, or I cell disease. In this condition the fibroblast cultures show coarse metachromatic inclusions, and the activity of a number of lysosomal enzymes, including beta-galactosidase, and alpha-L-fucosidase, is reduced.[295] Cretinism, another diagnostic alternative, may be distinguished from the mucopolysaccharidoses by determination of serum protein-bound iodine and I^{131} uptake.

Treatment

No therapy has proved successful. Fresh plasma or whole blood transfusions have been ineffective.[296] Long-term administration of corticosteroids results in a reduction of MPS output but does not alter the course of the disease. The finding of decreased sulfate fixation by chondrocytes in hypervitaminosis A did not prove to be clinically applicable, and administration of vitamin A increased seizure frequency and hepatosplenomegaly of patients with Hurler's syndrome.[297]

DISORDERS OF GLYCOPROTEIN METABOLISM

Familial Myoclonus Epilepsy

This condition, first described by Unverricht in 1895,[298] is manifested by progressive intellectual deterioration and myoclonic seizures. The latter are involuntary shocklike contractions of one or more muscles or parts of muscle appearing synchronously or asynchronously throughout the body.

Pathologic Anatomy

Many concentric amyloid (Lafora) bodies are found within the cytoplasm of ganglion cells throughout the neuraxis, particularly in the dentate nucleus, the substantia nigra, reticular substance, and hippocampus (Fig. 1–17). Histochemically these inclusions react as a protein-bound mucopolysaccharide. Similar amyloid material has been found in heart and liver.[299]

Isolation and hydrolysis of these organelles has shown them to consist of a glucose polymer, linked in the 1:4 and 1:6 positions, and chemically, but not structurally, related to glycogen. The protein content of isolated Lafora bodies varies from 7% in brain to 26% in liver.[300] The metabolic defect for the glycoprotein storage is unknown.

Clinical Manifestations

The disease appears between the ages 7 and 14 with the onset of grand mal and myoclonic seizures. At first, the latter are triggered by photic stimulation or proprioceptive impulses and are much more frequent when formal tests of coordination are attempted, simulating the intention tremor of cerebellar ataxia. The electroencephalogram is usually abnormal with numerous bilateral sharp waves and synchronous spike discharges. The interval between the bilateral sharp waves and the myoclonus is 15 msec in the upper extremities, and 25 msec in the lower extremities, suggesting that both cortical discharges and myoclonic seizures are secondary to a brain stem focus.

With progression of the disease, the major seizures become less frequent, myoclonus increases in intensity, and intellectual deterioration occurs. A terminal stage of dementia, spastic quadriparesis, and almost constant myoclonic seizures is reached within 4 to 10 years of the first symptoms.

Diagnosis

Myoclonic seizures occur in idiopathic epilepsy, and in a variety of degenerative diseases, most commonly the infantile and juvenile amaurotic idiocies. They are also found in the gray matter degenerative disorders and in subacute sclerosing panencephalitis (Dawson) (see Chapter 6). Finally, dentatorubral atrophy (Ramsay Hunt syndrome) must also be considered. As depicted by Hunt in 1921, the last is a progressive cerebellar ataxia accompanied by myoclonic seizures and atrophy of the dentate nucleus and superior cerebellar peduncles without the presence of amyloid bodies. It is not clear whether this disease represents a distinct entity (see Chapter 2).

The diagnosis of familial myoclonus epi-

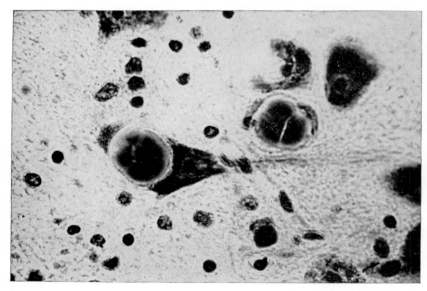

Fig. 1–17. Myoclonus epilepsy. Inclusion bodies in neurones of substantia nigra (Nissl stain). (From Merritt, H. H., *Textbook of Neurology*, 4th ed., 1970, courtesy of Lea and Febiger, Philadelphia, Pennsylvania.)

lepsy is confirmed by finding Lafora bodies in cortical biopsy specimens. No Lafora bodies are seen in a liver biopsy, but PAS-positive material is found in the extracellular spaces.[301] On electron microscopy the endoplasmic reticulum of liver is disrupted, and there are large vacuoles containing electron dense material. Biopsy of the skeletal muscle is normal.[302]

Treatment

No therapy has been found to arrest the progression of neurologic symptoms. The seizures are generally refractory to anticonvulsants.

Fucosidosis

This presumed defect in the metabolism of glycoproteins is characterized by progressive intellectual deterioration and spasticity commencing between two and six years of age.[303] Biochemically, there is an accumulation of a complex sphingolipid in a variety of organs including brain,[304] and a deficiency in alpha-L-fucosidase.[305] The stored sphingolipid structurally resembles the oligosaccharides of erythrocytes responsible for H and Lewis blood group activity.

Mannosidosis

A retarded child with radiologic abnormalities and vacuolated lymphocytes was found to have a deficiency of the lysosomal enzyme, alpha-mannosidase. This is believed to be responsible for the storage of mannose within neurons of the central nervous system including the spinal cord.[306]

DISORDERS MANIFESTED BY INTERMITTENT METABOLIC ACIDOSIS

A number of disorders of intermediary metabolism are manifested by intermittent episodes of vomiting, lethargy, acidosis, and the excretion of ketone bodies. Even though the enzymatic lesions responsible are not related, they are here grouped together for convenience. The conditions are summarized in Table 1–9.

Propionic Acidemia (Ketotic Hyperglycinemia)

Ketotic hyperglycinemia, the first of this group of disorders to be described, is charac-

TABLE 1-9.

CONDITIONS PRODUCING RECURRENT METABOLIC ACIDOSIS IN INFANCY AND CHILDHOOD

Condition	Reference
Glycogen storage disease (type I)	Howell et al.[307]
Propionic acidemia (ketotic hyperglycinemia)	Childs et al.[308]
Methylmalonic acidemia	Overholzer et al.[315]
Isovaleric acidemia	Budd et al.[325]
Lactic acidemia	Hartmann et al.[327]
Subacute necrotizing encephalomyelopathy	Leigh[333]
Renal tubular acidosis	
Intoxications	
Diabetes mellitus	

terized by intermittent episodes of vomiting, lethargy and ketosis, commencing within 18 hours of birth.[308] Marked intellectual retardation and a neurologic picture of a mixed pyramidal and extrapyramidal lesion ultimately become apparent. Attacks are precipitated by ingestion of proteins and various amino acids, notably leucine. Other findings include a persistent neutropenia and thrombocytopenia. Propionic acidemia is seen in all patients and both plasma and urinary glycine levels are markedly increased.[309] In the first reported patient, excretion of acetoacetic acid and acetone was high, and large amounts of other carbonyl compounds, such as methyl ethyl ketone, methyl isopropyl ketone, 2-pentanone, 3-pentanone, and a hexanone of uncertain structure were also detected.[310] Hsia et al. have shown a defect in propionyl CoA-carboxylase, the enzyme converting propionyl CoA to methylmalonyl CoA.[311] As a consequence of the metabolic block, long-chain ketones are formed from propionate precursors, methyl citrate results from the condensation of propionyl CoA and oxalacetate, and 3-hydroxypropionate is formed.[311a,311b]

Ketotic hyperglycinemia is distinct from familial glycinuria, described by deVries et al.,[312] a condition where serum glycine levels are normal, and the nervous system is unaffected. It should also be distinguished from iminoglycinuria,[197] and from nonketotic hyperglycinemia accompanied by a defect in the metabolism of glycine to CO_2 and hydroxymethyl tetrahydrofolate.[314] Isovaleric acidemia (vid. infr.) may also present with episodes of ketoacidosis and hyperglycinemia.[313]

Methylmalonic Acidemia

Although clinically similar to ketotic hyperglycinemia, methylmalonic acidemia is biochemically distinct. The patients present in early infancy with profound metabolic acidosis, intermittent lethargy or coma, and developmental retardation. Ingestion of a high protein diet precipitates ketoacidosis, long-chain ketonuria, and the excretion of large amounts of methylmalonic acid.[315] In some patients the blood levels of valine, threonine, isoleucine, and ammonia are increased.[316] The enzymatic defect has been localized to methylmalonyl CoA carbonyl mutase, the enzyme converting methylmalonyl CoA to succinyl CoA.[317,319] As a consequence of the metabolic block propionyl CoA accumulates, and promotes the formation of butanone and other long-chain ketones. The cause for the hyperglycinemia remains obscure. In some patients administration of vitamin B_{12} (1 mg/day), the cofactor for the mutase, reduces methylmalonic acid excretion to a significant degree, improves propionate and methylmalonate oxidation by leukocytes, and prevents attacks of ketosis.[320] In these patients the block is probably in the synthesis of 5'-deoxyadenosyl cobalamine, the coenzyme for methylmalonyl mutase, while in B_{12} unresponsive patients the primary abnormality is in the apoenzyme itself.[318,321]

Another variant of methylmalonic acidemia was reported by Levy et al.[322] Patients with this condition also have high serum levels of homocystine and cystathionine, and low levels of methionine. This condition results from defects in two cobalamine dependent reactions (methylation of homocysteine to methionine, and isomerization of methylmalonyl CoA to succinyl CoA), probably as a consequence of defective biosynthesis of the B_{12} cofactor.[321]

In a fourth variant of methylmalonic acidemia the defect is one of the racemase converting D-methyl malonyl-CoA to L-methylmalonyl-CoA.[321a] Methylmalonic acidemia can be suspected when urine treated with diazotized p-nitroaniline develops an emerald green color.[323] Patients with vitamin B_{12} deficiency will also excrete large amounts of methylmalonic acid. In children resistant to treatment with large doses of vitamin B_{12}, restriction of protein intake will prevent the severe acidosis.

Isovaleric Acidemia

A very striking odor of urine, perspiration, and exhaled air, resembling stale perspiration, is characteristic for patients with isovaleric acidemia. These infants, first described by Tanaka et al.,[324] present with recurrent acidosis and coma. Serum isovaleric acid concentrations are several hundred times normal, and the administration of L-leucine produces a sustained rise in isovaleric acid levels. Since the concentration of dimethyl acrylic acid is normal and since the oxidation of ^{14}C-labeled isovaleric acid is impaired in leucocytes of affected subjects, the defect can be localized to isovaleryl CoA dehydrogenase (step 3, Fig. 1–5).[325] The acidosis seen in this disease is due to an accumulation of ketone bodies rather than isovaleric acidemia. Inhibition of isovaleryl CoA dehydrogenase may also be seen following intoxication with ackee, the fruit inducing Jamaican Vomiting Sickness.[326] The condition, formerly known as "Sweaty Feet Syndrome," is probably also isovaleric acidemia.

Lactic Acidemia

In 1962 Hartmann and associates described a three-year-old mongoloid girl who since early infancy suffered from chronic acidosis due to an accumulation of blood lactate and pyruvate.[327] A number of other children with this condition have since been reported.[328,329] Features include mental retardation, hypotonia, obesity, seizures, and periods of impaired consciousness.

The metabolic defect underlying the accumulation of lactic and pyruvic acids is obscure, but infusions of sodium lactate result in an abnormally high rise and a very gradual fall of blood lactate. In contrast to the normal blood lactate of approximately 2mM per liter (18mg%) or less, fasting levels in these patients average 9mM per liter. Since the pyruvate: lactate ratio remains within normal limits, Israels and associates[328] have suggested that a partial block of pyruvate decarboxylation may produce this derangement of intermediary metabolism, while Skrede et al. have offered evidence for a diminished capacity for gluconeogenesis.[329] A similar metabolic block, but a completely different clinical picture is seen in pyruvate decarboxylase defect and hyperalaninemia. These children present with intermittent cerebellar ataxia and choreo-athetosis. Most attacks follow nonspecific febrile illnesses, and last from several hours up to one week. One such patient had optic atrophy and mental retardation; another was of normal intelligence.[330] Muscle fibers contain an excessive amount of neutral lipids. Pyruvic decarboxylase in cultured skin fibroblasts is less than 20 percent of normal. As a consequence of the enzyme defect serum levels of both lactic and pyruvic acids are elevated, and blood and urine alanine are also increased.[331] Treatment with prednisone will abort or abbreviate patients' attacks; thiamine and lipoic acid, cofactors for pyruvate decarboxylase, have been ineffective.[332]

Chronic lactic acidosis and hyperpyruvic acidemia is also seen in infants with subacute necrotizing encephalomyelopathy. This rare entity, first described in 1951 by Leigh,[333] presents as a familial gray matter degeneration characterized by foci of necrosis and capillary proliferation within the brain stem, particularly the periaqueductal, periventricular, and tegmental gray matter.[334] The pathologic picture bears some resemblance to Wernicke's encephalopathy, while the clinical course is one of a diffuse cerebral degenerative condition with onset of symptoms during early infancy. In the majority of infants blood lactate and pyruvate levels have been elevated. Hommes et al.[335] have found a marked reduction in pyruvate carboxylase, the enzyme converting pyruvate to oxalacetate. A deficiency of thiamine triphosphate, and an inhibition of thiamine triphosphate synthesis have also been demonstrated in a number of other infants with this

disorder.[336] Lipoic acid (0.7 mg/kg) reduced blood lactate levels to upper limits of normal and improved the general condition of at least one patient but apparently did not influence the developmental retardation.

Increased levels of blood lactic and pyruvic acids have also been found in patients with mitochondrial abnormalities in muscle (see Chapter 12).

Subacute necrotizing encephalomyelopathy may also present in older children and adults.

DISORDERS OF LIPID METABOLISM

This group of disorders includes a number of hereditary diseases characterized by an abnormal sphingolipid metabolism, which in most instances leads to the intracellular deposition of lipid material within the central nervous system. Clinically, these conditions assume a progressive course which varies only in the rate of intellectual and visual deterioration.

With the recent rapid advances in our knowledge of the composition, structure, and metabolism of cerebral lipids, these disorders are best classified according to the chemical nature of the storage material or, if known, the underlying enzymatic block. While such an arrangement will be adhered to in this section, the chemistry and metabolism of sphingolipids often prove to be too complex for the clinician who is not continuously involved in this field. To make matters more difficult, diseases with a similar phenotypic expression may be caused by completely different enzymatic blocks, and conversely an apparently identical biochemical defect may produce completely different clinical pictures.

A more practical grouping of the lipid storage diseases, intended to assist in the bedside diagnosis of these disorders, is presented in Table 1–10.

GANGLIOSIDOSES

In choosing the name "gangliosides," Klenk[337] emphasized the localization of these lipids within the ganglion cells of the neuraxis. His finding has since been amply confirmed by work indicating that gangliosides are found mainly in nuclear areas of gray matter and are present in myelin in only small amounts.

TABLE 1-10.
LIPID STORAGE DISEASES

Condition	Storage Material (in Brain)	Enzymatic Defect	Clinical Characteristics
Lipid storage disease without marked visceromegaly			
Tay-Sachs disease	G_{M2} ganglioside	(a) Hexosaminidase A (b) Hexosaminidase A and B (c) Unknown	Cherry red spot; onset first year of life
Late infantile amaurotic idiocy (LIAI) (Batten-Bielschowsky)			
LIAI with CL bodies	Unknown-EM: CL bodies	Unknown	Onset between second and sixth year of life; intellectual deterioration, ataxia, myoclonic seizures; retinal degeneration usually late
LIAI with LF bodies	Unknown-EM: LF bodies	Unknown	
Generalized gangliosidosis G_{M1}	G_{M1} ganglioside	β-Galactosidase	
"Juvenile" G_{M2} gangliosidosis	G_{M2} ganglioside	Hexosaminidase A (partial)	
Niemann-Pick (group C)	Unknown Sphingomyelin stored in viscera	Unknown	Similar course as other forms of LIAI; retinal cherry red spot common
Juvenile amaurotic idiocy (Spielmeyer-Vogt)			
	(a) Unknown-EM: LF bodies	(a) Unknown	Onset between sixth year and puberty; intellectual deterioration, visual deterioration, generalized seizures
	(b) Unknown-EM: pleomorphic bodies	(b) Unknown	

Disease	Stored material	Enzyme defect	Clinical features
Juvenile G_{M2} gangliosidosis Dystonic juvenile lipidosis	G_{M2} ganglioside Unknown-EM: variety of cytoplasmic inclusions	Hexosaminidase A (partial) Unknown	Dystonia prominent part of neurologic symptoms
Late onset lipidosis (Kufs)	Unknown-EM: LF material	Unknown	Mental deterioration in adult life; psychotic symptoms predominant in early stages
Lipid storage diseases with marked visceromegaly *Infantile onset* Generalized gangliosidosis G_{M1}	G_{M1} ganglioside	β-Galactosidase	Hurler's appearance; bony abnormalities; retinal cherry red spots common
Infantile Gaucher's disease	Unknown Ceramide glucose in spleen	Glucocerebrosidase	Bulbar signs common early in disease; occasional cherry red spot
Niemann-Pick (group A)	Sphingomyelin	Sphingomyelinase	Intellectual deterioration; anemia; hepatosplenomegaly
Juvenile onset Gaucher's disease, juvenile Niemann-Pick (group D)	G_{M3} ganglioside Slightly increased sphingomyelin in viscera	β-galactosidase Unknown (sphingomyelinase normal)	Slow intellectual deterioration, hepatosplenomegaly

Key. EM = electron microscopy, LF = lipofuscin, CL = curvilinear.

TABLE 1-11.

STRUCTURES OF MAJOR GANGLIOSIDES OF HUMAN BRAIN

Proposed Structure (Kuhn and Weigandt)	Symbol
Gal (1→3) GalNac (1→4) Gal (1→4) Glu (1→1) Ceramide 3 ↑ 2 NANA	G_{M1} (G_4)
Gal (1→3) GalNac (1→4) Gal (1→4) Glu (1→1) Ceramide 3 3 ↑ ↑ 2 2 NANA NANA	G_{D1a} (G_3)
Gal (1→3) GalNac (1→4) Gal (1→4) Glu (1→1) Ceramide 3 ↑ 2 NANA (8←2) NANA	G_{D1b} (G_2)
Gal (1→3) GalNac (1→4) Gal (1→4) Glu (1→1) Ceramide 3 3 ↑ ↑ 2 2 NANA NANA (8←2) NANA	G_{T1} (G_1)

The function of gangliosides is not completely understood. They have been isolated from a variety of cellular membranes where they may be involved in ion transport and in the binding of neurogenic amines. Gangliosides are composed of sphingosine, hexose, hexosamine, fatty acids, and neuraminic acid.

At least 10 different gangliosides have been isolated from brain. Of these, four are major components, accounting for over 90 percent of the total ganglioside fraction. The composition and structure of some of the major gangliosides are presented in Table 1–11.

The major gangliosides contain the skeleton ceramide-glucose-galactose-galactosamine-galactose. N-acetylneuraminic acid (NANA) is attached to the proximal galactose in the monosialoganglioside (Fig. 1–18), while in the two major disialo- species, an additional NANA unit is attached either to the terminal galactose or to the first NANA.[338,339]

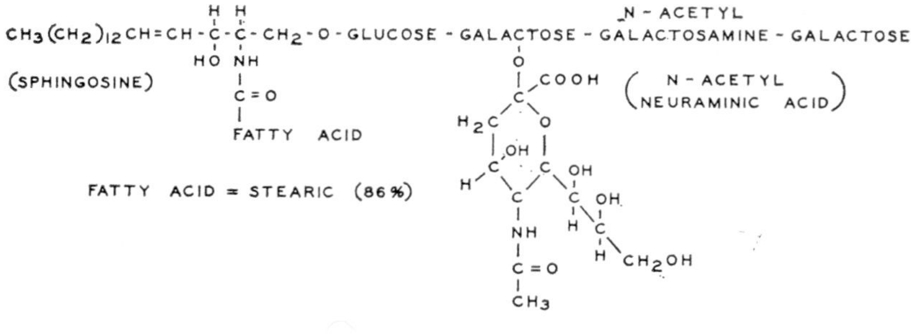

Fig. 1–18.   Structure of a monosialoganglioside.

Tay-Sachs Disease (G_{M2}-Gangliosidosis)

This, the most common of the gangliosidoses, was first described by Tay, who noted the retinal changes in 1881[350] and by Sachs in 1887.[341]

Pathology

The pathologic changes in Tay-Sachs disease are confined to the nervous system and represent the most florid of all the cerebral-retinal degenerations. Almost every neuron in the cerebral cortex is markedly distended, its nucleus displaced to the periphery, and the cytoplasm filled with lipid-soluble material (Fig. 1–19). A similar substance is stored in the apical dendrites of the pyramidal cells. As the disease progresses, the number of cortical neurons diminishes with only a few pyknotic cells remaining. The gliotic reaction is often quite extensive. In the white matter, myelination may become arrested, and in the terminal stages demyelination, accumulation of lipid breakdown products, and widespread status spongiosus are commonly observed. Similar alterations affect the cerebellar Purkinje cells and, to a somewhat lesser degree, the larger neurons of the brain stem and spinal cord. In the retina, the ganglion cells are distended with lipid, and at the margin of the fovea there is considerable reduction in their number and an accumulation of large phagocytic cells.

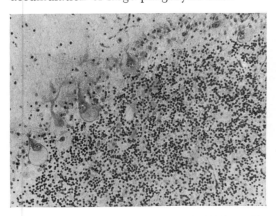

Fig. 1–19. Tay-Sachs disease. Purkinje cells, showing swollen cell bodies and an occasional "antler-like" dendrite. Generally, lipid storage in the cerebellum is less extensive than in the cerebral cortex. Cresyl violet × 150. (Courtesy of Dr. D. B. Clark, University of Kentucky, Lexington, Kentucky.)

On electron microscopic examination of the involved neurons the lipid is found in the "membranous cytoplasmic bodies," which are round, oval, 0.5 to 2.0 μ in diameter, and occupy a considerable portion of the ganglion cell cytoplasm (Fig. 1–20 A, B). The membranous bodies may also be located in axis cylinders, glial cells, and perivascular cells.[342] Membranous cytoplasmic bodies consist of aggregates of lipids (90 percent) and protein (10 percent). The composition of lipids is about one-third to one-half gangliosides, about 20 percent phospholipids, and 40 percent cholesterol. In vitro experiments show membranous cytoplasmic bodies to be formed in neurons as a consequence of high ganglioside concentrations in the presence of phospholipids and cholesterol.

Biochemical Pathology

On chemical analysis the most striking abnormality is the accumulation of G_{M2} ganglioside (Fig. 1–21) in cerebral gray matter and cerebellum. There is also an increased ganglioside level in white matter. Normally, the concentration of gangliosides in white matter is about one-fourth to one-tenth of that in gray matter; in Tay-Sachs disease a significantly higher ratio is found. The structure of G_{M2} ganglioside accumulating in Tay-Sachs disease is depicted in Figure 1–21. It consists of ceramide to which 1 mole each of glucose, galactose, N-acetylgalactosamine, and N-acetylneuraminic acid (NANA) has been attached.[343] Liver, spleen, and serum also contain increased amounts of G_{M2} ganglioside.[344,345]

Sialic acid-free derivatives, mainly ceramide trihexoside (ceramide-glucose-galactose-N-acetylgalactosamine), with lesser amounts of ceramide dihexoside and ceramide glucoside, are also markedly increased in gray matter.[346,347]

The enzymatic block responsible for these chemical abnormalities appears to be a defect in one of the two hexosaminidase components present in normal tissues (Fig. 1–21, step AII). Component A is absent from brain, blood, and viscera in the large majority of patients with Tay-Sachs disease.[348] Total hexosaminidase activity, however, is usually

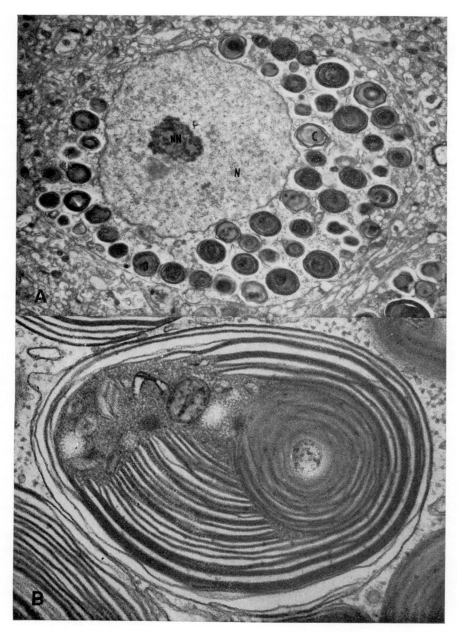

Fig. 1–20. Tay-Sachs disease, cortical biopsy. **A.** Neuron showing cytoplasmic granules. These are ganglioside in nature. Electron microscopic examination. $\times$ 10,000. (NN-nucleolus, N-nucleus, C-cytoplasmic granule.) **B.** Cytoplasmic granule showing lamellar arrangement. Lamellae are about 25 angstroms thick. Electron microscopic examination. $\times$ 90,000. (Courtesy of Dr. R. D. Terry, Albert Einstein College of Medicine, New York, and with the permission of the editors of *Journal of Neuropathology and Experimental Neurology.*)

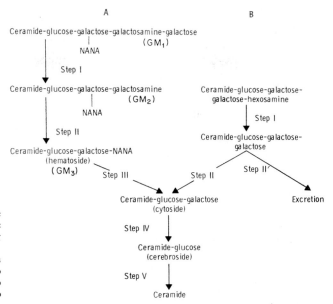

A
B

Ceramide-glucose-galactose-galactosamine-galactose
| (GM_1)
NANA

Step I

Ceramide-glucose-galactose-galactosamine
| (GM_2)
NANA

Ceramide-glucose-galactose-
galactose-hexosamine

Step I

Step II

Ceramide-glucose-galactose-
galactose

Ceramide-glucose-galactose-NANA
(hematoside)
(GM_3)   Step III   Step II   Step II'

Ceramide-glucose-galactose
(cytoside)   Excretion

Step IV

Ceramide-glucose
(cerebroside)

Step V

Ceramide

Postulated degradative pathways of sphingolipids

Fig. 1–21. Postulated degradative pathways for sphingolipids. Metabolic defects are located at the following points: generalized gangliosidosis GM_1—Step A I; Tay-Sachs disease and variants of generalized gangliosidosis GM_2—Step A II; juvenile Gaucher's disease—Step A III; adult Gaucher's disease—Step A V; Fabry's disease—Step B II. Enzymes for most of these reactions have been demonstrated in mammalian brain.

normal, and hexosaminidase B component is unable to hydrolyze ganglioside in vivo.

By means of enzymatic studies three other rare variants of GM_2 gangliosidosis have been uncovered.

In several cases of GM_2 gangliosidosis (Sandhoff's disease) both hexosaminidase components have been absent or reduced to about 10% of normal. These infants have been non-Jewish, have had a mild visceromegaly, and in contrast to infants with classical Tay-Sachs disease, these children accumulate globoside (ceramide-glu-gal-gal-galactosamine) rather than GM_2 ganglioside in their viscera.[349]

In another patient, both hexosaminidase components were present but inactive with respect to hydrolyzing GM_2.[350] Finally there are a few children who present with the clinical picture of late infantile or juvenile amaurotic idiocy (vid. infr.) who have been found to have GM_2 gangliosidosis, and a partial defect of hexosaminidase A.[351,352] The relationship between hexosaminidase A and B is obscure. Antisera against one cross-react against antisera against the other, but there is as yet insufficient evidence to

suppose that hexosaminidase B is a precursor of A.[353]

Clinical Manifestations

The classic form of Tay-Sachs disease usually occurs in Jewish families, particularly those of Eastern European background. It is transmitted as an autosomal recessive condition. In the United States the gene frequency is 1 in 40 among Jews and 1 in 380 among non-Jews.

At first the infants appear normal and until 3 to 10 months of age, growth and development are essentially unremarkable. Listlessness and irritability are usually the first indications of the illness, as well as hyperacusis in about half the infants. Soon thereafter an arrest in intellectual development and a loss of acquired abilities are observed. Examination at this time shows a generalized hypotonia, and what is termed a "cherry red spot" in both macular areas. This finding is characteristic of Tay-Sachs disease, although it is occasionally also observed in Niemann-Pick disease (group A and C), generalized GM_1 gangliosidosis, infantile Gaucher's disease and in a rare adult with myoclonic seizures. In Tay-Sachs disease it is invariably present by the time neurologic symptoms have developed.

There is no enlargement of liver or spleen. The neurologic symptoms progress rapidly to complete blindness and loss of all voluntary movements. Pupillary light reflexes remain intact, however. The hypotonia is replaced by spasticity and opisthotonus. Convulsions appear at this time, they may be generalized, focal, myoclonic, or gelastic. In the final stages a progressive enlargement of the head has been observed. This is invariably present if the disease has lasted longer than 18 months.[354] The condition terminates fatally by the second or third year of life.

Routine studies on the cerebrospinal fluid are normal, but aldolase, glutamic-oxalacetic transaminase, and lactic dehydrogenase activities may be elevated.

Diagnosis

The diagnosis of Tay-Sachs disease is easily made on clinical grounds in an infant with a progressive degenerative disease of the nervous system who has the characteristic retinal cherry red spot and lacks significant visceromegaly (Table 1–10). Hexosaminidase assay on serum will confirm the clinical impression and may also be used to detect the heterozygote. Prenatal diagnosis by assaying the hexosaminidase A content of fibroblasts cultured from amniotic fluid is possible during the first trimester of gestation.[262,355]

Treatment

There is no known effective treatment for this condition.

Generalized G_{M1} Gangliosidosis (Familial Neurovisceral Lipidosis, Pseudo-Hurler's Disease)

G_{M1} gangliosidosis occurs in two forms. Type 1, which is the more common, resembles Hurler's disease.

Although this condition is not too rare and has been known for several years either as a form of Tay-Sachs disease with visceral involvement[356] or as pseudo-Hurler's disease, it is only recently that the storage of a monosialoganglioside G_{M1} has been recognized as its basic defect (Fig. 1–21, step I) (Table 1–11).[357]

By contrast, the clinical presentation of type 2 generalized gangliosidosis resembles that of the other forms of late infantile amaurotic idiocy.

Pathologic Anatomy

The pathologic picture is that of neuronal storage resembling that of Tay-Sachs disease. The neurons are distended with PAS-positive lipid material, and on electron microscopy they contain a large number of membranous cytoplasmic bodies, similar to those seen in Tay-Sachs disease.[358] In addition, there are many unusual membrane-bound organelles which appear to be derived from lysosomes. Abnormalities are also seen in the extraneural tissues. In the kidneys there is a striking vacuolization of the glomerular epithelial cells and the cells of the proximal convoluted tubules. In the liver there is a marked histiocytosis associated with vacuolization of the parenchymal cells.

Biochemical Pathology

Total ganglioside content of brain and viscera is increased, and the stored G_{M1} ganglioside comprises up to 90 percent of total gray matter gangliosides. Its structure is depicted in Table 1–11. The ganglioside is also stored in liver and spleen.[345] However, the ultrastructure of the stored material in the liver is entirely different from the membranous cytoplasmic bodies found in neurons.[358] This has been attributed to the additional accumulation of a modified keratan sulfate and, to a lesser degree, of a sialomucopolysaccharide, which are also stored in viscera, probably as a result of defective catabolism of mucopolysaccharides in connective tissue.[359] It is the storage of these two compounds that accounts for the fact that hepatomegaly is seen in generalized G_{M1} gangliosidosis but not in Tay-Sachs disease (generalized G_{M2} gangliosidosis). A profound deficiency (2%–5% of normal) of β-galactosidase, the enzyme catalyzing the cleavage of the terminal galactose of G_{M1} (Fig. 1–21, step A-1), has been demonstrated in several tissues of patients with both types of gangliosidosis.[360,361] On electrophoresis three components can be demonstrated in tissue. In addition, differences in pH maximum have been observed. The major enzyme has a maximum between pH 4 to 5, while optimum activity of the minor component is at pH 6.6. In type 1, activity at both pH's is reduced, while in type 2, activity at pH 6.6 is nearly normal.[362,363]

Clinical Manifestations

Generalized gangliosidosis G_{M1} type 1 is a severe cerebral degenerative disease which may be clinically evident at birth. The infants are hypotonic, with a poor suck, and poor psychomotor development. Characteristic facial abnormalities include frontal bossing, a depressed nasal bridge, macroglossia, large low set ears, and marked hirsutism. Hepatosplenomegaly is usually present after six months of age. About 50 per cent of patients have cherry-red spots. The skeletal deformities (dysostosis multiplex) are similar to those of Hurler's syndrome.[288,364]

In type 2 generalized G_{M1} gangliosidosis the onset of neurologic symptoms occurs between 7 and 16 months of age. Hyperacusis may be striking, seizures occur in about half the instances, and there is a slowly progressive mental deterioration. Bony abnormalities and hepatosplenomegaly are absent, and optic atrophy, when present, is usually unaccompanied by a cherry-red spot.[365]

Diagnosis

In the infantile form of generalized gangliosidosis, the excretion of mucopolysaccharides is normal. The diagnosis is suggested by the early onset of clinical manifestations and rapid neurologic deterioration in a patient who has features and radiologic bone changes reminiscent of Hurler's disease, and from the absence of beta-galactosidase in leukocytes, skin, urine, or viscera. Since β-galactosidase is also deficient in Hurler's disease, analysis for this enzyme should be coupled with measurement of α-L-iduronidase activity. Enzyme assays on fibroblasts cultured from amniotic fluid will allow an antenatal diagnosis[262,365a] in offspring of known affected families.

Treatment

No treatment is available.

Generalized G_{M3} Gangliosidosis

This extremely rare condition is probably identical with juvenile Gaucher's disease. It is characterized by slowly progressive hepatosplenomegaly and intellectual deterioration. Intraneuronal lipid storage is marked, in contrast to the infantile and adult forms of Gaucher's diseases with which it has been grouped in the past.[366]

On chemical examination of the brain there is a definite increase in glycolipid content. The substances stored are ceramide dihexosides (ceramide-glucose-galactose), G_{M3} or hematosides (ceramide-glucose-galactose-NANA), and the Tay-Sachs ganglioside, (G_{M2}).[367] In spleen ceramide dihexoside is the principal glycolipid.[368]

In fibroblasts a deficiency of lactosylceramide galactosyl hydrolase has been observed, which localizes the enzymatic defect to step A IV (Fig. 1–21).[369]

GAUCHER'S DISEASE

This is a rare familial condition characterized by storage of cerebrosides in the reticuloendothelial system. It was first described by Gaucher in 1882.[370]

Three forms of the disease may be distinguished. The most common is chronic Gaucher's disease, a slowly progressive condition with marked visceral, but no nervous system involvement. Occasionally this form may appear at birth or during early childhood.

Infantile Gaucher's disease is a rare disorder, with a rapid downhill course and marked cerebral involvement. Juvenile Gaucher's disease is characterized by the storage of ganglioside (G_{M3}), and therefore was considered with the gangliosidoses.

Pathologic Anatomy

The outstanding feature of all forms of Gaucher's disease is the widespread presence of large numbers of Gaucher cells (Fig. 1–22). These are spherical or oval cells between 20 and 40 microns in diameter with a lacy, striated cytoplasm which contrasts with the vacuolated foam cells of Niemann-Pick disease. Gaucher cells appear in large clumps in the spleen, which may become tremendously

and hemorrhage are the usual neurologic complications.

The course of the illness is progressively downhill; death is usually due to renal failure.

Variants atypical through lack of cutaneous manifestations or isolated renal and corneal involvement (cornea verticillata) are fairly common.[391]

Diagnosis

The diagnosis of Fabry's disease is often made on renal biopsy of a child with suspected disseminated lupus. It is confirmed by finding a striking increase of ceramide trihexoside in urinary lipids,[392] and a marked reduction (15%–40% of normal) of alpha-galactosidase in leukocytes,[393] peripheral nerves, and skin fibroblasts. The hemizygote has two distinct clonal populations, one with enzymatic activity and the other enzyme deficient.[394]

Treatment

Treatment of the enzyme defect with plasma infusions has been attempted. Enzyme levels are maximum six hours after infusion and remain normal for about eight hours. The practicality of this therapy has not yet been demonstrated.[395] The use of kidney transplants has also been suggested.

NIEMANN-PICK DISEASE

This condition was first described in 1914 by Niemann.[396] It is now known to represent at least four groups of generalized lipid storage diseases characterized by an accumulation of sphingomyelin in the reticuloendothelial system.[397]

Pathologic Anatomy

The most characteristic alterations are due to the deposition of sphingomyelin in the foam cells of the reticuloendothelial system of liver, spleen, lungs, and bone marrow. Alterations in the brain are variable and range from no involvement (group B) to a picture of diffuse neuronal storage (groups A, C and D).

About 85% of patients fall into group A (classic Niemann-Pick disease) characterized by the onset of hepatosplenomegaly during the first year of life, intellectual deterioration,

and, in many instances, the presence of retinal cherry red spots. The essential pathologic changes in the brain and the retina in this condition are similar to those observed in Tay-Sachs disease: a massive and generalized deposition of foam cells, and the presence of ballooned ganglion cells in various areas of the brain, primarily the cerebellum, brain stem, and spinal cord.[398] Lipid storage also occurs in the endothelium of cerebral blood vessels, in arachnoid cells, and in the connective tissue of the choroid plexus.

In group B, the visceral or "chronic" form of Niemann-Pick disease, patients remain free of neurologic symptoms, despite massive visceral involvement.

Patients in group C have a slower progression of clinical symptoms, and central nervous system manifestations usually do not appear until two to four years of age (Table 1–10). In the central nervous system there is diffuse neuronal storage, but histochemical or chemical methods have not identified the nature of the storage product. In white matter there is more extensive myelin destruction and microglial swelling than can be explained by neuronal losses.[399]

In group D, termed the Nova Scotian Group, the clinical symptoms progress even more slowly, and neurologic abnormalities are not evident until early or middle childhood.

Biochemical Pathology

In all four entities there is tissue storage of sphingomyelin. This compound was first described in 1884 by Thudichum[500] and was found to have the structure depicted in Figure 1–23. Chemical and histochemical studies have shown sphingomyelin to be a major myelin constituent. It is also a normal component of spleen. An enzyme, sphingo-myelinase, which cleaves sphingomyelin into phosphatidylcholine and ceramide, is normally present in liver, kidney, and spleen.

Niemann-Pick Disease, Group A. In the viscera the accumulation of sphingomyelin is accompanied by a deposition of nonesterified cholesterol. The levels of cholesterol may even exceed those of sphingomyelin if values are compared on a molar basis. In addition, a nonpolar glycerol-phospholipid, lyso bis-

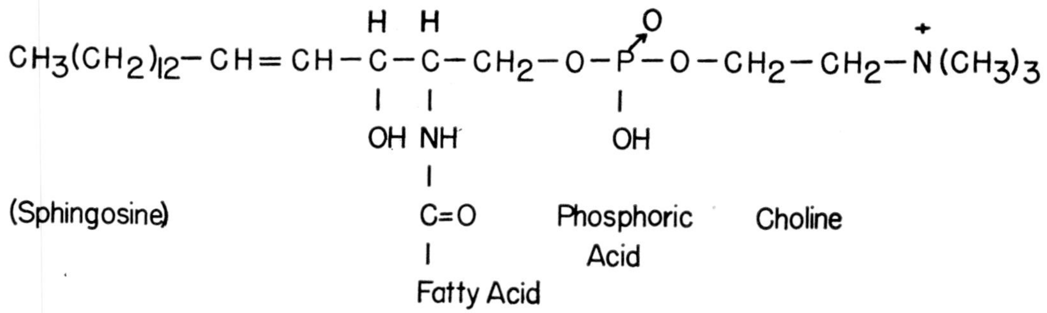

$$CH_3(CH_2)_{12}-CH=CH-\underset{\underset{OH}{|}}{C}-\underset{\underset{NH}{|}}{C}-CH_2-O-\underset{\underset{OH}{|}}{\overset{\overset{O}{\parallel}}{P}}-O-CH_2-CH_2-\overset{+}{N}(CH_3)_3$$

(Sphingosine) $\underset{\underset{Fatty\ Acid}{|}}{\underset{\underset{C=O}{|}}{}}$ Phosphoric Acid   Choline

Fig. 1–23: Structure of a sphingomyelin.

phosphatidic acid, has been found in a number of viscera.[401] Accumulation of sphingomyelin within the nervous system is relatively modest but may reach values as high as 10 times normal. In general, sphingomyelin deposition is more marked in gray matter. Examination of the sphingomyelin fatty acids has shown the proportion of stearic acid to be greater than normal, whereas that of the longer-chain fatty acids—normally found in sphingomyelin after completion of myelination—is decreased. The sphingomyelin cleaving enzyme, sphingomyelinase, normally present in liver, kidney, and spleen, is deficient in these organs.[402] Its absence can also be demonstrated in leukocytes,[403] and in tissue cultures derived from bone marrow or skin.[404]

Niemann-Pick Disease, Group B. A deficiency of visceral sphingomyelinase has been demonstrated in this entity, but although there is an increase in sphingomyelin in liver and spleen, the content of the phospholipid in brain is normal.

Niemann-Pick Disease, Group C. While there is a marked increase in sphingomyelin content of viscera, the concentration of the phospholipid in gray matter is normal. There is, however, an increase in gray matter glucocerebrosides, ceramide dihexosides, and G_{M2} and G_{M3} gangliosides. No deficiency in sphingomyelinase has as yet been demonstrated[402] in any of the organs examined.

Niemann-Pick Disease, Group D. These patients have an increase in cerebral sphingomyelin, but the visceral deposition of the phospholipid is minimal and is overshadowed by a six- to tenfold rise in nonesterified cholesterol.[405] Visceral sphingomyelinase activity is normal.[402,405a]

Clinical Manifestations

The classical form of the disease (group A) is transmitted as an autosomal recessive condition, with predilection for Jewish families.

Symptoms begin in the first year of life, with persistent early jaundice, enlarging abdomen and poor physical and intellectual development. In about one third of the patients, neurologic symptoms initially predominate, but few children survive beyond infancy without involvement of the nervous system, notably intellectual deterioration. Seizures, particularly myoclonic jerks, are often observed, and terminally there is marked spasticity. Retinal cherry red spots are found in about 25 percent of patients and may precede neurologic abnormalities.[397] The progression of the disease is variable but death usually ensues before five years of age.

The clinical course of patients classified into group C reflects the more chronic nature of the disease. Neurologic symptoms predominate and usually make their first appearance between the ages of two and four. Myoclonic or akinetic seizures and ataxia are common, as are macular cherry red spots.[399] Enlargement of liver and spleen is not as striking as in the classic form of the disease and may become less marked as the illness progresses.

Diagnosis

The presence of hepatosplenomegaly, anemia, and failure to thrive in children showing intellectual deterioration would lead one to suspect Niemann-Pick disease. This diagnosis is best confirmed by bone marrow aspiration, splenic or rectal biopsy,[406] or enzyme assay. The storage cells seen in Niemann-Pick disease differ from Gaucher cells in that they have a vacuolated rather than a striated cytoplasm. However, on occasion it is quite difficult to distinguish these two cells on histochemical evidence alone, and chemical analysis of the tissues may be necessary. While theoretically only the carbohydrate-containing Gaucher cerebrosides should give a positive periodic acid-Schiff test, sphingomyelin may stain positively as well under certain conditions. The phosphomolybdate reaction, originally believed to be specific for choline esters such as sphingomyelin, also does not distinguish between the two compounds.

A deficiency in sphingomyelinase activity will allow the diagnosis of the classic form (group A) of the disease and also of group B, but does not help to make the diagnosis in group C or group D patients. Sphingomyelinase activity has been found in cultured amniotic fibroblasts allowing an intrauterine diagnosis of group A or B.[262]

Therapy

X-ray therapy and antimetabolite drugs such as methotrexate and nitrogen mustards have been tried without altering the downhill course of the disease. Splenectomy is also of no avail.

OTHER DISORDERS OF LIPID METABOLISM

Refsum's Disease (Heredopathia Atactica Polyneuritiformis)

Although Refsum's disease has been known since 1944 when Refsum described two families with polyneuritis, muscular atrophy, ataxia, retinitis pigmentosa, diminution of hearing, and ichthyosis, an underlying disorder in lipid metabolism was uncovered only some 20 years later.[407,408]

In 1956 Cammermeyer[409] described depositions of lipids in swollen nerve cells and in areas of demyelination, with the formation of fatty macrophages.

The disease usually makes its appearance between ages four and seven, most commonly with a picture of partial, intermittent peripheral neuropathy. The cerebrospinal fluid shows an albumino-cytologic dissociation with a protein level between 100 and 600 mg percent. Electrocardiograms may reveal a prolongation of the QT segment and a widened QRS complex.

When the urinary sediment of a patient with Refsum's disease is stained for lipids, large amounts of fatty material can be detected. Fats are found both in free condition, in the form of droplets, and with epithelial cells. In all organs, including the brain, there are increased quantities of lipids. These contain, as one of their major fatty acids, a branched-chain compound, 3,7,11,15-tetramethylhexadecanoic acid (phytanic acid). Blood levels of phytanic acid range between 10 to 50 mg per 100 ml compared with normal values of 0.2 mg or less. Serum phytanic acid is partly in the form of cholesterol esters and partly as triglycerides. Three types of the latter have been isolated, containing one or two moles of phytanic acid.

Phytanic acid is primarily of exogenous origin and mainly derived from dietary phytol ingested in the form of nuts, spinach, or coffee. Patients with Refsum's disease have a block in the alpha-oxidation of phytanic to pristanic acid[410] (Fig. 1–24). When patients are placed on a phytol-free diet, blood phytanic acid falls slowly and within one year levels of about one-fourth of the original values are reached.[411] This is accompanied by increased nerve conduction time, return of reflexes, and improvement in sensation and in objective coordination. A dietary regimen is presented by Steinberg et al.[411]

The differential diagnosis of Refsum's disease includes other causes of intermittent polyneuritis, such as α-lipoprotein deficiency (Tangier disease), which can be diagnosed by examination of the plasma lipoproteins and by the low serum cholesterol levels. Other similar clinical entities are relapsing infectious polyneuritis, acute intermittent porphyria, recurrent exposures to toxins—particularly alcohol or lead—and less commonly a familial variant of relapsing hyper-

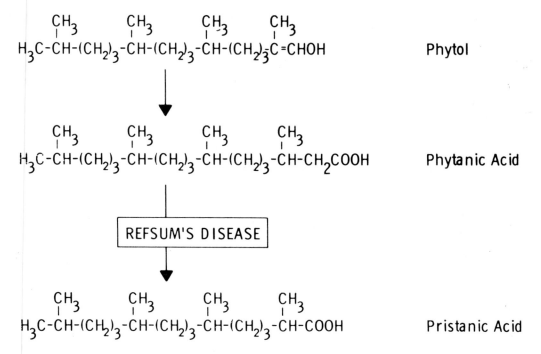

Fig. 1–24. Phytol metabolism. In Refsum's disease the metabolic block is located at the conversion of phytanic to pristanic acid.

trophic interstitial polyneuropathy (Dejerine-Sottas disease). A patient with ataxia, chorioretinitis, and peripheral neuropathy, resembling Hurler's disease, has been described by Shy. Neither mucopolysaccharide excretion nor serum phytanic acid levels were elevated.[412]

Cerebrotendinous Xanthomatosis

Although this rare but well-defined familial disease was first described by van Bogaert and associates in 1937,[413] its unique chemical feature, deposition of cholestanol (dihydrocholesterol) within the nervous system, was only uncovered in 1968 by Menkes and associates.[414] The disease is characterized by xanthomas of tendons and lungs, cataracts, slowly progressive cerebellar ataxia, and dementia. Symptoms usually are first noted in late childhood and progress slowly thereafter, in many instances not interfering with the normal lifespan of the affected individual. Serum cholesterol levels are normal but cholestanol concentrations in serum and erythrocytes are elevated.[415] On pathologic examination the brain stem and cerebellum are the two most affected areas within the nervous system. Here myelin destruction, a variable degree of gliosis, and xanthoma cells are visible.[416]

On chemical examination large amounts of free and esterified cholestanol are found stored within the nervous system. The sterol is located not only in affected areas such as the cerebellum, but also in histologically normal myelin. The content of cholestanol in the tendon xanthomas is increased, but here the predominant sterol is cholesterol. The underlying enzymatic defect is still unknown, but it is likely to result in an accentuation of the biosynthesis of cholestanol from cholesterol.[417]

Wolman's Disease

This condition was first described by Wolman and his group in 1956.[418] The clinical manifestations resemble those of the classic form of Niemann-Pick disease and include failure in weight gain, a malabsorption syndrome, and adrenal insufficiency. Lipoproteins and plasma cholesterol are reduced, and acanthocytes are in evidence.[419] There is a massive hepatosplenomegaly, and on roentgenographic examination the adrenals are found to be calcified. Neurologic symptoms are usually limited to a delayed intellectual development. On pathologic examination there is xanthomatosis of the viscera. Sudanophilic material is stored in the leptomeninges, retinal ganglion cells, and nerve cells of the myenteric plexus. Sudanophilic granules outline the cortical capillaries, and there is sudanophilic demyelination.[420]

On chemical examination of the affected tissues there is a striking accumulation of triglycerides and free and esterified cholesterol. Lipid accumulation is greatest in tissues which synthesize the most cholesterol esters. These include the adrenal cortex, liver, intestine, spleen, and lymph nodes.[421] The basic enzymatic defect is a deficiency in acid lipase, a lysosomal enzyme normally active against medium- and long-chain triglycerides, as well as cholesterol esters.[422]

Lipogranulomatosis

This rare disease was first described by Farber and associates.[423] The clinical features are unique and manifest themselves during the first few weeks of life. The infant becomes irritable, develops a hoarse cry, and nodular erythematous swelling of the wrists. Over subsequent months nodules develop in numerous sites, particularly in areas subject to trauma such as joints and the subcutaneous tissue of the buttocks. There is severe motor and mental retardation. Death usually ensues by two years of age.

The basic pathologic lesion is a granuloma formed by the proliferation and ballooning of mesenchymal cells, which ultimately become enmeshed in dense hyaline fibrous tissue. Within the central nervous system both neurons and glial cells are swollen and contain stored material.[424]

There is a striking increase in ceramides and gangliosides in affected tissues. The latter is particularly marked in subcutaneous nodules, which have the ganglioside concentration of normal gray matter. A defect in ceramidase has been demonstrated by Sugita et al.[425]

Cholesterol Storage Diseases

Several conditions characterized by intracerebral cholesterol deposition have been described. Only those which are due to a primary metabolic defect will be singled out for mention.

Involvement of the nervous system in Hand-Schüller-Christian disease (histiocytosis X), while rarely seen, has been well-documented. Most frequently there is an extension of the granulomatous lesion of the membranous bones of the skull into the tuber cinereum or about the cranial nerves at the base of the brain. Demyelination and perivascular lipid deposition are occasionally noted, particularly in the cerebellum. Feigin has also recorded a case in which cholesterol-containing nodules were deposited within the cerebral gray matter.[426]

A disease characterized by cerebral and cerebellar atrophy and deposition of crystalline cholesterol in the basal ganglia has been described by Jervis.[427]

Lipidoses of Unknown Etiology

In a number of progressive neurologic disorders the pathologic picture is that of a lipidosis. Neurons are distended with material which yields the histochemical reactions of a lipid, and in many instances gives a strong positive reaction with PAS, a feature which in the past has suggested that the stored material is a glycolipid, or possibly a ganglioside. Chemical studies on brain tissue from patients have failed to uncover any abnormality in ganglioside content for any of the disorders in this group, and their biochemical defect is still obscure. Classification of these diseases therefore still rests on their clinical and morphologic features.

Cerebral Retinal Degenerations

These entities, first described by Jansky in 1909[428] and subsequently by Bielschowsky,[429] Batten,[430] Spielmeyer,[431] and Kufs,[432] have in the past been differentiated according to the age at which neurologic symptoms first became evident. Tay-Sachs disease, a defect of ganglioside metabolism, is covered with the other disorders of lipid metabolism.

Late Infantile Amaurotic Idiocy
(Batten-Bielschowsky)

The onset of the clinical syndrome occurs later than that of Tay-Sachs disease; it does not affect Jewish children predominantly, its progression is slower, and patients lack the usual retinal cherry-red spot. The syndrome is characterized by normal mental and motor development for the first two to four years of life. The initial symptoms are seizures, often myoclonic. Ataxia develops subsequently, and is accompanied by a slowly progressive retinal degeneration, which is generally not obvious until the other neurologic symptoms have become well-established. Visual acuity is decreased and there is a florid degeneration in the macular and perimacular areas. The macular light reflex is defective, and a fine, brown pigment is deposited. The optic disk is pale. The electroretinogram is abnormal, showing decreased or absent scotopic responses. This is in contrast to the normal electroretinogram of Tay-Sachs disease.[433] Marked spasticity, as well as a Parkinsonian picture, may develop terminally. The condition progresses fairly slowly, and death does not occur until late childhood.

Laboratory studies may show a large number of vacuolated lymphocytes, and rarely an increase in cerebrospinal fluid protein. Jervis has noted that marked electroencephalographic abnormalities can precede even the slightest hint of neurologic disturbance.[434] Examination of the affected brain reveals generalized neuronal swelling, which however is less extensive than in Tay-Sachs disease. The intraneuronal material stains with PAS, but unlike the lipid stored in Tay-Sachs disease is nearly insoluble in lipid solvents.

Through ultrastructural examination two distinct disease entities have been described.

Late Infantile Neurovisceral Storage Disease with Curvilinear Bodies

In our experience this has been the most common type. Zeman and Donahue[435] first described cytoplasmic bodies with a granular and multiloculated appearance in this condition. With Watanabe, they described these structures in other patients and grouped them with similar clinical cases lacking this characteristic inclusion material.[435a] Duffy

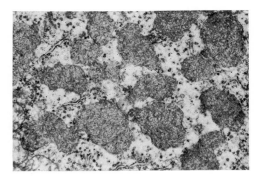

Fig. 1–25. Curvilinear body storage disease. Neuron containing numerous aggregates of curvilinear bodies in its cytoplasm. The endoplasmic reticulum and the osmiophilic granules representing the ribosomes lining it are clearly visible between the clumps of curvilinear bodies. × 11,200. (Courtesy of Dr. P. Cancilla, Department of Pathology, UCLA, Los Angeles, California.)

and associates[436] have referred to these inclusions as "curvilinear bodies" because of their morphologic appearance (Fig. 1–25). Storage of similar material has been seen in spleen, colon, exocrine sweat glands, and cutaneous nerves.[437] We have found lipid inclusions of different appearance in cytoplasm of skin fibroblasts.[438] The chemical identity of the stored material is still obscure. The content and distribution of gray matter gangliosides and the increased concentration of some of the polar glycolipids, notably ceramide trihexosides, that are found in this disorder probably do not reflect the primary biochemical lesion.[439]

Late Infantile Amaurotic Idiocy with Lipofuscin Storage

In another type of lipidosis the cytoplasmic inclusions are autofluorescent and give a positive histochemical reaction for ceroid or lipofuscin.[440] On electron microscopy the inclusions are membrane-bound and are composed of granular material (Fig. 1–26). It is possible that these inclusions are derived from subcellular membranes which are polymerized by-products of lipid peroxidation and bivalent metal ions. As they contain acid hydrolases, they may represent an intermediate stage in the transformation of lysosomelike bodies to lipofuscin. Similar inclusions can be seen in skeletal muscle, Schwann's

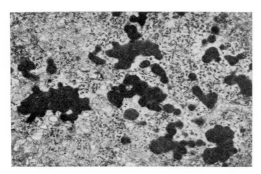

Fig. 1–26. Lipofuscin storage disease. Electron micrograph. × 12,000. Neuron, cytoplasm filled with large aggregates of amorphous material. Histochemically this is compatible with lipofuscin. (Courtesy of Dr. P. Cancilla, Department of Pathology, UCLA, Los Angeles, California.)

cells, and exocrine sweat glands.[437] An increased content of esterified cholesterol has been found in several such cases and may represent a part of the stored material.[441]

Other forms of late infantile amaurotic idiocy have known biochemical abnormalities and are outlined in Table 1–10.

Juvenile Amaurotic Idiocy (Spielmeyer-Vogt Disease)

This entity was first mentioned in 1893 by Freud[442] and subsequently by Spielmeyer[431] and Vogt.[443] As described in these classic monographs, visual and intellectual deterioration first becomes apparent between 6 and 14 years of age. Funduscopic examination at that time reveals abnormal amounts of peripheral retinal pigmentation and early optic atrophy. Loss of motor function becomes apparent subsequently. Ataxia and seizures are usually not seen. While many patients whose illness commences during the early school years follow this clinical pattern, variations do occur. For example, we have encountered one family in whom a boy followed the clinical course described by Spielmeyer, while his sister presented with ataxia and myoclonic seizures.

Lipofuscin Storage Disease

In this, the most common entity, morphologic studies show a decrease in cortical neurons but relatively little ballooning. The lipofuscin content of neurons is considerably increased, and on electron microscopy one may observe a variety of cytoplasmic inclusions. In part, these resemble the lipofuscin material found in one of the forms of late infantile amaurotic idiocy.

Other inclusions have been termed "membranous vesicular bodies" and "pleomorphic lipid bodies." These may represent stages in conversion of lysosomes into lipofuscin bodies and may reflect the chronicity of the storage process or the age of the patient.[444] A similar electron microscopic picture has been reported in Kufs's disease, the adult form of amaurotic idiocy.[445] Biochemical studies have failed to find any abnormality in gangliosides or to define the nature of the storage material.

Juvenile Dystonic Lipidosis

This rare entity is characterized by progressive dementia, dystonia, and a moderate degree of cerebellar ataxia. There is no amaurosis or visceromegaly. Unusual intraneuronal inclusions have been described by Elfenbein.[446]

Early Infantile Neurolipidosis with Failure of Myelination

This condition presents during the first year of life with deterioration in development and optic atrophy. Morphologic examination of the brain shows marked neuronal ballooning and failure of myelination. This condition may be identical with a congenital form of amaurotic idiocy and is similar to the Quaker and Jimpy forms of degenerative diseases encountered in inbred strains of mice. The biochemical lesion in this entity is still unknown.[447]

Diagnosis of Cerebroretinal Degenerations

While the classic case with relatively late onset of intellectual and visual deterioration and pigmentary degeneration of the retina offers few diagnostic problems, difficulty may be encountered in some children whose first symptom, at ages two to three, is loss of speech. The term Heller's disease has frequently been applied to such a case. Some of these children represent instances of late infantile amaurotic idiocy, others true childhood schizophrenia. Also, some children, mentally defective since birth, through parental enthusiasm learn to "speak" in a parrotlike manner. This achievement is often lost by the ages of two to three thus giving a superficial appearance of intellectual deterioration. Despite its present-day rarity, juvenile paresis, which is often accompanied by retinal degeneration, must always be included in the differential diagnosis. Enzymatic, biochemical, and morphologic studies are, however, necessary for a definitive diagnosis. These include assay of serum, leukocytes, and fibroblasts for hexosaminidase, and β-galactosidase, and a morphologic examination of more readily available tissue such as the bone marrow or lymph nodes. In the above entities biopsy of nerve tissue obtained from the central nervous system or the rectal myenteric plexus is commonly used as a diagnostic adjunct.

Rectal biopsy with histochemical examination of the sections may be employed to establish the diagnosis of the late infantile and juvenile amaurotic idiocies, but in general it is not helpful as in Tay-Sachs, Niemann-Pick or Wolman's diseases.[406]

Brain biopsy has the advantage that histologic, histochemical, and ultrastructural studies can be combined with chemical analysis of the cerebral lipids. Generally, the presence of progressive intellectual deterioration may be considered sufficient incentive to suggest the procedure for both prognostic and diagnostic purposes. Biopsies are usually taken from the frontal lobe. A single cube, at least 1.5 cm in dimension and including both gray and white matter, is removed and divided. One part is placed in 10 percent formalin-saline for histologic examination or is fixed in phosphate-buffered 5% glutaraldehyde for electron microscopy, while the other portion is frozen for chemical studies.

DISORDERS OF SERUM LIPOPROTEINS

Acanthocytosis (Beta-lipoprotein Deficiency, a-beta-lipoproteinemia)

This unusual disorder was first described by Bassen and Kornzweig in 1950.[448] The main clinical manifestations include acanthocytosis (large numbers of burr-shaped erythrocytes [Fig. 1–27]), hypocholesterolemia, progressive combined posterior column degenera-

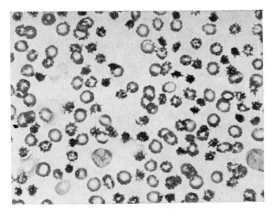

Fig. 1–27. Blood smear (Wright's stain) acanthocystosis. Acanthocytes may be distinguished by their burrlike projections. ×550. (Courtesy of Dr. A. M. DiGeorge, St. Christopher's Hospital, Philadelphia, Pennsylvania.)

tion, peripheral neuritis, mental retardation, retinitis pigmentosa, and steatorrhea. The disorder is transmitted in an autosomal recessive manner.

In the first year of life infants develop a typical celiac syndrome with abdominal distention, diarrhea, foul-smelling stools, decreased fat absorption, and occasionally osteomalacia. Neurologic symptoms are first noted between 2 and 17 years of age. Commonly, the initial sign is unsteadiness of gait. This is due to a combination of ataxia, proprioceptive loss, and muscle weakness. Deep tendon reflexes are generally absent, and a cutaneous sensory loss is often demonstrable.[449] The retinal degeneration is accompanied by decreased visual acuity and night blindness. The electroretinogram is often abnormal even in the early stages of the disease.

On autopsy, extensive demyelination of the posterior columns and spinocerebellar tracks can be observed as well as neuronal loss in the anterior horns, the cerebellar molecular layer, and the cerebral cortex.[450]

Characteristic laboratory findings include a low serum cholesterol, usually in the range of 30 to 80 mg percent, markedly depressed total serum lipids (80–285 mg%), serum triglycerides, and absent serum beta-lipoproteins.[451]

The pathogenesis of this disease is not clear. Ingestion of fat is normally followed by absorption of lipids by the mucosal cells, from which they are released in the form of chylomicrons and discharged into the lymphatic system. Isselbacher[452] observed that no fat was detectable in the lymphatic spaces of the small bowel and that no chylomicrons appeared in the plasma after fat loading in patients with a-beta-lipoproteinemia. He related the defect to the lipid transport from the mucosal cells into the lymphatic system, beta-lipoproteins apparently being necessary to chylomicrons. The manner by which neurologic symptoms are produced is not clear.

Analysis of erythrocyte lipids has revealed a decrease in linoleic acid and an abnormal distribution of phospholipids probably due to malabsorption of lipids by the intestine.[453] Sphingomyelin is the predominant phospholipid, in contrast to lecithin in the normal red cells. It is not known how these alterations result in acanthocytosis.

Infants with intestinal symptoms fare better on a low fat diet insofar as weight gain is concerned. However, no therapy instituted to date has arrested the progress of neurologic symptoms.

The occurrence of acanthocytes in peripheral blood is not limited to this condition. The phenomenon has also been seen occasionally in patients with anemia or advanced cirrhosis. It has also been present in patients with triglyceride hyperlipemia and in a family with Hallervorden-Spatz disease. Tolentino and associates have described an infant in whom acanthocytosis was accompanied by a celiac syndrome, retinal dystrophy, and hypocholesterolemia, but in whom beta-lipoproteins were normal.[454]

Several other families have been reported[455] in whom an extrapyramidal disorder, areflexia, and mental retardation were associated with the presence of acanthocytes, but in whom serum lipids were normal. In distinction from a-beta-lipoproteinemia, this condition appears to be transmitted as a dominant disorder with incomplete or inconstant penetrance.

Tangier Disease (Hypo-alpha-lipoproteinemia)

This is a hereditary disorder of lipid metabolism distinguished by almost complete absence of high-density plasma lipoproteins; reduction of low-density plasma lipoproteins, cholesterol, and phospholipids; and storage of cholesterol esters in the reticuloendothelial system of the liver, spleen, lymph nodes, tonsils, and cornea.

Symptoms are usually limited to enlargement of the affected organs. Retinitis pigmentosa and peripheral neuropathy have been observed.[456] The nature of the metabolic disorder is not clear. Fredrickson's group has shown the presence of small amounts of high-density lipoproteins by means of immunologic methods, indicating that although genetic information for the synthesis of the protein is present, it is not produced in adequate amounts.[456]

OTHER METABOLIC DISORDERS

WILSON'S DISEASE (HEPATOLENTICULAR DEGENERATION)

Wilson's disease is an inborn error in copper metabolism, associated with cirrhosis of the liver and degenerative changes in the basal ganglia.

During the second half of the nineteenth century, a condition termed "pseudosclerosis" was distinguished from multiple sclerosis by the lack of eye signs. In 1902, Kayser[457] observed green corneal pigmentation in one such patient; and Fleischer in 1903 commented on the association of the corneal rings with pseudosclerosis.[458] In 1912 Wilson gave the classic description of the disease and its pathologic anatomy.[459]

Since the derangement in copper metabolism is one of the important features of this condition, it is pertinent to review briefly our present knowledge of the field.[460]

The daily dietary intake of copper ranges between 2 and 5 mg. Less than one-tenth of this is absorbed, and this fraction enters the plasma where it is bound to albumin in the form of Cu^{++}. Within two hours the absorbed copper has become incorporated into a liver protein. It is then synthesized into ceruloplasmin which enters the circulation or is excreted into bile. More than 95 percent of normal serum copper is in the form of ceruloplasmin. Ceruloplasmin is an alpha globulin with a molecular weight of 120,000 and eight copper atoms per molecule.[460a]

In its crystalline state ceruloplasmin is a protein having a single, continuous polypeptide chain and reports depicting its fractionation into more than one distinct molecular species are probably the result of its relative instability.[460a]

There is considerable controversy as to the physiologic action of ceruloplasmin. While it shows definite oxidase activity toward certain polyphenols and polyamines but not to ascorbic acid, the significance of these properties is unknown. The extremely tight chemical bond of copper in ceruloplasmin makes it unlikely that it functions as a transport protein for copper.

The concentration of ceruloplasmin in plasma is normally between 30–40 mg/100 ml. It is elevated in a variety of circumstances, including pregnancy or other conditions with high estrogen concentrations, infections, cirrhosis, malignancies, hyperthyroidism, and myocardial infarction. The elevation described in autistic and schizophrenic patients is perhaps due to their poor nutrition and subsequent ascorbic acid deficiency. The concentration of ceruloplasmin is low in normal infants up to approximately two months of age and in children suffering from a combined iron and copper deficiency anemia. In the nephrotic syndrome, low levels are due to the vast renal losses of ceruloplasmin. Ceruloplasmin is also reduced in Kinky Hair disease as a consequence of impaired intestinal copper transport (see Chapter 2).

Several other copper-containing proteins have been isolated from mammalian tissues. Most prominently these include the enzymes cytochrome C oxidase and tyrosinase, neither of which is altered in Wilson's disease. Porter and his associates[461] have purified cerebrocuprein which is normally present in human brain. This substance, too, is a copper protein, differing from ceruloplasmin in having lower molecular weight and only two copper atoms per molecule. In cerebrocuprein, copper is bound to the protein moiety by means of a carboxyl group.

Biochemical Pathology

Knowledge of disturbed copper metabolism in Wilson's disease lay dormant for more than three decades. In 1913, one year after Wilson's report, Rumpel found unusually large amounts of copper in the liver of a patient with hepatolenticular degeneration.[462] Although this finding was confirmed, and an elevated copper concentration was also detected in the basal ganglia by Luthy,[463] the implication of these reports went unrecognized until 1945 when Glazebrook demonstrated abnormally high copper levels in serum, liver, and brain in a patient with this condition.[464] In 1952, five years after the discovery of the copper protein, several groups of workers simultaneously found that patients with Wilson's disease have low or absent ceruloplasmin. At first it appeared that the condition represented a simple deficiency of a serum protein. Actually the picture is much more complex.

While the vast majority of patients show markedly diminished ceruloplasmin concentrations, normal values have been recorded in several authentic cases. The concentrations of ceruloplasmin found in patients with nephrosis are often below the levels observed in hepatolenticular degeneration, yet cerebral or hepatic symptoms do not occur. Raising the level of ceruloplasmin by giving estrogens or the purified copper protein fails to affect the course of the disease.[465] On the other hand, many patients have been followed in whom marked ceruloplasmin deficiency antedated all other pathologic findings. This would suggest that a lack of the copper protein is part of the primary disease process, or that ceruloplasmin in patients with Wilson's disease is structurally abnormal. The latter possibility has been excluded by Holtzman and associates who found that the "finger printing" pattern of the peptides produced by tryptic hydrolysis of ceruloplasmin from patients with Wilson's disease is identical to that of normal ceruloplasmin.[466]

Another abnormal finding is the increased plasma level of nonceruloplasmin copper. The elevation of loosely bound copper may lead to its tissue deposition and be responsible for the marked cupriuria, particularly during the later stages of the disease, when levels averaging 15 times normal are reached.

Studies with radioisotopes suggest that the dynamic turnover of copper is disturbed.[467]

these may include indistinct speech and difficulty in swallowing. Minor intellectual impairment or emotional disturbances may also be observed but seizures or mental deterioration are not features of the disease. Before long the patient presents a characteristic appearance. A fixed smile is due to retraction of the upper lip, the mouth hangs open and drools. Speech is often severely impaired. Tremors are usually quite marked. These may often be unilateral during the early stages of the disease, but sooner or later they become generalized. They are present at rest but become exaggerated with movements and emotional disturbance. Initially fine, they gradually become coarse as the illness progresses until they assume a characteristic "wing-beating" appearance. Rigidity, contractures, and tonic spasms may involve the extremities and also advance steadily. Dementia may be severe in some cases, while others are merely emotionally labile. A nearly pure Parkinsonlike syndrome and cases with progressive choreo-athetosis have also been described.

On the basis of their response to chelation therapy, Denny-Brown has distinguished two types of cerebral symptomatology with each family tending to show a similar clinical course beginning at approximately the same age.[482] The first, pseudosclerosis, has as its characteristic features the presence of dysarthria and a flapping, wing-beating tremor. An asymptomatic cirrhosis invariably accompanies this form, and the untreated disease is but slowly progressive. The other form, termed the juvenile type or progressive lenticular degeneration, begins during childhood or early adolescence, commonly with overt hepatic involvement. The first signs are usually those of dystonia (i.e., the assumption of abnormal limb postures) and characteristic facies. A flapping tremor is rare in this type of Wilson's disease. In these patients the clinical course is marked by sudden severe relapses and periods of partial improvement. Without treatment, death ensues within one to three years of the onset of dystonia and is usually due to hepatic insufficiency.

The intracorneal, ring-shaped pigmentation first noted by Kayser and Fleischer may be evident to the naked eye or may only appear with slit lamp examination. The ring may be complete or incomplete and is present in most untreated children with hepatic or neurologic symptoms.[481] It appears gradually between six and nine years of age.

Diagnosis

The picture of Wilson's disease is fairly clear-cut when advanced. The important features are the family history of hepatic or neurologic involvement, progressive extrapyramidal symptoms commencing during the first or second decade of life, abnormal liver function, aminoaciduria, cupriuria, and absent or decreased ceruloplasmin. The presence of a Kayser-Fleischer ring is the single most important diagnostic feature. The absence of corneal pigmentation in untreated patients with neurologic symptoms rules out the diagnosis. The ring is not seen in presymptomatic patients or in some children with hepatic symptoms. While most patients with Wilson's disease have low or absent serum ceruloplasmin, more than a dozen cases have been reported in which the ceruloplasmin was normal. In affected families, the differential diagnosis between heterozygotes and presymptomatic homozygotes is of utmost importance, as it is generally accepted that the latter should be treated preventively.

Serum copper or ceruloplasmin levels are inadequate to make the distinction, and measurement of hepatic copper content may be required.[483] An alternative method, not yet fully explored, involves external monitoring of hepatic and muscle radioactivity following intravenous injection of Cu^{67}.[484]

Treatment

The variable clinical course of Wilson's disease makes evaluation of therapy extremely difficult. Treatment is directed at removing the copper deposited in tissues and toward minimizing the dietary intake.[485,486] D-penicillamine (alpha-amino-beta-mercaptoisovaleric acid) is the drug of choice for the purpose of forming a soluble complex with tissue copper. The drug (0.3 to 2 gm per day) is administered orally in divided doses, the exact amount given depending on the clinical response. The effectiveness of the drug can best be assessed by following the copper excretion. At the start of therapy, copper excretion is often increased five- to tenfold but the excretion rate returns to normal over the subsequent months. Raising the penicillamine dosage may again effect a transient outpouring of the metal.

Side reactions include fever, rash, adenopathy, a nephrotic syndrome, pyridoxine deficiency, and infrequently thrombocytopenia and leukopenia. These improve promptly with temporary interruption of therapy. Generally, the drug is given intermittently in courses of six to eight weeks' duration.

To minimize copper absorption, a low copper diet is prescribed.[486,487] Foods to be avoided include all forms of shellfish, liver, mushrooms, broccoli, cereals, chocolate, and nuts. A cation exchange resin or potassium sulfide (20 mg with each meal) is also prescribed. On this treatment there is often an improvement in neurologic symptoms. In 6 to 10 weeks the Kayser-Fleischer ring fades and disappears completely in a couple of years[488]; as shown by successive biopsies, the amount of copper deposited in the liver decreases. Both total serum copper and ceruloplasmin levels fall. The aminoaciduria and phosphaturia diminish. The hepatic defect, however, remains unchanged. According to Denny-Brown[482] chelation therapy greatly diminishes neurologic symptoms in the pseudosclerotic form of Wilson's disease but does not appear to influence the downhill course in the juvenile type of illness.

Other chelating agents, notably BAL and sodium diethyldithiocarbamate, have been used but show no advantage over penicillamine. Versene, although augmenting copper excretion, has little clinical effect. Ceruloplasmin substitution has proved ineffective.

A regimen of low copper diet and penicillamine has been recommended for asymptomatic children in whom a family history and laboratory data indicate the presence of presymptomatic hepatolenticular degeneration.[489]

Neurosurgical procedures have been found ineffective for the relief of extrapyramidal symptoms.

HYPERURICEMIA (LESCH-NYHAN SYNDROME)

The occurrence of hyperuricemia in association with spasticity, and severe choreoathetosis was first reported by Catel and Schmidt in 1959.[490] Since then the disease has been observed in a number of families, in whom it is transmitted as a sex-linked disorder.[491,492]

Biochemical Pathology

An abnormality of the enzyme hypoxanthine-guanine phosphoribosyl transferase has been demonstrated as the underlying defect.[493] In most instances the enzyme activity in a number of tissues, including fibroblast cultures, is less than 0.5% of normal, but in at least one patient enzyme assay in the presence of high magnesium concentrations increased the activity to between 8 and 34% of normal.[494] In another variant, a partial enzyme deficiency leads to excessive uric acid production, gouty arthritis, and mild neurologic symptoms—most commonly a spinocerebellar syndrome.[495] The residual enzyme in the classic form of Lesch-Nyhan syndrome and in the variant is activated by the normal transferase—a phenomenon which has not been clarified.[495a]

As a consequence of the defect, hypoxanthine cannot be reutilized, and whatever hypoxanthine is formed is either excreted or catabolized to xanthine and uric acid. In addition, guanylate, a known regulator of de novo purine synthesis, is depleted. For these reasons de novo uric acid production is markedly increased, and serum urine and cerebrospinal fluid uric acid levels are elevated. The excretion of other purines, such as xanthine and hypoxanthine, is also increased.

As would be expected from the Lyon hypothesis, the heterozygote female has two cell populations, one with full enzymatic activity, the other enzyme deficient.[496]

Pathologic Anatomy

The neuropathologic alterations seen with this disorder are sparse, and can be accounted by the uremia, which is often present terminally.[497]

Clinical Manifestations

Affected children appear normal at birth. During the first year of life psychomotor retardation becomes evident. Extrapyramidal movements are noted during the second year of life and persist until obliterated by progressive spasticity. A curious and unexplained feature of the disease is the involuntary self-destructive biting of fingers, arms, and lips. Children are disturbed by their compulsion to self-mutilation, and are happier when maintained in restraints. Hematuria and renal calculi are seen in the majority of individuals, and ultimately renal failure develops. Gouty arthritis and ureate tophi are also late complications. Mental retardation is never severe, and some individuals with marked extrapyramidal movements retain normal intelligence.

Diagnosis

The features of the illness, in particular, self-mutilation and extrapyramidal movements, make a diagnosis possible on clinical grounds. While serum uric acid is usually elevated, diagnostic confirmation is best obtained from the urinary uric acid content, with a urinary uric acid:creatine ratio of 2 being almost diagnostic.[498] Enzymatic analysis of blood, cultured skin fibroblasts, cultured amniotic fluid cells, or other tissue are easily carried out[499] and allow antenatal diagnosis.[262]

A rare entity manifested by mental retardation, dysplastic teeth, absent tears, and hyperuricemia, has been encountered.[500] Hypoxanthine-guanine activity was normal in erythrocytes of the patients.

Treatment

Allopurinol, a xanthine oxidase inhibitor, which blocks the last steps of uric acid synthesis, has been used in treatment. The fall in uric acid excretion induced by this drug is accompanied by a rise in hypoxanthine and xanthine. There is no evidence that neurologic symptoms are relieved or prevented by this form of therapy, although the urinary complications can be prevented. An attempt to reduce uric acid excretion by feeding precursors of known feedback inhibitors of purine synthesis has also been unsuccessful.[498]

PORPHYRIA

Of the various inherited disorders of porphyrin metabolism, only congenital erythropoietic porphyria is observed in childhood. It results in cutaneous photosensitivity and hemolytic anemia but is not accompanied by neurologic symptoms.

Acute intermittent porphyria is transmitted as an autosomal dominant trait with variable penetrance. Symptoms usually begin at puberty or shortly thereafter, are most pronounced in young adults, and commonly are aggravated or precipitated by the ingestion of barbiturates. They include intermittent colicky abdominal pain, and polyneuritis, which usually predominantly affects the motor nerves. The upper limbs are generally more involved, and the paralysis progresses to reach its maximum within several weeks. Mental disturbances are common, but there are no skin lesions.[501]

The metabolic defect is still unknown but is reflected in an overproduction of δ-aminolevulinic acid, resulting in the urinary excretion of increased amounts of porphobilinogen.

In variegate porphyria transient polyneuritis is accompanied by increased sensitivity of the skin to trauma and light.

EVALUATION OF THE PATIENT SUSPECTED OF A METABOLIC DISORDER

In many of the inborn metabolic errors, the clinical picture is nonspecific and the diagnosis must be made by demonstrating an abnormality of the enzymatic or chemical constituents in body fluids or tissues.

Routine screening of urine can usually detect all of the common disorders of amino acid and carbohydrate metabolism. We advocate the following five procedures:[502]

1. Ferric chloride test (see p. 6).

2. DNPH test: to 1.0 ml of urine, 0.2 ml of a 0.5% solution of 2,4-dinitrophenylhydrazine in 2 N hydrochloric acid is added by the drop. A definite yellow precipitate, forming within one minute, represents a positive reaction. The precipitate consists of the hydrazones of carbonyl compounds, including ketones such as acetone, and keto-acids such as phenylpyruvic, and alpha-ketoisocaproic acids.

TABLE 1-12.

SCREENING TESTS FOR METABOLIC DEFECTS

Condition	Ferric chloride	DNPH	Benedict's	Nitroprusside	CTAB
Phenylketonuria	Green	+	—	—	—
Maple syrup urine disease	Occasionally navy blue	+	—	—	—
Tyrosinosis	Pale green (transient)	+	±	—	—
Histidinemia	Green brown (permanent)	±	—	—	—
Propionic acidemia	Purple	+	—	—	—
Methylmalonic aciduria	Purple	+	—	—	—
Homocystinuria	—	—	—	+	—
Glutathioninuria	—	—	—	+	—
Cystinuria	—	—	—	+	—
Mucopolysaccharidoses	—	—	—	—	+
Galactosemia	—	—	+	—	—
Fructose intolerance	—	—	+	—	—

3. Benedict's test: for this purpose, Clinitest tablets (Ames Co., Inc., Elkhart, Indiana) are adequate. A positive reaction is usually obtained in patients with galactosemia, fructose intolerance, and in some children excreting large amounts of tyrosine and its metabolites.

4. Nitroprusside-cyanide test (see p. 18).

5. CTAB test (see p. 36).

The results obtained with these tests in the various common metabolic disorders are depicted in Table 1–12.

The disorders in the urea cycle are characterized by elevated concentrations of blood ammonia with the patient in the fasting state, or on a high-protein intake (4 gm/kg/day). A number of genetic disorders are characterized by hypoglycemia or intermittent acidosis. Determination of fasting blood sugar, serum pH, pCO_2, lactic and pyruvic acids is, therefore, indicated in a metabolic workup, and should the suspicion for a metabolic disorder be high, these determinations should be repeated with the child on a high protein intake. The presence of a macrocytic anemia suggests a disorder of B_{12} metabolism, such as is seen in some patients with methylmalonic acidemia. Other biochemical determinations required in the evaluation of a patient with a suspected metabolic defect include serum and urine uric acid, serum cholesterol, immunoglobulins, protein-bound iodine and magnesium.

Radiographic examination of the skull, vertebrae and long bones can be used to diagnose the mucopolysaccharidoses, Gaucher's disease, Niemann-Pick disease, and G_{M1} gangliosidosis.

In a number of metabolic disorders, notably the lipidoses and white matter degenerations, the diagnosis requires a combination of clinical evaluation and combined microscopic, ultrastructural, and biochemical studies on biopsied tissue.

Tissues which may be examined with a good likelihood of obtaining a diagnosis are as follows:

Lymphocytes: Battens, Spielmeyer-Vogt disease
                  Mucopolysaccharidoses

Rectal mucosa: Tay-Sachs disease
                  Niemann-Pick disease (group A)
                  Wolman's disease

Tonsils: Tangier disease
                  Niemann-Pick disease (group A)

Kidney: Hurler's disease
                  Generalized G_{M1} gangliosidosis
                  Fabry's disease

Peripheral nerve: Metachromatic leukodystrophy
                  Globoid cell leukodystrophy
                  Infantile neuroaxonal dystrophy
                  Fabry's disease
                  Refsum's disease
                  Tangier disease
                  ?Late infantile and juvenile amaurotic idiocy

Bone marrow: Niemann-Pick disease
                  Gaucher's disease
                  G_{M1} gangliosidosis

Brain: All lipidoses, and degenerative diseases of gray matter. All white matter
                  degenerations, with the possible exception of Pelizaeus-Merzbacher disease.
                  None of the disorders with primary basal ganglia symptoms, except
                  Huntington's chorea.

REFERENCES

1. Perry, T. L., et al.: Sucrosuria and mental deficiency: A coincidence, Pediatrics 24:774, 1959.
2. Lyon, I. C. T., Procopis, P. G., and Turner, B.: Cystathioninuria in a well-baby population Acta Paediat. Scand. 60:324, 1971.
3. Fontaine, G., Farriaux, J. P., and Dautrevaux, M.: L'hyperprolinemie de type I, Helv. Paediat. Acta 25:165, 1970.
4. Følling, A.: Uber Ausscheidung von Phenylbrenztraubensaure in den Harn als Stoffwechselanomalie in Verbindung mit Imbezillitat, Ztschr. Physiol. Chem. 227:169, 1934.
5. Berman, J. L., et al.: Causes for high phenylalanine with normal tyrosine, Amer. J. Dis. Child. 117:54, 1969.
6. Jervis, G. A.: Phenylpyruvic oligophrenia (phenylketonuria), A. Res. Nerv. Ment. Dis. Proc. (1953) 33:259, 1954.
7. Jervis, G. A.: Studies on phenylpyruvic oligophrenia: Position of metabolic error, J. Biol. Chem. 169:651, 1947.
8. Udenfriend, S. and Bessman, S. P.: Hydroxylation of phenylalanine and antipyrine in phenylpyruvic oligophrenia, J. Biol. Chem. 203:961, 1953.
9. Wallace, H. W., Moldave, K., and Meister, A.: Studies on conversion of phenylalanine to tyrosine in phenylpyruvic oligophrenia, Proc. Soc. Exp. Biol. Med. 94:632, 1957.
10. Kaufman, S. and Levenberg, B.: Further studies on the phenylalanine hydroxylation cofactor, J. Biol. Chem. 234:2683, 1959.
11. Tourian, A., Goddard, J., and Puck, T. T.: Phenylalanine hydroxylase activity in mammalian cells, J. Cell. Physiol. 73:159, 1969.
12. Barranger, J. A., et al.: Isozymes of phenylalanine hydroxylase, Science 175:903, 1972.
12a. Fisher, D. B., Kirkwood, R., and Kaufman, S.: Rat liver phenylalanine hydroxylase, an iron enzyme, J. Biol. Chem. 247:5161, 1972.
13. Lloyd, T., Mori, T., and Kaufman, S.: 6-methyltetrahydropteridin. Isolation and identification as the highly active hydroxylase cofactor from tetrahydrofolate, Biochemistry 10:2331, 1971.
14. Kaufman, S.: The structure of the phenylalanine hydroxylation cofactor, Proc. Nat. Acad. Sci. USA, 50:1085, 1963.
15. La Du, B. N.: "Genetic Variation in Metabolic Disorders," in Nyhan, W. L. (ed.): *Amino Acid Metabolism and Genetic Variation*, New York: McGraw-Hill Book Co., 1967.
16. Kaufman, S.: The phenylalanine hydroxylation cofactor in phenylketonuria, Science 128:1506, 1958.

17. Goodfriend, T. L. and Kaufman, S.: Phenylalanine metabolism and folic acid antagonists, J. Clin. Invest. 40:1743, 1961.

18. Jacubovic, A.: Phenylalanine hydroxylation system in the human fetus at different developmental ages, Biochim. Biophys. Acta 237:469, 1971.

19. La Du, B. N., et al.: A quantitative micromethod for the determination of phenylalanine and tyrosine in blood and its application in the diagnosis of phenylketonuria in infants, Pediatrics 31:39, 1963.

20. Menkes, J. H. and Avery, M. E.: The metabolism of phenylalanine and tyrosine in the premature infant, Bull. Hopkins Hosp. 113:301, 1963.

21. Allen, R. J., et al.: Phenylalanine hydroxylase activity in newborn infants, Pediatrics 33:512, 1964.

22. Taniguchi, K. and Armstrong, M. D.: The enzymatic formation of o-hydroxyphenylacetic acid, J. Biol. Chem. 238:4091, 1963.

23. Taniguchi, K., Kappe, T., and Armstrong, M. D.: Further studies on phenylpyruvic oxidase: Occurrence of side chain rearrangement and comparison with p-hydroxyphenylpyruvate oxidase, J. Biol. Chem. 239:3389, 1964.

23a. Fellman, J. H., et al.: The source of aromatic ketoacids in tyrosinaemia and phenylketonuria, Clin. Chim. Acta 39:243, 1972.

24. Jervis, G. A.: Studies on phenylpyruvic oligophrenia: Phenylpyruvic acid concentration of blood, Proc. Soc. Exp. Biol. Med. 81:715, 1952.

25. La Du, B. N. and Michael, P. J.: An enzymatic spectrophotometric method for the determination of phenylalanine in blood, J. Lab. Clin. Med. 55:491, 1960.

26. Armstrong, M. D., Shaw, K. N. F., and Robinson, K. S.: Studies on phenylketonuria: Excretion of o-hydroxyphenylacetic acid in phenylketonuria, J. Biol. Chem. 213:797, 1955.

27. Armstrong, M. D. and Robinson, K. S.: On the excretion of indole derivatives in phenylketonuria, Arch. Biochem. 51:287, 1954.

28. Bessman, S. P. and Tada, K.: Indicanuria in phenylketonuria, Metabolism 9:377, 1960.

29. Schreier, K. and Flaig, H.: Uber die Ausscheidung von Indolbrenztraubensaure im Urin von Gesunden und Patienten mit Follingscher Krankheit, Klin. Wschr. 34:1213, 1956.

30. Pare, C. M. B., Sandler, M., and Stacey, R. S.: Decreased 5-hydroxytryptophan decarboxylase activity in phenylketonuria, Lancet 2:1099, 1958.

31. Menkes, J. H.: The pathogenesis of mental retardation in phenylketonuria and other inborn errors of amino acid metabolism, Pediatrics 39:297, 1967.

32. Yarbro, M. T. and Anderson, J. A.: L-tryptophan metabolism in phenylketonuria, J. Pediat. 68:895, 1966.

33. Miyamoto, M. and Fitzpatrick, T. B.: Competitive inhibition of mammalian tyrosinase by phenylalanine and its relationship to hair pigmentation in phenylketonuria, Nature 179:199, 1957.

34. Malamud, N.: Neuropathology of phenylketonuria, J. Neuropath. Exp. Neurol., 25:254, 1966.

35. Coulson, W. F. and Bray, P. F.: An association of phenylketonuria with ulegyria, Dis. Nerv. Syst. 30:129, 1969.

36. Crome, L.: The association of phenylketonuria with leucodystrophy, J. Neurol. Neurosurg. Psychiat. 25:149, 1962.

37. Barden, H.: The histochemical relationship of neuromelanin and lipofuscin, J. Neuropath. Exp. Neurol. 28:419, 1969.

38. Partington, M. W.: The early symptoms of phenylketonuria, Pediatrics 27:465, 1961.

39. Low, N. L., Bosma, J. F., and Armstrong, M. D.: Studies on phenylketonuria: VI. EEG studies in phenylketonuria, Arch. Neurol. Psychiat. 77:359, 1957.

40. Watson, C. W., Nigam, M. P., and Paine, R. S.: Electroencephalographic abnormalities in phenylpyruvic oligophrenia, Neurology 18:203, 1968.

41. Fisch, R. O., et al.: Maternal phenylketonuria: Detrimental effects on embryogenesis and fetal development, Amer. J. Dis. Child. 118:847, 1969.

42. Allen, R. J., Fleming, L., and Spirito, R.: "Variations in Hyperphenylalaninemia," in Nyhan, W. L., (ed.): Amino Acid Metabolism and Genetic Variation, New York: McGraw-Hill Book Co., 1967, pp. 69–96.

43. Perry, T. L., et al.: A simple test for heterozygosity for phenylketonuria, Clin. Chim. Acta 15:47, 1967.

44. Kang, E. and Paine, R. S.: Elevation of plasma phenylalanine levels during pregnancies of women heterozygous for phenylketonuria, J. Pediat. 63:283, 1963.

45. Mabry, C. C., et al.: Maternal phenylketonuria: A cause of mental retardation in children without metabolic defect, New Eng. J. Med. 269:1404, 1963.

46. Mabry, C. C., Denniston, J. C., and Coldwell, J. G.: Mental retardation in children of phenylketonuric mothers, New Eng. J. Med. 275:1331, 1966.

47. Oldendorf, W. H., Sisson, W. B., and Silverstein, A.: Brain uptake of selenomethionine Se⁷⁵: II. Reduced brain uptake of selenomethionine Se⁷⁵ in phenylketonuria, Arch. Neurol. 24:524, 1971.

47a. Oja, S. S.: Incorporation of phenylalanine, tyrosine and tryptophan into protein of homogenates from developing rat brain: kinetics of incorporation and reciprocal inhibition, J. Neurochem. 19:2057, 1972.

48. La Du, B. N.: The importance of early diagnosis and treatment of phenylketonuria, Ann. Intern. Med. 51:1427, 1959.

49. Hudson, F. P., Dickinson, R. A., and Ireland, J. T.: Experiences in the detection and treatment of phenylketonuria, Pediatrics 31 :47, 1963.

50. Guthrie, R. and Susi, A.: A simple phenylalanine method for detecting phenylketonuria in large populations of newborn infants, Pediatrics 32 :338, 1963.

51. McCaman, M. W. and Robins, E.: Fluorometric method for the determination of phenylalanine in serum, J. Lab. Clin. Med. 59 :885, 1962.

52. Menkes, J. H. and Holtzman, N. A.: Neonatal hyperphenylalaninemia: A differential diagnosis, Neuropaediatrie 1 :434, 1970.

53. Woolf, L. I., et al.: Atypical phenylketonuria in sisters with normal offspring, Lancet 2 :464, 1961.

54. Justice, P., O'Flynn, M. E., and Hsia, D. Y. Y.: Phenylalanine hydroxylase activity in hyperphenylalaninemia, Lancet 1 :928, 1967.

55. Woolf, L. I., Cranston, W. L., and Goodwin, B. L.: Genetics of phenylketonuria, Nature 213 :882, 1967.

56. Woolf, L. I., et al.: A third allele at the phenylalanine-hydroxylase locus in mild phenylketonuria (hyperphenylalaninaemia), Lancet 1 : 114, 1968.

57. Auerbach, V. H., et al.: Delayed maturation of tyrosine metabolism in a full-term sibling of a child with phenylketonuria, J. Pediat. 62 :938, 1963.

58. Rouse, B. M.: Phenylalanine deficiency syndrome, J. Pediat. 69 :246, 1966.

58a.Knox, W. E.: Retrospective study of phenylketonuria. Treatment results in phenylketonuria in relation to phenylalanine levels, Phenylketonuria Newsletter #8 : 1, 1970.

59. Dodge, P. R., et al.: Hypoglycemia complicating treatment of phenylketonuria with a phenylalanine-deficient diet: Report of 2 cases, New Eng. J. Med. 260 :1104, 1959.

60. Royston, N. J. and Parry, T. E.: Megaloblastic anemia complicating dietary therapy of phenylketonuria in infancy, Arch. Dis. Child. 37 :430, 1962.

61. Hanley, W. B., et al.: Malnutrition with early treatment of phenylketonuria, Pediat. Res. 4: 318, 1970.

62. Centerwall, W. R., et al.: Phenylketonuria: I. Dietary management of infants and young children, J. Pediat., 59 :93, 1961.

63. Holtzman, N. A.: Dietary treatment of inborn errors of metabolism, Ann. Rev. Med. 21 :335, 1970.

64. Levy, H. L., et al.: Persistent mild hyperphenylalaninemia in the untreated state, New Eng. J. Med. 285 :424, 1971.

65. Knox, W. E.: An evaluation of the treatment of phenylketonuria with diets low in phenylalanine, Pediatrics 26 :1, 1960.

66. Birch, H. G. and Tizard, J.: The dietary treatment of phenylketonuria: Not proven? Develop. Med. Child Neurol. 9 :9, 1967.

67. Cohen, B. E., et al.: Evaluation of dietary treatment in phenylketonuria: A proposed methodology, Develop. Med. Child Neurol. 11 :96, 1969.

68. Fuller, R. N. and Shuman, J. B.: Phenylketonuria and intelligence: Trimodal response to dietary treatment, Nature 221 :639, 1969.

69. Hackney, I. M., et al.: Phenylketonuria: Mental development, behavior and termination of low phenylalanine diet, J. Pediat. 72 :646, 1968.

70. Solomons, G., Keleske, L., and Opitz, E.: Evaluation of the effects of terminating the diet in phenylketonuria, J. Pediat. 69 :596, 1966.

70a.Johnson, C. F.: What is the best age to discontinue the low phenylalanine diet in phenylketonuria? Clin. Pediat. (Phila.) 11 :148, 1972.

71. Fuller, R. and Shuman, J.: Treated phenylketonuria: Intelligence and blood phenylalanine levels, Amer. J. Ment. Defic. 75 :539, 1971.

72. La Du, B. N.: The enzymatic deficiency in tyrosinemia, Amer. J. Dis. Child. 113 :54, 1967.

73. Menkes, J. H., Hurst, P. L., and Craig, J. M.: A new syndrome: Progressive familial infantile cerebral dysfunction associated with unusual urinary substance, Pediatrics 14 :462, 1954.

74. Menkes, J. H.: Maple syrup disease: Investigations into the metabolic defect, Neurology 9 :826, 1959.

75. Bowden, J. A. and Connelly, J. L.: Branched-chain alpha-keto acid metabolism : II. Evidence for the common identity of alpha-ketoisocaproic acid and alpha-keto-beta-methyl valeric acid dehydrogenases, J. Biol. Chem. 243 :3526, 1968.

76. Goedde, H. W., et al.: Biochemical studies on branched-chain oxoacid oxidases, Biochim. Biophys. Acta 132 :524, 1967.

77. Dancis, J., Hutzler, J., and Cox, R. P.: Enzyme defect in skin fibroblasts in intermittent branched-chain ketonuria and in maple syrup urine disease, Biochem. Med. 2 :407, 1969.

78. Reed, L. J.: Pyruvate dehydrogenase complex, Current Topics in Cellular Regulation 1 :233, 1969.

79. Menkes, J. H.: Maple syrup disease: Isolation and identification of organic acids in the urine, Pediatrics 23 :348, 1959.

80. Norton, P. M., et al.: A new finding in maple-syrup-urine disease, Lancet 1 :26, 1962.

81. Crome, L., Dutton, G., and Ross, C. F.: Maple syrup urine disease, J. Path. Bact. 81 :379, 1961.

82. Prensky, A. L. and Moser, H. W.: Brain lipids, proteolipids, and free amino acids in maple syrup urine disease, J. Neurochem. 13 :863, 1966.

83. Menkes, J. H. and Solcher, H.: Effect of dietary therapy on cerebral morphology and chemistry in maple syrup disease, Arch. Neurol. 16 :486, 1967.

84. Dickinson, J. P., et al.: Maple syrup urine disease, Acta Paediat. Scand. 58 :341, 1969.

85. Donnell, G. N., et al.: Hypoglycemia in maple syrup urine disease, Amer. J. Dis. Child. 113 :60, 1967.

86. Dancis, J., Hutzler, J., and Rokkones, T.: Intermittent branched-chain ketonuria, New Eng. J. Med. 276:84, 1967.
87. Goedde, H. W., Langenbeck, U., and Brackertz, D.: Clinical and biochemical-genetic aspects of intermittent branched-chain ketoaciduria, Acta Paediat. Scand. 59:83, 1970.
88. Fischer, M. H. and Gerritsen, T.: Biochemical studies on a variant of branched chain ketoaciduria in a 19-year-old female, Pediatrics 48: 795, 1971.
89. Schulman, J. D., et al.: A new variant of maple syrup urine disease (branched chain ketoaciduria): Clinical and biochemical evaluation, Amer. J. Med. 49:118, 1970.
90. Scriver, C. R., et al.: Thiamine-responsive maple-syrup-urine disease, Lancet 1:310, 1971.
91. Appel, S. H.: Inhibition of brain protein synthesis: An approach to the biochemical basis of neurological dysfunction in the aminoacidurias, Trans. NY Acad. Sci. 29:63, 1966.
92. Snyderman, S. E.: The therapy of maple syrup urine disease, Amer. J. Dis. Child. 113:68, 1967.
93. Westall, R. G.: Dietary treatment of maple syrup urine disease, Amer. J. Dis. Child. 113:58, 1967.
94. Rey, F., et al.: Traitement d'urgence d'une forme aigue de leucinose par dialyse peritoneale, Arch. Franc. Pediat. 26:133, 1969.
95. Linneweh, F. and Solcher, H.: Ueber den Einflusz diatetischer Prophylaxe auf die Myelogenese bei der Leucinose (maple syrup urine disease), Klin. Wschr. 43:926, 1965.
96. Allan, J. D., et al.: A disease, probably hereditary, characterized by severe mental deficiency and a constant gross abnormality of amino acid metabolism, Lancet 1:182, 1958.
97. Levin, B.: Argininosuccinic aciduria, Amer. J. Dis. Child. 113:162, 1967.
98. Tomlinson, S. and Westall, R. G.: Argininosuccinic aciduria: Argininosuccinase and arginase in human blood cells, Clin. Sci. 26:261, 1964.
99. Kint, J. and Carton, D.: Deficient argininosuccinase activity in brain in argininosuccinic aciduria, Lancet 2: 635, 1968.
100. Crane, C. W., Gay, W. M. B., and Jenner, F. A.: Urea production from labeled ammonia in argininosuccinic aciduria, Clin. Chim. Acta 24:445, 1969.
101. Carton, D., et al.: Argininosuccinic aciduria: Neonatal variant with rapid fatal course, Acta Paediat. Scand. 58:528, 1969.
102. Lewis, P. D. and Miller, A. L.: Argininosuccinic aciduria, Brain 93:413, 1970.
103. Moser, H. W., et al.: Argininosuccinic aciduria: Report of two new cases and demonstration of intermittent elevation of blood ammonia, Amer. J. Med. 42:9, 1967.
104. Armstrong, M. D., Yates, K. N., and Stemmermann, M. G.: An occurrence of argininosuccinic aciduria, Pediatrics 33:280, 1964.
105. McMurray, W. C., et al.: Citrullinuria, Pediatrics 32:347, 1963.
106. Morrow, G., Barness, L. A., and Efron, M. L.: Citrullinemia with defective urea production, Pediatrics 40:565, 1967.
107. Tedesco, T. A. and Mellman, W. J.: Argininosuccinate synthetase activity and citrulline metabolism in cells cultured from a citrullinemia subject, Proc. Nat. Acad. Sci. USA 57:829, 1967.
107a. Scott-Emuakpor, A., Higgins, J. V., and Kohrman, A. F.: Citrullinemia: A new case, with implications concerning adaptation to defective urea synthesis, Pediat. Res. 6:626, 1972.
108. Van der Zee, S. P. M., et al.: Citrullinaemia with rapidly fatal neonatal course, Arch. Dis. Child. 46:847, 1971.
109. Milne, M. D., London, D. R., and Asatoor, A. M.: Citrullinuria in cases of cystinuria, Lancet 2:49, 1962.
110. Russell, A., et al.: Hyperammonaemia: A new instance of an inborn enzymatic defect of the biosynthesis of urea, Lancet 2:699, 1962.
111. Levin, B., et al.: Hyperammonaemia: A deficiency of liver ornithine transcarbamylase, Arch. Dis. Child. 44:152, 1969.
111a. Campbell, A. G. M., et al.: Ornithine transcarbamylase deficiency, New Eng. J. Med. 288:1, 1973.
112. Bruton, C. J., Corsellis, J. A. N., and Russell, A.: Hereditary hyperammonaemia, Brain 93:423, 1970.
113. Levin, B. and Russell, A.: Treatment of hyperammonemia, Amer. J. Dis. Child. 113:142, 1967.
114. Levin, B., et al.: Hyperammonaemia: A variant type of deficiency of liver ornithine transcarbamylase, Arch. Dis. Child. 44:162, 1969.
115. Freeman, J. M., et al.: Congenital hyperammonemia, Arch. Neurol. 23:430, 1970.
116. Hommes, F. A., et al.: Carbamylphosphate synthetase deficiency in an infant with severe cerebral damage, Arch. Dis. Child. 44:688, 1969.
116a. Ebels, E. J.: Neuropathological observations in a patient with carbamylphosphate-synthetase deficiency and in two sibs, Arch. Dis. Child. 47:47, 1972.
117. Burgi, W., Richterich, R., and Colombo, J. P.: L-Lysine dehydrogenase deficiency in a patient with congenital lysine intolerance, Nature 211:854, 1966.
118. Colombo, J. P., et al.: Congenital lysine intolerance with periodic ammonia intoxication: A defect in L-lysine degradation, Metabolism 16:910, 1967.
119. Kekomaki, M., Visakorpi, J. K., and Perheentupa, J.: Familial protein intolerance with deficient transport of basic amino acids: An analysis of 10 patients, Acta Paediat. Scand. 56:617, 1967.
120. Shih, V. E., Efron, M. L., and Moser, H. W.: Hyperornithemia, hyperammonemia and homocitrullinuria, Amer. J. Dis. Child. 117:83, 1969.

121. Kekomaki, M. P., Raiha, N. C. R., and Bickel, H.: Ornithine-ketoacid aminotransferase in human liver with reference to patients with hyperornithaemia and familial protein intolerance, Clin. Chim. Acta 23:203, 1969.

122. Landes, R. D., et al.: Propionyl-CoA carboxylase deficiency (propionic acidemia): Another cause of hyperammonemia, Pediat. Res. 6:394, 1972.

123. Rett, A.: *Uber ein Zerebral-atrophisches Syndrom bei Hyperamnonamie*, Wien: Verlag Bruder Hollinek, 1966.

124. Ghadimi, H., Partington, M. W., and Hunter, A.: A familial disturbance of histidine metabolism, New Eng. J. Med. 165:221, 1961.

125. Auerbach, V. H., et al.: Histidinemia, J. Pediat. 60:487, 1962.

126. La Du, B. N., Howell, R. R., and Jacoby, G. A.: Clinical and biochemical studies on 2 cases of histidinemia, Pediatrics 32:216, 1963.

127. Levy, H. L., Baden, H. P., and Shih, V. E.: A simple indirect method of detecting the enzyme defect in histidinemia, J. Pediat. 75: 1056, 1969.

128. Corner, H. D., et al.: A case of histidinemia controlled with a low histidine diet, Pediatrics 41:1074, 1968.

129. Gordon, N.: Delayed speech and histidinaemia, Develop. Med. Child Neurol. 12:104, 1970.

130. Woody, N. C., Snyder, C. H., and Harris, J. A.: Histidinemia, Amer. J. Dis. Child. 110:606, 1965.

131. Auerbach, V. H., DiGeorge, A. M., and Carpenter, C. G.: "Histidinemia," in Nyhan, W. L. (ed.): *Amino Acid Metabolism and Genetic Variation*, New York: McGraw-Hill Book Co., 1967, pp. 145–160.

132. Yoshida, T., et al.: Urocanic aciduria—A defect in the urocanase activity in the liver of a mentally retarded, Tohokushima J. Exp. Med. 104:305, 1971.

133. Arakawa, T., et al.: Formimino transferase deficiency syndrome: A new inborn error of folic acid metabolism. Ann. Paediat. 205:1, 1965.

134. Carson, N. A. J., Cusworth, D. C., and Dent, C. E.: Homocystinuria: A new inborn error of metabolism associated with mental deficiency, Arch. Dis. Child. 38:425, 1963.

135. Spaeth, G. L. and Barber, G. W.: Prevalence of homocystinuria among mentally retarded: Evaluation of specific screening test, Pediatrics 40:586, 1967.

136. Mudd, S. H., et al.: Homocystinuria: An enzymatic defect, Science 143:1443, 1964.

137. Brenton, D. P., Cusworth, D. C., and Gaull, G. E.: Homocystinuria: Metabolic studies on 3 patients, J. Pediat. 67:58, 1965.

138. Perry, T. L., et al.: Sulfur-containing amino acids in the plasma and urine of homocystinurics, Clin. Chim. Acta 15:409, 1967.

139. Applegarth, D. A., et al.: Excretion of s-adeno-sylmethionine and s-adenosylhomocysteine in homocystinuria, New Eng. J. Med. 285:1265, 1971.

140. Brenton, D. P., Cusworth, D. C., and Gaull, G. E.: Homocystinuria: Biochemical studies of tissues including a comparison with cystathioninuria, Pediatrics 35:50, 1965.

141. Seashore, M. R., Durant, J. L., and Rosenberg, L. E.: Studies of the mechanism of pyridoxine-responsive homocystinuria, Pediat. Res. 6:187, 1972.

142. Mudd, S. H., et al.: Homocystinuria associated with decreased methylenetetrahydrofolate reductase activity, Biochem. Biophys. Res. Commun. 46:905, 1972.

143. Goodman, S. I., et al.: Homocystinuria with methylmalonic aciduria. Two cases in sibship, Biochem. Med. 4:500, 1970.

144. Gibson, J. B., Carson, N. A., and Neill, D. W.: Pathological findings in homocystinuria, J. Clin. Path. 17:427, 1964.

145. Ratnoff, O. D.: Activation of Hageman factor by L-homocystine, Science 162:1007, 1968.

146. McCully, K. S.: Importance of homocysteine-induced abnormalities of proteoglycan structure in arteriosclerosis, Amer. J. Path. 59:181, 1970.

147. Henkind, P. and Ashton, N.: Ocular pathology in homocystinuria, Trans. Ophthal. Soc. UK 85:21, 1965.

148. Presley, G. D. and Sidbury, J. B.: Homocystinuria and ocular defects, Amer. J. Ophthal. 63:1723, 1967.

149. Schimke, R. N., et al.: Homocystinuria. Studies of 20 families with 38 affected members, JAMA 193:711, 1965.

150. Hurwitz, L. T., Chopra, J. S., and Carson, N. A. J.: Electromyographic evidence of a muscle lesion in homocystinuria, Acta Paediat. Scand. 57:401, 1968.

151. Brand, E., Harris, M. M., and Biloon, S.: Cystinuria: The excretion of a cystine complex which decomposes in the urine with the liberation of free cystine, J. Biol. Chem. 86:315, 1930.

152. Crawhall, J. C., et al.: Mercaptolactate-cysteine disulfide in the urine of a mentally retarded patient, Amer. J. Dis. Child. 117:71, 1969.

153. Uhlendorf, B. W. and Mudd, S. H.: Cystathionine synthetase in tissue culture derived from human skin: Enzyme defect in homocystinuria, Science 160:1007, 1968.

154. Carson, N. A. J. and Carre, I. J.: Treatment of homocystinuria with pyridoxine: A preliminary study, Arch. Dis. Child. 44:387, 1969.

155. Mudd, S. H.: Pyridoxine-responsive genetic disease, Fed. Proc. 30 (No. 3, pt 1): 970, 1971.

156. Harris, H., Penrose, L. S., and Thomas, D. H.: Cystathioninuria, Ann. Hum. Genet. 23:442, 1959.

157. Frimpter, G. W.: Cystathioninuria: Nature of the defect, Science 149:1095, 1965.

158. Lieberman, E., Shaw, K. N. F., and Donnell, G. N.: Cystathioninuria in galactosemia and certain types of liver disease, Pediatrics 40:828, 1967.

159. Perry, T. L., Hardwick, D. F., and Dixon, G. H.: Hypermethioninemia: A metabolic disorder associated with cirrhosis, islet cell hyperplasia, and renal tubular degeneration, Pediatrics 36:236, 1965.

160. Fritzell, S., Jagenburg, O. R., and Schnürer, L. B.: Familial cirrhosis of the liver, renal tubular defects with rickets and impaired tyrosine metabolism, Acta Paediat. 53:18, 1964.

161. Hooft, C., Timmermans, J., and Snoeck, J.: Methionine malabsorption in a mentally defective child, Lancet 2:20, 1964.

162. Schafer, I. A., Scriver, C. R., and Efron, M. L.: Familial hyperprolinemia, cerebral dysfunction and renal anomalies occurring in a family with hereditary nephropathy and deafness, New Eng. J. Med. 267:51, 1962.

163. Efron, M. L.: Familial hyperprolinemia, New Eng. J. Med. 273:1243, 1965.

164. Scriver, C. R., Efron, M. L., and Schafer, I. A.: Renal tubular transport of proline, hydroxyproline, and glycine in health and in familial hyperprolinemia, J. Clin. Invest. 43:374, 1964.

165. Woody, N. C., Snyder, C. H., and Harris, J. A.: Hyperprolinemia: Clinical and biochemical family study, Pediatrics 44:554, 1969.

166. Efron, M. L.: Familial hyperprolinemia: Report of a second case associated with congenital renal malformations, hereditary hematuria and mild mental retardation, with demonstration of an enzyme defect, New Eng. J. Med. 272:1243, 1965.

167. Simila, S.: Intravenous proline tolerance in a patient with hyperprolinemia type II and his relatives, Helv. Paediat. Acta 25:287, 1970.

168. Efron, M. L., Bixby, E. M., and Pryles, C. V.: Hydroxyprolinemia: A rare metabolic disease due to a deficiency of the enzyme "hydroxyproline oxidase," New Eng. J. Med. 272:1299, 1965.

169. Dancis, J., et al.: Familial hyperlysinemia with lysine-ketoglutarate reductase insufficiency, J. Clin. Invest. 48:1447, 1969.

170. Ghadimi, H., Binnington, V. I., and Pecora, P.: Hyperlysinemia associated with retardation, New Eng. J. Med. 273:723, 1965.

171. Harris, H., et al.: Phenotypes and genotypes in cystinuria, Ann. Hum. Genet. 10:57, 1955.

172. Whelan, D. T. and Scriver, C. R.: Hyperdibasicaminoaciduria: An inherited disorder of amino acid transport, Pediat. Res. 2:525, 1968.

173. Perheentupa, J. and Visakorpi, J. K.: Protein intolerance with deficient transport of basic amino acids, Lancet 2:813, 1965.

174. Malmquist, J., Jagenburg, R., and Lindstedt, G.: Familial protein intolerance: Possible nature of enzyme defect, New Eng. J. Med. 284:997, 1971.

175. Gatfield, P. D., Taller, E., and Hinton, G. G.: Hyperpipecolatemia, a new metabolic disorder associated with neuropathy and hepatomegaly: A case study, Canad. Med. Ass. J. 99:1215, 1968.

176. Carson, N. A. J., et al.: Saccharopinuria: A new inborn error of lysine metabolism, Nature 218:679, 1968.

176a. Simell, O., Visakorpi, J. K., and Donna, M.: Saccharopinuria, Arch. Dis. Child., 47:52, 1972.

177. Wada, Y., Tada, K., and Minagawa, A.: Idiopathic hypervalinemia: Probably a new entity of inborn error of valine metabolism, Tohokushima J. Exp. Med. 81:46, 1963.

178. Gerritsen, T. and Waisman, H. A.: Hypersarcosinemia, New Eng. J. Med. 275:66, 1966.

179. Scott, C. R., et al.: Clinical and cellular studies of sarcosinemia, J. Pediat. 77:805, 1970.

180. Scriver, C. R., Pueschel, S., and Davies, E.: Hyperbeta-alaninemia associated with beta-aminoaciduria and gamma-aminobutyricaciduria, somnolence, and seizures, New Eng. J. Med. 174:636, 1966.

181. Lonsdale, D., et al.: Intermittent cerebellar ataxia associated with hyperpyruvic acidemia, hyperalaninemia and hyperalaninuria, Pediatrics 43:1025, 1969.

182. Blass, J. P., Avigan, J., and Uhlendorf, B. W.: A defect in pyruvate decarboxylase in a child with an intermittent movement disorder, J. Clin. Invest. 49:423, 1970.

183. Perry, T. L., et al.: Carnosinemia, New Eng. J. Med. 277:1219, 1967.

183a. Terplan, K. L. and Cares, H. L.: Histopathology of the nervous system in carnosinase enzyme deficiency with mental retardation, Neurology (Minneap.) 22:644, 1972.

184. Stokke, O., et al.: New metabolic error in leucine degradation, Pediatrics 49:726, 1972.

185. Daum, R. S., et al.: A "new" disorder of isoleucine catabolism, Lancet 2:1289, 1971.

186. Kennaway, N. G. and Buist, N. R. M.: Metabolic studies in a patient with hepatic cytosol tyrosine aminotransferase deficiency, Pediat. Res. 5:287, 1971:

187. Baron, D. N., et al.: Hereditary pellagra-like skin rash with temporary cerebellar ataxia, constant renal aminoaciduria, and other bizarre biochemical features, Lancet 2:421, 1956.

188. Milne, M. D., et al.: The metabolic disorder in Hartnup disease, Quart. J. Med. 29:407, 1960.

189. Jepson, J. B.: "Hartnup Disease" in Stanbury, J. B., Wyngaarden, J. B., and Fredrickson, D. S., (eds.): The Metabolic Basis of Inherited Disease, 3rd ed., New York: McGraw-Hill Book Co., 1972, pp. 1486–1503.

190. Scriver, C. R.: Hartnup disease: A genetic modification of intestinal and renal transport of certain neutral alpha-amino acids, New Eng. J. Med. 273:530, 1965.

191. Borrie, P. F. and Lewis, C. A.: Hartnup disease, Proc. Roy. Soc. Med. 55:231, 1962.

192. Hill, W. and Sherman, H.: Acute intermittent familial cerebellar ataxia, Arch. Neurol. 18:350, 1968.

193. Tada, K., et al.: Congenital tryptophanuria with dwarfism: H-disease-like clinical features without indicanuria and generalized amino-aciduria, Tohokushima J. Exp. Med. 80:118, 1963.

194. Lowe, C. U., Terry, M., and MacLachlan, E. A.: Organicaciduria, decreased renal ammonia production, hydrophthalmos, and mental retardation: A clinical entity, Amer. J. Dis. Child. 83:164, 1952.

195. Richards, W., et al.: The oculo-cerebro-renal syndrome of Lowe, Amer. J. Dis. Child. 109:185, 1965.

196. Bartsocas, C. S., et al.: A defect in intestinal amino acid transport in Lowe's syndrome, Amer. J. Dis. Child. 117:93, 1969.

197. Scriver, C. R.: Membrane transport in disorders of amino acid metabolism, Amer. J. Dis. Child. 113:170, 1967.

198. Procopis, P. G. and Turner, B.: Iminoaciduria: A benign renal tubular defect, J. Pediat. 79:419, 1971:

199. Turner, B. and Brown, D. A.: Amino acid excretion in infancy and early childhood, Med. J. Aust. 1:11, 1970.

200. Berry, H. K.: Amino acid excretion in urine of normal infants and children: Paper chromatographic methods for amino acid analyses, Pediatrics 25:983, 1960.

201. Menkes, J. H., Richardson, F., and Verplanck, S.: Program for the detection of metabolic diseases, Arch. Neurol. Psychiat. 6:462, 1962.

202. Wright, S. W.: Investigations on mentally defective sibs: Studies on urinary amino acids, J. Ment. Defic. Res. 4:32, 1960.

203. Von Reuss, A.: Zuckerausscheidung im Sauglingsalter, Wien. Med. Wschr. 58:799, 1908.

204. Shih, V., et al.: Galactosemia screening of newborns in Massachusetts, New Eng. J. Med. 284:753, 1971.

205. Göppert, F.: Galaktosurie nach Milchzuckergabe bei angeborenem, familiarem chronischem Leberleiden, Berl. Klin. Wchnschr. 54:473, 1917.

206. Schwarz, V., et al.: Some disturbances of erythrocyte metabolism in galactosemia, Biochem. J. 62:34, 1956.

207. Kalckar, H. M., Anderson, E. P., and Isselbacher, K. J.: Galactosemia: A congenital defect in a nucleotide transferase, Biochim. Biophys. Acta 20:262, 1956.

208. Isselbacher, K. J., et al.: Congenital galactosemia: A single enzymatic block in galactose metabolism, Science 123:635, 1956.

209. Tedesco, T. A.: Human galactose-1-phosphate uridyl transferase, J. Biol. Chem. 247:6631, 1972.

210. Kirkman, H. N. and Bynum, E.: Enzymic evidence of a galactosemic trait in parents of galactosemic children, Ann. Hum. Genet. 23:117, 1959.

211. Russell, J. D. and DeMars, R.: UDP-glucose: Alpha-D-galactose-1-phosphate uridyltransferase activity in cultured human fibroblasts, Biochem. Genet. 1:11, 1967.

212. Segal, S. and Cuatrecasas, P.: The oxidation of C^{14} galactose by patients with congenital galactosemia, Amer. J. Med. 44:340, 1968.

212a. Bergren, W. R., et al.: Galactonic acid in galactosemia: Identification in the urine, Science 176:683, 1972.

213. Baker, L., et al.: Galactosemia: Symptomatic and asymptomatic homozygotes in one Negro sibship, J. Pediat. 68:551, 1966.

214. Segal, S., Rogers, S., and Holtzapple, P. G.: Liver galactose-1-phosphate uridyl transferase: Activity in normal and galactosemic subjects, J. Clin. Invest. 50:500, 1971.

215. Beutler, E., et al.: A new genetic abnormality resulting in galactose-1-phosphate uridyltransferase deficiency, Lancet 1:353, 1965.

216. Schapira, F. and Kaplan, J. C.: Electrophoretic abnormality of galactose-1-phosphate uridyl transferase in galactosemia, Biochem. Biophys. Res. Commun. 35:451, 1969.

217. Gitzelmann, R.: Hereditary galactokinase deficiency: A newly recognized cause of juvenile cataracts, Pediat. Res. 1:14, 1967.

218. Cook, J. G. H., Don, N. A., and Mann, T. P.: Hereditary galactokinase deficiency, Arch. Dis. Child. 46:465, 1971.

219. Schwarz, V. and Goldberg, L.: Galactose-1-phosphate in galactose cataract, Biochim. Biophys. Acta 18:310, 1955.

220. Sidbury, J. B., Jr.: The enzymatic lesions in galactosemia, J. Clin. Invest. 36:929, 1957.

221. Wells, W. W., et al.: The isolation and identification of galactitol from the brains of galactosemia patients, J. Biol. Chem. 240:1002, 1965.

222. Wells, W. W., et al.: Studies on myoinositol metabolism in galactosemia, Ann. NY Acad. Sci. 165:599, 1969.

223. Segal, S.: "Disorders of Galactose Metabolism," in Stanbury, J. B., Wyngaarden, J. B., and Fredrickson, D. S. (eds.): The Metabolic Basis of Inherited Disease, 3rd ed., New York: McGraw-Hill Book Co., 1972, pp. 174–195.

224. Smetana, H. F. and Olen, E.: Hereditary galactose disease, Amer. J. Clin. Path. 38:32, 1962.

225. Haberland, C., et al.: The neuropathology of galactosemia, J. Neuropath. Exp. Neurol. 30:431, 1971.

226. Crome, L.: A case of galactosemia with the pathological and neuropathological findings, Arch. Dis. Child. 37:415, 1962.

227. Walsh, F. B.: Clinical Neuro-ophthalmology, 2nd ed., Baltimore: Williams & Wilkins Co., 1957.

228. Huttenlocher, P. R., Hillman, R. E., and Hsia, Y. E.: Pseudotumor cerebri in galactosemia, J. Pediat. 76:902, 1970.

229. Franceschetti, A., Marty, F., and Klein, D.: Un syndrome rare: Heredoataxie avec cataracte congenitale et retard mental, Confin. Neurol. 16:271, 1956.

230. Beutler, E. and Baluda, M. C.: A simple spot screening test for galactosemia, J. Lab. Clin. Med. 68:137, 1966.
231. Donnell, G. N., et al.: The enzymatic expression of heterozygosity in families of children with galactosemia, Pediatrics 25:572, 1960.
232. Nadler, H. L.: Antenatal detection of hereditary disorders, Pediatrics 42:912, 1968.
233. Fishler, K., et al.: Psychological correlates in galactosemia, Amer. J. Ment. Defic. 71:116, 1966.
234. Cornblath, M. and Schwartz, R.: *Disorders of Carbohydrate Metabolism in Infancy*, Philadelphia: W. B. Saunders Co., 1966, pp. 275–278.
235. Gitzelmann, R. and Auricchio, S.: The handling of soya alpha-galactosides by a normal and a galactosemic child, Pediatrics 36:231, 1965.
236. Pompe, J. C.: Over idiopathische hypertrophie van het hart, Nederl. T. Geneesk. 76:304, 1932.
237. Cori, G. T.: Glycogen structure and enzyme deficiencies in glycogen storage disease, Harvey Lect. 48:145, 1952–1953.
238. Hers, H. G.: Alpha glucosidase deficiency in generalized glycogen storage disease (Pompe's disease), Biochem. J. 86:11, 1963.
239. Baudhuin, P., Hers, H. G., and Loeb, H.: An electronmicroscopic and biochemical study of type II glycogenosis, Lab. Invest. 13:1139, 1964.
240. Crome, L., Cumings, J. N., and Duckett, S.: Neuropathological and neurochemical aspects of generalized glycogen storage disease, J. Neurol. Neurosurg. Psychiat. 26:422, 1963.
241. DiSant'Agnese, P. A., Andersen, D. H., and Mason, H. H.: Glycogen storage disease of the heart: Critical review of the literature, Pediatrics 6:607, 1950.
242. Childs, A. W., Crose, R. F., and Henderson, P. H.: Glycogen storage disease of the heart: Report of 2 cases occurring in siblings, Pediatrics 10:208, 1952.
243. Swaiman, K. F., Kennedy, W. R., and Sauls, H. S.: Late infantile acid maltase deficiency, Arch. Neurol. 18:642, 1968.
244. Angelini, C. and Engel, A. G.: Comparative study of acid maltase deficiency. Biochemical differences between infantile, childhood, and adult types, Arch. Neurol. 26:344, 1972.
244a. Dreyfus, J. C. and Alexandre, Y.: Electrophoretic characterization of acidic and neutral 1-4-glucosidase (acid maltase) in human tissues and evidence for two electrophoretic variants in acid maltase deficiency, Biochem. Biophys. Res. Commun. 48:914, 1972.
245. Huijing, F., van Creveld, S., and Losekoot, G.: Diagnosis of generalized glycogen storage disease (Pompe's disease), J. Pediat. 63:984, 1963.
246. Hug, G., Schubert, W. K., and Soukup, S.: Ultrastructure and enzymatic deficiency of fibroblast cultures in type II glycogenosis, Pediat. Res. 5:107, 1971.
247. Hirschhorn, K., Nadler, H. L., and Waithe, W. I.: Pompe's disease: Detection of heterozygotes by lymphocyte stimulation, Science 166:1632, 1969.
248. Hug, G., Schubert, W. K., and Schwachman, H.: Imbalance of liver phosphorylase and accumulation of hepatic glycogen in a girl with progressive disease of the brain, J. Pediat. 67:741, 1965.
249. Chambers, R. A. and Pratt, R. T. C.: Idiosyncrasy to fructose, Lancet 2:340, 1956.
250. Rennert, O. M. and Greer, M.: Hereditary fructosemia, Neurology 20:421, 1970.
251. Lindemann, R., et al.: Amino acid metabolism in hereditary fructosemia, Acta Paediat. Scand. 59:141, 1970.
252. Nikkila, E. A., et al.: Hereditary fructose intolerance: An inborn deficiency of liver aldolase complex, Metabolism 11:727, 1962.
253. Jeune, M., et al.: Hereditary intolerance to fructose: Apropos of a case, Pediatrie 16:605, 1961.
254. Schapira, F. and Dreyfus, J. C.: L'aldolase hepatique dans l'intolerance au fructose, Rev. Franc. Etude. Clin. Biol. 12:486, 1967.
255. Kranhold, J. F., Loh, D., and Morris, R. C., Jr.: Renal fructose-metabolizing enzymes: Significance in hereditary fructose intolerance, Science 165:402, 1969.
256. Phillips, M. J., Little, J. A., and Ptak, T. W.: Subcellular pathology of hereditary fructose intolerance, Amer. J. Med. 44:910, 1968.
257. Bickel, H.: Mellituria: A paper chromatographic study, J. Pediat. 59:641, 1961.
258. Hunter, C.: A rare disease in two brothers, Proc. Roy. Soc. Med. 10:104, 1917.
259. Hurler, G.: Uber einen Typ multipler Abartungen, vorwiegend am Skelett-system, Z. Kinderheilk. 24:220, 1919.
260. Ellis, R. W. B., Sheldon, W., and Capon, N. B.: Gargoylism, Quart. J. Med. 5:119, 1936.
261. Neufeld, E. F. and Fratantoni, J. C.: Inborn errors of mucopolysaccharide metabolism, Science 169:141, 1970.
262. Milunsky, A., et al.: Prenatal genetic diagnosis, New Eng. J. Med. 283:1370, 1441, 1498, 1970.
263. Varadi, D. P., Cifonelli, J. A., and Dorfman, A.: The acid mucopolysaccharides in normal urine, Biochim. Biophys. Acta 141:103, 1967.
264. Pedrini, V., Lennzi, L., and Zambotti, V.: Isolation and identification of keratosulfate in urine of patients affected by Morquio-Ullrich disease, Proc. Soc. Exp. Biol. Med. 110:847, 1962.
265. Sanfilippo, S. J., et al.: Mental retardation associated with acid mucopolysacchariduria (heparitin sulfate type), J. Pediat. 63:837, 1963.
266. Scheie, H. G., Hambrick, G. W., Jr., and Barness, L. A.: A newly recognized forme fruste of Hurler's disease (gargoylism), Amer. J. Ophthal. 53:753, 1962.
267. Maroteaux, P., et al.: Une nouvelle dysostose avec elimination urinaire de chondroitinsulfate B, Presse Med. 71:1849, 1963.

268. Spranger, J. W., Schuster, W., and Freitag, F.: Chondroitin-4-sulfate mucopolysaccharidosis, Helv. Paediat. Acta 26:387, 1971.

269. Stumpf, D. A. and Austin, J. H.: Sulfatase B deficiency in the Maroteaux-Lamy syndrome (Mucopolysaccharidoses—VI) Trans. Amer. Neurol. Ass. 97:29, 1972.

270. Spranger, J.: The systemic mucopolysaccharidoses, Ergebn. Inn. Med. Kinderheilk. 32:165, 1972.

271. Linker, A. and Hovingh, P.: The enzymatic degradation of heparitin sulfate: II. Isolation and characterization of non-sulfated oligosaccharides, Biochim. Biophys. Acta 165:89, 1968.

272. Bella, A., Jr. and Danishefsky, L.: The dermatan sulfate-protein linkage region, J. Biol. Chem. 243:2660, 1968.

273. Telser, A., Robinson, H. C., and Dorfman, A.: The biosynthesis of chondroitin sulfate, Arch. Biochem. 116:458, 1966.

274. Hilz, H. and Lipmann, F.: The enzymatic activation of sulfate, Proc. Nat. Acad. Sci. USA 41:880, 1955.

275. Knecht, J., Cifonelli, J. A., and Dorfman, A.: Structural studies on heparitin sulfate of normal and Hurler tissues, J. Biol. Chem. 242:4652, 1967.

276. Fratantoni, J. C., Hall, C. W., and Neufeld, E. F.: Hurler and Hunter's syndromes: Mutual correction of the defect in cultured fibroblasts, Proc. Nat. Acad. Sci. USA 60:699, 1968.

277. Bach, G., et al.: The defect in the Hurler and Scheie syndromes: Deficiency of α-L-Iduronidase, Proc. Nat. Acad. Sci. USA 69:2048, 1972.

278. MacBrinn, M., et al.: Beta galactosidase deficiency in the Hurler syndrome, New Eng. J. Med. 281:338, 1969.

279. Jervis, G. A.: Familial mental deficiency akin to amaurotic idiocy and gargoylism, Arch. Neurol. Psychiat. 47:943, 1942.

280. Ledeen, R., et al.: Structure comparison of the major monosialogangliosides from brains of normal human, gargoylism and late infantile systemic lipidosis, J. Neuropath. Exp. Neurol 24:341, 1965.

281. Meyer, K., et al.: Sulfated mucopolysaccharides of urine and organs in gargoylism (Hurler's syndrome): Additional studies, Proc. Soc. Exp. Biol. Med. 102:587, 1959.

281a. Cantz, M., et al.: The Hunter corrective factor. Purification and preliminary characterization, J. Biol. Chem. 247:2456, 1972.

282. Wiesmann, U. and Neufeld, E. F.: Scheie and Hurler syndromes: Apparent identity of the biochemical defect, Science 169:72, 1970.

282a. O'Brien, J. S.: Sanfilippo syndrome; profound deficiency of alpha-acetylglucosaminidase activity in organs and skin fibroblasts from Type B patients, Proc. Nat. Acad. Sci. USA 69:1720, 1972.

282b. Figura, K. von, and Kresse, H.: The Sanfilippo B corrective factor. A N-acetyl-α-D-Glucosaminidase, Biochem. Biophys. Res. Commun. 48:262, 1972.

283. Lindsay, S., et al.: Gargoylism: Study of pathologic lesions and clinical review of 12 cases, Amer. J. Dis. Child. 76:239, 1948.

284. Jervis, G. A.: Gargoylism (lipochondrodystrophy), Arch. Neurol. Psychiat. 63:681, 1950.

285. Lagunoff, D., Ross, R., and Benditt, E. P.: Histochemical and electron microscopic study in a case of Hurler's disease, Amer. J. Path. 41:273, 1962.

286. Van Hoof, F. and Hers, H. G.: L'ultrastructure des cellules hepatiques dans la maladie de Hurler (gargoylisme), C. R. Acad. Sci. (Paris) 259:1281, 1964.

287. McKusick, V. A.: *Hereditable Disorders of Connective Tissue*, 3rd ed., St. Louis: C. V. Mosby Co., 1966, pp. 325–399.

288. Caffey, J.: Gargoylism: Prenatal and postnatal bone lesions and their early postnatal evolution, Amer. J. Roentgen. 67:715, 1952.

289. Belcher, R. W.: Ultrastructure and cytochemistry of lymphocytes in the genetic mucopolysaccharidoses, Arch. Path. 93:1, 1972.

290. Levin, S.: A specific skin lesion in gargoylism, Amer. J. Dis. Child. 99:444, 1960.

291. Craig, W. S.: Gargoylism in a twin brother and sister, Arch. Dis. Child. 29:293, 1954.

292. Robins, M. M., Stevens, H. F., and Linker, A.: Morquio's disease: An abnormality of mucopolysaccharide metabolism, J. Pediat. 62:881, 1963.

293. Renuart, A. W.: Screening for inborn errors of metabolism associated with mental deficiency or neurologic disorders or both, New Eng. J. Med. 274:384, 1966.

294. Langer, L. D., Kronenberg, R. S., and Gorlin, R. J.: A case simulating Hurler's syndrome of unusual longevity without abnormal mucopolysaccharides, Amer. J. Med. 40:448, 1966.

295. Leroy, J. G., et al.: I-Cell disease. Biochemical studies, Pediat. Res. 6:752, 1972.

296. Dekaban, A. S., Holden, K. R., and Constantopoulos, G.: Effects of fresh plasma or whole blood transfusions on patients with various types of mucopolysaccharidosis, Pediatrics 50:688, 1972.

297. Madsen, J. A. and Linker, A.: Vitamin A and mucopolysaccharidosis: A clinical and biochemical evaluation, J. Pediat. 75:843, 1969.

298. Unverricht, H.: *Die Myoklonie*, Leipzig and Vienna: Franz Deuticke, 1891.

299. Harriman, D. G. F. and Millar, J. H. D.: Progressive familial myoclonic epilepsy in three families: Its clinical features and pathological basis, Brain 78:325, 1955.

300. Sakai, M., et al.: Studies in myoclonus epilepsy (Lafora body form): II. Polyglucosans in the systemic deposits of myoclonus epilepsy and in corpora amylacea, Neurology 20:160, 1970.

301. Janeway, R., et al.: Progressive myoclonus epilepsy with Lafora inclusion bodies. I. Clinical genetic, histopathologic and biochemical aspects, Arch. Neurol. 16:565, 1967.

302. Odor, D. L., et al.: Progressive myoclonus epilepsy with Lafora inclusion bodies. II. Studies of ultrastructure, Arch. Neurol. 16:583, 1967.

303. Loeb, H., et al.: Biochemical and ultrastructural studies in a case of mucopolysaccharidosis F (fucosidosis), Helv. Paediat. Acta 24:519, 1969.

304. Durand, P., et al.: Fucosidosis, Lancet 1:1198, 1968.

305. Van Hoof, F. and Hers, H. G.: Mucopolysaccharidosis by absence of alpha-fucosidase, Lancet 1:1198, 1968.

306. Kjellman, B., et al.: Mannosidosis: A clinical and histopathologic study, J. Pediat. 75:366, 1969.

307. Howell, R. R., Ashton, D. M., and Wyngaarden, J. B.: Glucose-6-phosphatase deficiency glycogen storage disease, Pediatrics 29:553, 1962.

308. Childs, B., et al.: Idiopathic hyperglycinemia and hyperglycinuria: A new disorder of amino acid metabolism, Pediatrics 27:522, 1961.

309. Ando, T., et al.: Propionic acidemia in patients with ketotic hyperglycinemia, J. Pediat. 78:827, 1971.

310. Menkes, J. H.: Idiopathic hyperglycinemia: Isolation and identification of three previously undescribed urinary ketones, J. Pediat. 69:413, 1966.

311. Hsia, Y. E., Scully, K. J., and Rosenberg, L. E.: Inherited propionyl-CoA deficiency in "ketotic hyperglycinemia," J. Clin. Invest. 50:127, 1971.

311a. Ando, T., et al.: Isolation and identification of methyl citrate, a major metabolic product of propionate in patients with propionic acidemia, J. Biol. Chem. 247:2200, 1972.

311b. Ando, T., et al.: 3-hydroxypropionate: Significance of β-oxidation of propionate in patients with propionic acidemia and methylmalonic acidemia, Proc. Nat. Acad. Sci. USA 69:2807, 1972.

312. de Vries, A., et al.: Glycinuria: A hereditary disorder associated with nephrolithiasis, Amer. J. Med. 23:408, 1957.

313. Ando, T., et al.: Isovaleric acidemia presenting with altered metabolism of glycine, Pediat. Res. 5:478, 1971.

314. Gerritsen, T., et al.: Metabolism of glyoxylate in nonketotic hyperglycinemia, Pediat. Res. 3:269, 1969.

315. Overholzer, V. G., et al.: Methylmalonic aciduria: Inborn error of metabolism leading to chronic metabolic acidosis, Arch. Dis. Child. 42:492, 1967.

316. Halvorsen, S., Stokke, O., and Eldjarn, L.: Abnormal patterns of urine and serum amino acids in methylmalonic acidemia, Acta Paediat. Scand. 59:28, 1970.

317. Pincus, J. H., et al.: Subacute necrotizing encephalomyelopathy: Effects of thiamine and thiamine propyl disulfide, Arch. Neurol. 24:511, 1971.

318. Mahoney, M. J. and Rosenberg, L. E.: Inherited defects of B12 metabolism, Amer. J. Med. 48:584, 1970.

319. Rosenberg, L. E., Lilljeqvist, A. C., and Hsia, Y. E.: Methylmalonic aciduria, New Eng. J. Med. 278:1319, 1968.

320. Hsia, Y. E., Lilljeqvist, A. C., and Rosenberg, L. E.: Vitamin B12-dependent methylmalonic aciduria: Amino acid toxicity, long chain ketonuria, and protective effect of Vitamin B12, Pediatrics 46:497, 1970.

321. Mahoney, M. T., et al.: Defective metabolism of vitamin B12 in fibroblasts from children with methylmalonic aciduria, Biochem. Biophys. Res. Commun. 44:375, 1971.

321a. Kang, E. S., Snodgrass, P. J., and Gerald, P. S.: Methylmalonic coenzyme A racemase defect. Another cause of methylmalonic aciduria, Pediat. Res. 6:875, 1972.

322. Levy, H. L., et al.: A derangement of B12 metabolism associated with homocystinemia, cystathioninemia, hypomethioninemia and methylmalonic aciduria, Amer. J. Med. 48:390, 1970.

323. Giorgio, A. J. and Plant, G. W. E.: Method for colorimetric determination of urinary methylmalonic acid in pernicious anemia, J. Lab. Clin. Med. 66:667, 1965.

324. Tanaka, K., et al.: Isovaleric acidemia: A new genetic defect of leucine metabolism, Fed. Proc. 25:710, 1966.

325. Budd, M. A., Tanaka, K., and Holmes, L. B.: Isovaleric acidemia, New Eng. J. Med. 277:321, 1967.

326. Tanaka, K., Isselbacher, K. T., and Shih, V.: Isovaleric and α-methyl butyric acidemias induced by hypoglycin A: Mechanism of Jamaican vomiting sickness, Science 175:69, 1972.

327. Hartmann, A. F., Sr., et al.: Lactate metabolism: Studies of a child with a serious congenital deviation, J. Pediat. 61:165, 1962.

328. Israels, S., et al.: Chronic acidosis due to an error in lactate and pyruvate metabolism: Report of 2 cases, Pediatrics 34:346, 1964.

329. Skrede, S., et al.: Fatal congenital lactic acidosis in two siblings: II. Biochemical studies in vivo and in vitro, Acta Paediat. Scand. 60:138, 1971.

330. Lonsdale, D., et al.: Intermittent cerebellar ataxia associated with hyperpyruvic acidemia, hyperalaninemia, and hyperalaninuria, Pediatrics 43:1025, 1969.

331. Blass, J. P., Avigan, J., and Uhlendorf, B. W.: A defect in pyruvate decarboxylase in a child with an intermittent movement disorder, J. Clin. Invest. 49:423, 1970.

332. Blass, J. P., Kark, R. A. P., and Engel, W. K.: Clinical studies of a patient with pyruvate decarboxylase deficiency, Arch. Neurol. 25:449, 1971.

333. Leigh, D.: Subacute necrotizing encephalo-myelopathy in an infant, J. Neurol. Neurosurg. Psychiat. 14:216, 1951.

334. Dayan, A. D., Oegenden, B. G., and Crome, L.: Necrotizing encephalomyelopathy of Leigh: Neuropathological findings in 8 cases, Arch. Dis. Child. 45:39, 1970.

335. Hommes, F. A., Polman, H. A., and Reerink, J. D.: Leigh's encephalomyelopathy: An inborn error of gluconeogenesis, Arch. Dis. Child. 43:423, 1968.

336. Pincus, J. H.: Subacute necrotizing encephalo-myelopathy (Leigh's disease): A consideration of clinical features and etiology, Develop. Med. Child Neurol. 14:87, 1972.

337. Klenk, E.: Beitrage zur Chemie der Lipoido-sen: Niemann-Picksche Krankheit und amauro-tische Idiotie, Ztschr. physiol. Chem. 262:128, 1939.

338. Ledeen, R.: The chemistry of gangliosides: A review, J. Amer. Oil Chem. Soc. 43:57, 1966.

339. Shapiro, D.: *Chemistry of Sphingolipids*, Paris: Hermann, 1969.

340. Tay, W.: Symmetrical changes in the region of the yellow spot in each eye of an infant, Trans. Ophthal. Soc. UK 1:55, 1880–1881.

341. Sachs, B.: On arrested cerebral development, with special reference to its cortical pathology, J. Nerv. Ment. Dis. 15:541, 1887.

342. Terry, R. D. and Weiss, M.: Studies in Tay-Sachs disease: Ultrastructure of cerebrum, J. Neuropath. Exp. Neurol. 22:18, 1963.

343. Svennerholm, L.: The chemical structure of normal human brain and Tay-Sachs ganglio-sides, Biochem. Biophys. Res. Commun. 9:436, 1962.

344. Sastry, P. S. and Stancer, H. C.: Blood gangliosides in infantile amaurotic idiocy, Clin. Chim. Acta 20:487, 1968.

345. Suzuki, K.: Cerebral GM_1 gangliosidosis: Chemical pathology of visceral organs, Science 159:1471, 1968.

346. Korey, S. R. and Stein, A.: Studies in Tay-Sachs disease: Biochemistry, catabolism of gangliosides and related compounds, J. Neuro-path. Exp. Neurol. 22:67, 1963.

347. Suzuki, K. and Chen, G. C.: Brain ceramide hexosides in Tay-Sachs disease and generalized gangliosidosis (GM_1-gangliosidosis), J. Lipid Res. 8:105, 1967.

348. Okada, S. and O'Brien, J. S.: Tay-Sachs disease: Generalized absence of a beta-D-N-acetylhexosaminidase component, Science 165:698, 1969.

349. Sandhoff, K., Andreae, V., and Jatzkewitz, H.: Deficient hexosaminidase activity in an excep-tional case of Tay-Sachs disease with additional storage of kidney globoside in visceral organs, Life Sci. 7:283, 1968.

350. Sandhoff, K., et al.: Enzyme alterations and lipid storage in three variants of Tay-Sachs disease, J. Neurochem. 18:2469, 1971.

351. Suzuki, K., et al.: Juvenile GM_2-ganglio-sidosis: Clinical variant of Tay-Sachs disease or new disease, Neurology 20:190, 1970.

352. Menkes, J. H., et al.: Juvenile GM_2 ganglio-sidosis. Biochemical and ultrastructural studies on a new variant of Tay-Sachs disease, Arch. Neurol. 25:14, 1971.

353. Robinson, D. and Carroll, M.: Tay-Sachs disease—interrelation of hexosaminidases A and B, Lancet 1:322, 1972.

354. Aronson, S. M., et al.: The megaloencephalic phase of infantile amaurotic familial idiocy: Cephalometric and pneumoencephalographic studies, Arch. Neurol. Psychiat. 79:151, 1958.

355. O'Brien, J. S., et al.: Tay-Sachs disease: Detection of heterozygotes and homozygotes by serum hexosaminidase assay, New Eng. J. Med. 283:15, 1970.

356. Norman, R. M., et al.: Tay-Sachs disease with visceral involvement and its relationship to Niemann-Pick disease, J. Path. Bact. 78:409, 1959.

357. O'Brien, J. S., et al.: Generalized ganglio-sidosis: Another inborn error of ganglioside metabolism? Amer. J. Dis. Child., 109:338, 1965.

358. Suzuki, K., Suzuki, K., and Chen, G. C.: Morphological histochemical and biochemical studies on a case of systemic late infantile lipidosis (generalized gangliosidosis), J. Neuropath. Exp. Neurol. 27:15, 1968.

359. MacBrinn, M. C., et al.: Generalized ganglio-sidosis: Impaired cleavage of galactose from a mucopolysaccharide and a glycoprotein, Science 163:946, 1969.

360. Okada, S. and O'Brien, J. S.: Generalized gangliosidosis: Beta-galactosidase deficiency, Science 160:1002, 1968.

361. Suzuki, Y., Crocker, A. C., and Suzuki, K.: GM_1-gangliosidosis: Correlation of clinical and biochemical data, Arch. Neurol. 24:58, 1971.

362. O'Brien, J. S.: "GM_1 Gangliosidoses," in Stanbury, J. B., Wyngaarden, J. B., and Fredrickson, D. S. (eds.): *The Metabolic Basis of Inherited Diseases*, 3rd ed., New York: McGraw-Hill Book Co., 1972, pp. 639–662.

363. Pinsky, L. and Powell, E.: GM_1-gangliosidosis types 1 and 2: Enzymatic differences in cultured fibroblasts, Nature 228:1093, 1971.

364. O'Brien, J. S.: Generalized gangliosidosis, J. Pediat. 75:167, 1969.

365. Wolfe, L. S., et al.: GM_1-gangliosidosis without chondrodystrophy or visceromegaly, Neurology 20:23, 1970.

365a. Lowden, J. A., et al.: Prenatal diagnosis of GM_1-gangliosidosis, New Eng. J. Med. 288:225, 1973.

366. Jervis, G. A., Harris, R. C., and Menkes, J. H.: "Cerebral Lipidosis of Unclear Nature," in Aronson, S. M., and Volk, B. W. (eds.): *Cerebral Sphingolipidoses*, New York: Academic Press, 1962, p. 101.

367. Pilz, H., Sandhoff, K., and Jatzkewitz, H.: Eine Gangliosidstoffwechselstorung mit Anhaufung von Ceramid-Lactosid, Monosialoceramid-Lactosid und Tay-Sachs-Gangliosid im Gehirn, J. Neurochem. 13:1273, 1966.

368. Rosenberg, A.: "The Sphingolipids From the Spleen of a Case of Lipidosis," in Aronson, S. M., and Volk, B. W. (eds.): Cerebral Sphingolipidoses, New York: Academic Press, 1962, p. 119.

369. Dawson, G., Matalon, R., and Stein, A. O.: Lactosylceramidosis: Lactosylceramide galactosyl hydrolase deficiency and accumulation of lactosylceramide in cultured skin fibroblasts, J. Pediat. 79:423, 1971.

370. Gaucher, P.: De l'epithelioma primitif de la rate. These de Paris, 1882.

371. Lee, R. E.: The fine structure of the cerebroside occurring in Gaucher's disease, Proc. Nat. Acad. Sci. USA 61:484, 1968.

372. Banker, B. Q., Miller, J. Q., and Crocker, A. C.: "The Cerebral Pathology of Infantile Gaucher's Disease," in Aronson, S. M., and Volk, B. W. (eds.): Cerebral Sphingolipidoses, New York: Academic Press, 1962, p 73.

373. Lieb, H. and Mladenovic, M.: Cerebrosidspeicherung bei Morbus Gaucher, Ztschr. physiol. Chem. 181:208, 1929.

374. Philippart, M., Rosenstein, B., and Menkes, J. H.: Isolation and characterization of the main splenic glycolipids in the normal organ and in Gaucher's disease: Evidence for the site of metabolic block, J. Neuropath. Exp. Neurol. 24:290, 1965.

375. Brady, R. O., et al.: Demonstration of a deficiency of glucocerebroside-cleaving enzyme in Gaucher's disease, J. Clin. Invest. 45:1112, 1966.

376. Statler, M. and Shapiro, B.: Studies on the etiology of Gaucher's disease: I. Catabolism of glycolipids by rat liver in vivo, Israel J. Med. Sci. 1:514, 1965.

377. Ho, M. W. and O'Brien, J. S.: Gaucher's disease: Deficiency of "acid" β-glucosidase and reconstitution of enzyme activity in vitro, Proc. Nat. Acad. Sci. USA 68:2810, 1971.

378. Philippart, M. and Menkes, J. H.: "Isolation and Characterization of the Principal Cerebral Glycolipids in the Infantile and Adult Forms of Gaucher's Disease," in Aronson, S. M., and Volk, B. W. (eds.): Inborn Errors of Sphingolipid Metabolism, Oxford and New York: Pergamon Press, 1966, pp. 389–400.

379. Rodgers, C. L. and Jackson, S. H.: Acute infantile Gaucher's disease: Case report, Pediatrics 7:53, 1951.

380. Meyer, R.: Syndrome neurologique et diagnostic clinique de la maladie de Gaucher du nourisson, Rev. Franç. Pediat. 8:559, 1932.

381. Crocker, A. C. and Landing, B. H.: Phosphatase studies in Gaucher's disease, Metabolism 9:341, 1960.

382. Hers, H. G. and van Hoof, F.: "Genetic Abnormalities of Lysosomes," in Dingle, J. T. and Fell, H. B. (eds.): Lysosomes in Biology and Pathology, Amsterdam: North Holland Publishing Co., 1969, vol. 2, p. 19.

383. Beutler, E. and Kuhl, W.: Detection of the defect of Gaucher's disease and its carrier state in peripheral blood leucocytes, Lancet 1:612, 1970.

384. Beutler, E., et al.: Detection of Gaucher's disease and its carrier state from fibroblast cultures, Lancet 2:369, 1970.

385. Wise, D., Wallace, H. J., and Jellinek, E. H.: Angiokeratoma corporis diffusum, Quart. J. Med. 31:177, 1962.

386. Rahman, A. N. and Lindenberg, R.: The neuropathology of hereditary dystopic lipidosis, Arch. Neurol. 9:373, 1963.

387. Christensen-Lou, H. O. and Reske-Nielsen, E.: The central nervous system in Fabry's disease. A clinical, pathological, and biochemical investigation, Arch. Neurol. 25:351, 1971.

388. Sweeley, C. C. and Klionsky, B.: Fabry's disease: Classification as a sphingolipidosis, and partial characterization of a novel glycolipid, J. Biol. Chem. 238:3148, 1963.

389. Kint, J. A.: Fabry's disease: Alpha-galactosidase deficiency, Science 167:1268, 1970.

390. Loeb, H., et al.: Etude clinique, biochimique et ultra structurelle de la maladie de Fabry chez l'enfant, Helv. Paediat. Acta 23:269, 1968.

391. Franceschetti, A. T., Philippart, M., and Franceschetti, A.: A study of Fabry's disease: I. Clinical examination of a family with cornea verticillata, Dermatologica 138:209, 1969.

392. Philippart, M., Sarlieve, L., and Manacorda, A.: Urinary glycolipids in Fabry's disease, Pediatrics 43:201, 1969.

393. Kint, J. A.: The enzyme defect in Fabry's disease, Nature 227:1173, 1970.

394. Romeo, G. and Migeon, B. R.: Genetic inactivation of the alpha-galactosidase locus in carriers of Fabry's disease, Science 170:180, 1970.

395. Mapes, C. A., Anderson, R. L., and Sweeley, C. C.: Enzyme replacement in Fabry's disease: An inborn error of metabolism, Science 169:987, 1970.

396. Niemann, A.: Ein unbekanntes Krankheitsbild, Jahrb. Kinderheilk. 79:1, 1914.

397. Crocker, A. C. and Farber, S.: Niemann-Pick disease: A review of 18 patients, Medicine (Baltimore) 37:1, 1958.

398. Ivemark, B. I., et al.: Niemann-Pick disease in infancy: Report of two siblings with clinical, histologic, and chemical studies, Acta Paediat. 52:391, 1963.

399. Philippart, M., et al.: Niemann-Pick disease: Morphologic and biochemical studies in the visceral form with late central nervous system involvement (Crocker's Group C), Arch. Neurol. 20:227, 1969.

400. Thudichum, J. L. W.: A Treatise on the Chemical Constitution of the Brain, Based Throughout Upon Original Researches, London: Bailliere, Tindall and Cox, 1884.

401. Rouser, G., et al.: Accumulation of a glycerol-phospholipid in classical Niemann-Pick disease, Lipids 3:287, 1968.

402. Schneider, P. T. and Kennedy, E. P.: Sphingomyelinase in normal human spleens and in spleens from subjects with Niemann-Pick disease, J. Lipid Res. 8:202, 1967.

403. Kampine, J. P., et al.: Diagnosis of Gaucher's disease and Niemann-Pick disease with small samples of venous blood, Science 155:86, 1967.

404. Sloan, H. R., et al.: Deficiency of sphingomyelin-cleaving enzyme activity in tissue cultures derived from patients with Niemann-Pick disease, Biochem. Biophys. Res. Commun. 34:582, 1969.

405. Fredrickson, D. S. and Sloan, H. R.: "Sphingomyelin Lipidoses: Niemann-Pick Disease," in Stanbury, J. B., Wyngaarden, J. B., and Fredrickson, D. S. (eds.): *The Metabolic Basis of Inherited Disease*, 3rd ed., New York: McGraw-Hill Book Co., 1972, pp. 783–807.

405a. Vethamany, V. G., Welch, J. P., and Vethamany, S. K.: Type D Niemann-Pick disease (Nova Scotia variant), Arch. Path. 93:537, 1972.

406. Nakai, H. and Landing, B. H.: Suggested use of rectal biopsy in the diagnosis of neural lipidoses, Pediatrics 26:225, 1960.

407. Refsum, S., Salomonsen, L., and Skatvedt, M.: Herodopathia atactica polyneuritiformis in children: Preliminary communication, J. Pediat. 35:335, 1949.

408. Richterich, R., van Mechelen, P., and Rossi, E.: Refsum's disease (heredopathia atactica polyneuritiformis): An inborn error of lipid metabolism with storage of 3, 7, 11, 15-tetramethyl hexadecanoic acid, Amer. J. Med. 39:230, 1965.

409. Cammermeyer, J.: Neuropathologic changes in hereditary neuropathies: Manifestation of the syndrome heredopathia atactica polyneuritiformis in the presence of interstitial hypertrophic polyneuropathy, J. Neuropath. Exp. Neurol. 15:340, 1956.

410. Mize, C. E., et al.: Localization of the oxidative defect in phytanic acid degradation in patients with Refsum's disease, J. Clin. Invest. 48:1033, 1969.

411. Steinberg, D., et al.: Phytanic acid in patients with Refsum's syndrome and response to dietary treatment, Arch. Intern. Med. 125:75, 1970.

412. Shy, G. M., Silberberg, D. H., and Appel, S. H.: A generalized disorder of nervous system, skeletal muscle and heart resembling Refsum's disease and Hurler's syndrome, Amer. J. Med. 42:163, 1967.

413. van Bogaert, L., Scherer, H. J., and Epstein, E.: *Une Forme Cerebrale de la Cholesterinose Generalisee*, Paris: Masson & Cie, 1937.

414. Menkes, J. H., Schimschock, J. R., and Swanson, P. D.: Cerebrotendinous xanthomatosis: The storage of cholestanol within the nervous system, Arch. Neurol. 19:47, 1968.

415. Salen, G.: Cholesterol deposition in cerebrotendinous xanthomatosis, Ann. Intern. Med. 75:843, 1971.

416. Schimschock, J. R., Alvord, E. C., and Swanson, P. D.: Cerebrotendinous xanthomatosis: Clinical and pathological studies, Arch. Neurol. 18:688, 1968.

417. Salen, G. and Polito, A.: Biosynthesis of 5α-cholestan-3β-ol in cerebrotendinous xanthomatosis, J. Clin. Invest. 51:134, 1972.

418. Abramov, A., Schorr, S., and Wolman, M.: Generalized xanthomatosis with calcified adrenals, Amer. J. Dis. Child. 91:282, 1956.

419. Eto, Y. and Kitagawa, T.: Wolman's disease with hypolipoproteinemia and acanthocytosis: Clinical and biochemical observations, J. Pediat. 77:862, 1970.

420. Wolman, M.: Involvement of nervous tissue in primary familial xanthomatosis with adrenal calcification, Path. Europ. 3:259, 1968.

421. Lough, J., Fawcett, J., and Weigensberg, B.: Wolman's disease, Arch. Path. 89:103, 1970.

422. Patrick, A. D. and Lake, B. D.: Deficiency of an acid lipase in Wolman's disease, Nature 222:1067, 1969.

423. Farber, S., Cohen, J., and Uzman, L. L.: Lipogranulomatosis: A new lipoglycoprotein "storage" disease, J. Mount Sinai Hosp. NY 24:816, 1957.

424. Abul-Haj, S. K., et al.: Farber's disease: Report of a case with observations on its histogenesis and notes on the nature of the stored material, J. Pediat. 61:221, 1962.

425. Sugita, M., Dulaney, J. T., and Moser, H. W.: Ceramidase deficiency in Farber's disease (lipogranulomatosis), Science 178:1100, 1972.

426. Feigin, I.: Xanthomatosis of nervous system, J. Neuropath. Exp. Neurol. 15:400, 1956.

427. Jervis, G. A.: Degenerative encephalopathy of childhood, J. Neuropath. Exp. Neurol. 16:308, 1957.

428. Jansky, J.: Uber einen noch nicht beschriebenen Fall der familiaren amaurotischen Idiotie mit Hypoplasie des Kleinhirns, Z. Erforsch. Behandl. Jugendlich. Schwachsinns 3:86, 1909 (abst.).

429. Bielschowsky, M.: Uber spatinfantile familiare amaurotische Idiotie mit Kleinhirnsymptomen, Deutsch. Z. Nervenheilk. 50:7, 1914.

430. Batten, F. E.: Family cerebral degeneration with macular change (so-called juvenile form of family amaurotic idiocy), Quart. J. Med. 7:444, 1914.

431. Spielmeyer, W.: Ueber eine besondere Form von familiaerer amaurotischer Idiotie, Neurol. Zbl. 25:51, 1906.

432. Kufs, M., Uber eine Spatform der amaurotischen Idiotie und ihre heredofamiliaren Grundlagen, Z. Ges. Neurol. Psychiat. 95:169, 1925.

433. Copenhaver, R. M. and Goodman, G.: The electroretinogram in infantile, late infantile, and juvenile amaurotic idiocy, Arch. Ophthal. 63:559, 1960.

434. Jervis, G. A.: Juvenile amaurotic idiocy, Amer. J. Dis. Child. 97:663, 1959.
435. Zeman, W. and Donahue, S.: Fine structure of the lipid bodies in juvenile amaurotic idiocy, Acta Neuropath. 3:144, 1963.
435a. Donahue, S., Zeman, W., and Watanabe, I.: "Electron Microscopic Observations in Batten's Disease," in Aronson, S. N. and Volk, B. W.: *Inborn Disorders of Sphingolipid Metabolism*, Oxford, Pergamon Press, 1967, pp. 3–22.
436. Duffy, P. E., Kornfeld, M., and Suzuki, K.: Neurovisceral storage disease with curvilinear bodies, J. Neuropath. Exp. Neurol. 27:351, 1968.
437. Carpenter, S., Karpati, G., and Andermann, F.: Specific involvement of muscle, nerve and skin in late infantile and juvenile amaurotic idiocy, Neurology 22:170, 1972.
438. Tellez-Nagel, I. and Menkes, J. H.: Unpublished studies.
439. Andrews, J. M., et al.: Late infantile neurovisceral disease with curvilinear bodies, Neurology 21:207, 1971.
440. Zeman, W. and Dyken, P.: Neuronal ceroid-lipofuscinosis (Batten's disease): Relationship to amaurotic family idiocy, Pediatrics 44:570, 1969.
441. Ryan, G. B., et al.: Lipofuscin (ceroid) storage disease of the brain: Neuropathological and neurochemical studies, Brain 93:617, 1970.
442. Freud, S.: Ueber familiaere Formen von cerebralen Diplegien, Neurol. Centralbl. 12:512, 542, 1893.
443. Vogt, H.: Ueber familiaere amaurotische Idiotie und verwandte Krankheitsbilder, Monatsschr. Psychiat. Neurol. 18:161, 310, 1905.
444. Odor, D. L., Pearce, L. A., and Janeway, R.: Juvenile amaurotic idiocy: An electron microscopic study, Neurology 16:496, 1966.
445. Kornfeld, M.: Generalized lipofuscinosis (generalized Kuf's disease), J. Neuropath. Exp. Neurol. 31:668, 1972.
446. Elfenbein, I. B.: Dystonic juvenile idiocy without amaurosis, a new syndrome: Light and electron microscopic observations of cerebrum, Johns Hopk. Med. J. 123:205, 1968.
447. Haberland, C. and and Brunngraber, E. G.: Early infantile neurolipidosis with failure of myelination, Arch. Neurol. 23:481, 1970.
448. Bassen, F. A. and Kornzweig, A. L.: Malformation of erythrocytes in cases of atypical retinitis pigmentosa, Blood 5:381, 1950.
449. Schwartz, J. F., et al.: Bassen-Kornzweig syndrome: Deficiency of serum β-lipoprotein, Arch. Neurol. 8:438, 1963.
450. Sobrevilla, L. A., Goodman, M. L., and Kane, C. A.: Demyelinating central nervous system disease, muscular atrophy, and acanthocytosis (Bassen-Kornzweig syndrome), Amer. J. Med. 37:821, 1964.
451. Salt, H. B., et al.: On having no beta-lipoprotein: A syndrome comprising a-beta-lipoproteinaemia, acanthocytosis, and steatorrhoea, Lancet 2:325, 1960.
452. Isselbacher, K. J.: Metabolism and transport of lipid by intestinal mucosa, Fed. Proc. 24:16, 1965.
453. Phillips, G. B. and Dodge, J. T.: Phospholipid and phospholipid fatty acid and aldehyde composition of red cells of patients with abetalipoproteinemia, J. Lab. Clin. Med. 71:629, 1968.
454. Tolentino, P., Spirito, L., and Jannuzzi, C.: Celiac syndrome, retinal dystrophy, acanthocytosis, without defect of beta-lipoprotein, Ann. Paediat. 203:178, 1964.
455. Critchley, E. M. R., Clark, D. B., and Wikler, A.: Acanthocytosis and neurological disorder without beta-lipoproteinemia, Arch. Neurol. 18:134, 1968.
456. Engel, W. K., et al.: Neuropathy in Tangier disease, Arch. Neurol. 17:1, 1967.
457. Kayser, B.: Ueber einen Fall von angeborener grunlicher Verfarbung der Cornea, Klin. Mbl. Augenheilk. 40: II, 22, 1902.
458. Fleischer, B.: Uber eine der "Pseudosklerose" nahestehende bisher unbekannte Krankheit, Deutsch. Z. Nervenheilk. 44:179, 1912.
459. Wilson, S. A. K.: Progressive lenticular degeneration: A familial nervous disease associated with cirrhosis of the liver, Brain 34: 295, 1912.
460. Walshe, J. M.: The physiology of copper in man and its relation to Wilson's disease, Brain 90:149, 1967.
460a. Ryden, L.: Single-chain structure of human ceruloplasmin, Europ. J. Biochem. 26:380, 1972.
461. Porter, H.: Cerebrocuprein I copper in the brain in Wilson's disease, Arch. Neurol. 5:197, 1961.
462. Rumpel, A.: Uber das Wesen und die Bedeutung der Leberveranderungen und der Pigmentierungen bei den damit verbundenen Fällen von Pseudosklerose, zugleich ein Beitrag zur Lehre der Pseudosklerose (Westphal-Strumpell), Deutsch. Z. Nervenheilk. 49:54, 1913.
463. Luthy, F.: Uber die hepato-lentikulare Degeneration (Wilson-Westphal-Strumpell), Deutsch. Z. Nervenheilk. 123:101, 1931.
464. Glazebrook, A. J.: Wilson's disease, Edinburgh Med. J. 52:83, 1945.
465. German, J. L., III and Bearn, A. G.: Effect of estrogens on copper metabolism in Wilson's disease, J. Clin. Invest. 40:445, 1961.
466. Holtzman, N. A., et al.: Ceruloplasmin in Wilson's disease, J. Clin. Invest. 46:993, 1967.
467. Sass-Kortsak, A., et al.: Observations on ceruloplasmin in Wilson's disease, J. Clin. Invest. 38:1672, 1959.
468. Gibbs, K. and Walshe, J. M.: Studies with radioactive copper (^{64}Cu and ^{67}Cu); the incorporation of radioactive copper into caeruloplasmin in Wilson's disease and in primary biliary cirrhosis, Clin. Sci. 41:189, 1971.

HUNTINGTON'S CHOREA

Huntington's chorea is a chronic progressive degenerative disease characterized by choreiform movements, mental deterioration, and an autosomal dominant transmission. Although its essential features were first described by Waters[1] in 1841, Huntington provided its most accurate and graphic description in residents of East Hampton, Long Island.[2]

The incidence of Huntington's chorea in the general population has been estimated as and homovanillic acid concentrations in the caudate nucleus are diminished. γ-Aminobutyric acid (GABA) and homocarnosine are also reduced in the caudate nucleus, as well as in the substantia nigra and putamen.[4c] While these abnormalities may well be secondary to cell death in these regions, they may be responsible for the involuntary movements. These improve when patients are treated with reserpine and alpha-methyl-p-tyrosine, which decrease the concentration of dopamine in the brain. Haloperidol, which blocks dopamine receptors,

469. O'Reilly, A., Pollycove, M., and Bank, W. T.: Iron metabolism in Wilson's disease, Neurology 18:634, 1968.

470. Ragan, H. A., et al.: Effect of ceruloplasmin on plasma iron in copper-deficient swine, Amer. J. Physiol. 217:1320, 1969.

471. Stein, W. H., Bearn, A. G., and Moore, S.: Amino acids in Wilson's disease, J. Clin. Invest. 33:410, 1954.

472. Bearn, A. G., Yü, T. K., and Gutman, A. B.: Renal function in Wilson's disease, J. Clin. Invest. 36:1107, 1957.

473. Porter, H.: Tissue copper proteins in Wilson's disease: Intracellular distribution and chromatographic fractionation, Arch. Neurol. 11:341, 1964.

474. Schaffner, F., et al.: Hepatocellular changes in

489. Sternlieb, I. and Scheinberg, I. H.: Prevention of Wilson's disease in asymptomatic patients, New Eng. J. Med. 278:352, 1968.

490. Catel, W. and Schmidt, J.: Uber familiare gichtische Diathese in Verbindung mit zerebalen und renalen Symptomen bei einen Kleinkind, Deutsch. Med. Wschr. 84:2145, 1959.

491. Lesch, M. and Nyhan, W. L.: A familial disorder of uric acid metabolism and central nervous system function, Amer. J. Med. 36:561, 1964.

492. Hoefnagel, D., et al.: Hereditary choreoathetosis, self-mutilation and hyperuricemia in young males, New Eng. J. Med. 273:130, 1965.

493. Seegmiller, J. E., Rosenbloom, F. M., and

tolenticular degeneration, Arch. Ophthal. 80: 622, 1968.

also improves chorea. Increasing dopamine concentrations, as by the administration of L-dopa, worsens the chorea. Increasing the level of acetylcholine within the brain through the administration of physostigmine, a centrally active anticholinesterase, will improve some of the choreic symptoms. These observations suggest an imbalance of dopamine/acetylcholine within the central nervous system of patients with Huntington's chorea.[5]

The pathologic findings are limited to the brain.[6] Grossly, there is gyral atrophy affecting the frontal lobes most extensively, and generalized and symmetric dilatation of the lateral ventricles. In almost every case the striatum (caudate nucleus and putamen) is markedly shrunken (Fig. 2–1). Under the microscope the principal damage is found in the cortex and basal ganglia, particularly the caudate nucleus and the middle portion of the putamen, although the thalamus, cerebellum, and subthalamic nuclei may also be affected. In both areas there is gross neuronal depletion affecting primarily the small internuncial neurons which show pyknosis and cytoplasmic loss. In the most severely affected areas, the larger neurons are also affected. Astrocytosis can often be striking and tends to be most extensive in the caudate nucleus. The lipofuscin content of cytoplasm is far greater than in control brains of comparable

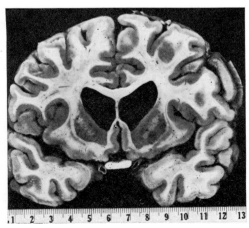

Fig. 2–1. Huntington's chorea. There is gross atrophy of the caudate nucleus giving the lateral ventricles a butterfly appearance. (Courtesy of Dr. J.A.N. Corsellis, The Maudsley Hospital, London.)

age. There is little demyelination except secondary to nerve cell loss. Electron microscopic examination of cortical biopsies shows prominent lipofuscin material, and an increase in the smooth endoplasmic reticulum and Golgi apparatus. Dense degenerating mitochondria with increased granular densities in the matrix, and occasional myelin figures are also seen.[7] Chemical analyses of lipids obtained from the caudate nucleus show a reduction in total lipids and total protein, the outcome of tissue atrophy. A relative increase in the concentration of sphingomyelin probably reflects sparing of myelinated fibers.[8]

Clinical Manifestations

Although the usual onset of symptoms is between 35 and 40 years, about 5 percent of patients are under 14 years of age.[9] Often anticipation is seen in choreic families, implying that the disease develops at an earlier age in children than in their parents. However, when families are examined in whom the onset of the disease is known over the course of three generations, anticipation is no longer seen.

These observations suggest that the spurious phenomenon of anticipation as seen in Huntington's chorea and a number of other heredodegenerative diseases is due to one of five causes:[10]

1. Selection of affected parents in whom the onset of the disease is late.

2. Selection of affected offspring in whom the onset of the disease is early.

3. Selection of families with simultaneous onset of the disease in parents and offspring.

4. Weakness of a real correlation of onset ages in parents and offspring.

5. A general variability in the age of onset.

The clinical picture in children differs from that of adults. In general, it is one of hypokinesia, rigidity, seizures, and mental deterioration.[11] Cases of childhood Huntington's chorea tend to occur in families, and in about 70% of instances the child has received the gene by transmission from his father.[12]

The clinical picture as seen in childhood is summarized in Table 2–1.[11,13]

In children, mental symptoms are the earliest signs. Rigidity, decreased facial ex-

TABLE 2-1.
CLINICAL FEATURES OF HUNTINGTON'S
CHOREA OF CHILDHOOD (28 CASES)*

	Number of Patients
Age of onset	
Less than 5 years	7
5 to 10 years	21
Hyperkinesia or choreo-athetosis	13
Rigidity	19
Seizures	13
Mental deterioration	22
Cerebellar symptoms	5

* Jervis[11] and Markham and Knox.[13]

pression, and reduction of voluntary movements are prominent in the majority and are more common than the choreo-athetosis seen in adult patients.[14,15] The latter movements are similar in character to those observed in Sydenham's chorea but have a greater affinity for the trunk and proximal girdle muscles. They are increased by voluntary physical activity and excitement and cease during sleep. Seizures are rare in adults with Huntington's chorea but affect about 50 percent of children; in some cases it is the most prominent neurologic symptom. They are usually grand mal attacks, although myoclonic attacks have been reported. Cerebellar signs may occasionally be a major feature and include incoordination, ataxia, and intention tremor. Oculomotor apraxia, an abnormality of lateral gaze, can in some cases be striking.[13] Mental deterioration is almost invariable and may be present early in life. The disease progresses rapidly in children, with an average duration in the reported cases of less than eight years.

Laboratory studies are all within normal limits, although the EEG is often abnormal, and the cerebrospinal fluid protein concentration is sometimes elevated. A pneumoencephalogram often shows dilatation of the lateral ventricles, particularly evident in the region of the caudate nucleus.

Diagnosis

Without family history, Huntington's chorea is difficult to differentiate from a variety of other progressive basal ganglia diseases of childhood. These include dystonia musculorum deformans, Hallervorden-Spatz disease, Wilson's disease, and postencephalitic Parkinsonism. When intellectual deterioration and seizures are the chief features, the disease must be differentiated from various gray matter degenerations and lipidoses. Huntington's chorea and Sydenham's chorea differ in the distribution of the choreiform movements. In the former, these principally affect proximal and trunk muscles and are rarely asymmetric, while in the latter they may be asymmetric and involve the distal parts of the extremities. Benign nonprogressive familial chorea, also transmitted as a dominant trait, is unassociated with seizures or intellectual deterioration. It begins during the first two decades and continues unchanged throughout life.[16]

Treatment

There is no effective treatment. Reserpine and phenothiazines may alleviate the choreiform movements but are ineffective against the mental deterioration. Anti-Parkinsonian drugs may provide temporary benefit in the rigid form of the disease.

DYSTONIA MUSCULORUM DEFORMANS

This progressive extrapyramidal disorder, characterized by slow spasmodic twisting and turning of the spine and limbs, was first described by Schwalbe in 1908[17] as a variant of hysteria. Although in the past, cases of dystonia musculorum deformans were thought of as Wilson's disease or as the consequence of perinatal trauma, there is now no doubt that this disease represents as many as two genetic entities, with autosomal recessive and dominant forms of inheritance.[18]

Pathology

The pathologic alterations are limited to the nervous system. They are scanty and in many instances have not been clearly distinguished from agonal changes due to anoxia or terminal infections.[19] Most commonly there is gross atrophy of the caudate nuclei, and microscopically the number of large ganglion cells in this area and in the putamen and dentate nuclei is reduced.

iron metabolism has been demonstrated, and no treatment is available.

FAMILIAL CALCIFICATION OF BASAL GANGLIA (FAHR'S DISEASE)

This condition, first described by Fahr in 1930, is characterized by the deposition of large quantities of calcium within the walls of the cerebral blood vessels, particularly those of the lenticular and dentate nuclei (Fig. 2–3). The disease is transmitted as an autosomal dominant disorder.

Symptoms appear early in life and include mental deterioration, convulsions, and generalized rigidity. The calcifications within the basal ganglia are visible upon radiographic examination; they may even be present in asymptomatic cases.[33] A normal blood calcium and phosphorus level distinguishes this condition from the cerebral calcifications due to hypoparathyroidism. Pseudohypoparathyroidism may also result in the cerebral deposition of calcium but the presence of long-bone changes and a failure in urinary

$3',5'$-AMP response to parathormone serves to distinguish the former from Fahr's disease.[34,35]

HEREDITARY TREMOR

This common but benign familial degenerative process is transmitted as an autosomal dominant with a tendency for anticipation in successive generations. Symptoms usually become evident around puberty although patients five years or younger have been observed.

The tremor is rhythmic, with a variable oscillation. It increases with movement, is present with the limb at rest but disappears with sleep. It initially affects one or both of the upper extremities but usually does not interfere with fine coordination. With progression there may be head nodding. The lower extremities are unaffected and intelligence, speech, gait, and strength remain normal.[36]

While the disease is progressive during its early stages, it becomes arrested during much

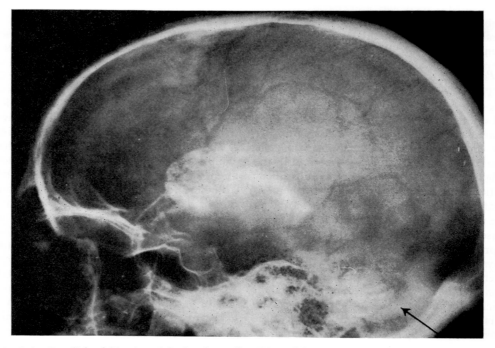

Fig. 2–3. Familial calcification of the basal ganglia. The calcifications include the head and part of the tail of the caudate nucleus. Arrow indicates calcification of the dentate nucleus. (Courtesy of Dr. M. A. Moskowitz, Boston Children's Hospital.)

of adult life and interferes little with the patient's daily activity. However, in later life the condition may suddenly become aggravated, and "senile tremor" may be a late manifestation of essential tremor.

The pathology of essential tremor has not been studied, although similarity of this condition to the tremor associated with midbrain lesions suggests an abnormality of the red nucleus or its projections.[37]

The diagnosis of essential tremor rests on the exclusion of other disorders of the basal ganglia, particularly dystonia musculorum deformans, which may present as a tremor in the dominant variant, Wilson's disease, and Huntington's chorea. A family history of the disorder or, preferably, examination of the parents and other family members is helpful.

Treatment

No treatment is available for this condition.

JUVENILE PARALYSIS AGITANS

In 1917 Hunt described four unrelated adolescent patients with a rapidly progressive degenerative disease manifested by tremor and rigidity.[38] Autopsy on one of them revealed severe atrophy of the large neurons within the globus pallidus and, to a lesser degree, in the caudate nucleus and putamen.[39] Although sporadic and familial cases of "juvenile paralysis agitans" have since been recorded,[40] it is uncertain whether this condition is distinct from atypical Wilson's disease, Huntington's chorea, or postencephalitic Parkinsonism.

HEREDODEGENERATIVE DISEASES OF THE CEREBELLUM, BRAIN STEM, AND SPINAL CORD

All these diseases involve a slow, progressive deterioration of one or more of the functions subserved by the cerebellum, brain stem, or spinal cord, due to a neuronal atrophy within the affected tract or tracts, commencing at the axonal periphery and advancing in a centripetal manner. The usual pattern is one of a markedly familial distribution. Within each family unit, the disease picture tends to be stereotyped and can usually be assigned to one of the clinical and pathologic entities. Yet several factors prevent a complete classification of these heredodegenerative processes. One is the commonly observed presence in affected families of stigmata such as mental deficiency, deafmutism, and retinitis pigmentosa, which may appear singly or in association with the degenerative disease. Another is the existence of atypical families in some of whom a hybrid disease pattern may be found, while in others two or even more clinical entities may flourish side by side. The cause of these illnesses is completely unknown and speculatively is attributed to enzymatic defects with variable modes of expression.

FRIEDREICH'S ATAXIA (SPINOCEREBELLAR ATAXIA)

The most common of the heredodegenerative conditions, this was first distinguished from syphilitic locomotor ataxia by Friedreich in 1863.[41] Characterized by ataxia, nystagmus, kyphoscoliosis, and pes cavus, it is distributed among all racial and national entities, either as an autosomal recessive or as an autosomal dominant trait, which affects both sexes equally. The recessive disease has its onset between 11 and 12 years of age, and is ten times as frequent as the dominant form. Consanguinity is present in 18 percent of affected families.[42] The dominant form has its onset between 18 and 22 years of age.[42]

Pathology

The cause of Friedreich's ataxia is unknown. Determination of serum enzymes, urinary and serum amino acids, and excretion of tryptophan metabolites have revealed no significant or consistent abnormalities. Hyperinsulinism has been found in a large proportion of nonobese patients with Friedreich's ataxia, even in the absence of overt diabetes.[43] The significance of this interesting observation is still obscure. In a patient with the recently described late form of necrotizing encephalopathy and hyperalaninemia, possibly due to a defect in pyruvate metabolism, the clinical features were suggestive but hardly typical of Friedreich's ataxia.[44]

The essential pathologic process in Friedreich's ataxia as well as in the other cerebellar degenerations, is a dying back of neurons in

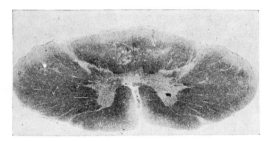

Fig. 2–4. Friedreich's ataxia. Section of spinal cord stained for myelin. The area of myelination involves the posterior columns, and the lateral and ventral spinocerebellar tracts. The corticospinal tracts are relatively spared, although demyelination is more extensive than would be expected from the clinical picture at the time of demise. (Courtesy of Dr. K. E. Earle, Armed Forces Institute of Pathology, Washington, D.C.)

certain systems from the periphery to the center with eventual disappearance of the cell body.[45] The principal cerebral lesions are found in the long ascending and descending tracts[46] (Table 2–2) (Fig. 2–4). The peripheral nerves may also be affected, as well as the brain stem and less often the cerebellum. In all these areas there is axonal degeneration, demyelination, and a compensatory gliosis. Degenerative cellular changes are most striking in Clark's column, and to a lesser extent in a variety of nuclei of the lower

brain stem and in the Purkinje cells. Other areas of gray matter are usually unaffected. A reduction in glycolytic enzymes and an increase in oxidative and hydrolytic enzymes have been found on histochemical examination of the posterior columns of the spinal cord. Aside from the expected loss of proteolipids that accompanies demyelination, no lipid abnormalities have been documented in affected tracts.[47,48]

Examination of the viscera frequently reveals cardiomegaly and the presence of myocarditis.

Clinical Manifestations

In most families the onset of the disease occurs at the same period of life without evidence for anticipation. The recessive and dominant forms show similar clinical manifestations. These are outlined in Table 2–3. Children may be slow in learning to walk, or may begin to stumble frequently. Less commonly, abnormal speech or incoordination of hand movements are the initial complaints.

Neurologic symptoms advance relentlessly. While in a few children the disease evolves rapidly, progression is slow in the vast majority, and occasionally there are long stationary periods. Intercurrent infections fre-

TABLE 2-2.
STRUCTURES INVOLVED IN VARIOUS TYPES OF CEREBELLAR DEGENERATIONS*

Site of Pathologic Changes	Friedreich's Ataxia	Olivopontocerebellar Degeneration	Menzel's Cerebellar Ataxia (Cerebellipetal)	Holmes's Cerebellar Ataxia (Cerebellifugal)
Cerebellar afferents:				
In brain stem	0	4+	4+	1+
In spinal cord	4+	0	4+	0
Intracerebellar fibers	0	2+	2+	4+
Cerebellar efferents	0	0	1+	2+
Other structures: cranial nerve nuclei, basal ganglia, cerebral cortex, corticospinal tract, anterior horn cells, dorsal, ventral roots	2+	0	2+	0

* Adapted from Locke and Foley.[46]

TABLE 2-3.
FREQUENCY OF NEUROLOGIC SYMPTOMS
IN 74 PATIENTS
WITH FRIEDREICH'S ATAXIA[49]

Symptom	Percent Incidence
Truncal ataxia	100
Positive Romberg	95
Dysmetria of upper extremities	89
Disturbed speech	84
Deformities of feet	82
Impaired deep sensations	81
Absent ankle reflexes	80
Deformities of spine	77
Nystagmus	76
Absent patellar reflexes	76
Weakness of extremities	72
Ataxia of lower extremities	70
Extensor plantar reflexes	66
Muscle atrophy	64

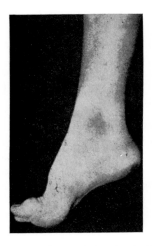

Fig. 2–5. Typical foot deformity in Friedreich's ataxia. (From Ford, F. R.: *Diseases of the Nervous System in Infancy, Childhood and Adolescence,* 5th ed., 1966, courtesy of Charles C Thomas Publisher, Springfield.)

quently aggravate existing symptoms, and bring new ones to light. The patient with fully developed Friedreich's ataxia has an immature, dysmorphic appearance. There are a number of skeletal deformities, some of which may even stem from birth. In about three-quarters of the patients, the feet have a high arch (pes cavus), hammer toes, and wasting of the small muscles of the sole (Fig. 2–5). In patients who have this abnormality at birth, it may for many years represent the only sign of Friedreich's ataxia. Kyphoscoliosis is present in about 80 percent of subjects.[49]

The most prominent sign, however, is ataxia. As might be expected from the pathologic lesions, this is due to a combination of cerebellar asynergia and loss of posterior column sensation. Ataxia is usually more marked in the legs than in the arms and is most evident when the child's gait or station is examined. Speech is also involved and acquires a staccato or explosive character— the result of an incoordination of respiration and phonation. Nystagmus is seen in more than half the cases. It is usually bilateral, and present only on lateral movements of the eyes. Nystagmus on upward gaze is rare.[45] Sjögren saw optic atrophy in 12 percent of patients.[49] This may be congenital, or have its onset during early infancy, progressing

rapidly after its inception. Occasionally there is also pigmentary retinal degeneration.[50] Vestibular involvement, including loss of caloric reactions and attacks of vertigo, were already described by Friedreich[41] and often appear early.

Weakness of the distal musculature of the lower limbs and wasting of the small muscles of the hands and feet are common and are out of proportion to the degree of disuse. There is a loss of vibratory and proprioceptive sensation, and in the advanced cases, the other sensory modalities are also likely to be affected, notably in the distal portions of the extremities.[45] Pains, cramps, and paresthesias are common. The knee and ankle reflexes are usually absent, and in two-thirds of patients the plantar responses are extensor. Bladder and bowel control is not infrequently impaired, even as an early symptom. Mental deficiency or deterioration occurs in more than one-half of patients, especially in the recessive form. It may be seen in subjects unaffected by ataxia. Electrocardiographic evidence of myocarditis has been found in as many as 90 percent of patients, and T-wave abnormalities and congenital heart block are particularly common.[51,52] An unusually high incidence of diabetes (23%) has been recorded in both forms of spinocerebellar degeneration.[52]

The patient with an advanced case of Friedreich's ataxia is bedridden, with dysphagia and other bulbar signs. Death is due to inanition, or myocarditis with intractable congestive failure.

Diagnosis

In the typical patient the diagnosis rests upon the presence of progressive ataxia and skeletal deformities in conjunction with a positive family history of a similar condition, or the skeletal stigmata. Ataxia-telangiectasia (Chapter 10) is the second most common cause for progressive ataxia commencing in childhood. It is distinguished by the presence of cutaneous telangiectases, a history of frequent serious respiratory infections, absent or marked reduction of IgA globulins, and a lack of skeletal deformities and sensory signs. Atypical cases existing within the same family as patients with the classic form of spino-

cerebellar ataxia are not rare. These possess only a fragment of the clinical picture, such as the pes cavus, scoliosis, mental retardation, optic atrophy, deafness, or merely absent deep tendon reflexes in the legs.

Cases intermediate between Friedreich's ataxia and the other heredodegenerative conditions have been described. These syndromes are depicted in Figure 2–6. Most common is mixed spinocerebellar degeneration and peroneal muscular atrophy (Lévy-Roussy syndrome), and spinocerebellar disease with progressive spastic paraplegia, also termed spastic ataxia.

All laboratory studies except the electrocardiogram have been normal.

Treatment

Children with spinocerebellar ataxia should remain active for as long as possible and participate in physical therapy and programmed remedial exercises. Orthopedic surgery for skeletal deformities is contraindicated, for

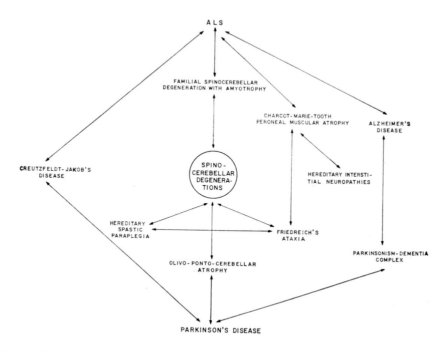

Fig. 2–6. Schematic outline of the relationships in the continuum of degenerative disorders of the nervous system. (ALS—Amyotrophic lateral sclerosis.) (From Cooke, R. E.: *The Biologic Basis of Pediatric Practice*, 1968, courtesy of McGraw-Hill Book Co., New York, and Dr. N. C. Myrianthopolus, National Institutes of Health, Bethesda, Maryland.)

postoperative immobilization will aggravate existing symptoms.

OLIVOPONTOCEREBELLAR ATROPHY

This rare condition, first delineated by Dejerine and Thomas in 1900,[53] is manifested by progressive cerebellar ataxia, Parkinsonian-like rigidity, resting tremor, and impairment of speech. Both autosomal recessive and dominant transmissions have been reported.

Pathologically there is loss of neurons in the cerebellar cortex, basis pontis, and inferior olivary nucleus.[49] In contrast to Friedreich's ataxia there are no spinal cord abnormalities (Table 2–2).

While the disease usually begins in adult life,[54] a dominant form with associated retinal degeneration may develop neurologic symptoms, usually ataxia of gait and visual impairment, as early as the first year.[55]

HEREDITARY CEREBELLAR ATAXIA

Familial degeneration of the cerebellum with the onset of symptoms during childhood is extremely rare, and in families like those first described by Menzel,[56] and Holmes,[57] onset is only rarely as early as adolescence. Exceptions were described by Norman[58] and Jervis,[59] in which cerebellar ataxia, hypotonia, nystagmus, and mental deficiency were evident during infancy. A small posterior fossa was seen on radiologic examination. The main pathologic finding was atrophy of the granular cell layer of the cerebellum. Progression was slow, and one suspects a familial congenital defect of the nervous system, rather than true heredodegeneration.

A number of forms of cerebellar degenerations are seen during adult life. In all the Purkinje cells bear the brunt. A cerebel-lipetal atrophy, that is involvement of afferent tracts from the spinal cord and the brain stem to the cerebellum, also known as Menzel's cerebellar ataxia,[56] is characterized by the appearance of unsteady gait and dysarthria during the second to sixth decade.[46,49] Pathologic changes involve the pons, brachium pontis, olivary nuclei, and cerebellum (Table 2–2). In the type of cerebellar degeneration described by Gordon Holmes[57] (cerebello-olivary degeneration), the clinical picture is identical, but the atrophic changes are centered on the cerebellum, and to a lesser extent on the efferent tracts and the olivary nuclei (Table 2–2).

In the child with progressive ataxia the differential diagnosis depends on the rapidity with which the symptoms have appeared. When they are of short duration, the ataxia is most likely to be of neoplastic, toxic, or infectious nature. If the ataxia is slowly progressive, posterior fossa tumors must be excluded. Structural anomalies of the upper cervical spine and foramen magnum, as for instance platybasia, may present with ataxia, as does hydrocephalus due to partial obstruction at the aqueduct of Sylvius (Chapter 4). The lipidoses, particularly the group of late infantile amaurotic idiocies, may present a primarily cerebellar picture (Chapter 1). Of the familial cerebellar degenerations, Friedreich's ataxia and ataxia-telangiectasia are the most common. A rare condition which is manifested by cerebellar ataxia, mental deficiency, cataracts, impaired physical growth, and various skeletal anomalies has been described by Sjögren, Marinesco, Garland[60,61] and others. Refsum's disease, or heredopathia atactica polyneuritiformis, is characterized by cerebellar ataxia, deafness, retinitis pigmentosa, and polyneuritis. It is produced by a defect in the oxidation of branched-chain fatty acids (Chapter 1). A sex-linked, progressive cerebellar ataxia associated with myoclonic epilepsy and extra-pyramidal signs has been reported by Malamud and Cohen.[62] Finally, sporadic cerebellar degenerations of childhood may also be due to toxins such as lead or organic mercury compounds.[63]

DENTATORUBRAL ATROPHY (RAMSAY HUNT SYNDROME)

This was first described by J. Ramsay Hunt in 1921 in a family presenting with myoclonus epilepsy and cerebellar ataxia.[64] Autopsy showed well-marked degeneration of the spinocerebellar tracts, atrophy of the dentate nucleus, and pallor of the superior cerebellar peduncle, including the dentatorubral tract. The Ramsay Hunt syndrome probably represents a heterogeneous group of patients. Many patients with myoclonus epilepsy from a variety of causes appear to have cerebellar ataxia. In some this is clearly the result of severe rhythmic myoclonus exaggerated by the proprioceptive stimulation of voluntary movements. In Ramsay Hunt syndrome mental functions deteriorate slowly or not at all. In this respect the condition is distinct from Unverricht's myoclonus epilepsy characterized by myoclonic seizures and mental deterioration. In this disorder there is an accumulation of polyglucosan-containing amyloid bodies throughout the nervous system (Chapter 1). Myoclonic seizures, ataxia and mental deterioration are also seen in the lipidoses, particularly the late infantile amaurotic idiocies, and in Huntington's chorea.

FAMILIAL SPASTIC PARAPLEGIA

Characterized by progressive spastic paraplegia, and first described by Seeligmüller in 1876,[65] this exhibits a variable mode of inheritance, and families have been reported in whom the condition is transmitted in dominant, sex-linked, and most commonly, autosomal recessive manner.[42]

Pathology

The major changes are in the spinal cord. Here there is always degeneration of the pyramidal tracts, most evident below the cervical level. Other tracts may also be involved, in particular the posterior columns and the spinocerebellar fibers, and the cells of the dorsal root ganglion which may degenerate and show satellitosis.[66] In affected tracts the myelin sheath is lost, and the axis cylinder disappears.

Clinical Manifestations

In the recessive variant of familial spastic paraplegia the average age of onset of symptoms is 11.5 years; in the dominant form it is 18.5 years.[42] Children may be slow in learning to walk, and then their gait is stiff and awkward, and the legs are scissored. Muscle tone is increased, the deep tendon reflexes are hyperactive, and the plantar responses are extensor. There is no muscular atrophy, and despite the pathologic involvement of the posterior columns, usually no impairment of position or vibratory sensation. Bladder and bowel control is retained during the early stages of the illness. The disease progresses slowly. Often the upper extremities remain virtually unaffected and are only involved terminally. In some families wasting of the small muscles of the hand and the lower legs accompanies the spasticity.[67,68] In other kinships, ataxia, nystagmus, and dysarthria are present, and the mixture of spinocerebellar degeneration and familial spastic paraplegia (Fig. 2–6) has been termed spastic ataxia. Extrapyramidal signs, mental retardation, and optic atrophy accompany spastic paraplegia in yet other families.[69] In some pedigrees blindness is particularly common.

Diagnosis

In the absence of a family history, the diagnosis of familial spastic paraplegia is one of exclusion. Progression of symptoms speaks against spastic diplegia of perinatal origin (Chapter 5). Neither sensory deficits nor sphincter disturbances, which usually accompany spinal cord tumors, are seen in the patient with familial spastic paraplegia. Nevertheless, in the absence of a convincing family history, a lumbar myelogram is required to exclude a spinal cord neoplasm.

Treatment

In view of the slow progression of symptoms an active physiotherapy program should be designed. Orthopedic surgery, unless essential to relieve contractures, should be discouraged.

FAMILIAL AMYOTROPHIC LATERAL SCLEROSIS

This rare condition, sometimes termed Fazio-Londe disease, is probably heterogeneous and distinct from Werdnig-Hoffmann disease (Chapter 12) and from amyotrophic lateral sclerosis—the latter a sporadic degeneration of the anterior horn cells and pyramidal fibers confined to adult life.

The clinical picture reflects a progressive deterioration of the anterior horn cells, particularly those of the bulbar musculature and of the pyramidal tracts. Symptoms begin at a variable age; in the family we have encountered symptoms began during early childhood. They progress fairly rapidly and lead to death within about a decade.[70,71,72]

In some patients the degree of pyramidal tract involvement is minimal and may be limited to extensor plantar responses; the clinical picture is therefore essentially that of the late appearing form of Werdnig-Hoffmann disease.[73] In other families, clinical or pathologic evidence of posterior column deficit relates this particular form of heredodegenerative disease to the spinocerebellar group.[74] When anterior horn cell involvement is exclusively distal, is accompanied by significant spasticity, and progression is slow, the condition can be related to familial spastic paraplegia.[67,68] This variant may be transmitted as a recessive or dominant trait.

In a few families, progressive degeneration of the anterior horn cells and pyramidal tracts appears after the age of twenty. This includes a large series of cases among the Chamorro tribe of Guam and is frequently associated with Parkinsonism and dementia. A slow virus infection has been documented in the latter group of patients.[75]

In diagnosis, tumors of the brain stem must be excluded. When pyramidal tract signs are not striking, myasthenia gravis or an ocular muscle dystrophy should be excluded.

Treatment

There is no treatment.

CHARCOT-MARIE-TOOTH DISEASE (PERONEAL MUSCULAR ATROPHY)

Virchow[76] in 1855, and subsequently in 1886 Charcot and Marie[77] working in France and Tooth[78] in England described this familial degenerative disease as a peroneal type of progressive muscular atrophy. It is relatively common and exhibits every type of inheritance, most often an autosomal dominant.[79]

Pathology

Only a few postmortem examinations are available and the pathogenesis is unknown. As a rule degenerative lesions are found in the peripheral nerves, the ventral roots, and the anterior horn cells. Analogous changes on the afferent limb of the spinal cord are almost as common, and involve atrophy of the dorsal roots, diminution of neurons in the dorsal root ganglia, and atrophy of the posterior columns. Within the peripheral nerves fiber reduction is particularly prominent in the muscular branches, and there is an excess of interstitial connective tissue, probably secondary to the fiber loss. Degenerative changes in skeletal muscles are secondary to damage of the peripheral nerves.

Clinical Manifestations

Symptoms develop between five and twenty years, with earlier onset in the recessive form. Generally, the peroneal muscles are involved first, and a slapping storklike gait may bring the child to his physician. In the upper extremities weakness and atrophy are at first limited to the small muscles of the hand but later spread to the forearm. The face, trunk, and proximal musculature is usually spared.

In the fully developed condition examination reveals a marked club foot or pes cavus deformity,[80] and contractures of the wrist and fingers which have produced a claw hand. There is striking atrophy and weakness of the distal musculature, which contrasts with the preservation of the bulk and strength of the proximal parts. Sensation, particularly vibratory and position sense, is reduced over the distal portions of the extremities. Vasomotor signs are common and include flushing and cyanosis or marbling of the skin. The ankle reflexes are generally lost; other deep tendon reflexes are preserved. The plantar responses may be difficult to elicit. Some authors have considered thickened peripheral nerves to be characteristic.[79]

The classic case lacks cerebellar signs, nystagmus, or deformities of the spine.

Progression of the disease is slow, and spontaneous arrests are common. The cerebrospinal fluid protein level is occasionally elevated but there are no other abnormalities. Peripheral conduction velocities, such as in the ulnar, median, and peroneal nerves, are almost always diminished. Low conduction velocities may be recorded prior to any clinical manifestations, or in nerves such as the facial, which remain uninvolved.[81]

Diagnosis

The diagnosis of Charcot-Marie-Tooth disease is made on the basis of familial incidence, the characteristic distal distribution of the slowly progressive muscular wasting and weakness, and the reduced peripheral nerve conduction velocities. The sensory deficits distinguish this disease from the slowly progressive distal myopathies.

A number of clinical variants of Charcot-Marie-Tooth disease have been described which link this condition to hereditary interstitial neuropathy and Friedreich's ataxia.

In the more severe cases of peroneal muscular atrophy the distal portions of the peripheral nerves may be thickened to palpation. In part this reflects an increase in interstitial tissue of the peripheral nerves, in part muscular atrophy permits easier palpation of nerves. This clinical form merges with hypertrophic interstitial neuritis (Dejerine-Sottas) where early nerve enlargement may only involve the more proximal portions and is less apparent distally. Pupillary abnormalities, a common finding in Dejerine-Sottas disease, are not seen in peroneal muscular atrophy.

A syndrome, clinically intermediate between peroneal muscular atrophy and Friedreich's ataxia, was described by Roussy and Lévy,[82] and Symonds and Shaw in 1926.[83] It is characterized by a clumsy gait, atrophy of the peroneal and hand muscles, impairment of vibratory sensibility, and a tremor of the hands. Characteristic cerebellar signs or nystagmus are absent. The disease progresses slowly if at all. Conduction velocities in the peripheral nerves are reduced, and Yudell et al. have suggested that Lévy-Roussy syndrome is identical to Charcot-Marie-Tooth disease with superimposed familial essential tremor, both dominant traits.[84] However, families with some members having well-defined Charcot-Marie-Tooth disease and others showing a clinical picture akin to Friedreich's ataxia have been encountered.[85,86]

Treatment

Aside from orthopedic measures designed to prevent the disabling deformities, no specific therapy is available.

HEREDODEGENERATIVE DISEASES OF THE PERIPHERAL AND CRANIAL NERVES

HYPERTROPHIC INTERSTITIAL NEURITIS

This rare familial progressive disorder was first described by Dejerine and Sottas in 1893.[87] A dominant trait with variable penetrance, it is characterized by a progressive picture of a chronic peripheral and sensory neuropathy with firm enlarged nerves.

Pathology

Different disease entities produce a pathologic and clinical picture of hypertrophic interstitial neuritis, with the underlying disorder in each of them affecting primarily the Schwann cell or the axon itself. Refsum's disease, a recessive disorder due to impaired metabolism of phytanic acid (Chapter 1), may present a similar pathologic picture.

Pathologically there is gross enlargement of the proximal portions of the peripheral nerves, the plexi, and the roots, with lesser involvement of the distal peripheral nerves and the cranial nerves. This results from proliferation of the sheath of Schwann and endoneurium, and an increase in collagen around the individual fibers. Because of their appearance on transverse section, the concentric lamellae surrounding the nerve fibers were first termed "onion bulbs" by Dejerine and Sottas.[87,88,89] On electron microscopy these can be shown to contain only Schwann cells and their processes, and probably reflect a nonspecific regenerative response of the Schwann cells to axonal loss.[89] Demyelination is segmental or complete, and there may be axonal degeneration. Biochemical changes in the peripheral nerves are compatible with an active peripheral demyelinating process, such as has been produced in experimental Wallerian degeneration.[90] Within the central nervous system, the degenerative changes are in keeping with the loss of peripheral nerves.

Clinical Manifestations

The condition appears insidiously during late childhood or adolescence, often as a disturbance in gait or weakness of the hands. As the disease progresses, distal weakness and atrophy become evident. Distal sensory impairment is usual and tends particularly to affect vibration. Pupillary abnormalities are seen in about 25 percent of patients[88] and include a progressively impaired reaction to light. There was nystagmus in Dejerine's original family[87] and slurred speech also occurs. Kyphoscoliosis or foot deformities are seen in over one-third of patients. The feature of hypertrophic interstitial neuritis, which gives the condition its name, is a diffuse and uniform enlargement of many of the superficial nerves, which become firm to palpation.

In most instances symptoms progress slowly and the disease may not reduce the average life span.

Laboratory findings include an occasional elevated CSF protein content and abnormal nerve conduction times.[91] Electromyography shows widespread evidence of peripheral denervation, with frequent fibrillation potentials at rest.

Diagnosis

The diagnosis of Dejerine-Sottas disease should be considered in any chronic progressive peripheral neuropathy of childhood.[92] Enlargement of nerves must be distinguished from nerves made easily visible by muscular atrophy. Other conditions that produce chronic polyneuropathy are metachromatic leukodystrophy, Refsum's disease, and chronic polyneuropathy secondary to nonspecific infections. In the latter, family history is negative, while both metachromatic leukodystrophy and Refsum's disease are transmitted as a recessive trait, contrasting with the usual dominant transmission of Dejerine-Sottas disease. The presence of "onion bulbs" on biopsy of peripheral nerves is not specific for this condition but reflects the chronicity of the polyneuritis.

Clinical forms intermediate between hypertrophic interstitial neuritis and Charcot-Marie-Tooth disease have been reported.

Treatment

Aside from orthopedic measures, and consistent, active physiotherapy, there is no specific treatment. Steroids have been ineffective.

HEREDITARY SENSORY NEUROPATHY

This is a rare entity with dominant transmission, characterized by a sensory deficit in the distal portion of the lower extremities, chronic perforating ulcerations of the feet, and progressive destruction of the underlying bones. It may be identical with familial lumbosacral syringomyelia. There is degeneration of the dorsal root ganglia and the dorsal roots[93] of the spinal cord segments supplying the lower limbs.

Symptoms appear in late childhood, or early adolescence, although onset has been

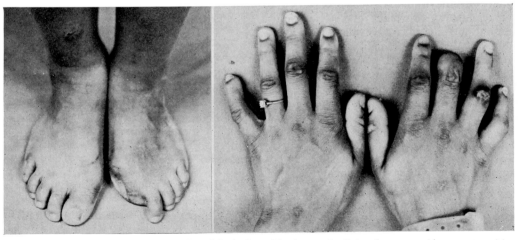

Fig. 2–7. Hereditary sensory neuropathy. Marked trophic changes in digits of upper and lower extremities. (Courtesy of Dr. K. E. Astrom, Massachusetts General Hospital, Boston.)

myelin sheaths are lacking in the mesencephalic roots of the trigeminal nerve. These changes are slowly progressive, without neuronophagia or evidence of myelin breakdown.

The primary enzymatic lesion is unknown. Smith, Taylor, and Wortis[111] have demonstrated an abnormality in catecholamine metabolism, which could, in part, explain the clinical picture. The excretion of vanillylmandelic acid (VMA) is generally decreased, and that of homovanillic acid increased.[112] These alterations are often slight and inconsistent.[113] At best, there is considerable overlap in the pattern of catecholamine excretion of normal and dysautonomic children.[114] While synthesis of norepinephrine and VMA from dihydroxyphenylalanine (L-dopa) is normal in the disease, norepinephrine turnover is unusually rapid.[115] This suggests a normal rate of norepinephrine production, but reduced norepinephrine stores. These findings may reflect depletion of functioning adrenergic neurons, rather than the essential defect.

Clinical Manifestations

Familial dysautonomia is characterized by symptoms referable to the autonomic nervous system. No single feature but rather their association points to the diagnosis.

Usually nervous system dysfunction is evident from birth as decreased muscle tone, poor cry, and a poor Moro reflex. Nursing difficulties result in frequent regurgitation.[116] Retarded physical development, poor temperature control, and motor incoordination become prominent during early childhood, and subsequently other clinical features are detected, as outlined in Table 2–4.[117] These include inability to produce overflow tears with the usual stimuli, absent or hypoactive deep tendon reflexes, absent corneal reflexes, postural hypotension, relative indifference to pain, and absence of the fungiform papillae on the tongue,[118,119] in association with a marked diminution in taste sensation. Many patients have serious feeding difficulties, including cyclic vomiting and recurrent pneumonia. In part these may be attributed to absent or decreased lower esophageal peristalsis, a dilated esophagus, and impaired gastric

TABLE 2-4.
CLINICAL FEATURES OF
FAMILIAL DYSAUTONOMIA

Disturbances of Autonomic Nervous System:

Reduced or absent tears	+++
Peripheral vascular disturbances	
Hypertension with excitement	++
Postural hypotension	+++
Skin blotching with excitement or with eating	++
Cold hands and feet	+++
Excessive perspiration	+++
Erratic temperature control	++
Disturbed swallowing reflex	+++
Drooling beyond usual age	++
Cyclic vomiting	++

Disturbances of Voluntary Neuromuscular System:

Absent or hypoactive deep tendon reflexes	+++
Poor motor coordination	+++
Dysarthria	+++
Convulsions	+
Abnormal EEG	++

Sensory Disturbances:

Relative indifference to pain	+++
Corneal anesthesia	++

Psychologic Disturbances:

Apparent mental retardation	++
Breath-holding spells in infancy	++
Emotional lability	+++

Other Disturbances:

Absence of fungiform papillae	+++
Corneal ulcerations	++
Frequent bronchopneumonia	++
Retardation of body growth	++
Scoliosis	++

+	Common
++	Occurs frequently but not required for the diagnosis
+++	Probably present in all cases

motility.[120] Scoliosis is frequent and becomes more marked with age.

Although many patients succumb to the disease during infancy or childhood, usually through aspiration pneumonia or gastric hemorrhage secondary to prolonged vomiting, long survival has been reported,[117] and perhaps some symptoms, particularly cyclic vomiting and the relative indifference to pain, become less marked with age.

Other clinical aspects of this systemic

disease including ophthalmologic abnormalities, the anesthetic hazards, and the various emotional problems encountered, are discussed by Goldberg et al.,[121] McCaughey,[122] and Freedman et al.[123]

Diagnosis

The diagnosis of dysautonomia rests on the patient's history, genetic background, and on the clinical features of the condition. Of the various tests designed to elicit autonomic dysfunction, the intradermal histamine test has been the most reliable in our hands. In normal subjects intradermal injection of histamine phosphate (0.03–0.05 ml of a 1:1000 solution) produces a local wheal, and a red erythematous flare extending 1 to 3 cm beyond the wheal. In dysautonomic patients the flare response is absent. A similar response may be produced in atopic dermatitis, and in some disorders of the spinal cord or peripheral nerves as, for instance, progressive sensory neuropathy.

The urinary excretion of catecholamines is too variable to assist in the diagnosis.

Treatment

This is symptomatic. Recurrent bouts of vomiting may be treated with chlorpromazine (0.5 mg–2.0 mg/kg given intramuscularly) and parenteral fluids for rehydration. Aspiration pneumonia is prevented by maintaining the head in an elevated position. Feeding and swallowing difficulties in the infant may necessitate gavage. Hypertensive crises are treated with sedation and chlorpromazine.

DIFFUSE CEREBRAL DEGENERATIVE DISEASES

Various hereditary diseases affecting the central nervous system in a nonselective manner are included under this heading. Though there is evidence of a defect in cerebral metabolism in a number of these conditions the relationship between the enzymatic defect and the neurologic abnormalities has not yet been defined.

Diseases With Degeneration Affecting Primarily White Matter

Hereditary widespread demyelination of the cerebral white matter can be grouped by the histochemical characteristics of the myelin breakdown products. The following entities are distinguished: 1) sudanophilic cerebral sclerosis; 2) Pelizaeus-Merzbacher disease; 3) spongy degeneration of white matter (Canavan's sclerosis); 4) Alexander's disease; 5) metachromatic leukodystrophy; and 6) Krabbe's disease (globoid cell sclerosis).

SUDANOPHILIC CEREBRAL SCLEROSIS

This entity is characterized by visual and intellectual impairment, seizures, spasticity, and a more or less rapid progression to a fatal termination. From histochemical and genetic studies it has become clear that a number of distinct diseases have been included within this term, the most common of which has been named sudanophilic diffuse sclerosis.[124]

Sudanophilic diffuse sclerosis may assume at least three forms. One, sporadic, is probably related to multiple sclerosis, and is considered in Chapter 7. Familial cases are usually transmitted as a sex-linked recessive trait, accompanied by Addison's disease and adrenal atrophy. Less often the condition presents as an autosomal recessive disorder.[125] The pathologic lesions in the sporadic and genetic forms are similar and are described in Chapter 7. The etiology for the genetic disorder is unknown. The myelin composition is abnormal, with a decrease in galactolipids and an increase in cholesterol—both nonspecific alterations.[126]

Clinical Manifestations

In the sex-linked disorder, onset is usually between five and eight years of age, with a gradual disturbance in gait and slight intellectual impairment. Sometimes abnormal pigmentation or classic adrenal insufficiency has preceded neurologic abnormalities by several years while in other cases adrenal cortical atrophy was asymptomatic during life.[127,128] Early seizures of a variety of types are common, as well as attacks of crying and screaming. Visual complaints are initially rare, while swallowing is disturbed in about one-third of the children. On occasion, hemiplegia may develop, more frequently in adults. Progression is fairly rapid. Spastic contractures of the lower extremities appear, and not infrequently the child becomes ataxic. Extrapyramidal symptoms may also be observed. Cutaneous melanosis or evidence of Addison's disease can often be detected.[126] The spinal fluid protein may be elevated, and there may be a mild lymphocytosis. The excretion of adrenal androgens and corticosteroids is decreased, and ACTH stimulation fails to produce a rise in the 17-hydroxycorticoid excretion.[128] We have not been able to confirm the presence of an abnormal steroid in demyelinating white matter.

Adrenal insufficiency, if present, is pathognomonic. When absent, diagnosis usually necessitates examination of the brain. Biochemical studies on the brain biopsy, while valuable, still cannot replace careful histologic and histochemical examination.

PELIZAEUS-MERZBACHER DISEASE

This rare, slowly progressive, demyelinating condition, first described by Pelizaeus[129] in 1885 and Merzbacher in 1910,[130] takes two forms.[131] One appears in infancy and is transmitted in a sex-linked recessive manner. The families described by Pelizaeus and Merzbacher fall into this category, as do the more modern cases of Seitelberger. The second form has a later onset and dominant transmission.[132]

Pathology

The pathologic picture resembles that of sudanophilic diffuse sclerosis, but there is little neutral fat in white matter. Loss of myelin is not as extensive, and islands of myelination, particularly around small blood vessels, are characteristic. The axons in a demyelinated area are covered by their lipid sleeves which give histochemical reactions for sphingolipids. Chemical examination of the brain shows a reduction in all lipids in cerebral white matter. In contrast to sudanophilic diffuse sclerosis, cholesterol esters are absent from the demyelinated areas.[133]

Seitelberger has noted a phosphorus-free glyceride in patients with this disease[134] by virtue of which he assumes a disorder of glycerophosphatide metabolism. But probably increased amounts of triglycerides reflect the very slow myelin destruction. White matter in cerebrovascular infarcts shows a similar chemical picture. The amounts of triglycerides are increased with relatively high concentrations of polyunsaturated fatty acids, originally bound to phosphatidyl ethanolamine or phosphatidyl serine.

Clinical Manifestations

The sex-linked recessive form is the more common variant.[135] The clinical course differs from the other leukodystrophies only by the presence, prior to three months of age, of arrhythmically trembling and roving eye movements. Head control is poor and cerebellar ataxia, including intention tremor and scanning speech, is frequent. Over the years, involuntary movements and spasticity become apparent. The disease progresses slowly, with many plateaus. The spinal fluid is normal, as are other laboratory studies.

Diagnosis

In the absence of other affected members of the family, the diagnosis cannot be made with certainty during the patient's lifetime. Ocular and cerebellar symptoms of extremely slow progression and the sex-linked recessive transmission tend to differentiate Pelizaeus-Merzbacher disease from other degenerative conditions, while the absence of remissions and early onset distinguish it from multiple sclerosis.

Treatment

There is no known effective treatment.

SPONGY DEGENERATION OF THE CEREBRAL WHITE MATTER (CANAVAN'S SCLEROSIS)

This is a rare familial degenerative disease of cerebral white matter first described by Canavan in 1931.[136] Symptoms appear during the second and third months of life and include failure of intellectual development, optic atrophy, and hypotonia. Subsequently seizures appear in about half of the infants, and there is progressive increase in muscular tone. Choreo-athetotic movements are occasionally noted. A significant and progressive enlargement of the head, observed in all instances, is often evident by six months of age. Death usually ensues prior to two years of age.[137]

The main pathologic findings are in white matter—particularly of the convolutional areas—which is replaced by a fine network of fluid-containing cystic spaces giving the characteristic spongy appearance. The central portions and the internal capsule remain relatively spared. Edema fluid collects in the cytoplasm of astrocytes and in intra-myelinic vacuoles which result from splitting of the myelin sheath at the intraperiod lines.[138] Products of myelin degradation cannot be found.[139] Chemical analyses have shown an increase in water content, and a marked diminution of all lipid fractions in affected white matter with the exception of ceramide dihexoside the concentration of which in white matter is abnormally high. There is axonal degeneration of the peripheral nerves, with clumping and granular disintegration of axonal material.[139a] In cultured skin fibroblasts there is an elevation in the activities of the lysosomal enzymes alpha-galactosidase, beta-glucosidase, and xylosidase.[140] The significance of this observation is still obscure. Myelin isolated from affected white matter has a low content of proteolipid protein and phospholipids, and a compensatory increase in cholesterol.[141] It is likely that the primary defect is chronic cerebral edema, perhaps the consequence of mitochondrial dysfunction leading to a defect in the permeability of the plasma membrane to ions and water. This may cause myelin destruction or a failure in myelin maturation.

ALEXANDER'S DISEASE

First described by Alexander in 1949,[142] this entity presents within the first year of life with intellectual deterioration, macrocephaly, spasticity, and seizures. Eosinophilic material, resembling neurokeratin, is deposited along the pial surface of the brain, the peri-vascular spaces, and sometimes in cytoplasm of astrocytes. There is usually an accompanying leukodystrophy. The nature of the deposits or of the disease itself is unknown.[143,144]

METACHROMATIC LEUKODYSTROPHY

Greenfield in 1933 described this as a form of diffuse sclerosis in which oligodendroglial degeneration was characteristic.[145]

Pathology

Diffuse demyelination and accumulation of metachromatically staining granules are the outstanding pathologic features. (Metachromatic staining implies that the tissue-dye complex has an absorption spectrum sufficiently different from the original dye to produce an obvious contrast in color. The spectral shift is caused by the polymerization of the dye, induced by negative charges such as RSO_3^- present in close proximity to one another within the tissue.) This material is present either free in the tissues or stored within glial cells (Figs. 2–9 and 2–10). Almost always it is also found in neuronal cytoplasm, distending the cell body as in Tay-Sachs disease but to a lesser extent. Electron microscopy demonstrates cytoplasmic inclusions and alteration in the lamellar structure of myelin (Fig. 2–10). Demyelination is diffuse but with emphasis on those tracts which myelinate during the latter part of infancy. In all the involved areas there is loss of oligodendroglia. Metachromatic granules are also found in the renal tubules, the bile duct epithelium, gall bladder, islet cell and ductal epithelium of pancreas, reticular zone of adrenal cortex, and the liver. They have been shown to contain cholesterol, phospholipids and galactolipids, mostly sulfatides, in an equimolar ratio.[146]

In 1960 Austin showed the metachromatic material to be a sulfatide, or a sulfuric acid

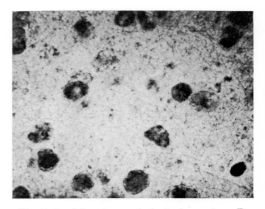

Fig. 2–9. Metachromatic leukodystrophy. Dentate nucleus with an accumulation of orange-brown metachromatic material in neurons and interstitium. Cresyl violet stain. (Courtesy of Dr. E. P. Richardson, Massachusetts General Hospital, Boston.)

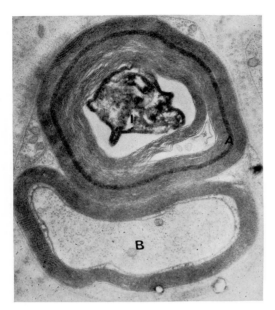

Fig. 2–10. Metachromatic leukodystrophy. Sural nerve biopsy. Within the myelin loop there is a circular band of increased density (**A**). Large cytoplasmic inclusions (**I**) corresponding in size and distribution to metachromatic material observed in frozen sections of the same nerve can be seen. The adjacent axon and myelin are normal (**B**). Electron microscopic examination × 18,400. (Courtesy of Dr. H. De F. Webster, National Institutes of Health, Bethesda, Maryland.)

deposition of sulfatides and demyelination, the latter leading to a reduction in all lipid fractions, most predominantly cholesterol, C_{24} sphingomyelins, and cerebrosides.[150] Since the reduction in cerebroside content is counterbalanced by an accumulation of sulfatides, values for the total hexose content tend to be normal, or even higher than normal, and the ratio of sulfatides to cerebrosides is greater than 1, compared to normal values of about 0.3. A similar reversal of the sulfatide:cerebroside ratio has been found in sciatic nerve.

Austin et al.[151] and Jatzkewitz and Mehl[152] have shown that the basic enzymatic defect is an inactivity of a heat-labile cerebroside sulfatase. Immunologic studies have shown the enzyme to be present, but functionally abnormal.[153] This defect results in the blocked hydrolysis of sulfatides to cerebrosides (Fig. 2–11). The diminution, but not complete absence of arylsulfatase A activity, a sulfatase hydrolyzing aromatic sulfate, has been found in gray and white matter of brain, kidney, liver, urine and leukocytes.[154]

Clinical Manifestations

In the late infantile form, a gradual "stiffening" of gait and strabismus occurs at age two. Impairment of speech, spasticity, and

ester of cerebroside with the sulfate group linked to a galactose at the C_3 position. Sulfatides comprise about one-third of total myelin glycolipids.[147] Sulfatides stored in metachromatic leukodystrophy have a structure similar to those isolated from normal white matter, although minor structural alterations have been noted in sulfatides stored in the late infantile variant. In the juvenile form of the disease, sulfatides accumulating in demyelinated white matter have fatty acids with a shorter chain length than normal and also contain higher proportions of odd-numbered fatty acids.[148] Sulfatides stored in affected kidneys also differ from normal in having a lower content of monounsaturated fatty acids and a higher proportion of hydroxy acids and of C_{22} fatty acids.[149]

Alterations in cerebral lipid composition reflect two distinct pathologic processes, the

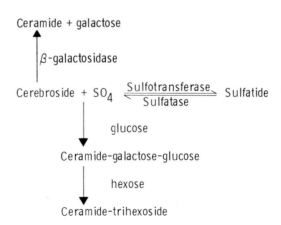

Fig. 2–11. Glycolipid metabolism in brain. In metachromatic leukodystrophy, sulfatase is defective. In globoid cell leukodystrophy there is a deficiency of sulfotransferase and of cerebroside beta-galactosidase. There is also a secondary increase in ceramide di- and tri-hexosides.

intellectual deterioration appear gradually, and occasionally there are coarse tremors or athetoid movements of the extremities. Deep tendon reflexes in the legs are reduced or even absent. Unexplained bouts of fever or severe abdominal pain may develop as the disease advances. Optic atrophy becomes apparent. Seizures are never prominent, although they may appear terminally.[155] Progression is inexorable with death within six months to four years after the onset of symptoms. The cerebrospinal fluid protein is elevated. The conduction velocity in the peripheral nerves is decreased, and the electroretinogram—in contrast to juvenile amaurotic idiocy—is normal.

The juvenile form of metachromatic leukodystrophy is rarer. It was described by Scholz,[156] and subsequently by others.[148,155] Neurologic symptoms become evident between five and seven years of age and progress slowly. Adult metachromatic leukodystrophy presents with an organic mental syndrome and progressive corticospinal, corticobulbar, cerebellar or, rarely, extrapyramidal signs.[157] A deficiency in arylsulfatase A has been documented in these variants also. The reason for the slower progression is still a matter of speculation.[157]

Diagnosis

The time of onset, presence of ataxia, spasticity, and particularly depressed deep tendon reflexes with elevated cerebrospinal fluid protein suggests the diagnosis. Confirmatory tests include a slowed nerve conduction time and a nonfunctioning gall bladder. Large quantities of metachromatic bodies in urine are pathognomonic but this diagnostic test has been superseded by an assay of urinary or leukocyte arylsulfatase A activity.[158,159] Brown metachromatic bodies may also be found on biopsy of various peripheral nerves as early as 15 months after the onset (Fig. 2–10).[160] Segmental demyelination of peripheral nerves is encountered in other leukodystrophies, including globoid cell leukodystrophy, Canavan's spongy degeneration,[161] and, rarely, Tay-Sachs disease and the juvenile amaurotic idiocies (Spielmeyer-Vogt disease).[162]

The assay of leukocyte arylsulfatase A ac-

tivity can also be used for the biochemical identification of heterozygotes.[159]

Treatment

No treatment has been effective. The intravenous or intrathecal infusion of arylsulfatase A raises hepatic enzyme activity to normal, but the enzyme does not enter the brain.

GLOBOID CELL LEUKODYSTROPHY (KRABBE'S DISEASE)

This condition was first described by Beneke in 1908,[163] and more definitively by Krabbe in 1916,[164] who noted the characteristic globoid cells in affected white matter.

Pathology[165]

The white matter of the cerebrum, the cerebellum, the spinal cord, and the cortical projection fibers is extensively demyelinated, with only minimal sparing of the subcortical arcuate fibers. In the areas of recent demyelination, mononuclear epitheloid cells and large (20 to 50 microns) multinucleated globoid cells are seen around the smaller blood vessels (Fig. 2–12). The globoid cells are believed to arise from vascular adventitia. Histochemical reactions and chemical analyses on globoid cell-rich fractions prepared by differential centrifugation show that a protein-bound cerebroside is stored within them. The appearance of globoid cells is believed

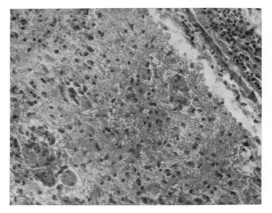

Fig. 2–12. Globoid cell leukodystrophy. Cerebral white matter. Aggregates of globoid cells are seen in vicinity of a blood vessel. There is a considerable increase in cellularity in the demyelinated area. Hematoxylin and eosin × 280.

to be stimulated by the release of cerebrosides from myelin, as a similar cellular response can be produced in experimental animals through intracerebral injection of both natural and synthetic cerebrosides.[166]

Small clusters of globoid cells occur in a number of degenerative diseases of myelin and the distinguishing feature of Krabbe's disease is not the mere presence of these cellular elements but rather their vast number. Ultrastructural examination reveals intra- and extracellular crystalline inclusions, most commonly seen within the globoid cells, which correspond to the PAS-positive material.[167] The peripheral nerves show segmental demyelination and marked endoneurial fibrosis.[168] The presence of globoid cells has also been noted in lungs, spleen, and lymph nodes.[169]

Biochemical Pathology

In contrast to the phospholipid and cholesterol concentrations, which are lower than normal, the amount of cerebroside is normal or slightly increased and there is an increased ratio of cerebrosides to sulfatides. In part this is due to increased amounts of cytosides (ceramide dihexosides).[170] Isolated myelin has a normal composition, however.[171] Bachhawat, Austin, and Armstrong documented a deficiency of cerebroside sulfotransferase activity, preventing the conversion of cerebrosides to sulfatides[172] (Fig. 2–11). More recently Malone[173] and Suzuki and Suzuki[174] have demonstrated a deficiency of galactocerebroside beta-galactosidase in leukocytes, brain, liver, kidney, and spleen of patients (Fig. 2–11). A third enzyme, psychosine galactosidase, is also deficient.[174a] Other sphingolipid hydrolases are either slightly elevated, or show no marked deficiency.[175] It is still not clear how these enzymatic deficiencies result in the pathologic picture, or whether indeed they represent the primary defect, which we feel lies in a disorder of axonal metabolism.[167] Suzuki has postulated that the enzymatic defect results in early cessation of cerebroside synthesis due to disappearance of oligodendroglia, the site of cerebroside formation,[171,176] and that the known cytotoxic effects of psychosine are responsible for the loss of oligodendroglia.[174a]

The disease begins acutely at four to six months of age with restlessness, irritability, and progressive stiffness. Convulsions may develop later. Frequently, these are tonic spasms, induced by light, noise, or touch. Infants show increased muscular tone, with few spontaneous movements. Optic atrophy and hyperacusis are often seen. The deep tendon reflexes are characteristically difficult to elicit, and may be absent in the legs. Terminally, infants are flaccid and develop bulbar signs.

Laboratory studies reveal a consistently elevated cerebrospinal fluid protein. Conduction velocity of motor nerves is reduced.[168]

Diagnosis

Various degenerative conditions present a picture akin to Krabbe's disease. In general, Tay-Sachs disease can be distinguished by its characteristic retinal changes. Juvenile amaurotic idiocy and metachromatic leukodystrophy have a somewhat later onset. In the rare progressive degenerations of the gray matter, seizures tend to appear earlier and more frequently. The most salient diagnostic feature for globoid cell leukodystrophy is peripheral nerve involvement: depressed deep tendon reflexes, elevated CSF protein, and delayed nerve conduction, in a deteriorating infant. The deficiency of leukocyte beta-galactosidase is probably the most definitive test, and by means of this enzymatic assay, ante-natal diagnosis may be made.

Treatment

No known therapy has proved effective.

Two rare entities which may represent demyelinating diseases should be mentioned at this point.

COCKAYNE'S SYNDROME

This condition, probably transmitted as an autosomal recessive trait, was first described by Cockayne in 1936.[177] It is characterized by failure of growth first manifested in the second year of life, slowly progressive intellectual deterioration, lack of subcutaneous fat, retinal degeneration, and hypersensitivity of skin to sunlight.[178] Radiographic examinations reveal thickening of the skull bones and kyphoscoliosis. In the brain there may be perivascular calcification in the basal ganglia and cerebellum, and a patchy demyelination, somewhat akin to that seen in Pelizaeus-Merzbacher's disease (see p. 102).[179] A peripheral neuropathy has also been demonstrated.[180]

CHEDIAK-HIGASHI SYNDROME

This syndrome, first described by Chediak in 1952,[181] is characterized by partial albinism, photophobia, nystagmus, hepatosplenomegaly, lymphadenopathy, and the presence of giant, peroxidase-positive granules in the polymorphonuclear leukocytes. A variety of neurologic symptoms may be found. These include cranial and peripheral neuropathies, a progressive spinocerebellar degeneration and mental retardation.[182,183] Intracytoplasmic inclusions within the neurons and perivascular infiltrations are found throughout the nervous system, most prominently in the pons and cerebellum. Similar infiltrations are seen in peripheral nerves.[184] The etiology of the condition is still obscure.

Diseases With Degeneration Affecting Primarily Gray Matter

Degenerative conditions which primarily affect cerebral gray matter are less common than those affecting white matter. Although it is unlikely that these entities represent a single genetic condition, they are generally grouped as Alpers' disease.[185]

Pathology

Grossly, the cerebral cortical gray matter is markedly reduced, and in some areas may not even be identifiable.[186] Microscopically, the cortical cytoarchitecture is severely disturbed, and there is extensive cellular loss with astrocytosis and neuronophagia.

Clinical Manifestations

Onset is usually prior to six years of age, and convulsions, particularly myoclonic seizures, appear early. Intellectual deterioration soon becomes evident, and spasticity or opisthotonus is invariable.[187] Clinically, however, these conditions cannot be differentiated from the leukodystrophies. While generally severe seizures point to a gray matter degeneration, and prominent spasticity indicates a leukodystrophy, this is not necessarily so. Neither etiology nor treatment has been suggested.

A few rare entities which primarily affect the gray matter have had a clinical picture sufficiently distinctive to permit a presumptive diagnosis during life. A focal degenerative disorder of gray matter named "kinky hair disease" and transmitted in a sex-linked manner was first reported by Menkes et al.[188] The cases are distinguished by their peculiar white hair, early and severe growth retardation, seizures, and focal cerebral and cerebellar atrophy. Danks et al.[189] have demonstrated reduced serum copper and ceruloplasmin levels and have suggested that defective copper absorption represents the basic biochemical lesion. This observation would explain the clinical features and a diminution in the proportion of the highly unsaturated fatty acids in gray matter previously noted by O'Brien and Sampson.[190]

A degenerative disorder of the nervous system, of early onset, mixed upper and lower motor neuron signs, with widespread axonal swelling has been designated as infantile neuroaxonal dystrophy.[191] This condition is characterized by a slowly progressive weakness, hypotonia, and muscular atrophy accompanied by evidence of corticospinal tract involvement. Tendon reflexes are usually hyperactive, urinary retention is common, as are disturbances of ocular mobility and optic atrophy. Convulsions are rare. The diagnosis can be made by biopsy of the peripheral nerves which demonstrate globular swellings along the course of axons.[192] Although the pathologic picture resembles that of experimental vitamin E deficiency, its etiology is still unknown.[193] The relationship of this condition to Hallervorden-Spatz disease (p. 87) is a matter of speculation.

Many other variants of gray or white matter degenerations have been recorded in which the pathologic picture is unique for one reason or another. These entities are undoubtedly very rare, although collectively they probably constitute an appreciable percentage of the total reported cases of cerebral degenerative conditions.

REFERENCES

1. Cited by Bruyn, G. W.: "Huntington's Chorea—Historical, Clinical and Laboratory Synopsis" in Vinken, P. J. and Bruyn, G. W. (eds.): *Diseases of the Basal Ganglia*, Amsterdam: North-Holland Publishing Co., 1968.
2. Huntington, G.: On chorea, Med. Surg. Reporter 26:317, 1872.
3. Reed, T. E. and Chandler, J. H.: Huntington's chorea in Michigan, Amer. J. Hum. Genet. 10:201, 1958.
4. Stevens, D. and Parsonage, M.: Mutation in Huntington's chorea, J. Neurol. Neurosurg. Psychiat. 32:140, 1969.
4a.Cowie, V. A.: "Serum Protein Changes (Particularly Gamma-Globulins) in Huntington's Chorea," in Barbeau, A. and Brunette, J. R. (eds.): *Progress in Neuro-genetics*, Amsterdam: Excerpta Medica Foundation, 1969.
4b.Barbeau, A., Chase, T. N., and Paulson, G. W.: *Huntington's Chorea 1872–1972*, New York: Raven Press, 1973.
4c.Perry, T. L., Hansen, S., and Kloster, M.: Huntington's chorea. Deficiency of γ-aminobutyric acid in brain, New Eng. J. Med. 288: 337, 1973.
5. Klawans, H. L. and Rubovits, R.: Central cholinergic-anticholinergic antagonism in Huntington's chorea, Neurology (Minneap.) 22:107, 1972.
6. McCaughey, W. T. E.: Pathologic spectrum of Huntington's chorea, J. Nerv. Ment. Dis. 133:91, 1961.
7. Tellez-Nagel, I.: Barbeau, A., Chase, T. N., and Paulson, G. W. (eds.): *Huntington's Chorea 1872–1972*, New York: Raven Press, 1973.
8. Borri, P. F., et al.: Biochemical studies in Huntington's chorea, Neurology (Minneap.) 17:172, 1967.
9. Bell, J.: Huntington's chorea, Treasury of Human Inheritance 4:1, 1934.
10. Penrose, L. S.: The problem of anticipation in pedigrees of dystrophia myotonia, Ann. Eugenics 14:125, 1947–49.
11. Jervis, G. A.: Huntington's chorea in childhood, Arch. Neurol. 9:244, 1963.
12. Barbeau, A.: Parental ascent in the juvenile form of Huntington's chorea, Lancet 2:937, 1970.
13. Markham, C. H. and Knox, J. W.: Observations in Huntington's chorea, J. Pediat. 67:46, 1965.
14. Bittenbender, J. B. and Quadfasel, F. A.: Rigid and akinetic forms of Huntington's chorea, Arch. Neurol. 7:275, 1962.
15. Hansotia, P., Cleeland, C. S., Chun, R. W. M.: Juvenile Huntington's chorea, Neurology (Minneap.) 18:217, 1968.
16. Pincus, J H. and Chutorian, A.: Familial benign chorea with intention tremor: Clinical entity, J. Pediat. 70:724, 1967.
17. Schwalbe, M. W.: Eine eigentümliche, tonische Krampfform mit hysterischen Symptomen. Inaug. Dissert. Berlin, G. Schade, 1908.
18. Eldridge, R.: The torsion dystonias: Literature review and genetic and clinical studies, Neurology (Minneap.) 20(pt. 2):1, 1970.
19. Davison, C. and Goodhart, S. P.: Dystonia musculorum deformans: A clinicopathologic study, Arch. Neurol. Psychiat. 39:939, 1938.
20. Zeman, W.: Pathology of the torsion dystonias (dystonia musculorum deformans), Neurology (Minneap.) 20(pt. 2):79, 1970.
21. Cooper, I. S.: Dystonia musculorum deformans. Natural history and neurosurgical alleviation, J. Pediat. 74:585, 1969.
22. Larsson, T. and Sjögren, T.: Dystonia musculorum deformans, Acta Neurol. Scand. 42 Suppl.: 17, 1966.
23. Johnson, W., Schwartz, G., and Barbeau, A.: Studies on dystonia musculorum deformans, Arch. Neurol. 7:301, 1962.
24. Hansen, R. A., Berenberg, W., and Byers, R. K.: Changing motor patterns in cerebral palsy, Develop. Med. Child Neurol. 12:309, 1970.
25. Cooper, I. S.: Neurosurgical treatment of dystonia, Neurology (Minneap.) 20 (pt. 2):133, 1970.
26. Mandell, S.: The treatment of dystonia with L-dopa and haloperidol, Neurology (Minneap.) 20 (pt. 2):103, 1970.
27. Hallervorden, J. and Spatz, H.: Eigenartige Erkrankung im System mit besonderer Beteilung des Globus Pallidus und der Substantia Nigra, Z. Ges. Neurol. Psychiat. 79:254, 1922.
28. Nakai, H., Landing, B. H., and Schubert, W. K.: Seitelberger's spastic amaurotic axonal idiocy; report of a case in a 9-year-old boy with comment on visceral manifestations, Pediatrics 25:441, 1960.
29. Jervis, G. A.: Hallervorden-Spatz disease associated with atypical amaurotic idiocy, J. Neuropath. Exp. Neurol. 11:4, 1952.
30. Swisher, C. N. et al.: Coexistence of Hallervorden-Spatz disease with acanthocytosis, Trans. Amer. Neurol. Ass. 97:212, 1972.
31. Sacks, O. W., Aguilar, M. J., and Brown, W. J.: Hallervorden-Spatz disease; its pathogenesis and place among the axonal dystrophies, Acta Neuropath. 6:164, 1966.
32. Koenig, H.: Acute axonal dystrophy caused by fluorocitrate: The role of mitochondrial swelling, Science 164:310, 1969.
33. Babbitt, D. P., et al: Idiopathic familial cerebrovascular ferrocalcinosis (Fahr's disease) and review of differential diagnosis of intracranial calcification in children, Amer. J. Roentgen. 105:352, 1969.
34. Foley, J.: Calcification of the corpus striatum and dentate nuclei occurring in a family, J. Neurol. Neurosurg. Psychiat. 14:253, 1961.
35. Moskowitz, M. A., Winickoff, R. N., and Heinz, E. R.: Familial calcification of the basal ganglions: A metabolic and genetic study, New Eng. J. Med. 285:72, 1971.

36. Critchley, M.: Observations on essential (heredofamilial) tremor, Brain 72:113, 1949.
37. Holmes, G.: On certain tremors in organic cerebral lesions, Brain 27:327, 1904.
38. Hunt, J. R.: Progressive atrophy of the globus pallidus. (Primary atrophy of the pallidal system.) A system disease of the paralysis agitans type, Brain 40:58, 1917.
39. Van Bogaert, L.: Contribution clinique et anatomique a l'étude de la paralysie agitante juvenile primitive, Rev. Neurol. (Paris) 2:315, 1930.
40. Martin, W. E., Resch, J. A., and Baker, A. B.: Juvenile Parkinsonism, Arch. Neurol. 25:494, 1971.
41. Friedreich, N.: Ueber degenerative Atrophie der spinalen Hinterstraenge, Virchow. Arch. Path. Anat. 26:391, 1863.
42. Bell, J. and Carmichael, E. A.: On hereditary ataxia and spastic paraplegia, Treasury of Human Inheritance 4:141, 1939.
43. Joffe, B. I., Segal, I., and Keller, P.: Insulin levels in hereditary ataxias, New Eng. J. Med. 283, 1410, 1970.
44. Dunn, H. G. and Dolman, C. L.: Necrotizing encephalomyelopathy, Neurology (Minneap.) 19:536, 1969.
45. Greenfield, J. G.: *The Spino-Cerebellar Degenerations*, Blackwell, Oxford, 1954.
46. Locke, S. and Foley, J. M.: A case of cerebellar ataxia with a discussion of classification, Arch. Neurol. 3:279, 1960.
47. Robinson, N.: Friedreich's ataxia: A histochemical study. I. Enzymes of carbohydrate metabolism, Acta Neuropath. 6:25, 1966.
48. Robinson, N.: Chemical changes in the spinal cord in Friedreich's ataxia and motor neurone disease, J. Neurol. Neurosurg. Psychiat. 31:330, 1968.
49. Sjögren, T.: Klinische und erbbiologische Untersuchungen über die Heredoataxien, Acta Psych. et Neurol. Suppl. 27, 1943.
50. André-van-Leeuwen, M.: Sur deux cas familiaux de maladie de Friedreich avec atrophie optique précoce globale et grave. Rev. Neurol. (Paris) 81:941, 1949.
51. Boyer, S. H., Chisholm, A. W., and McKusick, V. A.: Cardiac aspects of Friedreich's ataxia, Circulation 25:493, 1962.
52. Hewer, R. L.: Study of fatal cases of Friedreich's ataxia, Brit. Med. J. 3:649, 1968.
53. Dejerine, J. and Thomas, A.: L'atrophie olivoponto-cerebelleuse, Nouv. Icon. Salpet. 13:330, 1900.
54. Critchley, M. and Greenfield, J. G.: Olivoponto-cerebellar atrophy, Brain 71:343, 1948.
55. Weiner, L. P., et al.: Hereditary olivopontocerebellar atrophy with retinal degeneration, Arch. Neurol. 16:364, 1967.
56. Menzel, P.: Beitrag zur Kenntnis der hereditaeren Ataxie und Kleinhirnatrophie, Arch. Psychiat. Nervenkr. 22:160, 1891.
57. Holmes, G. M.: A form of familial degeneration of the cerebellum, Brain 30:466, 1907.
58. Norman, R. M.: Primary degeneration of the granular layer of the cerebellum: An unusual form of familial cerebellar atrophy occurring in early life, Brain 63:365, 1940.
59. Jervis, G. A.: Early familial cerebellar degeneration, J. Nerv. Ment. Dis. 111:398, 1950.
60. Garland, H. and Moorhouse, D.: An extremely rare recessive hereditary syndrome including cerebellar ataxia, oligophrenia, cataract, and other features, J. Neurol. Neurosurg. Psychiat. 16:110, 1953.
61. Andersen, B.: Marinesco-Sjögren syndrome: Spinocerebellar ataxia, congenital cataract, somatic and mental retardation, Develop. Med. Child Neurol. 7:249, 1965.
62. Malamud, N. and Cohen, P.: Unusual form of cerebellar ataxia with sex-linked inheritance, Neurology (Minneap.) 8:261, 1958.
63. Hunter, D. and Russell, D. S.: Focal cerebral and cerebellar atrophy in a human subject due to organic mercury compounds, J. Neurol. Neurosurg. Psychiat. 17:235, 1954.
64. Hunt, J. R.: Dyssynergia cerebellaris myoclonica, Brain, 44:490, 1921.
65. Seeligmüller, A.: Sklerose der Seitenstränge des Rückenmarks bei 4 Kindern derselben Familie, Deutsch. Med. Wschr. 2:185, 1876.
66. Schwarz, G. A. and Liu, C.: Hereditary spastic paraplegia, Arch. Neurol. Psychiat. 75:144, 1956.
67. Silver, J. R.: Familial spastic paraplegia with amyotrophy of hands, J. Neurol. Neurosurg. Psychiat. 29:135, 1966.
68. Refsum, S. and Skillicorn, S. A.: Amyotrophic familial spastic paraplegia, Neurology (Minneap.) 4:41, 1954.
69. Rhein, J. H. W.: Family spastic paralysis, J. Nerv. Ment. Dis. 44:115, 1914.
70. Van Bogaert, L.: La sclerose laterale amyotrophique et la paralysie bulbaire progressive chez l'enfant, Rev. Neurol. (Paris) 1:180, 1925.
71. Markand, O. N. and Daly, D. D.: Juvenile type of slowly progressive bulbar palsy: Report of a case, Neurology (Minneap.) 21:753, 1971.
72. Gomez, M. R., Clermont, V., and Bernstein, J.: Progressive bulbar paralysis in childhood (Fazio-Londe's disease), Arch. Neurol. 6:317, 1962.
73. Pearce, J. and Harriman, D. G. F.: Chronic spinal muscular atrophy, J. Neurol. Neurosurg. Psychiat. 29:509, 1966.
74. Engel, K., Kurland, L. T., and Klatzo, I.: An inherited disease similar to amyotrophic lateral sclerosis with a pattern of posterior column involvement: An intermediate form?, Brain 82:203, 1959.
75. Hirano, A., Arumugasamy, N., and Zimmerman, H. M.: Amyotrophic lateral sclerosis. A comparison of Guam and classical cases, Arch. Neurol. 16:357, 1967.

76. Virchow, R.: Ein Fall von progressiver Muskelatrophie, Virchow. Arch. Path. Anat. 8:537, 1855.

77. Charcot, J. M. and Marie, P.: Sur une forme particuliere d'atrophie musculaire progressive: souvent familial debutant par les pieds et les jambes, et atteignant plus tard les mains, Rev. Med. (Paris) 6:97, 1886.

78. Tooth, H. H.: *The Peroneal Type of Progressive Muscular Atrophy*, Cambridge University Thesis, London: H. K. Lewis, 1886.

79. Bell, J.: On the peroneal type of progressive muscular atrophy, Treasury of Human Inheritance 4:69, 1935.

80. Tyrer, J. H. and Sutherland, J. M.: The primary spinocerebellar atrophies and their associated defects, with a study of the foot deformity, Brain 84:289, 1961.

81. Dyck, P. J., Lambert, E. H., and Mulder, D. H.: Charcot-Marie-Tooth disease: Nerve conduction and clinical studies of a large kinship, Neurology (Minneap.) 13:1, 1963.

82. Roussy, G. and Lévy, G.: Sept cas d'une maladie familiale particuliere. Troubles de la marche, pieds bots, et areflexie tendineuse generalisee, avec, accessoirement, legere maladresse des mains, Rev. Neurol. (Paris) 1:427, 1926.

83. Symonds, C. P. and Shaw, M. E.: Familial claw-foot with absent tendon jerks: A "forme fruste" of the Charcot-Marie-Tooth disease, Brain 49:387, 1926.

84. Yudell, A., Dyck, P. J., and Lambert, E. H.: A kinship with Roussy-Lévy syndrome, Arch. Neurol. 13:432, 1965.

85. Roth, M.: On a possible relationship between hereditary ataxia and peroneal muscular atrophy; with a critical view of the problem of "intermediate forms" in the degenerative disorders of the central nervous system, Brain 71:416, 1948.

86. Spillane, J. D.: Familial pes cavus and absent tendon jerks. Its relationship with Friedreich's disease and peroneal muscular atrophy, Brain 63:275, 1940.

87. Dejerine, J. and Sottas, J.: Sur la nevrite interstitielle hypertrophique et progressive de l'enfance, Soc. Biol. Compt. Rend. (Paris) 5:63, 1893.

88. Austin, J. H.: Observations on the syndrome of hypertrophic neuritis (the hypertrophic interstitial radiculo-neuropathies), Medicine (Baltimore) 35:187, 1956.

89. Webster, H. deF., et al.: Role of Schwann cells in formation of "onion bulbs" found in chronic neuropathies, J. Neuropath. Exp. Neurol. 26:276, 1967.

90. Koeppen, A. H., Messmore, H., and Stehbens, W. E.: Interstitial hypertrophic neuropathy: Biochemical study of the peripheral nervous system, Arch. Neurol. 24:240, 1971.

91. Bradley, W. G. and Aguayo, A.: Hereditary chronic polyneuropathy: Electrophysiologic and pathologic studies in affected family, J. Neurol. Sci. 9:131, 1969.

92. Tasker, W. and Chutorian, A. M.: Chronic polyneuritis of childhood, J. Pediat. 4:699, 1969.

93. Denny-Brown, D.: Hereditary sensory radicular neuropathy, J. Neurol. Neurosurg. Psychiat. 14:237, 1951.

94. Pinsky, L. and DiGeorge, A. M.: Congenital family sensory neuropathy with anhidrosis, J. Pediat. 68:1, 1968.

95. Munro, M.: Sensory radicular neuropathy in a deaf child, Brit. Med. J. 1:541, 1956.

96. Leber, T.: Ueber hereditare und kongenital angelegte Sehnervenleiden, Arch. Ophthal. 4:266, 1871.

97. Kwittken, J. and Barest, H. D.: The neuro-ophthalmology of hereditary optic atrophy (Leber's disease): The first complete anatomic study, Amer. J. Path. 34:185, 1958.

98. Wallace, D. C.: A new manifestation of Leber's disease and a new explanation for the agency responsible for its unusual pattern of inheritance, Brain 93:121, 1970.

99. Adams, J. H., Blackwood, W., and Wilson, J.: Further clinical and pathological observations on Leber's optic atrophy, Brain 89:15, 1966.

100. Osuntokun, B. O., Aladetoyinbo, A., and Adeuja, A. O. G.: Free cyanide levels in tropical ataxic neuropathy, Lancet 2:372, 1970.

101. Bruyn, G. W. and Went, L. N.: A sex-linked heredodegenerative neurological disorder associated with Leber's optic atrophy, J. Neurol. Sci. 1:59, 1964.

102. Kjer, P.: Hereditary infantile optic atrophy with dominant transmission, Danish Med. Bull. 3:135, 1956.

103. Wartenberg, R.: Progressive facial hemiatrophy, Arch. Neurol. Psychiat. 54:75, 1945.

104. Merritt, K. K., Faber, H. K., and Bruch, H.: Progressive facial hemiatrophy. A report of two cases with cerebral calcification, J. Pediat. 10:374, 1937.

105. Rosenberg, R. N. and Chutorian, A.: Familial opticoacoustic nerve degeneration and polyneuropathy, Neurology (Minneap.) 17:827, 1967.

106. Franceschetti, A. and Klein, D.: Heredo-ataxies par degenerescence spinoponto-cerebelleuse. Les manifestatiens tapeto-retiniennes, Rev. Otoneuroophtal. 20:109, 1948.

107. Konigsmark, B. W.: Hereditary deafness in man, New Eng. J. Med. 281:713, 774, 827, 1969.

108. Riley, C. M., et al.: Central autonomic dysfunction with defective lacrimation, Pediatrics 3:468, 1949.

109. Mahloudji, M., Brunt, P. W., and McKusick, V. A.: Clinical neurological aspects of familial dysautonomia, J. Neurol. Sci. 11:383, 1970.

110. Brown, W. J., Beauchemin, J. A., and Linde, L. M.: A neuropathological study of familial dysautonomia (Riley-Day syndrome) in siblings. J. Neurol. Neurosurg. Psychiat. 27:131, 1964.

111. Smith, A. A., Taylor, T., and Wortis, S. B.: Abnormal catecholamine metabolism in familial dysautonomia, New Eng. J. Med. 268:705, 1963.

112. Smith, A. A. and Dancis, J.: Catecholamine release in familial dysautonomia, New Eng. J. Med. 277:61, 1967.

113. Greer, M. and Williams, C. M.: Sympathetic neurohormones in pheochromocytoma, neuroblastoma and dysautonomia, Trans. Amer. Neurol. Ass. 88:223, 1963.

114. Gitlow, S. E., et al.: Excretion of catecholamine metabolites by children with familial dysautonomia, Pediatrics 46:513, 1960.

115. DeQuattro, V. and Linde, L.: Intact synthesis and increased turnover of norepinephrine ^{3}H after L-DOPA-^{3}H in dysautonomia, Clin. Res. 17:237, 1969.

116. Geltzer, A. I., et al: Familial dysautonomia: Studies in newborn infant. New Eng. J. Med. 271:436, 1964.

117. Yatsu, F. and Zussman, W.: Familial dysautonomia (Riley-Day Syndrome), Arch. Neurol. 10:459, 1964.

118. Riley, C. M.: Familial dysautonomia, Advances Pediat. 9:157:1957.

119. Pearson, J., Finegold, M. J., and Budzilovich, G.: The tongue and taste in familial dysautonomia, Pediatrics 45:739, 1970.

120. Linde, L. M. and Westover, J. L.: Esophageal and gastric abnormalities in dysautonomia, Pediatrics 29:303, 1962.

121. Goldberg, M. F., Payne, J. W., and Brunt, P. W.: Ophthalmologic studies of familial dysautonomia: Riley-Day syndrome, Arch. Ophthal. 80:732, 1968.

122. McCaughey, T. J.: Familial dysautonomia as anesthetic hazard, Canad. Anaesth. Soc. J. 12:558, 1965.

123. Freedman, A. M., et al.: Psychiatric aspects of familial dysautonomia, Amer. J. Orthopsychiat. 27:96, 1957.

124. Poser, C. M.: The differential diagnosis of diffuse scleroses in children, AMA J. Dis. Child. 100:380, 1960.

125. Einarson, L., Neel, A. V., and Strömgren, E.: On the problem of diffuse brain sclerosis with special reference to the familial forms, Acta Jutlandica 16:1, 1944.

126. Aguilar, M. J., O'Brien, J. S., and Taber, P.: "The Syndrome of Familial Leukodystrophy, Adrenal Insufficiency and Cutaneous Melanosis," in Aronson, S. M. and Volk, B. W. (eds.): Inborn Disorders of Sphingolipid Metabolism, London: Pergamon Press, 1967.

127. Hoefnagel, D., van der Noort, S., and Ingbar, S. H.: Diffuse cerebral sclerosis with endocrine abnormalities in young males, Brain 85:553, 1962.

128. Forsyth, C. C., Forbes, M., and Cumings, J. N.: Adrenocortical atrophy and diffuse cerebral sclerosis, Arch. Dis. Child. 46:273, 1971.

129. Pelizaeus, F.: Ueber eine eigentümliche Form spastischer Lähmung mit Cerebralerscheinungen auf hereditärer Grundlage, Arch. Psychiat. Nervenkr. 16:698, 1885.

130. Merzbacher, L.: Eine eigenartige familiär-hereditäre Erkrankungsform. Z. Ges. Neurol. Psychiat. 3:1, 1910.

131. Zerbin-Rüdin, E. and Peiffer, J.: Ein genetischer Beitrag zur Frage der Spätform der Pelizaeus-Merzbachschen Krankheit, Humangenetik 1:107, 1964.

132. Camp, C. D. and Lowenberg, K.: An American family with Pelizaeus-Merzbacher disease, Arch. Neurol. Psychiat. 45:261, 1941.

133. Zeman, W., DeMyer, W., and Falls, H. F.: Pelizaeus-Merzbacher's disease; a study in nosology, J. Neuropath. Exp. Neurol. 23:334, 1964.

134. Seitelberger, F.: "Contribution to Pelizaeus-Merzbacher's Disease," in Folch-Pi, J. and Bauer, H., (eds.): Brain Lipids and Lipoproteins and the Leucodystrophies, New York: Elsevier Publ. Co., 1963.

135. Tyler, H. R.: Pelizaeus-Merzbacher disease. Arch. Neurol. Psychiat. 80:162, 1958.

136. Canavan, M. M.: Schilder's encephalitis periaxialis diffusa, Arch. Neurol. Psychiat. 25:299, 1931.

137. Hogan, G. R. and Richardson, E. P., Jr.: Spongy degeneration of the nervous system (Canavan's disease), Pediatrics 35:284, 1965.

138. Gambetti, P., Mellman, W. J., and Gonatas, N. K.: Familial spongy degeneration of the central nervous system. (Van Bogaert-Bertrand Disease), Acta Neuropath. 12:103, 1969.

139. Banker, B. Q., Robertson, J. T., and Victor, M.: Spongy degenerations of the central nervous system in infancy, Neurology (Minneap.) 14:981, 1964.

139a. Adornato, B. T., et al.: Cerebral spongy degeneration of infancy. A biochemical and ultrastructural study of affected twins, Neurology (Minneap.) 22:202, 1972.

140. Milunsky, A., et al.: Elevated lysosomal enzyme activities in Canavan's disease, Pediat. Res. 6:425, 1972.

141. Kamoshita, S., et al.: Spongy degeneration of the brain, Neurology (Minneap.) 18:975, 1968.

142. Alexander, W. S.: Progressive fibrinoid degeneration of fibrillary astrocytes associated with mental retardation in hydrocephalic infant, Brain 72:373, 1949.

143. Friede, R. L.: Alexander's disease, Arch. Neurol. 11:414, 1964.

144. Sherwin, R. M. and Berthrong, M.: Alexander's disease with sudanophilic leukodystrophy, Arch. Path. 89:321, 1970.

145. Greenfield, J. G.: A form of progressive cerebral sclerosis in infants associated with primary degeneration of the interfascicular glia, J. Neurol. Psychopath. 13:289, 1933.

146. Suzuki, K., Suzuki, K., and Chen., G. C.: Isolation and chemical characterization of metachromatic granules from a brain with MLD, J. Neuropath. Exp. Neurol. 26:537, 1967.

147. Eichberg, J., Hauser, G., and Karnovsky, M.: "Lipids of Nervous Tissue," in Bourne, G. H. (ed.): *The Structure and Function of Nervous Tissue*, vol. 3, New York: Academic Press, 1969.

148. Menkes, J. H.: Chemical studies of two cerebral biopsies in juvenile metachromatic leukodystrophy: The molecular composition of cerebrosides and sulfatides, J. Pediat. 69:422, 1966.

149. Martensson, E., Percy, A., and Svennerholm, L.: Kidney glycolipids in late infantile metachromatic leucodystrophy, Acta Paediat. Scand. 55:1, 1966.

150. Hagberg, B., Sourander, P., and Svennerholm, L.: Sulfatide lipidosis in childhood: Report of a case investigated during life and at autopsy, Amer. J. Dis. Child. 104:664, 1962.

151. Austin, J. H., Balasubramanian, A. S., and Pattabiraman, T. N.: A controlled study of enzymic activities in three human disorders of glycolipid metabolism, J. Neurochem. 10:805, 1963.

152. Jatzkewitz, H. and Mehl, E. L.: Cerebrosidesulphatase and arylsulphatase: A deficiency in metachromatic leukodystrophy, J. Neurochem. 16:19, 1969.

153. Stumpf, D., et al.: Metachromatic leukodystrophy, X. Immunological studies of the abnormal sulfatase A, Arch. Neurol. 25:427, 1971.

154. Percy, A. K. and Brady, R. O.: Metachromatic leukodystrophy: Diagnosis with samples of venous blood, Science 161:594, 1968.

155. Austin, J. H.: "Mental Retardation. Metachromatic Leucodystrophy," in Carter, C. H. (ed.): *Medical Aspects of Mental Retardation*, Springfield: Charles C Thomas, Publisher, 1965, pp. 768–812.

156. Scholz, W.: Klinische, pathologische anatomische und erbiologische Untersuchungen bei familiarer diffuser Hirnsklerose im Kindesalter, Z. Ges. Neurol. Psychiat. 99:651, 1925.

157. Austin, J. H., Armstrong, D., and Fouch, S.: Metachromatic leukodystrophy (MLD): VIII. MLD in adults: Diagnosis and pathogenesis, Arch. Neurol. 18:225, 1968.

158. Austin, J., et al.: Metachromatic form of diffuse cerebral sclerosis: VI. A rapid test for the sulfatase: A deficiency in metachromatic leukodystrophy (MLD) urine, Arch. Neurol. 14:259, 1966.

159. Bass, N. H., Witmer, J., and Dreifuss, F. E.: A pedigree study of metachromatic leukodystrophy: Biochemical identification of the carrier state, Neurology 20:52, 1970.

160. Hagberg, B., Sourander, P., and Thoren, L.: Peripheral nerve changes in the diagnosis of metachromatic leucodystrophy, Acta Paediat. Scand. 51 (Suppl. 135):63, 1962.

161. Suzuki, K.: Peripheral nerve lesion in spongy degeneration of the central nervous system, Acta Neuropath. 10:95, 1968.

162. Carpenter, S., Karpati, G., and Andermann, F.: Specific involvement of muscle, nerve, and skin in late infantile and juvenile amaurotic idiocies, Neurology 22:170, 1972.

163. Beneke, R.: Ein Fall hochgradigster ausgedehnter Sklerose des Zentralnervensystem, Arch. Kinderheilk. 47:420, 1908.

164. Krabbe, K.: A new familial infantile form of diffuse brain sclerosis, Brain 39:74, 1916.

165. Norman, R. M., Oppenheimer, D. R., and Tingey, A. H.: Histological and chemical findings in Krabbe's leucodystrophy, J. Neurol. Neurosurg. Psychiat. 24:223, 1961.

166. Austin, J. H. and Lehfeldt, D.: Studies in globoid (Krabbe) leukodystrophy: Significance of experimentally produced globoid-like elements in rat white matter and spleen, J. Neuropath. Exp. Neurol. 24:265, 1965.

167. Andrews, J. H., et al: Globoid cell leukodystrophy (Krabbe's disease): Morphological and biochemical studies, Neurology 21:337, 1971.

168. Hogan, G. R., Gutmann, L., and Chou, S. M.: The peripheral neuropathy of Krabbe's (globoid) leukodystrophy, Neurology 19:1094, 1969.

169. Hager, H. and Oehlert, W.: Diffuse brain sclerosis of the Krabbe type as an inflammatory general disease, Z. Kinderheilk. 80:82, 1957.

170. Menkes, J. H., Duncan, C., and Moossy, J.: Molecular composition in the major glycolipids in globoid cell leukodystrophy, Neurology 16:581, 1966.

171. Suzuki, K. and Suzuki, Y.: Globoid cell leukodystrophy (Krabbe's disease): Deficiency of galactocerebroside beta-galactosidase, Proc. Nat. Acad. Sci. USA 66:302, 1970.

172. Bachhawat, B. K., Austin, J., and Armstrong, D.: A cerebroside sulphotransferase deficiency in a human disorder of myelin, Biochem. J. 104:15c, 1967.

173. Malone, M.: Deficiency in a degradative enzyme system in globoid leukodystrophy, Trans. Amer. Soc. Neurochem. 1:56, 1970.

174. Suzuki, Y. and Suzuki, K.: Krabbe's globoid cell leukodystrophy: Deficiency of galactocerebrosidase in serum, leukocytes and fibroblasts, Science 171:73, 1971.

174a. Miyatake, T. and Suzuki, K.: Globoid cell leukodystrophy: Additional deficiency of psychosine galactosidase, Biochem. Biophys. Res. Commun. 48:539, 1972.

175. Austin, J., Suzuki, K., and Armstrong, D.: Studies in globoid (Krabbe) leukodystrophy (GLD): V. Controlled enzymic studies in ten human cases, Arch. Neurol. 23:502, 1970.

176. Suzuki, K.: Renal cerebroside in globoid cell leukodystrophy (Krabbe's disease), Lipids 6:433, 1971.

177. Cockayne, E. A.: Dwarfism with retinal atrophy and deafness, Arch. Dis. Child. 11:1, 1936.

178. Macdonald, W. B., Fitch, K. D., and Lewis, I. C.: Cockayne's syndrome, Pediatrics 25:997, 1960.

179. Moossy, J.: The neuropathology of Cockayne's syndrome, J. Neuropath. Exp. Neurol. 26:654, 1967.

180. Moosa, A. and Dubowitz, V.: Peripheral neuropathy in Cockayne's syndrome, Arch. Dis. Child. 45:674, 1970.

181. Chediak, M.: Nouvelle anomalie leucocytaire de caractere constitutionnel et familial, Rev. Hemat. 7:362, 1952.

182. Donohue, W. L. and Bain, H. W.: Chediak-Higashi syndrome, Pediatrics 20:416, 1957.

183. Sheramata, W., Kott, S., and Cyr, D. P.: The Chediak-Higashi-Steinbrinck syndrome, Arch. Neurol. 25:289, 1971.

184. Sung, J. H., et al.: Neuropathological changes in Chediak-Higashi disease, J. Neuropath. Exp. Neurol. 28:86, 1969.

185. Alpers, B. J.: Diffuse progressive degeneration of the cerebral gray matter, Arch. Neurol. Psychiat. 25:469, 1931.

186. Laurence, K. M. and Cavanagh, J. B.: Progressive degeneration of the cerebral cortex in infancy, Brain 91:261, 1968.

187. Ford, F. R., Livingston, S., and Pryles, C. V.: Familial degeneration of the cerebral gray matter in childhood, with convulsions, myoclonus, spasticity, cerebellar ataxia, choreoathetosis, dementia, and death in status epilepticus; differentiation of infantile and juvenile types, J. Pediat. 39:33, 1951.

188. Menkes, J. H., et al.: A sex-linked recessive disorder with growth retardation, peculiar hair, and focal cerebral and cerebellar degeneration, Pediatrics 29:764, 1962.

189. Danks, D. M., et al.: Menkes' kinky hair syndrome: Defect in copper absorption, Pediatrics 50:188, 1972.

190. O'Brien, J. S. and Sampson, E. L.: Kinky hair disease, II.. Biochemical studies, J. Neuropath. Exp. Neurol. 25:523, 1966.

191. Cowen, D. and Olmstead, E. V.: Infantile neuroaxonal dystrophy, J. Neuropath. Exp. Neurol. 22:175, 1963.

192. Duncan, C., et al.: Peripheral nerve biopsy as an aid to diagnosis in infantile neuroaxonal dystrophy, Neurology 20:1024, 1970.

193. Herman, M. M., Huttenlocher, P. R., and Bensch, K. G.: Electron microscopic observations in infantile neuroaxonal dystrophy, Arch. Neurol. 20:19, 1969.

Chromosomal
Anomalies

CHAPTER 3

The single most common neurologic associate of chromosomal anomalies is impaired intellectual function. This is not unexpected since rearrangement of genetic material to such a degree as to be visible as altered chromosomal morphology must involve numerous genetic loci and interfere extensively with growth and differentiation of the developing human zygote. Mental retardation associated with autosomal chromosomal aberrations is accompanied either by gross anatomic or by microscopic malformations of the central nervous system.

As with inborn errors of metabolism, the incidence of mental defect in chromosomal abnormalities is difficult to ascertain because of the strong bias in the sample of population surveyed for chromosomal abnormalities. Many of the abnormal sex chromosome constitutions have been ascertained by surveys of the institutionally retarded, using sex chromatin analysis as the screening device. Abnormalities of the autosomes have been sought almost exclusively in children with multiple congenital anomalies and mental retardation. A better evaluation of the relationship of abnormal sex chromosome composition to intellectual defect is possible through follow-up studies on infants found to have abnormal chromosome patterns in surveys of newborn populations.[1] The use of fluorescent and heterochromatin staining to identify each

homologous pair of chromosomes will increase the incidence of detectable translocations and minor chromosome abnormalities. Studies in other species as well as our own[2] have shown that major duplications or deficiencies in the autosomes are frequently lethal. If the organism survives, trisomy usually causes severe and multiple congenital malformations. The improved sensitivity of cytogenetic diagnosis has led to the detection of minor chromosomal abnormalities in neurologically handicapped children. These findings must however be interpreted in the light of studies on normal population which have revealed chromosomal variants in the absence of obvious physical or intellectual defects.[3,4,5]

For the basic principles of cytogenetics, the reader may choose one of several excellent texts.[6,7] There are also reviews of aberrations involving autosomes,[8,9] sex chromosomes,[10] and mongolism.[11,12,13]

AUTOSOMAL ABNORMALITIES

MONGOLISM (DOWN'S SYNDROME)

By far the most common autosomal anomaly is associated with mongolism. Because of its frequency the cytogenetics of mongolism have been well worked out; this condition has served as prototype for the various aberrations and the genetic transmission of other autosomal abnormalities. The condition was differentiated from other forms of mental retardation by Down[14] and Seguin[15] in 1866.

Etiology and Pathogenesis

Mongolism is associated with either an extra number 21* chromosome,[16] or an effective trisomy for this chromosome by its translocation to another chromosome, usually a number 14 (D/G) or a number 21/22 (G/G). One cannot distinguish clinically between mongoloids with "regular" trisomy 21 from those with an effective trisomy translocation. The association of phenotypic mongoloids with a normal karyotype has been reported, although mosaicism can never be completely excluded,[17,18] and newer methods of cytogenetic diagnosis may uncover various chromosomal abnormalities.[19] The incidence of mongolism among newborn infants ranges from 1 in 478 to 1 in 1428,[1,20] and the condition accounts for some 10 to 20 percent of inmates of state hospitals.

The frequency of "regularly" trisomic mongols increases with maternal age[21] reaching an incidence of 1 in 54 births to mothers aged 45 or more.[22] About 1 in 40 of spontaneous abortions have a mongoloid karyotype. But the incidence of translocation mongolism is independent of maternal age. Most translocations producing mongolism arise de novo in the affected child and are not associated with familial mongolism. Data obtained from the study of 227 mongols of mothers aged 15 to 29 show 92 percent "regular" trisomy to 8 percent with translocation.[23] Of the 18 translocation mongols, 13 involved a translocation between the number 21 chromosome and the D† group, while five showed a translocation involving two G* group chromosomes. In only four of the translocation mongoloids, all of them 14/21 (D/G), were the mothers carriers of the translocation, so that the incidence of translocation carriers in families of mongoloids is low.

Rare families have been reported in which there are more than one "regularly" trisomic mongoloid.[24] In some of these families there

* Denver classification.
† According to group nomenclature of Patau.

may be a transmittable tendency to meiotic errors with multiple occurrence of aneuploidy in their offspring.[25] The factors producing nondisjunction are poorly understood. They include such known associations as maternal age and a familial tendency to nondisjunction and possible external influences such as infections by viruses or other organisms[26] and exposure to radiation.

How the presence of a small acrocentric chromosome in triplicate produces the mongoloid phenotype is still unknown. Patients with normal or nearly normal intelligence have been found to have atypical cytogenetic features, including partial trisomy[27] or mosaicism.[28]

Numerous attempts to map the number 21 chromosome have been unsuccessful. The activity of a number of enzymes, including alkaline phosphatase,[29] galactose-1-phosphate uridyl transferase,[30] and glucose-6-phosphate dehydrogenase,[31] is inconsistently increased in the leukocyte of mongols, but these abnormalities may represent a generalized disturbance of enzyme regulation. The demonstration of reduced serotonin in the whole blood of "regularly" trisomic mongoloids and normal levels in translocation mongoloids, is due to reduced platelet levels of the monoamine. The conversion of tryptophan to 5-hydroxyindoleacetic acid is normal, as is monoamine oxidase activity in platelets.[32] Metabolism of serotonin in brain is normal.

Pathology

Malformation affects principally the heart and the great vessels. About 20%–60% of mongoloids suffer from congenital heart disease. Defects in the atrioventricular septum were the most common abnormalities encountered by Rowe and Uchida[33] in 36% of their patients, most of whom were under two years of age. A ventricular septal defect was present in 33%, and a patent ductus arteriosus in 10% of patients. Among the other malformations, gastrointestinal anomalies are the most common. These include duodenal stenosis or atresia, anal atresia, and megacolon. Malformations of the spine, particularly of the upper cervical region, may occasionally produce neurologic symptoms.[34]

Gross and microscopic abnormalities within

the nervous system are minor, inconsistent, and nonspecific. Grossly, the brain is small and spherical, and the frontal lobes, brain stem, and cerebellum are smaller than normal. The secondary sulci are generally reduced in number and the superior temporal gyrus is poorly developed. A number of microscopic abnormalities have also been described.[35,36] These include a diffuse or patchy reduction of nerve cells in the third cortical layer, fibrillary gliosis of the central white matter, and persistence of the tuber flocculi, an accumulation of undifferentiated fetal cells in the cerebellum. In a few patients, particularly those dying in infancy, demyelinated patches are observed in the periventricular white matter, where they are accompanied by fat-filled granular cells. The most usual neuropathologic finding is the premature development of senile changes unassociated with cerebral arteriosclerosis. These are found in nearly all subjects dying after 35 years and may already be evident during the first decade.[37] Microscopic alterations include pigmentary degeneration of neurons, Alzheimer's neurofibrillary changes, senile plaques, and calcium deposits within the basal ganglia and cerebellar folia.

The relation of these pathologic findings to the clinical picture cannot be determined. A number of mongoloid children die of congenital heart disease or sepsis, processes which may readily result in some of the minor microscopic alterations. On the other hand, failure in gyral development and aplasia of the brain stem and cerebellum represent structural anomalies which may be the direct result of the chromosome disorder itself.

No major abnormalities in the constitution of the brain lipids have been noted.[38]

Clinical Manifestations

The clinical picture of Down's syndrome is protean and consists of an unusual combination of anomalies, rather than of unusual anomalies.[12,20]

Most important is the mental and physical retardation. The birth weight of mongoloid infants is less than normal, and 20% weigh $5\frac{1}{2}$ lbs. or less.[39] Neonatal complications are more common than normal, physical growth is consistently delayed, and the adult mongoloid is significantly retarded in height.[40] There is considerable variability in the mental age which is ultimately achieved. In part this is related to environmental factors, including age of institutionalization, degree of intellectual stimulation, and the early evolution of presenile dementia even prior to puberty. As a rule the developmental quotient (DQ) is higher than the intelligence quotient (IQ) and decreases with age (Table 3–1). Most of the older patients with Down's syndrome have IQs between 25 and 49, with the average about 43. The social adjustment tends to be about three years ahead of that expected for the mental age.[12]

At present there is no evidence that when mongolism is phenotypically evident the prognosis for intellectual function in mosaicism is better than in complete trisomy.[41]

Aside from mental retardation, specific neurologic signs are rare and are limited to generalized muscular hypotonia and hyperextensibility of the joints. This is particularly evident during infancy and presents to a significant degree in 44 percent of subjects under nine years of age.[42]

In addition to these neurologic abnormalities, patients with Down's syndrome exhibit a number of stigmata. None of these are invariably present, nor are they consistently absent in the normal population, but their conjunction contributes to the characteristic appearance of the mongoloid.

The eyes show numerous abnormalities. The palpebral fissures are oblique and narrow

Table 3-1. Intellectual Functioning of Children with Down's Syndrome*

Age (yrs.)		Mean	Standard Deviation	Range
0–1	DQ	65	±15	27–100
1–2	DQ	51	±11	23–73
2–3	DQ	46	± 8	32–55
3–4	IQ	43	±16	10–55
4–9	IQ	43	± 7	10–61

* After Loeffler, F. and Smith, G. F., cited in Penrose and Smith.[12]

laterally; there is a persistence of a complete median epicanthal fold, a fetal characteristic rarely present in normal children over 10 but observed in 47 percent of mongoloids aged 5–10 and in 30 percent of older subjects.[43] The Brushfield spots are an accumulation of fibrous tissue in the superficial layer of the iris. They appear as slightly elevated light spots encircling the periphery of the iris (Fig. 3-1).

According to Donaldson they are present in 85 percent of mongols, as compared with 24 percent of control subjects.[44] Blepharitis and conjunctivitis are common, as are lenticular opacifications, particularly in older subjects.

Anomalies of the external ear are common. The ear is low-set, while the helix is angular, the tragus hypoplastic, and the cartilage often deficient. The lips have radial furrows

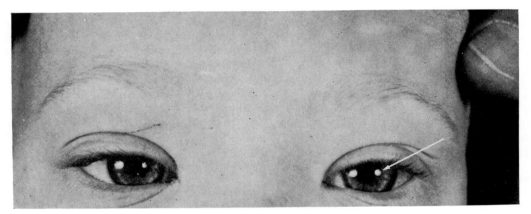

Fig. 3–1.   Five-year-old child with Down's syndrome demonstrating Brushfield spots (arrow). (Courtesy of Dr. H. Zellweger, Department of Pediatrics, University of Iowa.)

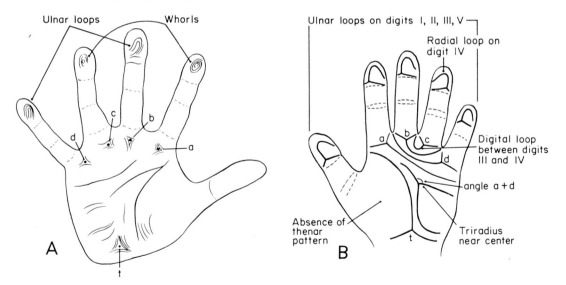

Fig. 3–2.   Outlines of the digital, palmar, and plantar configurations. **A.** Normal child. The triradii are *a*, *b*, *c*, *d*, and *t*—the meeting point of sets of parallel ridges; *t* is located near the base of the fourth metacarpal bone at some point on its axis. **B.** Child with Down's syndrome. There is a transverse palmar crease, fingers tend to have a loop pattern, the triradius *t* subtends an angle of about 80° with points *a* and *d* instead of the normal 45°. (After Penrose, L. S., Nature, 227:933, 1963.)

and, as a consequence of the generalized hypotonia, the tongue, often fissured, tends to protrude. A typical finding, particularly evident in infants, is a roll of fat in the nape of the neck.

The extremities are short. The little finger is incurved, and the middle phalanx hypoplastic. As a consequence, its distal interphalangeal crease is proximal to the proximal interphalangeal crease of the ring finger. The simian fold, a transverse palmar crease, is present bilaterally in 45% of patients[37] (Fig. 3–2). In the feet a diastasis between the first and second toe is the most characteristic anatomic abnormality.

The dermatoglyphic pattern of the mongoloid shows several abnormalities. Of these a distally displaced triradius, the palmar meeting point of three differently aligned crease lines, is seen in 88% of mongoloids but in only 10% of nonmongoloid subjects.[12] Dermatoglyphic abnormalities of the finger print patterns are equally characteristic[12, 45,45a] (Fig. 3–2).

Abnormalities of the skin are common. Xeroderma and localized chronic hyperkeratotic lichenification are seen in 90% and 75% of subjects respectively.

A number of factors have contributed to a reduced life expectancy which is currently about 18 years. In order of importance, these are a high susceptibility to infectious diseases, a high incidence of major cardiovascular malformations, an incidence of leukemia which is fifteen times that of the general population,[46] and the early appearance of dementia.

Diagnosis

The diagnosis of Down's syndrome is made by an examination of the chromosome pattern. Quinacrine fluorescence microscopy allows differentiation between chromosomes 21 and 22 and specific identification of the chromosomes involved in translocation Down's syndrome.[46a]

While radiographic abnormalities are not pathognomonic for Down's syndrome, they assist in the diagnosis. Typically, the skull is brachycephalic, and the anterior fontanelle and the metopic suture close late. The iliac wings and bodies are widened, resulting in a

more acute acetabular angle in at least 80 percent of patients, measured according to Caffey and Ross.[47] Cytogenetic studies of amniotic fluid can be used for the antenatal diagnosis of Down's syndrome as early as the third month of gestation although the detection of mosaicism may present considerable problems.[48,48a]

Treatment

Despite the number of vigorously and fervently advocated regimens, none have proven successful in improving the mental deficit of the mongoloid child. Currently, medical intervention is limited to prophylaxis against infections and, if possible, correction of the congenital heart disease or other significant malformations.

The early administration of 5-hydroxytryptophan, a 5-hydroxytryptamine (serotonin) precursor, appears to reverse the muscular hypotonia characteristically present in the mongoloid infant,[49] and may in some instances accelerate motor milestones. It is unlikely, however, that this form of treatment will have any effect on the ultimate level of intelligence.

The treatment of the mentally retarded mongoloid is that of children retarded due to any causes and having the same potential of intellectual and social function. The subject is discussed in Chapter 13.

Trisomy of an apparent group G chromosome (trisomy 22) has been reported in the absence of mongolism in males or females. Trisomy 22 is associated with mental retardation, while a 47, XYY complement may be found with increased height only.[20,50]

OTHER ABNORMALITIES OF AUTOSOMES

Trisomies involving the other, larger chromosomes are associated with multiple severe malformations of the brain and viscera, and affected children usually do not survive infancy. The two entities most commonly encountered are trisomies of chromosomes 13 and 18.

CHROMOSOME 13 (D₁) TRISOMY (PATAU'S SYNDROME)

This anomaly occurs in one out of 5000 births. The clinical picture is characterized

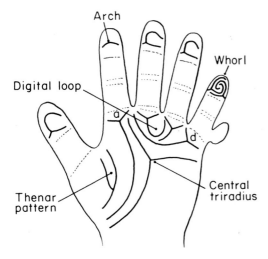

Fig. 3–3. Dermatoglyphics in trisomy 13. Polydactyly is present. The *a-t-d*-angle is almost 90°. Unlike in Down's syndrome, both arches and whorls may be present. (After Penrose, L. S., Nature, 227: 933, 1963.)

by feeding difficulties, apneic spells during early infancy, and striking developmental retardation.[51,52,53,54] Subjects have varying degrees of median facial anomalies, including hairlip or cleft palate, and micrognathia. The ears are low-set and malformed, and many infants appear deaf. Polydactyly, flexion deformities of the fingers, and a horizontal palmar crease are common. The dermatoglyphics are abnormal and often diagnostic (Fig. 3–3). Eighty percent of patients have cardiovascular anomalies, most commonly a patent ductus arteriosus, or a ventricular septal defect. About one-third of patients have polycystic kidneys. Microcephaly is present in 83 percent and microphthalmus in 74 percent.[52]

The major neurologic abnormality is arhinencephaly, a complex group of malformations which have in common absence of the olfactory bulbs and tracts with the presence of other cerebral anomalies. The cerebral malformations vary in severity from simple agenesis of the superficial olfactory pathways to a cyclopian brain with a single ventricle. On autopsy there are a number of microscopic malformations including heterotopic nerve cells in the cerebellum and in the subcortical white matter.[55] This anomaly while seen in about two-thirds of patients with chromosome 13 trisomy is not completely specific. Absent olfactory apparatus also occurs with a normal karyotype, and with deletion of the short arm of chromosome 18 and in the 18 (E₁) trisomy syndrome.[56] The prognosis for children with chromosome 13 trisomy is poor. About half die during the first month of life, and only 20 percent survive into the second year.

CHROMOSOME 18 (E₁) TRISOMY (EDWARD'S SYNDROME)

This anomaly occurs with a frequency of about 1 in 4500. The clinical picture is highlighted by a long narrow skull, low-set malformed ears, a webbed neck, and marked physical and mental retardation.[52,53,57] The second finger characteristically overlies the third, and distally implanted, retroflexible thumbs are frequently encountered. As in chromosome 13 trisomy, polycystic kidneys and congenital heart disease are common. A striking dermatoglyphic pattern, relatively less common in other autosomal anomalies, is the presence of simple arches in all fingers.

No consistent central nervous system malformation is associated with the trisomy 18 syndrome. The brain is grossly normal; microscopically, heterotopias of white matter are often seen, but not with the frequency encountered in trisomy 13.[55] The prognosis for children with chromosome 18 trisomy is poor, and 90 percent die by one year of age.

Other trisomies have been found in spontaneous human abortions.[58]

STRUCTURAL AUTOSOMAL ANOMALIES

Major structural autosomal anomalies are much less frequent than trisomies. The most common entity is cri du chat syndrome, a deletion of the short arm of the number 5 chromosome. This condition is seen with a frequency of 1 in 50,000 to 100,000 births.[59]

A low birth weight and failure in physical growth is associated with a characteristic cry likened to that of a meowing kitten. Infants have microcephaly, large corneas, moon-shaped faces, ocular hypertelorism, epicanthal folds, a transverse palmar (Simian) crease, and generalized muscular hypotonia.

The brain, though small, is grossly and microscopically normal, representing a rare example of true microcephaly[60] (see Chapter 4).

The other structural autosomal anomalies associated with neurologic symptoms are summarized in Table 3–2.

It is necessary to point out that in some instances the association of multiple congenital anomalies with a structural chromosomal anomaly may be fortuitous. Structural variants of autosomes, as for example deletion of the short arm of chromosome 5, may be asymptomatic and familial.[70]

When a battery of currently available techniques is used to screen a population of developmentally retarded children, minor structural chromosomal abnormalities are seen in 10%–20%. Often these are small differences in the length of the chromosomal arms and only evident upon examination of the homologues. In the normal population the incidence of these defects is much lower, but their significance in terms of being associated with physical abnormalities is still far from established.[71]

Table 3-2. Some Structural Autosomal Anomalies Associated with Neurologic Symptoms

Chromosomal Anomaly	Clinical Picture	Reference
Deletion short arm of no. 5	Microcephaly, kitten cry	Lejeune, et al.[59]
	Hypertelorism, epicanthal folds	Solitare[60]
Deletion short arm of no. 4	Midline deficits, mental retardation, ptosis	Warburton, et al.[61]
Partial deletion short arm of no. 4	Mental retardation, microcephaly, hypotonia, hypertelorism, broad base of nose, ptosis, carp mouth, normal cry	Miller, et al.[62]
Deletion short arm of no. 18	Congenital ptosis, microcephaly, hypertelorism, epicanthal folds	Nitowsky, et al.[63]
Deletion long arm of no. 18	Hypoplasia of nasomaxillary region, microcephaly, carp mouth	Wertelecki, et al.[64]
Deletion long arm of no. 5	Mental retardation, microphthalmos	Lele, et al.[65]
Ring 18 chromosome*	Mental retardation, bilateral atresia external auditory meatus	deGrouchy, et al.[66]
Ring D chromosome*	Microcephaly, absent thumbs, coloboma of iris, nystagmus	Sparkes, et al.[67]
Ring C chromosome*	Antimongoloid slant of palpebral fissures, longish nose, large ears, elongated skull	Turner, et al.[68]
Ring 22 chromosome*	Retardation of growth and development, depressed bridge of nose	Hoefnagel, et al.[69]

* Phenotypic expression of ring chromosomes may be variable.

SEX CHROMOSOME ABNORMALITIES

As determined by surveys of the newborn population[1,10] or of amniotic sex chromatin patterns in placentas,[72] the incidence of sex chromosome abnormalities is about 0.8 to 2.1 per 1000 for phenotypic males and 1.6 to 2.2 per 1000 for phenotypic females. Although there appears to be considerable geographic variation, the most common abnormality in the male is XXY or Klinefelter's syndrome.[1] The great majority of the abnormalities (75%) in females involve the triple X syndrome (XXX), with less than 25% being X monosomies (Turner's syndrome) or variants thereof.[1,73]

KLINEFELTER'S SYNDROME

This clinical condition was first described by Klinefelter in 1942 in male patients who suffered from increased development of breasts, lack of spermatogenesis, and an increased excretion of follicle stimulating hormone. The chromosomal constitution of XXY, present in most subjects, was elucidated in 1959.

Although electroencephalographic abnormalities including spike and spike and wave discharges are common,[74] the principal neurologic deficit encountered in Klinefelter's syndrome is mental retardation.

Surveys of male inmates in mental institutions reveal a greater incidence of XXY males (5.4 per 1000) than in the newborn population.[73]

But using a small, selected sample, Money has shown that Klinefelter's syndrome is not invariably associated with an intellectual deficit and that the IQ distribution of patients with this disease approximates the normal curve.[75] When retardation does occur in the XXY karyotype it usually is not severe. Many patients are hospitalized for psychoses and antisocial behavior.

XYY KARYOTYPE

The XYY karyotype is the second most common chromosomal anomaly encountered in the phenotypical male, with a frequency as high as 4 per 1000 male newborns.[75a]

The XYY karyotype has been associated with unusually tall stature and antisocial behavior, the frequency of the latter being still unascertained.[76] As a rule, patients are not mentally retarded. Neurologic abnormalities include intention tremor, mild motor incoordination,[77] and limitation of motion at the elbows, secondary to radio-ulnar synostoses.[78]

Since the subjects, in general, have been ascertained by surveys in prison populations, the validity of the phenotype-karyotype correlation remains to be seen.[79]

The XYYY child reported by Townes and associates was only mildly retarded,[80] while all of the twelve XXXYY males reviewed by Schlegel[81] had major intellectual deficit with IQs varying from 35 to 74.

In the XXXY syndrome there are severe mental retardation, small testes, microcephaly, and a variety of minor deformities.[82] The XXXXY chromosomal anomaly is characterized by mental retardation, hypotonia, and a facial appearance reminiscent of Down's syndrome. The palpebral fissures are slanted, there are epicanthal folds, excess posterior cervical skin, and widely separated eyes. The fifth digits are usually short and incurved.[83]

TURNER'S SYNDROME

In 1938 Turner described a syndrome of sexual infantilism, cubitus valgus, and webbed neck in women of short stature. Ford, in 1959, found this condition to be generally associated with the XO chromosomal structure. At least 80% of subjects are sex-chromatin negative and have the XO karyotype, while the remainder are chromatin-positive and have an XO/XX karyotype or, less commonly, other mosaicisms.

While the clinical and endocrinologic picture of Turner's syndrome is complex, we confine ourselves to the neurologic symptoms. As a rule, absence of the X chromosome is not associated with an intellectual deficit,[75] and the incidence of Turner's syndrome is no greater in the institutionalized retarded than in the newborn.[73] But the majority of patients have a right-left disorientation and a defect in perceptual organization,[84] leading to a deficit in achievement on performance as compared to verbal items on the Wechsler intelligence tests.

A syndrome, phenotypically similar to Turner's, but in karyotypically normal females and males (pseudo-Turner's syndrome) is commonly associated with eighth-nerve deafness and mental retardation.[85]

The presence in the female of more than two X chromosomes may be associated with mental retardation. Although there is no specific clinical pattern for females with XXX sex chromosome complement, some are mildly retarded although this may reflect the method of ascertainment. As a consequence the frequency of this karyotype among institutionalized retarded is 4.3 per 1000, over three times more than in the normal newborn.[1,86] The tetrasomic and pentasomic X females are usually mentally retarded.[87]

THE ROLE OF CYTOGENETICS IN NEUROLOGIC DIAGNOSIS

It is usually not feasible to apply the battery of currently available cytogenetic techniques for the diagnosis of the neurologically handicapped child. Rather, the physician must select the patient for whom such time-consuming and expensive studies have the greatest likelihood of yielding a diagnosis.

It has been our practice to suggest cytogenetic studies in children with developmental retardation who have congenital anomalies, particularly when these involve mesodermal and endodermal germ layers. Other clinical features which prompt us to request chromosomal studies are small stature, abnormalities in the configuration of the face or extremities, unusual dermatoglyphics, microcephaly, and the syndrome of muscular hypotonia with brisk deep tendon reflexes ("atonic cerebral palsy").

REFERENCES

1. Hamerton, J. L., et al.: Chromosome studies in a neonatal population, Canad. Med. Ass. J. 106:776, 1972.
2. Carr, D. H.: Chromosome studies in abortuses and stillborn infants, Lancet 2:603, 1963.
3. Migeon, B. R.: Familial variant autosomes: New human cytogenetic markers, Bull. Hopkins Hosp. 116:396, 1965.
4. Jacobs, P. A.: In Harris, R. J. C. (ed.): Cytogenetics of Cells in Culture, New York: Academic Press, 1964.
5. Court-Brown, W. M. and Smith, P. G.: Human population cytogenetics, Brit. Med. Bull. 25:74, 1969.
6. Hamerton, J. L.: Human Cytogenetics, New York: Academic Press Inc., 1971.
7. Engel, E.: "The Chromosome Basis of Human Heredity," in Stanbury, J. B., Wyngaarden, J. B., and Fredrickson, D. S. (eds.): The Metabolic Basis of Inherited Disease, New York: McGraw-Hill Book Co., 1972, pp. 52–82.
8. Polani, P. E.: Chromosome anomalies, Ann. Rev. Med. 15:93, 1964.
9. Polani, P. E.: Autosomal imbalance and its syndromes, excluding Down's, Brit. Med. Bull. 25:81, 1969.
10. Jacobs, P. A.: Structural abnormalities of the sex chromosomes, Brit. Med. Bull. 25:94, 1969.
11. Wolstenholme, G. E. W. and Porter, R. (eds.): Mongolism, Ciba Foundation Study Group No. 25, London: Churchill, 1967.
12. Penrose, L. W. and Smith, G. F.: Down's Anomaly, London: Churchill, 1966.
13. Apgar, V. (ed.): Down's Syndrome (mongolism), Ann. NY Acad. Sci. 171:303, 1970.
14. Down, J. L. H.: Observation on an ethnic classification of idiots, Clin. Lect. Rep., London Hosp. 3:259, 1866.
15. Seguin, E.: Idiocy: Its Treatment by the Physiological Method, New York: William Wood Co., 1866.
16. Lejeune, J., Gautier, M., and Turpin, R.: Genetique—etude des chromosomes somatiques de neuf enfants mongoliens, C. R. Acad. Sci. (Paris) 248:1721, 1959.
17. Hall, B.: Down's syndrome with normal chromosomes, Lancet 2:1026, 1962.
18. Sergovich, F. R., et al.: Mongolism (Down's syndrome) with atypical clinical and cytogenetic features, J. Pediat. 65:197, 1964.
19. Uchida, I. A. and Lin, C. C.: Identification of partial 12 trisomy by quinacrine fluorescence, J. Pediat. 82:269, 1973.
20. Zellweger, H.: Mongolismus—Down's syndrome, Ergebn. Inn. Med. Kinderheilk. 22:268, 1965.
21. Penrose, L. S.: Maternal age in familial mongolism, J. Mental Sci. 97:738, 1951.
22. Penrose, L. S.: Mongolism, Brit. Med. Bull. 17:184, 1961.
23. Petersen, C. D. and Luzzatti, L.: The role of chromosome translocation in the recurrence risk of Down's syndrome, Pediatrics 35:463, 1965.
24. Hamerton, J. L., et al: Chromosome studies in detection of parents with high risk of second child with Down's syndrome, Lancet 2:788, 1961.
25. Turner, B., den Dulk, G. M., and Watkins, G.: The 17–18 trisomy and 21 trisomy syndromes in siblings, J. Pediat. 64:601, 1964.
26. Nichols, W. W.: Viruses and chromosomal abnormalities, Ann. NY Acad. Sci. USA 171:478, 1970.
27. Dent, T., Edwards, J. H., and Delhanty, J. D. A.: A partial mongol, Lancet 2:484, 1963.
28. Clarke, C. M., Edwards, J. H., and Smallpiece, E. V.: 21-Trisomy/normal mosaicism in an intelligent child with some mongoloid characters, Lancet 1:1028, 1961.

29. Alter, A. A., et al.: Leukocyte alkaline phosphatase in mongolism; a possible chromosome marker, J. Clin. Invest. 41:1341, 1962.

30. Brandt, N. J., et al.: Galactosemia locus and the Down's syndrome chromosome, Lancet 2:700, 1963.

31. Mellman, W. J., et al.: Leucocyte enzymes in Down's syndrome, Lancet 2:674, 1964.

32. Lott, I. T., Murphy, D. L., and Chase, T. N.: Down's syndrome. Central monoamine turnover in patients with diminished platelet serotonin, Neurology (Minneap.) 22:967, 1972.

33. Rowe, D. R. and Uchida, I. A.: Cardiac malformation in mongolism, Amer. J. Med. 31:726, 1961.

34. Dzenitis, A. J.: Spontaneous atlanto-axial dislocation in a mongoloid child with spinal cord compression, J. Neurosurg. 25:458, 1966.

35. Meyer, A. and Jones, T. B.: Histologic changes in the brain in mongolism, J. Mental Sci. 85:206, 1939.

36. Davidoff, L. M.: The brain in mongolian idiocy, Arch. Neurol. Psychiat. 20:1229, 1928.

37. Olson, M. I. and Shaw, C. M.: Presenile dementia and Alzheimer's disease in mongolism, Brain 92:147, 1969.

38. Stephens, M. C. and Menkes, J. H.: Cerebral lipids in Down's syndrome, Devel. Med. Child Neurol. 11:346, 1969.

39. Levinson, A., Friedman, A., and Stamps, F.: Variability of mongolism, Pediatrics 16:43, 1955.

40. Cowie, V. A.: *A Study of the Early Development of Mongols*, Oxford: Pergamon Press, 1970.

41. Kohn, G., et al.: Mosaic mongolism. I. Clinical correlations, J. Pediat. 76:874, 1970.

42. Loesch-Mdzewska, D.: Some aspects of the neurology of Down's syndrome, J. Ment. Defic. Res. 12:237, 1968.

43. Eissler, R. and Longenecker, L. P.: The common eye findings in mongolism, Amer. J. Ophthal. 54:3984, 1962.

44. Donaldson, D. D.: The significance of spotting of the iris in mongoloids, Arch. Ophthal. 65:26, 1961.

45. Holt, S. B.: Fingerprint patterns in mongolism, Ann. Hum. Genet. 27:279, 1964.

45a. Reed, T. E., et al.: Dermatoglyphic nomogram for the diagnosis of Down's syndrome, J. Pediat. 77:1024, 1970.

46. Krivit, W. and Good, R. A.: Simultaneous occurrence of mongolism and leukemia, Amer. J. Dis. Child. 94:289, 1957.

46a. Alfi, O. S., Donnell, G. N., and Derencsenyi, A.: Identification of the G. chromosomes in Down's syndrome by quinacrine fluorescence microscopy, J. Pediat. 79:656, 1971.

47. Caffey, J. and Ross, S.: Pelvic bones in infantile mongoloidism, Amer. J. Roentgen. 80:458, 1958.

48. Nadler, H. L. and Gerbie, A. B.: Amniocentesis in the intrauterine detection of genetic disorders, New Eng. J. Med. 282:596, 1970.

48a. Kardon, N. B., et al.: Pitfalls in prenatal diagnosis resulting from chromosomal mosaicism, J. Pediat. 80:297, 1972.

49. Bazelon, M., et al.: Reversal of hypotonia in infants with Down's syndrome by administration of 5-hydroxytryptophan, Lancet 1:1130, 1967.

50. Hsu, L. Y. F., et al.: Trisomy 22: A clinical study, J. Pediat. 79:12, 1971.

51. Patau, K., et al.: Multiple congenital anomaly caused by an extra autosome, Lancet 1:790, 1960.

52. Taylor, A. I.: Patau's, Edwards' and Cri du chat syndromes: A tabulated summary of current findings, Develop. Med. Child Neurol. 9:78, 1967.

53. Taylor, A. I.: Autosomal trisomy syndromes: A detailed study of 27 cases of Edward's syndrome and 27 cases of Patau's syndrome, J. Med. Genet. 5:227, 1968.

54. Snodgrass, G. J. A., et al.: The "D" (13–15) trisomy syndrome: An analysis of seven examples, Arch. Dis. Child. 41:250, 1966.

55. Norman, R. M.: Neuropathological findings in trisomies 13–15 and 17–18 with special reference to the cerebellum, Develop. Med. Child Neurol. 8:170, 1966.

56. Migeon, B. R. and Young, W. J.: Reciprocal D:E translocation: Euploid transmission in three generations, Bull. Hopkins Hosp. 115:379, 1964.

57. Edwards, J. H., et al.: A new trisomic syndrome, Lancet 1:787, 1960.

58. Szulman, A. E.: Chromosomal aberrations in spontaneous human abortions, New Eng. J. Med. 272:811, 1965.

59. Lejeune, J., et al.: Three cases of partial deletion of the short arm of chromosome 5, C. R. Acad. Sci. (Paris) 257:3068, 1964.

60. Solitare, G. B.: The cri du chat syndrome: Neuropathologic observations, J. Ment. Defic. Res. 11:267, 1967.

61. Warburton, D., et al.: Distinction between chromosome 4 and chromosome 5 by replication pattern and length of long and short arms, Amer. J. Hum. Genet. 19:399, 1967.

62. Miller, O. J., et al.: Partial deletion of the short arm of chromosome no. 4 (4p–): Clinical studies in five unrelated patients, J. Pediat. 75:792, 1970.

63. Nitowsky, H. M., et al.: Partial 18 monosomy in the cyclops malformation, Pediatrics 37:260, 1966.

64. Wertelecki, W., Schindler, A. M., and Gerald, P. S.: Partial deletion of chromosome 18, Lancet 2:641, 1966.

65. Lele, K. P., Penrose, L. S., and Stallard, H. B.: Chromosome deletion in a case of retinoblastoma, Ann. Hum. Genet. 27:171, 1963.

66. de Grouchy, J., Herrault, A., and Cohen-Solal, J.: Une observation de chromosome 18 en anneau (18r), Ann. Genet. (Paris) 11:33, 1968.

67. Sparkes, R. S., Carrel, R. E., and Wright, S. W.: Absent thumbs with a ring D_2 chromosome. A new deletion syndrome, Amer. J. Hum. Genet. 19:644, 1967.

68. Turner, B., et al.: A self-perpetuating ring chromosome, Med. J. Aust. 49:56, 1962.

69. Hoefnagel, D., et al.: A child with group G ring chromosome, Humangenetik 4:52, 1967.

70. Migeon, B. R.: Familial variant autosomes. New human cytogenetic markers, Bull. Hopkins Hosp. 116:396, 1965.

71. Lubs, H. A., Ewing, L., and Merrick, S.: How useful are the new cytogenetic technics? Pediat. Res. 6:330, 1972

72. Eller, E., et al.: Prognosis in newborn infants with X-chromosomal abnormalities, Pediatrics 47:681, 1971.

73. Miller, O. J.: The sex chromosome anomalies, Amer. J. Obstet. Gynec. 90:1078, 1964.

74. Dumermuth, G.: EEG Untersuchungen beim jugendlichen Klinefelter-syndrom, Helv. Paediat. Acta 16:702, 1961.

75. Money, J.: Two cytogenetic syndromes: Psychologic comparisons. I. Intelligence and specific factor quotients, J. Psychiat. Res. 2:223, 1964.

75a. Sergovich, F., et al.: Chromosome aberrations in 2159 consecutive newborn babies, New Eng. J. Med. 280:851, 1969.

76. Court-Brown, W. M.: Males with an XYY sex chromosome complement, J. Med. Genet. 5:341, 1968.

77. Daly, R. F.: Neurological abnormalities in XYY males, Nature 221:472, 1969.

78. Arias, D. and Smith, G. F.: Radio-ulnar synostosis, behavioral disturbance and XYY chromosomes, J. Pediat. 74:103, 1969.

79. Money, J., Gaskin, R. J., and Hall, H.: Impulse, aggression, and sexuality in the XYY syndrome, St. John's Law Rev. 44:220, 1970.

80. Townes, P. L., Ziegler, N. A., and Lenhard, L. W.: A patient with 48 chromosomes (XYYY), Lancet 1:1041, 1965.

81. Schlegel, R., et al.: Studies on a boy with XXYY chromosome constitution, Pediatrics 36:113, 1965.

82. Zollinger, H.: XXXY Syndrome: Two new observations at early age and review of literature, Helv. Paediat. Acta 24:589, 1969.

83. Zaleski, W. A., et al.: The XXXXY chromosome anomaly: Report of three new cases and review of 30 cases from the literature, Canad. Med. Ass. J. 94:1143, 1966.

84. Alexander, D., Walker, H. T., and Money, J.: Studies in direction sense. I. Turner's syndrome, Arch. Gen. Psychiat. (Chicago) 10:337, 1964.

85. Noonan, J. A.: Hypertelorism with Turner phenotype: New syndrome with associated congenital heart disease, Amer. J. Dis. Child. 116:373, 1968.

86. Barr, M. L., et al.: The triplo-X female, Canad. Med. Ass. J. 101:247, 1969.

87. Brody, J., Fitzgerald, M. G., and Spiers, A. S. D.: A female child with five X chromosomes, J. Pediat. 70:105, 1967.

Malformations of the Central Nervous System

Ronald S. Gabriel

CHAPTER 4

INTRODUCTION

The embryologic creation of brain and spinal cord from a prosaic fragment of tissue—the axial medullary plate—is a wondrous event. The faithful transmission of form in this creation, a unique occasion for each biologic species, remains an enigma. However, the various mysteries of transmission of substance have gradually yielded to the impatient violation of succeeding generations of biologists. Thus today almost all defects of CNS ontogenesis can be explained in terms of evolving anatomy of fetal brain, from the initial induction of the neural tube by primordial mesenchyme to the ultimate migration and organization of cellular and subcellular constituents, and elaboration of neuropil with synapse and myelin formation.

To summarize the ontogenetic development of the human nervous system during fetal life (Table 4–1) both the simultaneity and the sequence of events must be emphasized. Many different events happen at the same time and the concept of "critical period" or vulnerability in utero relative to a given noxious stimulus, i.e., degree of organ susceptibility when an insult strikes, accounts for the modern study of teratology.[1] The

sequence of embryonic events in man and the ability to modify them with noxious stimuli in experimental animals has led to the construction of biologic time tables of human fetal growth and has provided insight as to when major defects of embryogenesis are most likely to occur. It has illustrated two concepts: the increasing vulnerability with increasing cephalization of primates as they ascend the evolutionary scale; and "biologic Freudianism"[2] as it applies to fetal life, i.e. the origin determines the end. One of medicine's great challenges will be to exploit our expanding knowledge of teratology and apply it to preventive medicine.

In this respect neural ontogeny is critical since 75% of fetal deaths and 40% of deaths within the first year of life are secondary to CNS malformations.[3] CNS malformations comprise one-third of all congenital malformations identified in the perinatal period. Ninety percent are defects of neural tube closure and include anencephaly, spina bifida cystica, and hydrocephalus.[4] To the extent that the human birth process is unimportant for the development of the nervous system; to the extent that adult brain is relatively impervious to the wide variety of exogenous factors

These are cells from whence spring the dorsal root ganglia of spinal nerves, ganglia of cranial nerves V, VII, VIII, IX, X, sympathetic nervous system, and Schwann cells. Also during the fourth week mesoderm elaborates into vascular primordia and into somites, reaching a total of 40. The latter subdivide into three anlagen: myotome (muscle), dermatome (subcutaneous tissue), and sclerotome (vertebrae and skull). This is dependent upon neural tube induction of adjacent mesoderm and represents the third time-specific inductive process; this time ectoderm activates mesoderm.

During the fourth week autoradiographic studies of the neural tube using tritiated thymidine, a DNA precursor, demonstrate 100% labelling of premitotic cells of the germinal neural epithelium (neuroblasts) composing the neural tube.[10] This very active period of mitosis must be completed before cellular migration and organization can occur. At this time a fourth inductive process involves the elaboration of foregut entoderm to form anlagen for facial structures. This process is activated by rostral neural tube, the anlage for telencephalon, and by cephalic mesoderm, the anlage for facial bone and skull.

Failure in the facial-forebrain inductive process leads to disorders qualitatively different from disorders involving the other three inductive events. Thus, there is an interdependence of germ layers requiring mutual induction in at least four time-specific stages. These inductive processes occur in conjunction with and presumably as a consequence of transfer of substances between cells of different germ layers, a phenomenon unique to embryologic tissue.[11] Interference with growth during this period gives rise to a series of inductive failures, either dorsal (dysraphic) or anterior (facio-telencephalic).

CELLULAR PROLIFERATION AND MIGRATION (ONE MONTH TO POSTNATAL PERIOD)[8,12]

By 30 days human gestation, the major inductive processes are complete and cellular differentiation begins. The undifferentiated germinal cells of the neural tube, comprising the medullary epithelium, begin to proliferate at their locus of origin, the ependymal matrix zone, forming the borders of the embryonic ventricular system. These germinal cells include medulloblasts, precursors for neurons and oligodendroglia; spongioblasts, precursors for astrocytes and ependyma; and cell precursors for choroidal and pineal tissue. They are in various stages of active mitosis. Their dynamics can be studied both by colchicine which arrests mitosis and by radioactive thymidine which labels DNA. As cells cease mitosis they are no longer labelled and begin migration away from the matrix zone to form the surrounding mantle zone (gray matter). The mantle zone cells then develop cellular processes which extend laterally to form the marginal zone (white matter).

By seven weeks there is a second migration of post-mitotic cells from the medullary epithelium across both the mantle and the marginal zones to form cerebral cortex (gray matter). This "inside-out" sequence of cellular migration applies both to the zones of white and gray matter, and to the formation of cortical laminations, with earlier cells forming deeper layers and later arrivals passing through the deep layers to form superficial regions. By 12 weeks the cerebral cortex is highly cellular. Unique features of this cellularity are both the polarization of the neuron to allow uniform connectivity via axons and dendrites, and the fact that neurons originate before glial cells, and large pyramidal neurons before small granule or Golgi type I cells.

The same sequence of events occurs in the cerebellum, beginning somewhat later. A zone of germinal cells in the roof of the fourth ventricle arises by the 32nd day and enlarges through cellular proliferation. Between 60 to 80 days outward cell migrations begin, initially forming the cerebellar plate,[13] followed by successive waves of migration accounting for the roof nuclei (gray matter), the external cellular processes (white matter), and finally the surrounding cortex composed of Purkinje and granular cells (gray matter).

By 25 weeks gestation the adult number of neurons is reached, and neuronal proliferation in the cerebral cortex of man probably ceases. However, experimental animal models suggest that neuron production may occur postnatally in both the hippocampus and brain stem nuclei. Neuronal (Purkinje and granular cell) production in the cerebellar cortex of man and animals continues into the eleventh postnatal month and accounts for the vulnerability of this organ to a variety of postnatal insults. Successive generations of migrating cells continue to appear on the cortical landscape into the sixth postnatal month in the cerebrum and as long as the second postnatal year in the cerebellum. Clearly then, morphogenesis involves orderly and reproducible patterns of spatial and temporal events, in which the phylogenetically older brain has an earlier ontogenesis. Or more elegantly, "ontogeny recapitulates its phylogeny." The Aristotelian cosmos—patterns within patterns—finds its final expression in man's private cosmos, his head.

During this stage the pageant of rapid brain growth unfolds. At 30 days gestation bilateral cleavage in the telencephalic outpouching of forebrain heralds future cerebral hemispheres. Cerebral circulation is elaborated and eye development proceeds with cleft optic cups and ectoderm invagination of future lens. At 32 days the cerebellar plate primordium is evolving and at 35 days the brain is defined by five cerebral vesicles, accounting for all major subdivisions of the central nervous system. Optic and facial structures are further elaborated and choroid plexi appear. At 40 days the embryonic period ends. By 50 days the cerebral hemispheres, basal ganglia, thalamus, sympathetic and parasympathetic nerves, eyes, and cerebral blood vessels are well-differentiated. Between two to four months the cerebral cortex has a smooth outer surface and encloses a large ventricular system. Muscle becomes functional at this time. The corpus callosum is evident by three months and becomes the largest and most important fiber tract connecting the two cerebral hemispheres. This fiber tract, comprising a substantial portion of the marginal zone, is critical in guiding succeeding waves of migrating neurons and glial cells to their ultimate cortical destination. At five months, primary fissures demarcate the major cortical sensory and motor areas. The spinal cord ends at the third lumbar segment. Between seven and nine months secondary sulci appear and cortical gray matter develops its laminar characteristics. Just before birth tertiary sulci emerge, lamination nears completion, and neuron migration and glial cell production proceed in the cerebral cortex until the sixth postnatal month.

Insults to morphogenesis after one month gestation give rise to disorders of cellular proliferation and migration.[3,14] Proliferative disorders are often genetically determined, with an autosomal dominant transmission affecting multiple body organs. They may involve single or multiple cell types of the central or peripheral nervous system. Examples of abnormal cell proliferation resulting in benign tumor formation include tuberous sclerosis, Sturge-Weber syndrome, and von Recklinghausen's disease (Chapter 10). Migration disorders occur when cells fail to reach their predetermined destination which results in abnormal cortical laminar structure, gray matter heterotopias, and cerebral hypoplasia. These latter disorders are a pathologic cellular response to a wide variety of toxic insults and do not represent specific disease entities. Infections, irradiation, and drugs account for a substantial percentage of such insults.

CELLULAR ARCHITECTONICS— SYNAPTIC DEVELOPMENT—MYELIN FORMATION (25 WEEKS TO TWO YEARS)

By twenty-five weeks human gestation, the CNS has reached its full complement of neurons and recognizable electric activity occurs. Thereafter begins the rapid growth of neuronal processes, dendrites, and axons, with synapse formation. The radial and columnar (vertical) arrangement of cells and processes is juxtaposed with the earlier horizontal layering of cells by the "inside-out" migration and heralds the functional organization of the mature cerebral cortex. Hence, orderly synaptic (axodendritic and axosomatic) development depends upon earlier cell migration and continues into the first two postnatal years.[15] Proper polarization of the neuron during migration accounts for the patterned growth of axon and dendrites and for the organization of synaptic connections. Thus, neural induction not only determines organogenesis of the CNS in the first thirty days of fetal life but also defines the elaboration of neuropil during the last trimester and the first two postnatal years. An increase in glia correlates with increasing functional activity without further increase in neurons. By birth there is a striking proliferation of oligodendroglia which presages postnatal myelination.

Infections, genetically determined metabolic diseases affecting either white or gray matter, hormonal disturbances, placental insufficiency and perinatal hypoxia and trauma are the primary destructive agents during this period. Unlike disorders incurred during the first two stages of morphogenesis, profound neurologic dysfunction is accompanied by relatively subtle but more conventional pathologic changes seen in the mature cortex.

EMBRYOGENIC-INDUCTION DISORDERS (0-4 WEEKS GESTATION)

These disorders represent a failure in the mutual induction of mesoderm and neuroectoderm. The primary defect is a failure of the neural folds to fuse and form the neural tube (ectoderm) with secondary maldevelopment of skeletal structures enclosing the CNS (mesoderm). The defects range from anencephaly to sacral meningomyelocele in the cephalic to caudal direction of the neural tube, and from holoprosencephaly to craniospinal rachischisis (midline posterior splitting of skull and vertebral column) in the anterior to posterior direction. For convenience they are divided into posterior and anterior midline defects. The former is named dysraphism to indicate the persistent continuity between posterior neuroectoderm and cutaneous ectoderm. The latter is called faciotelencephalopathy to connote the fusion failure of anterior neural tube, cephalic mesoderm, and adjacent foregut entoderm, the anlagen for facial structures.[3]

POSTERIOR MIDLINE CNS-AXIAL SKELETAL DEFECTS: DYSRAPHISM

ANENCEPHALY

This process is the paradigm of the various dysraphic disorders. While affected infants rarely survive early infancy, insight into the mechanics of neural ontogenesis provided by this disorder is enormous.

Pathogenesis and Pathology

The defect is time-specific in that the insult probably occurs after the onset of neural fold development (16 days) but before closure of the anterior neuropore (26 days). It is stimulus nonspecific because a variety of genetic,[16] infectious,[17] metabolic,[18] chemical[19,19a,20] and irradiation insults[21,22] have been implicated. These result in a failure of the cephalic neural folds to fuse into a neural tube. This, in turn, leads to degeneration of all forebrain germinal cells and an inability of mesoderm to differentiate into somites and hence into sclerotome, the latter being the anlagen for skull and vertebrae. Thus, mutual induction between the three germ layers fails at time-specific stages, resulting in deformities of both nervous tissue and supporting axial bone.[23]

Recent studies on human embryos have suggested that splitting of an already closed neural tube may account for this and other dysraphic entities.[24] Open areas of the tube are fully covered by cutaneous ectoderm, a condition for which a previous neural tube closure is presumed to be necessary. Splitting of a closed neural tube (neuroschisis) may in part be due to an abnormal increase in cerebrospinal fluid pressure during the first trimester.[25] It is possible that some cases of anencephaly and other dysraphic states indeed may occur via this mechanism after the major inductive period. Muscle differentiates normally in anencephaly despite disruption of motor innervation. This suggests that the latter occurred after muscle development, and therefore after embryogenesis and neural tube closure.[25a]

On examination of the nervous system the spinal cord, brain stem, and cerebellum are small. Descending tracts within the spinal cord are absent. Above this level there is nothing save a few tangles of glial and vascular tissue and remnants of midbrain. The pituitary is absent with secondary adrenal hypoplasia. The optic nerves are absent but the eyes are normal indicating that the anterior cephalic end of the neural tube, from whence the optic vesicles spring, closed and diverticulated properly.

The calvaria fails to develop and the frontal, occipital, and parietal bones are partially absent. Malformations of the foramen magnum and cervical vertebrae are frequent. Fifty percent of cases exhibit rachischisis of cranium and vertebrae, resulting in exposure and herniation of cerebral tissue (exencephaly). The deformed forehead lends a rather odd appearance to the face with relatively large ears and eyes. However, all facial structures are normally developed, except for an occasional lateral cleft lip or palate.

Clinical Picture

Anencephaly is the most common major CNS malformation in the Western world.[26] Its incidence varies from 0.65 per 1000 births in Japan to more than 3 per 1000 in the British Isles.[26a,26b] During the world depression years of 1929 through 1932, the incidence increased to 7 per 1000 births in Ireland.[27] There is a decisive ethnic difference in prevalence. It is more frequent in the Western world, rarer in the Eastern. Females are affected twice as frequently as males. There is a three- to five-percent recurrence rate in families with an affected child and the incidence increases with maternal age. The transmission appears to be matrilineal; there is no relationship to consanguinity, no concordance in monozygotic twins, and the recurrence rate for a maternal half-sibling is the same as for a full sibling. These factors are against a simple polygenetic inheritance pattern and are more consistent with environmental factors producing defects in germ plasm which are maternally transmitted.[16]

Anencephalic subjects do not survive infancy. During their few weeks of life they exhibit slow stereotyped movements and frequent decerebrate posturing. Head, facial, and limb movements may be spontaneous or pain induced. Some brain stem functions and automatisms such as sucking, rooting, and righting responses, and the Moro reflex, are present and are more readily and more reproduceably elicited than in normal infants. This reflects the absence of cortical inhibitory influences on subcortical and brain stem function.[28]

The presence of anencephaly may be predicted during the second half of pregnancy by finding a low maternal urinary excretion of estriol.[29] This is presumably due to fetal adrenal hypoplasia secondary to pituitary agenesis. This assay should be performed in mothers who have had a previous anencephalic infant.

SPINA BIFIDA AND CRANIUM BIFIDUM

These entities result from a failure in fusion of the posterior midline of the skull (cranium bifidum) or the vertebral column (spina bifida). The result is a bony cleft through which varying quantities of brain or spinal cord tissue protrude. In cranium bifidum the neural herniation is termed encephalocele, and may consist of brain parenchyma and meninges, or only meninges. These form the wall of a saclike cyst filled with cerebrospinal fluid. In spina bifida the herniation is called meningocele or meningomyelocele (myelomeningocele) according to whether the meninges herniate alone, or in concert with spinal cord parenchyma and nerve roots.

Spina bifida occulta represents a fusion failure of the posterior vertebral arches, unaccompanied by herniation of meninges or neural tissue. Spina bifida cystica is a term used to collectively designate meningocele and myelomeningocele (Fig. 4–2 A,B).

A similar terminology has been used for cranium bifidum. Rachischisis connotes complete posterior splitting of the craniovertebral bone with exposure of the brain, spinal cord, and meninges. Encephalocele connotes the various mass lesions associated with cranium bifidum.

Pathogenesis

Spina bifida and cranium bifidum are not only disorders of induction but are also associated with major abnormalities of cellular migration, and secondary mechanical deformities of the nervous system. On the basis of anatomic studies showing preserved continuity between neural and cutaneous ectoderm, the primary defect is believed to be a failure in neural tube closure.[23]

The argument that this continuity is illusory, and that the primary defect is a cleavage of a neural tube that has already fused (neuroschisis) has been used in this type of a defect as well as in anencephaly.[24] Whether the primary defect is one of fusion failure or neuroschisis or both, it is clear that the defects in bone formation are secondary. Failure

of neural tube closure prevents fusion of the surrounding axial skeletal structure.[30]

Like anencephaly, these defects are time-specific and stimulus nonspecific. The insult, assuming it to be a fusion failure of the mid- or caudal-neural tube,[31] must occur before 28 days gestation—the time of closure of the posterior neuropore (Table 4–1). A com-

52

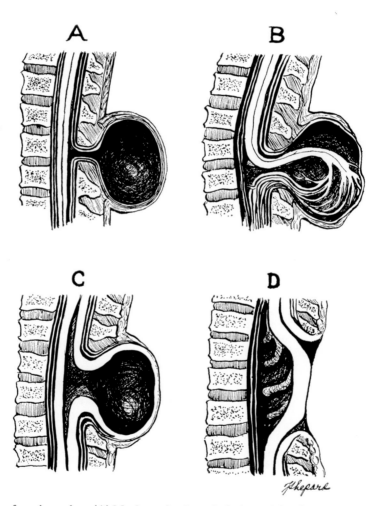

Fig. 4–2. Diagram of meningoceles. (**A**) Meningocele: through the bony defect (spina bifida) the meninges herniate and form a cystic sac filled with spinal fluid. The spinal cord does not participate in the herniation and may or may not be abnormal. (**B**) Myelomeningocele: spina bifida with meningocele; the spinal cord is herniated into the sac and ends there or may continue in an abnormal way further downward. (**C**) Myelocystocele or syringomyelocele: the spinal cord shows hydromyelia; the posterior wall of the spinal cord is attached to the ectoderm and undifferentiated. (**D**) Myelocele: the spinal cord is araphic; a cystic cavity is in front of the anterior wall of the spinal cord. (From Benda, C. E.: "*Developmental Disorders of Mentation and Cerebral Palsies*, 1952, courtesy of Grune & Stratton, Inc., New York.)

TABLE 4-2.

SPINA BIFIDA CYSTICA—SITE OF LESION*

Level	Number of Patients	
Cervical	51	
Thoracic	103	
Thoracolumbar	137	
Lumbar	583	
Lumbosacral	382	
Sacral	119	
Anterior	6	
Thoracic		3
Pelvic		3
Undesignated	9	
TOTAL	1390	

Level of the meningeal sac in 1390 consecutive patients treated for spina bifida cystica in the Boston Children's Medical Center.

* From Matson.[34]

bination of genetic and environmental factors are believed to act in conjunction. The latter include irradiation,[32] insulin, a deficiency of riboflavin or folic acid, and either an excess or a deficiency of vitamin A.[33]

Pathology

Spina Bifida Cystica. Of the defects collectively termed spina bifida cystica 75% are myelomeningoceles and 25% are meningoceles. Locations of the defect are depicted in Table 4–2. A lumbar or lumbosacral defect is most common, while cervical lesions are the least frequent posterior defects. The caudal spinal cord is favored because this is the location of the posterior neuropore, the last portion of the neural tube to close. Anterior midline defects of the vertebral arches are uncommon and constituted less than 0.5% of cases in the experience of Matson.[34] Cervical and thoracic meningomyeloceles have narrow bases and are usually not associated with hydrocephalus. By contrast 90% of lumbosacral myelomeningoceles are accompanied by hydrocephalus and Chiari malformations types 2 and 3.

In 95% of children with lumbar or lumbosacral meningomyelocele the spinal cord demonstrates abnormalities of the cervical region.

In 40% of instances there is hydromyelia, and in 20% syringomyelia, diplomyelia, or winged and dorsally slit cords.[35,36] In over 70% the medulla overrides the cervical cord dorsally, in association with type 2 Chiari malformation (Fig. 4–3). Seventy percent show defects in the posterior arch of the atlas, which is bridged by a firm fibrous band, suggesting that congenital atlantoaxial dislocation may be a mild expression of an induction disorder.[37] Examination of the parenchyma of the spinal cord reveals atrophic or poorly developed anterior horn cells, absent or abnormal corticospinal and sensory tracts, incomplete posterior horns, and exceedingly small and deranged anterior and posterior root fibers. These changes result in muscle

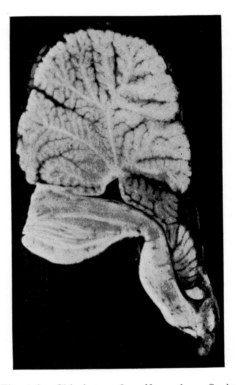

Fig. 4–3. Chiari, type 2 malformation. Sagittal section through the cerebellum and brain stem in an extreme case of Chiari malformation. Note the kinking of medulla, elongation of 4th ventricle, displacement of cerebellar tonsils caudad to foramen magnum level, and narrowing of aqueduct. (From Matson, D. D.: *Neurosurgery of Infancy and Childhood*, 2nd ed., 1969, courtesy of Charles C Thomas Publisher, Springfield.)

denervation during fetal life, and ultimately produce limb deformities and joint contractures.

Defects of cellular migration in the cerebral hemispheres include gray matter heterotopias, schizencephaly, gyral anomalies, and mesodermal heterotopias leading to teratomas and dermoids.[14]

The pathologic picture of spina bifida cystica is complicated by mechanical factors. In the normal fetus by the fourth fetal month, the vertebral column, now closed, is equal to the spinal cord in length. Thereafter, the column grows caudally more rapidly than the cord, and since the latter is anchored cranially, its distal end approximates the third to fourth lumbar vertebra at birth and the first lumbar vertebra in adulthood. In spina bifida cystica a tethering has been postulated to occur between the cord and the vertebral column at the site of the lesion. The differential growth of the column results in downward traction of intracranial contents to which the cord is attached. Therefore, the medulla and cerebellum are pulled partially through the foramen magnum producing mechanical distortion of cervical cord, medulla, vermis, and midbrain. The resulting impaction at the foramen magnum and aqueductal kinking produces hydrocephalus. Pressure disturbances in turn result in intrinsic cord damage characterized by syringomyelia and hydromelia.[38,39] This traction hypothesis,[40,41] debated for some years, has been given recent experimental support[42] as one of several factors responsible for the clinical picture of spina bifida cystica, Chiari malformation type 2, and hydrocephalus.

Accompanying these ectodermal defects there are a number of mesodermal lesions. These include splitting of the vertebral arches, and other dysplasias of bone such as double ribs and defects in the base of the skull.

Spina Bifida Occulta. This lesion usually involves the fifth lumbar and first sacral vertebrae and represents the benign end of the continuum of dysraphic disorders. Occasionally spina bifida occulta is accompanied by other congenital defects of the neuraxis. These include diastematomyelia, diplomyelia, subdural or epidural tumors such as lipomas, teratomas or dermoids, syringomyelia, Chiari

malformations type 1, and midline dermal sinuses in the sacrococcygeal region.[43]

Cranium Bifidum. Like anencephaly, cranium bifidum is a cephalic dysraphic disorder but of smaller magnitude. In the Western world about 85% of these lesions are dorsal defects involving the occipital bone. Parietal, frontal, or nasal encephaloceles are far less common. In the Far East the majority of encephaloceles are anterior and involve the frontal, nasal, and orbital bones.[34,44,44a] Other defects of the cerebral hemispheres are a frequent accompaniment. These include schizencephaly,[14] microgyria, agenesis of the corpus callosum, heterotopias of gray matter and accompanying dorsal encephaloceles, Chiari malformations type 2, and hydrocephalus.

Clinical Picture

Spina Bifida Cystica is one of the most common anomalies of the nervous system, with an incidence that ranges from 0.2 per 1000 live births in Japan to 4.2 per 1000 live births in Ireland.[44b,45] A recurrence rate of 5% is seen in affected families. At birth, the defect may assume a variety of appearances. These range from complete exposure of neural tissue to a flat, partially epithelialized membrane. Most commonly, there is a saclike structure that may be located at any point along the spinal column. Most often the sac is covered by a fine membrane, which is prone to tears through which the cerebrospinal fluid leaks. In other instances the defect is covered by skin, by meninges, or by dura. In the latter cases it will epithelialize rapidly and spontaneously. If the cystic mass is soft and can be completely transilluminated it is most likely a meningocele. In this case, although the nerve roots are displaced, motor, sensory, reflex, and sphincter functions are usually normal. Seventy-five percent of defects are myelomeningoceles and produce neurologic dysfunction corresponding to their anatomic level.[46]

Some 80% of myelomeningoceles are localized to the lumbar and lumbosacral region (Table 4–2). These produce a variety of conus, epiconus, and cauda equina syndromes. When the lesion is below the second lumbar vertebra, the cauda equina bears the brunt of the damage. Children exhibit varying degrees of flaccid, areflexic paraparesis, and sensory deficits from the third or fourth lumbar dermatome distally. The sphincter and detrusor tone of the bladder is compromised, and there is overflow incontinence. An absent anal skin reflex and poor tone of the rectal sphincter is often apparent and may result in rectal prolapse. Lesions below the third sacral vertebra cause no motor impairment but may result in bladder and anal sphincter paralysis, and saddle anesthesia involving the third through fifth sacral dermatomes. Electromyographic studies and conduction velocities obtained in the lower extremities of affected newborns suggest that the paralysis is the outcome of a combined upper and lower motor neuron lesion.[47] Upper motor neuron lesions, resulting from involvement of the corticospinal tracts, are, however, usually obscured by the more severe involvement of the nerve roots, cauda equina, and anterior horn cells.

Cauda equina lesions produce muscular denervation in utero resulting in joint deformities of the lower limbs. Most commonly these are flexion or extension contractures, valgus or varus contractures, hip dislocations, and lumbosacral scoliosis. The expression of the contracture depends on the extent and severity of dermatome involvement.

Hydrocephalus, associated with types 2 and 3 Chiari malformations, complicates 90% of lumbosacral myelomeningoceles.[48] It is manifest at birth in 50%–75% of cases. In the remainder, the ventricles are dilated at birth but the head circumference is normal, suggesting that hydrocephalus almost always precedes operative closure of the myelomeningocele sac.[49]

Thoracic and cervical myelomeningoceles are usually not associated with neurologic deficits or hydrocephalus. Occasionally lesions of the higher spinal cord segments may involve the spinal cord in conjunction with the cauda equina.

Radiographs of the spine will reveal the extent of the nonfused vertebrae. The relationship between the cord segment and the vertebral bodies is abnormal. While at birth the terminal segments of the normal cord lie between the vertebral bodies of T_{11} and L_1, in infants with myelomeningocele the cord may extend as far down as L_5. The position of the spinal cord segments remains normal in the lower cervical and upper thoracic levels.[50]

Spina bifida cystica is also associated with malformations of the craniobasal bones, resulting in a short neck, or in the cervical rib syndrome. A variety of congenital tumors of the brain or spinal cord may also be present. These include lipomas, teratomas, and sacrococcygeal dermoids. These may masquerade as a skin-covered meningomyelocele but their presence and extent can be assessed by oil myelography.

Malformations and infections of the genitourinary tract occur in 90% of newborns with spina bifida cystica. Most commonly, there is a disturbance in bladder function. One group, representing one-third of patients, shows more or less constant dribbling, and the bladder content is easily expressed manually. Direct cystometry reveals absent detrusor activity.[50a] In another, larger group of patients, detrusor contractions are weakly present, but bladder emptying is inefficient, and there is outlet obstruction at the level of the external sphincter. This is believed to be the result of impaired coordination between detrusor and sphincter function. Bladder sensation may be intact in these children. This type of a defect results in a high incidence of bladder trabeculation, an elevated resting bladder pressure, and dilatation of the upper urinary tract, which often reaches enormous proportions.[51] The second type of abnormality appears to correlate best with lesions in the higher lumbar or low thoracic lesions, the site of the efferent sympathetic fibers. Continence appears to depend more upon preservation of detrusor activity than sphincter function.

As a consequence of these lesions persistent bacteriuria is seen in 50% of two-year-olds, with hydronephrosis being found in 25%.[52] After three years of age, renal disease is the most common cause for morbidity and mortality.[53] Therefore, early and constant monitoring of the urinary tract with intravenous pyelograms, colony counts, and cystography is an essential part of any therapeutic program.

Spina Bifida Occulta. This defect is extremely common and is found in 25% of hospitalized children and in 10% of the general pediatric population. It generally involves the posterior arches of fifth lumbar and first sacral vertebrae. While usually asymptomatic and an incidental finding on x-ray examination, the skin of the low mid back region may manifest a hairy tuft, dimple, a dermal sinus, or a mass due to a subcutaneous lipoma or teratoma.[43a,44] In the child who presents with a neurogenic bladder or a variety of neurologic deficits of the lower limbs, spina bifida occulta may suggest an underlying malformation of the spinal cord.[44] In these patients the presence of neurologic deficits, even in the absence of urinary tract or cutaneous abnormalities, is an indication for diagnostic studies including myelography.[34] In some instances spina bifida occulta is associated with any combination of the many defects of neural tube closure, the most serious of which are the Chiari malformations, hydrocephalus and anencephaly.

Cranium Bifidum. The incidence of cranium bifidum is about one-sixth that of spina bifida cystica. In this country the vast majority present as encephaloceles in the occipital region. The encephalocele usually contains herniated neural tissue and often compromises cerebral spinal fluid drainage resulting in hydrocephalus. The degree of neurologic and developmental damage depends upon the quantity of herniated tissue, the degree of hydrocephalus and the extent of hind brain lesions or cerebral hemisphere dysplasias resulting from the associated disorder of cellular migration and organization.[14]

Often no functional impairment is noted until childhood, by which time mild mental retardation, spastic diplegia and impaired cognitive function or seizures may be evident. In the newborn, the mass must be distinguished from cephalohematoma, inclusion cysts of the scalp, cystic hygromas, caput succedaneum and in the case of anterior defects, nasal polyps. Its location along the midline, a pulsatile quality synchronous with heart rate, and absence of periosteal new bone formation distinguishes it from these other conditions. Skull x rays will reveal the bony defect and air encephalograms will define the ventricular system and quantity of neural tissue within the sac.

Treatment[34]

Spina Bifida Cystica. The management of spina bifida cystica was given new energy by English orthopedic surgeons in the early 1960s.[54,55] Their studies suggested that skin closure within 24 hours of birth reduces mortality and morbidity due to meningitis and ventriculitis. They argue that early closure not only prevents local infection and trauma to the exposed neural tissue but also avoids stretching of additional nerve roots likely to occur as the cystic sac expands over the first 24 hours. As a consequence, further deterioration of lower limb function and sphincter control is prevented and motor power of the legs is improved. Given the need for repair in the first instance, hydrocephalus does not appear to be a more disabling complication as a consequence of early closure. Skin grafts are employed to repair the lesion without either dissecting neural elements from the sac or removing any portion of the sac. Skin closure prior to the infant's first feeding, while meconium is still sterile, prevents fecal contamination of the lesion, a major cause of meningitis. The incidence of postoperative meningitis has been reduced by local application of triple antibiotic spray consisting of neomycin, polymyxin, and bacitracin.[56]

At the present time advocates of early closure of both meningocele and myelomeningoceles in all patients regardless of neurologic deficits, recommend intervention in the first 12 to 18 hours of life as an emergency procedure.[30,57] Children seen after the first 24 hours are repaired as promptly as possible unless infection requires prior antibiotic therapy. Rapidly enlarging hydrocephalus may have to be shunted before repair of the spina bifida cystica, and spinal rachischisis may be technically impossible to repair until enough skin is available and the lesion is epithelialized.

Matson and others have recommended selection of patients and suggest that infants with total paraplegia and sphincter paralysis not be operated upon in the first few months of life.[34,58] Patients with extensive paralysis below L 1, gross kyphosis, major associated congenital defects, or a head circumference that is at least 2 cm above the ninetieth percentile, fare poorly despite modern operative, antibiotic, and rehabilitative techniques.[58a] Patients who survive infancy without significant hydrocephalus and with some intellectual capacity are repaired at two to six years to facilitate ambulation. Gellis recommends with qualifications that the selection process be put into effect after surgery.[59] This can be done by determining how intensively pneumonia and GU tract infections are treated in those children clearly destined to be severely mentally retarded and totally paralyzed. These decisions should not be made during the neonatal period.

Complicating hydrocephalus usually becomes manifest after meningomyelocele closure.[60] This condition is treated according to the principles outlined elsewhere. Contracture deformities of the lower limbs require physical therapy, leg braces, and stabilization of dislocated hips. Muscle or tendon transplants and joint arthrodeses may be necessary in the ambulating child.

Disorders of the excretory system are the most common cause of morbidity and mortality in patients surviving beyond two years. Careful upper and lower urinary tract evaluation beginning in the newborn period should include colony counts, creatinine clearance, a cystourethrogram, and an IVP. Acute urinary tract infection demands prompt and appropriate antibiotics, as chronic infection inevitably leads to upper tract dilatation signified by persistent vesicourethral reflux.[53] This may necessitate urinary diversion, particularly an ileal loop bladder procedure.[53,61] Incontinence with hypotonic bladder may respond to cholinergic agents such as bethanechol (Urecholine). Incontinence due to a spastic bladder may respond to parasympatholytic agents such as propantheline (Probanthine). In lumbosacral spina bifida cystica only a small minority of patients attains urinary continence[53] and if it is not achieved by three years of age it is unlikely ever to develop.[61a]

Spina Bifida Occulta. Spina bifida occulta deserves surgical exploration if the neurologic deficits are progressive[62] or when there is an associated tumor, or neurodermal sinus.[34]

Cranium Bifidum Cysticum. Cranium bifidum cysticum should be repaired urgently if there is leaking cerebrospinal fluid or if the defect is not covered by skin. When the defect is completely epithelialized, closure is done prior to the infant's discharge from the hospital. Posterior encephaloceles are often associated with posterior fossa malformations leading to hydrocephalus. Therefore, an air encephalogram should be done prior to surgery in all cases. If indicated, posterior fossa exploration is done prior to defect closure. Anterior encephaloceles should be repaired by a neurosurgeon working with a plastic surgeon.

Prognosis

Untreated, 45% of infants with spina bifida cystica die by three months and 84% by two years, most often as a consequence of central nervous system infection or hydrocephalus.[48,60,63] Infants who have been subjected to early surgical repair of the spinal defect and correction of hydrocephalus have a two-year survival rate of 65%.[64] The quality of survival with surgery is another problem, since a large number of infants with significant mental retardation and neurologic deficits survive as a consequence of modern surgical techniques. From 30 to 50 percent of children with myelomeningocele are left with a total flaccid paraplegia and incontinence, while the remainder have significant locomotor problems. Hydrocephalus is seen in 70%–80% of infants. If treated successfully, half of these are educationally retarded or better.[30] After early childhood, death is usually the result of urinary tract infection with sepsis and renal failure. Less often, it is the consequence of pulmonary disease resulting from progressive kyphoscoliosis.

Although better quality of survival will occur with improved techniques for control of hydrocephalus and urinary tract infection, as for instance, stimulation of bladder function by the use of electronic implants, the essence of treatment will be prevention. This will require major advances in the identification and prevention of environmental factors jeopardizing the fetus in the first month of gestation.

CHIARI MALFORMATIONS TYPES 1, 2, 3

The third major expression of dysraphism was originally and completely described by Chiari in 1891.[65,66,67] This disorder is characterized by cerebellar elongation and protrusion through the foramen magnum into the cervical spinal cord. Primary anomalies of hind brain and skeletal structure with consequent mechanical deformities account for three variants:

Type 1

The medulla is displaced caudally into the spinal canal, with the inferior pole of the cerebellar hemispheres herniated through the foramen magnum in the form of two parallel, tonguelike processes. This herniation may extend as far down as the third cervical vertebra. Malformations at the base of the skull and the upper cervical spine are almost invariably present. These include platybasia, basilar impression, atlas assimilation, atlantoaxial dislocation, asymmetric small foramen magnum and Klippel-Feil syndrome.[68] Hydromyelia, syringomyelia, syringobulbia, and diastematomyelia are frequently present; spina bifida cystica is less common.[66]

The Chiari malformation type 1 is often asymptomatic in childhood and only presents in adolescence or adulthood with hydrocephalus, resulting from aqueductal stenosis, or obstruction of the fourth ventricle at the outlet foramina or at the foramen magnum. With obstruction at the foramen magnum, torticollis, opisthotonus, and signs of cervical cord compression are evident. Headache, vertigo, and progressive cerebellar signs may be accompanied by lower cranial nerve deficits which are often asymmetric.[68a]

Type 2

In this variant, which is the most common of the Chiari malformations, any combination of features of type 1 malformation may be associated with obstructive hydrocephalus and lumbosacral spina bifida. These defects are responsible for mechanical factors which modify the primary embryologic lesions. While in type 1 malformation the caudal displacement of the cerebellum is due solely to adhesions between it and the posterolateral region of the brain stem, these adhesions occur in type 2 as well, but in addition, hydrocephalus exerts downward pressure and spina bifida cystica, which is responsible for a cord tethered in the lumbosacral region, exerts downward traction. These forces become particularly evident during the third trimester as a result of differential growth of the vertebral column and the spinal cord. They produce a cerebellar pressure cone, which displaces the fourth ventricle into the spinal canal as far down as the fifth cervical vertebra. The medulla and pons are ventrally kinked and juxtaposed (Fig. 4-3). The pons and cranial nerves are elongated and the cervical roots compressed and forced to course upward, rather than downward, to exit through their respective foramina. Cervical-thoracic hydromyelia and syringomyelia may result from the mechanical effect produced by the pulsations of the choroid plexus, transmitted through the central canal of the spinal cord, rather than through the outlets of the fourth ventricle, and the basal cisterns. Both the foramina of Luschka and Magendie and the basal cisterns are occluded as a result of impaction of the foramen magnum or atresia of the foramina outlets.[69]

With subsequent neural overgrowth the premature fusion of the bilateral cerebellar primordia within an abnormally small posterior fossa contributes to cerebellar herniation.[24] In addition to these gross abnormalities, there are also developmental arrests of the cerebellar and brain stem structures, and heterotopias of cerebral gray matter, polygyria, and microgyria. The latter point to an additional defect in cerebral cellular migration.[69a]

In 90% of patients type 2 Chiari malformation presents as a complex problem of spina bifida cystica with hydrocephalus and any combination of the assorted defects of type 1.[69b] Conversely, all subjects with spina bifida cystica and hydrocephalus will exhibit the type 2 defect.

Type 3

This variant may have any of the features of the first two, with the additional presence of occipital cranium bifidum with encephalocele or cervical spina bifida cystica. Hydrocephalus is regularly seen and is the result of differing degrees of atresia of the fourth ventricle foramina, aqueductal stenosis, or impaction at the foramen magnum.

Management

The clinical condition and therapeutic regimen for types 2 and 3 of the Chiari syndrome are described in other sections, i.e., spina bifida cystica, cranium bifidum, and hydrocephalus. In the older patient with Chiari type 1 and a slowly progressive increase of intracranial pressure, a direct decompression through an occipital craniectomy and cervical laminectomy may be adequate. If the aqueduct is seen to be occluded, either on preoperative air encephalogram or at the time of surgery, a shunting procedure will be necessary.[34]

Other Dysraphic States

DIPLOMYELIA AND DIASTEMATOMYELIA

Diplomyelia represents a reduplication of the spinal cord, usually in the low thoracic-lumbar region, and occasionally extending for as many as 10 segments or more. It may be associated with extensive spina bifida cystica, or tumors of the spinal cord, but may also occur in the absence of any neurologic deficits.

Diastematomyelia is a cleft in the spinal cord, which becomes divided longitudinally by a septum of bone and cartilage emanating from the posterior vertebral arch and extending anteriorly. Each half of the cord has its own dural covering. The cord or cauda equina becomes impaled by the bony spur and differential growth between vertebral column and spinal cord results in stretching of the cord above its point of fixation. In over 90% of subjects diastematomyelia is confined to the low thoracic-lumbar region, extending for as many as 10 segments.[34,70]

Diastematomyelia is a relatively mild expression of a neural tube fusion disorder with displaced mesoderm intruding into the neural tube during early induction and resulting in ectopic bone surrounded by neuroectoderm. Spina bifida occulta often overlies[34,70] the defect, and cutaneous lesions are found in about 75% of subjects. Most commonly these are tufts of hair, or skin dimples, but occasionally there are subcutaneous lipomas, vascular malformations, or dermal sinuses. Anomalies of the craniobasal bones are seen, as well as syringomyelia and hydromyelia (Fig. 4–2,C). A neurenteric cyst may be located in the cleft portions of the spinal cord.[71]

The defect is seen three times more often in girls than in boys. The presenting complaint is usually impaired gait, weakness of the lower extremities, or incontinence of bladder or bowel. A combination of upper and lower motor neuron signs in the lower extremities is associated with atrophy of the leg muscles and skeletal deformities of the feet.[72] Spinothalamic and posterior column sensory deficits correspond with the level of the lesion. With suspicion aroused by cutaneous anomalies and neurologic dysfunction of the lower limbs and sphincters, diagnosis may almost always be made by means of tomography of the lumbosacral spine or oil myelography.

Surgical removal of the bony spur allows the cord to become freely movable and favors neurologic improvement, or at least prevents further progression of symptoms. The more recent the neurologic deficit the more likely it is to be reversible.[34,70] Prophylactic surgery for the infant or young child without neurologic deficit is therefore indicated.

SYRINGOMYELIA AND HYDROMYELIA

These disorders should be considered different expressions of the same pathologic process, and intermediate stages are common. Hydromyelia is the pathologic dilatation of the spinal cord central canal (Fig. 4–2,C). Syringomyelia is random single or multiple cavity formation within spinal cord parenchyma, lined by ependyma or proliferating glial tissue. A syrinx often communicates with the central canal. Both types of lesions primarily affect the cervical cord and may extend into the brain stem (syringobulbia).

Syringomyelia usually accompanies one of the major forms of dysraphism. In the uncomplicated case these defects are inevitably associated with spina bifida occulta, or skeletal anomalies of the craniobasal bones. Within the spinal cord gray and white matter are disorganized and displaced—a gross microscopic picture that is analogous to schizencephaly of the cerebral cortex. Thus, syringomyelia represents a combined dysraphic disorder (embryogenesis) and disarrayed cellular migration (histogenesis).

Syringomyelia and hydromyelia are anatomically and clinically progressive for three reasons. First, they are associated with hydrocephalus and anomalies of the craniobasal bones. Secondly, almost 20% will develop intramedullary neoplasms.[73] Thirdly, as the force of the normal cerebrospinal fluid pulse is prevented from becoming expended through the foramina of Luschka and Magendie, which are often atretic, it is directed to the central canal and the communicating syrinx, causing their progressive dilatation.[38]

When uncomplicated, these entities are usually asymptomatic until the second or third decade. Since the cavities are more central than eccentric, they damage fibers crossing through central white matter of the cord, and thus compromise temperature and pain sensation, sparing sensory modalities mediated by the posterior columns. This disassociated anesthesia is responsible for trophic, sudomotor, and vasomotor disorders of skin, including painless ulcerations, coldness, cyanosis, and hyperhidrosis. It is responsible for the painless arthropathies such as "Charcot joints" similar to those seen in tabes dorsalis but involving joints of the upper rather than the lower extremities.

Involvement of anterior horn cells, pyramidal tracts, and posterior columns in the cervical region leads to segmental asymmetric lower motor neuron signs in the upper limbs with the formation of joint contractures, and in the lower extremities spasticity, hyperreflexia, and loss of position and vibratory sense. In children the first sign may be a rapidly progressive scoliosis.[74] Syringobulbia presents with asymmetric lower cranial nerve palsies and is almost always associated with anomalies of the craniobasal bones.

Diagnosis is best made by air myelography which visualizes the enlarged segment of affected cord. Radiation therapy to the affected segments has been recommended but is probably of limited value. Decompression by ventricular shunting procedures or by opening the atretic foramina of Luschka and Magendie has provided temporary or lasting improvement.[38,39]

SACRAL AGENESIS

Agenesis of the sacrum and coccyx is usually associated with anomalous development of the lumbosacral cord. Neurologic signs are those of sphincter incontinence, and motor and sensory deficits of the lower limbs. The defect has been associated with other congenital anomalies[75] and is more frequent in offspring of diabetic mothers.

NEURODERMAL SINUS[34]

The vast majority of dermal sinuses, as for instance the pilonidal sinus, do not connect with the central nervous system and are therefore of limited neurologic importance.

Neurodermal sinuses are a communication lined by stratified squamous epithelium between skin and any portion of the neuraxis. Most commonly the defects are in the lumbosacral region and the occiput, the former occurring about nine times as frequently as the latter. These two points represent the posterior and anterior neuropores respectively, the terminal closure sites of the neural tube.

The sinus is often surrounded by a small mound of skin, the dimple, or by other cutaneous lesions such as tufts of hair or angiomata. It often overlies a spina bifida occulta. It may expand into an epidermoid or dermoid cyst at its proximal end, thus causing segmental neurologic deficits, either through mass effect or by traction on the neuraxis. Cerebellar and brain stem signs or, on occasion, hydrocephalus may be produced by a neurodermal sinus in the occipital region. The presence of an open sinus tract may allow drainage of cerebrospinal fluid or provide a portal of entry for bacterial infections. A neurodermal sinus is one of the most common causes for recurrent meningitis. When the lesion is in the lumbosacral region, coliform bacteria and staphylococci are the most common invaders; a sinus tract in the occiput is more likely to produce recurrent staphylococcal meningitis. Such defects must be scrupulously sought for in any case of central nervous system infection.[76] Any dermal sinus whose ending is not clearly visualized should be traced with plain radiography and myelography.

These lesions require surgical exploration

and complete excision of the sinus before the development of symptoms. Treatment for an occipital sinus is primary excision of the entire sinus tract and of the proximal cyst if it be present. In Matson's experience surgical results are poorer when performed after the development of infection, and death may result from chronic meningitis or hydrocephalus.[34]

DEVELOPMENTAL ANOMALIES OF THE BASE OF THE SKULL AND UPPER CERVICAL VERTEBRAE

PLATYBASIA

Platybasia is a familial disorder characterized by a deformity of the osseous structures at the base of the skull producing an upward displacement of the floor of the posterior fossa, and a narrowing of the foramen magnum. The condition is transmitted as an autosomal dominant trait, with occasional lack of penetrance.[77]

Neurologic symptoms are progressive and due to compression of the cervical spinal cord. As a rule they do not appear until the second or third decade of life. Commonly, they include progressive spasticity, incoordination, and nystagmus, with weakness of the lower cranial nerves. Platybasia may be associated with other malformations of the central nervous system, including the Chiari malformations and aqueductal stenosis.

The diagnosis is suggested by the presence of a short neck, and is confirmed by radiographs of the skull. These reveal an odontoid process which extends above a line drawn from the dorsal lip of the foramen magnum to the dorsal margin of the hard palate.

Treatment is by surgical decompression of the posterior fossa and upper cervical cord.[78]

KLIPPEL-FEIL SYNDROME

This condition, first described in 1912 by Klippel and Feil,[79] is characterized by a fusion or reduction in the number of cervical vertebrae.

On examination children have a short neck and a low hair line. Passive and active movements of the neck are limited. Neurologic symptoms are variable. Progressive paraplegia due to compression of the cervical cord may appear early in life. Some children are retarded or show learning deficits. An association with mirror movements has been reported. This may reflect the "soft signs" seen in children with mild intellectual deficits, or result from an inadequate decussation of the pyramidal tracts or dorsal closure of the cord.[80] Associated malformations are common. They include spina bifida, syringomyelia, congenital deafness, or congenital heart disease.[81,82]

The diagnosis of Klippel-Feil syndrome rests on the demonstration by radiologic examination of fused cervical or cervical-thoracic vertebrae, hemivertebrae, or atlanto-occipital fusion.

When there is clinical evidence for compression of the cervical cord, laminectomy is indicated.

CLEIDOCRANIAL DYSOSTOSIS

This condition is transmitted as an autosomal dominant trait, and is characterized by rudimentary clavicles, a broad head, delayed or defective closure of the anterior fontanelle, mental deficiency, and a variety of cerebral malformations.[83] Other skeletal malformations are common. These include spina bifida, short and wide fingers, and delayed ossification of the pelvis.

ANTERIOR MIDLINE DEFECTS (FACIOTELENCEPHALOPATHY)

HOLOPROSENCEPHALY

Just as anencephaly is the most catastrophic dysraphism, so this process is the most devastating of the anterior anomalies. It is due to induction failure of three germ layers: cephalic mesoderm, adjacent neuroectoderm, and the entodermal anlage for facial structures. Like anencephaly, it is time-specific and stimulus nonspecific. Normally, induction probably occurs prior to 23 days gestation, just before the elaboration of the optic vesicles (24 days). Thus, of the major induction malformations, it has the shortest vulnerable period, which accounts for its relative rarity.[84] Associated chromosomal abnormalities are frequent, including nondisjunction leading to 13–15 trisomy and deletion of the short arm of chromosome 18 (see Chapter 3).[85] The malformation is also associated with such maternal disorders as diabetes mellitus, syphilis, cytomegalic inclusion disease, and toxoplasmosis.[86] It is likely that the toxic stimulus, probably environmental, accounts for both the embryogenic failure as well as the chromosome defects. Siblings of affected patients have a considerably higher incidence of a similar defect, but adequate statistics are not available.

The defect is one of failure of the primary cerebral vesicle (telencephalon) to cleave and expand bilaterally.[87] Various degrees of severity are recognized.[88,89] In its most complete expression the brain is characterized by a single large ventricular cavity encompassed within an undivided prosencephalic vesicle (Fig. 4–4). The thalamus remains un-divided, the inferior frontal and temporal regions are often absent, and the remainder of the isocortex is rudimentary, with only the primary motor and sensory cortex present. The olfactory diverticuli and rhinencephalon are absent, but the brain stem and cerebellum are present and fully differentiated. Gray matter heterotopias and agenesis of the septum pellucidum[90] point to subsequent abnormal cellular migration.

In the less severe forms there is partial or complete division of the hemispheres, and the olfactory bulbs and tracts are absent or hypoplastic (arhinencephaly).[89] Skeletal changes include anomalous development of the orbital, nasal, maxillary, and ethmoid bones. In the most extreme form, the face is overwhelmed by cyclopia, a single median orbital

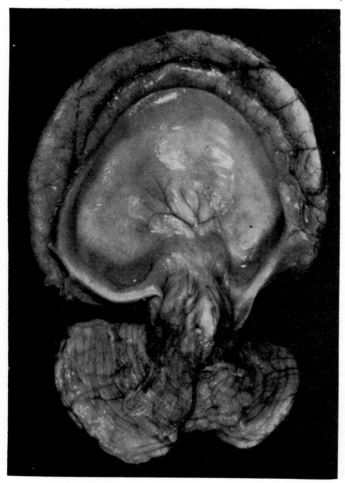

Fig. 4–4. Holoprosencephaly. The dorsal view shows the undivided lateral ventricle. The corpus striatum below it is fused. Note that the brain stem and cerebellum are well-formed. (Courtesy of Dr. W. De-Myer, Indiana University Medical Center, Indianapolis and the National Foundation; from Birth Defects, Original Article Series, vol. 7, p. 961, 1971.)

fossa and eye with protruding noselike appendage above the orbit. Other constitutional dysplastic features include polydactyly and ventricular septal defect.

In the less extensive malformations there is hypotelorism, a median cleft lip, and a nose that lacks its bridge, columella, or septum.

The neurologic picture is characterized by severe mental retardation, seizures, rigidity, apnea, temperature imbalance, and rarely hydrocephalus. Diagnostic studies should include skull and facial x rays which show deformed anterior craniobasal bones, dermatoglyphics and air encephalogram for definitive evaluation of the central nervous system. When the patient has many extracephalic anomalies, a chromosomal anomaly is likely, while in their absence the karyotype is usually normal.

OTHER FACIOTELENCEPHALOPATHIES

Cleft Median Face Syndromes[88]

This group of disorders, the visible common denominator of which is the median cleft lip and palate, is of two types. The first includes subjects with orbital hypotelorism, who represent a less severe form of holoprosencephaly. These less striking facial and ocular anomalies occur in the form of cebocephaly. In this entity, the proboscis is laid down on its side and there is orbital hypotelorism.[86] Many patients have a fairly normal neocortex and often survive with relatively little or no neurologic dysfunction. Some, however, have a fully developed holoprosencephaly with severe neurologic impairment, often exhibiting abnormal karyotypes.

The second type displays hypertelorism and may be associated with anterior cranium bifidum, a dysraphism.

In both types, the facial and brain structures exhibit varying degrees of induction anomalies, together with histogenetic disorders of cellular proliferation such as lipomas or teratomas.[88]

Non-Cleft Median Face Syndrome

This group includes several syndromes familiar to pediatricians, such as Treacher Collins', Crouzon's, and Apert's. They also embrace the chromosomal trisomies 18 and 21. The facial deformities are mild but stereotyped, characterized by mongoloid and antimongoloid slants, and hypo- or hypertelorism. The brain reveals maldevelopment of the neocortex with frequent migration anomalies causing defective cortical lamination, and occasional failure of inductive diverticulation.

DISORDERS OF CELLULAR MIGRATION AND PROLIFERATION (1 TO 7 MONTHS GESTATION)

While it is recognized that disorders of organ induction will produce secondary histogenic migration or proliferation anomalies, this section confines itself to those disorders of cellular migration which are unassociated with defects of embryogenesis. The proliferative anomalies, notably the phakomatoses and various congenital tumors of the nervous system, while frequently accompanied by migration defects, are discussed in Chapter 10.

Migration disorders occur when neurons of the ependymal matrix zone, which lines the ventricular cavity, fail to reach their intended destination in the cerebral cortex. This results in focal or generalized structural deformities of the cerebral hemispheres. These will be discussed in sequence of their ontogenetic chronology.

SCHIZENCEPHALY

This anomaly of morphogenesis is characterized by clefts, placed symmetrically within the cerebral hemispheres, and extending from the cortical surface to the underlying ventricular cavity (Fig. 4–5).[14,91] The cerebral region which harbors the cleft is usually hypoplastic, and the axis of the cleft is oriented along the normal primary fissures. Yakovlev has termed the continuity between cortical surface and ventricular lining the "pia-ependymal seam."[14]

Like syringomyelia, schizencephaly may be associated with induction disorders and hence initiated by a toxic stimulus during the first 30 days of gestation. It may also be due to impairment of subsequent cellular migration and diverticulation. Unlike syringomyelia, however, schizencephaly most often is unaccompanied by mesodermal or ento-

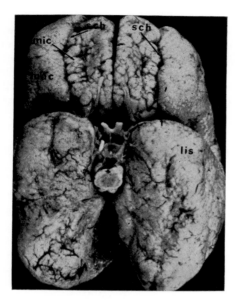

Fig. 4–5. Schizencephaly. Ventral view of the brain in a 10-year-old, severely retarded boy. In addition to the symmetric clefts in the orbital walls of the frontal lobes, the brain also shows failure of sulcation (lissencephaly), and microgyria of the frontal lobes. (Courtesy of Yakovlev, P. I. and Wadsworth, R. C., Journal of Neuropathology and Experimental Neurology, 1946, and courtesy of Adams, R. D. and Sidman, R. L.: *Introduction to Neuropathology*, 1968, McGraw-Hill Book Co., New York.)

dermal anomalies, suggesting that the teratogenic stimulus usually strikes after the 30-day induction period and before the onset of primary sulcation at 60 days. Other major errors in migration occur. These include gray matter heterotopias, disorganized white matter, and defects in gyral patterns.

This anomaly should be distinguished from a porencephalic cyst caused by a variety of vascular or infectious insults to the brain during the late fetal or early infantile life.[14] The latter results from the dissolution of necrotic regions of brain with cavitation and cyst formation within the parenchyma of the cerebral hemispheres. Porencephalic cysts frequently do not communicate with the ventricular system or with the cerebral cortical surface. Most importantly, they are asymmetric, not aligned with the primary fissures, and unassociated with major cerebral migration defects.

The clinical picture of schizencephaly is characterized by profound neurologic and developmental defects. Symmetric spastic and rigid quadriparesis occurs with generalized seizure and decerebration. Porencephaly differs in that there is often a well-defined destructive event, and the neurologic deficits are often focal, asymmetric, or silent, or even compatible with relatively normal development.

Unlike schizencephaly, a porencephalic cyst may present as a one-way ball valve type communication with the ventricular system. It may enlarge progressively and behave like an expanding lesion impinging on the ventricular system to produce hydrocephalus.[34]

LISSENCEPHALY (AGYRIA)

Lissencephaly, a term coined in the 19th century, literally means "smooth brain."[92] The cerebral hemispheres approximate the smooth two- to four-month fetal cerebral cortex, with the absence of sulcation. The insult is believed to occur before the end of three months gestation and prevents succeeding waves of migrating neurons from reaching the cerebral cortex. Thus, gray matter heterotopias, macrogyri, micropolygyri, and schizencephaly together with defective cortical lamination are often associated (Fig. 4–6).[14] The defect is rare and clinically characterized by spastic quadriplegia with

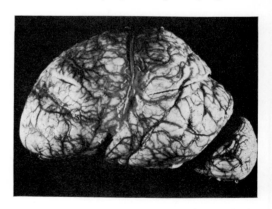

Fig. 4–6. Lissencephaly. Eight-year-old with severe retardation. There is a developmental arrest of the cerebrum, with few primitive gyral markings present. (Courtesy of Dr. Abraham Towbin, Laboratory of Neuropathology, Danvers State Hospital, Hathorne, Massachusetts.)

decerebration, microcephaly, severe mental retardation and seizures, or "atonic diplegia."[93],[94]

MACROGYRIA (PACHYGYRIA)

In this anomaly the gyral patterns are too coarse and too few (Fig. 4–7). More common than lissencephaly, the toxic stimuli inducing it may occur up to the fifth month of gestation by which time the primary sulci have already become elaborated. Thus, secondary sulcation is abortive and tertiary sulcation is prevented. Other migration anomalies are associated and the clinical picture is similar to that seen in lissencephaly. Since the anomalies tend to be more asymmetric, the neurologic deficits are often lateralized (see Chapter 5).

MICROPOLYGYRIA

This defect results from an insult to the nervous system sustained prior to the fifth month of gestation. The brain resembles a chestnut kernel and is characterized by an excess of secondary and tertiary sulci, resulting in gyri that are both too small and too many (Fig. 4–5).[66] In addition to the gyral anomalies there are other migration defects, gray matter heterotopias, defective cortical cell polarization, and abnormal cellular lamination. Microscopically the brain resembles that of a four- to five-months fetus.

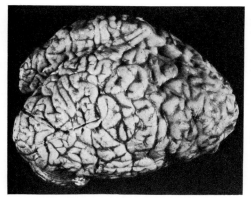

Fig: 4–7. Macrogyria (pachygyria). In this developmental disturbance of the convolutional pattern, there are thickened, irregular convolutions in the frontal lobes. The patient was a 13-year-old with spastic quadriplegia. (Courtesy of Dr. Abraham Towbin, Laboratory of Neuropathology, Danvers State Hospital, Hathorne, Massachusetts.)

There are four cellular layers of cerebral cortex, compared to the normal six, and the layering is irregular and more columnar than laminar. The reduced number of migrating cells results in a decreased amount of white matter, and in hypoplastic pyramidal tracts. The anomaly may be generalized or only affect focal areas of the cerebral cortex. The cerebellum also shows deformities, with a failure in the development of a normal folial pattern. Gray matter heterotopias occur along the brain stem and cerebellar axis. The abnormal cellular architecture serves to distinguish this anomaly from microgyri seen as a consequence of perinatal destructive lesions.

The clinical picture in micropolygyria is generally one of mental retardation and spasticity, or hypotonia with active deep tendon reflexes ("atonic cerebral palsy") (see Chapter 5).

AGENESIS OF THE CORPUS CALLOSUM

This condition takes one of two forms. In one type, agenesis of the corpus callosum is accompanied solely by defects of contiguous and phylogenetically related structures. Abnormalities include a disturbance in the convolutional pattern of the medial wall of the hemisphere, which assumes a radiate arrangement. A complete or partial absence of the cingulate gyrus and of the septum pellucidum may also be observed. The most striking feature in these brains is the presence of a longitudinal bundle, which includes those fibers which having been unable to cross to the opposite hemisphere via the corpus callosum continue their way ipsilaterally. In this type of agenesis of the corpus callosum significant neurologic abnormalities may be absent, or nonspecific, and include seizures or mild to moderate mental retardation.[94a]

In the second form, agenesis of the corpus callosum is accompanied by numerous abnormalities of cellular proliferation, including micropolygyria and heterotopias of gray matter. In these patients, including families in which the trait is transmitted by an X-linked gene,[95] there are severe intellectual retardation and seizures.

The development of the cavum septum pellucidum depends upon and follows the

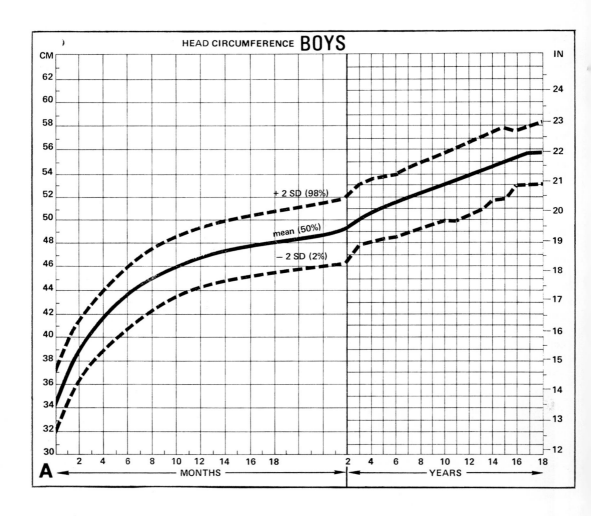

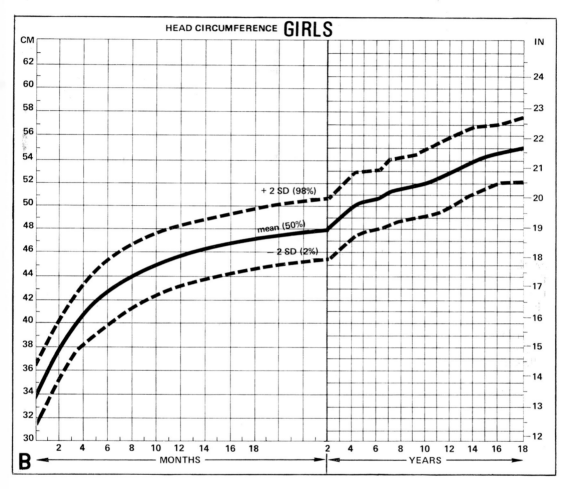

Fig. 4–8. Composite international and interracial head circumference graph. (**A**) boys; (**B**) girls. (Courtesy, Dr. G. Nellhaus, Division of Pediatric Neurology, University of Colorado School of Medicine, Denver.)

Clinical Picture

It is clear that both types of microcephaly display a broad spectrum of neurologic disorders. This ranges from decerebration to a mild impairment of fine motor coordination, from complete nonresponsiveness to educational mental retardation, and from severe autistic behavior to mild hyperkinesis.

Diagnosis

In the diagnostic evaluation of the microcephalic child various possible causes must be considered. Serologic studies for intrauterine infections, dermatoglyphics and karyotype, amino acid screening, skull x rays for intracranial calcifications, and spine films for bony dysraphisms should be considered. Craniosynostosis can be distinguished by the presence at birth of bony union between sutures. In the experience of Matson[34] no case of craniosynostosis was encountered in whom the affected suture was open at birth but closed subsequently.

Although a relationship between microcephaly and decreased intelligence was first noted over 40 years ago,[107] formal analysis correlating head circumference and mental retardation showed almost 100% of microcephalic children to be mentally retarded. In children with or without growth failure, the presence of a head circumference which is two standard deviations or more below the norm is usually indicative of mental retardation.[108] A direct linear relationship between intelligence and the severity of microcephaly has been demonstrated.[109] One can therefore expect that 90% or more of all noninstitutionalized children with a head circumference two or more standard deviations below the mean will be mentally retarded, with or without neurologic deficits.[110]

CRANIOSYNOSTOSIS

Introduction and Anatomy

This disorder was first described by Homer in the person of Thersites, "whose skull went up to a point . . . fluent orator though . . . the ugliest man who came beneath Ilion." Virchow in 1851 provided a more complete clinical resume.[111]

Craniosynostosis is defined as the premature closure at birth of one or more cranial sutures. The pathologic closure of sutures is primary and not the result of impaired brain growth. By contrast to microcephaly, craniosynostosis prejudices normal skull expansion and results in variable cosmetic deformities due to asymmetric skull growth and frequent neurologic abnormalities due to constriction of brain growth.

In the normal newborn, all sutures are separated by several millimeters except the metopic which closes antenatally. By three months the posterior fontanelle is closed. By six months there is fibrous union of suture lines and serrated edges interlock. By 20 months the anterior fontanelle is closed. At eight years, there is complete ossification of craniobasal bones and by 12 years the sutures cannot be separated by raised intracranial pressure. Solid bony union of all sutures is complete by the eighth decade.

Pathology and Etiology

There is no histologic abnormality of the prematurely fused sutures and the cause of the defect is unknown. One proposal suggests a fundamental germ layer disturbance involving the mesenchymal matrix in which bone is laid.[112] The bone itself is considered an innocent bystander, uniting only when mesenchyme has disappeared or undergone transformation. This mesenchymal defect may reflect deficient enzymatic inhibition of ossification, and may express itself either as premature cessation of mesenchymal proliferation or abnormal ossification centers within mesenchyme. In support of this concept, there are a number of familial dysmorphic syndromes, some with autosomal recessive or dominant inheritance, in which craniosynostosis plays an important part.[102,113] These syndromes comprise about 10% of patients with craniosynostosis.

Another hypothesis implicates a genetic defect of hormonal or mineral metabolism, resulting in ossification centers at abnormal sites. The finding of secondary craniosynostosis in one-third of 59 patients with vitamin D deficient or resistant rickets suggests an "osteogenic rebound" due to treatment or remission.[114] A number of generalized metabolic disorders are accompanied by premature or delayed ossification of cranial bones. These include hypophosphatasia, hypophosphatemic rickets, hypercalcemia, cleidocranial dysostosis, hyperthyroidism, and Conradi's disease.[115,116]

Mechanical factors also appear to play a role in craniosynostosis: in microcephaly and following reduction of increased intracranial pressure as occurs with surgical treatment of hydrocephalic infants, there is a secondary premature fusion of sutures. Whatever the causes of craniosynostosis, it is reasonable to assume that since both autosomal recessive and dominant transmission have been observed, the condition represents more than a single metabolic disorder of embryogenesis.

Clinical Picture

The incidence of craniosynostosis is less than five per 10,000 births, and males are affected twice as often as females.

The classification of craniosynostosis depends upon the description of head contour or upon the suture or sutures involved. The final skull shape depends upon which sutures close, the duration and order of the closure process, and the success or failure of other sutures to compensate by expansion. As a rule, skull growth is inhibited in a direction at right angles to the closed sutures. The frequency of the various types of synostosis is depicted in Table 4–3.

TABLE 4-3.

DISTRIBUTION OF SUTURE INVOLVEMENT IN 519 PATIENTS WITH CRANIOSYNOSTOSIS*

Suture or Combination of Sutures Involved	Term	Percent of Patients
Sagittal	Dolichocephaly Scaphocephaly	56
One coronal	Plagiocephaly	13
Both coronals	Acrocephaly	12
Any three	Plagiocephaly	6.9
Four or more	Oxycephaly	5.8
Metopic only	Trigonencephaly	4.0
Any two unpaired sutures	—	1.9
One lamboid only	—	1.3
Both lamboids only	—	1.0

* From Matson.[34]

6

Premature closure of the sagittal suture, the most common form of craniosynostosis, results in elongation of the skull in the anterior-posterior direction. Associated anomalies are seen in 26% of patients, and 4.8% of children are retarded. When the coronal suture fuses prematurely, expansion of the brain occurs in a lateral direction. In this condition the incidence of associated anomalies is higher, being 33% with involvement of one, and 59% with involvement of both coronal sutures.[34]

Of all types of craniosynostosis, oxycephaly may produce the most severe CNS involvement. Increased intracranial pressure, divergent strabismus, optic atrophy, anosmia, and bilateral pyramidal tract signs may occur because there are insufficient nonfused sutures to allow for expansion of the brain.

Psychomotor retardation may result from prolonged increased intracranial pressure but more often is due to associated cerebral malformations or concurrent hydrocephalus.[116a]

In Crouzon's disease (craniofacial dysostosis) premature closure of multiple sutures is associated with hypertelorism, micrognathia, choanal atresia, prognathism, beaked nose, high arched palate, but usually with normal intellect. The condition tends to be hereditary or familial.[117] In Apert's syndrome (acrocephalosyndactylism) the head is abnormally high, the orbits are shallow with resulting exophthalmos, and there is syndactyly or polydactyly. Hydrocephalus occurs commonly.

Diagnosis

In the small infant the diagnosis may be suspected in the presence of an abnormally shaped head or face. Skull x rays are diagnostically definitive. They reveal the extent of premature fusion and show an increased density of the fused suture. If the sagittal suture is involved the anterior fontanelle is obliterated. With raised intracranial pressure skull x rays after six months of age may show demineralization and thinning of bone with increased digital impressions. An air encephalogram will be necessary if hydrocephalus is suspected.

The most important differential diagnosis is that of microcephaly. Oxycephaly in particular may mimic primary microcephaly. Deformity of skull contour, closure of suture at birth or during the neonatal period, and the presence of raised intracranial pressure characterized oxycephaly.

Treatment

The indications for surgery are twofold: in cases with multiple suture closure—to limit the extent of brain damage resulting from chronic increased intracranial pressure; in children with synostosis of only one suture—to effect a good cosmetic result.

There is a unanimity of opinion regarding the need for surgery in the presence of raised intracranial pressure.[117a] However, there has been considerable debate regarding the need in the second condition, particularly in scaphocephaly. Some feel that the latter is rarely complicated by intellectual or neurologic dysfunction and that skull surgery is not justified for cosmetic reasons alone.[118] They refer to a high morbidity and poor cosmetic result in some hospitals. Matson and others point out, however, that surgery carried out late or done poorly will indeed have poor results. They argue that a significant number of sagittal fusions are associated with the late development of disabling neurologic and cognitive abnormalities[34] including intracranial hypertension and ocular abnormalities.

The relatively simple surgical procedure was developed almost 30 years ago. At that time it consisted of a linear craniectomy— that is, excision of long bars of bone along the fused suture or parallel to the suture if the sagittal was involved. Today, a polyethylene or silicone coated film is placed at the craniectomy site to prevent recalcification and osseus bridging during the growing stages.[34,119,120] If multiple sutures are fused with attendant neurologic dysfunction, surgery is performed as promptly as possible. Otherwise, as in the case of premature closure of the sagittal suture, surgery within the first six months of life will insure optimal results. Today operative mortality is 0.4% with the need for re-operation less than 15% in children with closure of a single suture, and up to 40% if multiple sutures are involved. Zenker's solution has been used following craniotomy

as a tissue fixative applied to the outer layer of dura mater to delay bone regrowth and reduce the need for re-operation.[120a] Morbidity consists of local hematoma, wound infection, or the development of a leptomeningeal cyst, and permanent morbidity is less than 1%.[121]

MACROCEPHALY

Macrocephaly is defined as a head circumference which is more than two standard deviations above the mean for age, sex, race, and gestation (Fig. 4–8). It is not a disease but a syndrome of diverse causes, most of which are discussed in other portions of this book. Clinically, it is a most vexing exercise in etiologic diagnosis. Table 4–4 outlines the most important diagnostic considerations appropriate for each age group.

Hydrocephalus and megalencephaly, each an important cause of macrocephaly, deserve special mention. The former represents enlarged ventricles due to increased cerebrospinal fluid pressure. The latter is due to an increase in brain substance abounding in excessive amounts of normal constituents, cellular proliferation, or storage of metabolites.

In true megalencephaly the increase in all neural elements is usually accompanied by overgrowth, abnormal migration, abnormal organization of some or all cellular and fiber elements of gray and white matter, giant neurons, gray matter heterotopias and defective cortical lamination.[66] The brain, which normally weighs 350 grams at birth, and 1250 to 1400 grams at maturity, may be twice as heavy as expected for the age. True megalencephaly is primarily a proliferation disorder of embryogenic origin, hamartomatous in nature with occasional malignant transformation, and therefore related to such phakomatoses as tuberose sclerosis and von Recklinghausen's disease (see Chapter 10).

The clinical picture is one of mental retardation, seizures and mild pyramidal tract and cerebellar deficits. These symptoms are occasionally progressive. The skull bones are thin, the anterior fontanelle large, and sutures slow in closing. The head reveals neither frontal bossing suggestive of hydrocephalus, nor lateral bulging seen so often with infantile subdural fluid collections. The head size, height, and weight are often large at birth and there are multiple minor congenital anomalies including abnormal dermatoglyphics and high arched palate.

Numerous instances of megalencephaly without abnormalities of cortical architecture, and with normal intellect have been reported.[122] This condition is often familial and may be transmitted as an autosomal dominant trait.

Differential Diagnosis

The differential diagnosis of macrocephaly takes into account the various conditions found to be the most likely for age of the patient. The history must answer three important questions: Was the patient abnormal from birth, or was there a period of normal growth and development before deterioration set in? Is there a family history of neurologic or cutaneous abnormalities? Is there a history of central nervous system trauma or infection?

The patient and family should be examined for cutaneous lesions such as angiomata, café-au-lait spots, vitiligo, shagreen patches, telangiectasia, and subcutaneous nodules. The fontanelle, if open, is palpated for increased intracranial pressure and its size is measured. The ranges of normal size have been recorded by Popich and Smith.[122a] Persistent enlargement of the fontanelle is not only seen in hydrocephalus, but also in athyrotic hypothyroidism, achrondroplasia, cleidocranial dysostosis, Down's syndrome, trisomies 13 and 18, and the rubella syndrome. In addition to examination of the fontanelle, the skull should be auscultated for intracranial bruits. In the infant the skull is transilluminated to assess for subdural fluid, porencephalic cysts, and hydranencephaly. An abnormal degree of transillumination may occur in hydrocephalics if the cortical mantle is less than 1 cm wide. The fundi must be evaluated for macular degeneration seen in the lipidoses, for choreoretinitis and cataracts produced by intra-uterine infections and for optic nerve tumors due to phakomatoses.

Skull, vertebral, and long bone x rays are essential to assess the presence of increased intracranial pressure, cranial or spinal dysraphisms, and intracranial calcifications produced by prenatal infections, hypoparathyroidism, or parasitic cysts. Increased cortical thickness of long bones will suggest primary skeletal disturbances and fractures in different stages of healing will suggest the diagnosis of a battered infant and a subdural hematoma.

Echoencephalography and brain scan serve as preliminary screens for ventricular size and provide evidence for a mass lesion such as a neoplasm, vascular malformation, subdural fluid collections, or porencephalic cysts.

Additional studies depend upon diagnostic expectations for each age group (Table 4–4).

HYDROCEPHALUS

Hydrocephalus is neither a disease nor a syndrome. It is a morbid entity with multiple causes, characterized by an increased amount of cerebrospinal fluid (CSF) which usually is under increased pressure as a consequence of obstructed drainage. The variation in the pathologic picture, including the nature and the extent of CSF pathway dilatation and the amount of brain damage, depends primarily on the site of obstruction, while the clinical evolution depends on the time when obstruction develops.

Physiology of the CSF

An account of the embryology, physiology, and anatomy of CSF dynamics and ventricular and subarachnoid spaces is necessary to illustrate best the spectrum of pathology. As we have discussed earlier, closure of the neural tube and primordial cephalization occur by 28 days. In man the cerebral vesicles with a central lumen develop from the cephalic end of the neural tube. These represent the major brain subdivisions and the tentatively defined ventricles, both of which become further elaborated as certain regions constrict and others expand to form the basic pattern of the ventricular system.[123]

During the second month choroid plexi primordia develop, first as a mesenchymal invagination of the roof of the fourth ventricle, then followed by a similar invaginations of the lateral and third ventricles. By the third month the plexi fill 75% of the lateral ventricle and then begin to decrease in size.

During the third trimester the plexi become very cellular and glycogen-rich. Following birth the glycogen is lost as the cell begins aerobic oxidation.[124]

As the plexi develop in the second month, the fetal ventricles are very large relative to the thickness of the cortical wall, and with further development of white and gray matter this relative dilatation disappears. It is not clear when CSF secretion is initiated, but it is certain that complete circulation from ventricle to the subarachnoid spaces cannot occur until after two months gestation.[125]

At this time the fourth ventricle exit foramina develop. These are the foramina of Luschka, two lateral apical roof apertures leading to the pontine cistern, and the foramen of Magendie, a single median posterior roof aperture leading to the cisterna magna. The fully developed choroid plexi are outpouchings into the ventricular cavity of ependyma-lined blood vessels of the pia mater. Thus this specialized epithelial layer is highly vascularized. It produces an ultrafiltrate of plasma in a stroma separated from the ventricular cavity by ependyma. CSF is then secreted across the ependyma into the ventricular cavity. These ependymal lined tufts occupy an area of 1 m². In man, probably over 90% of CSF comes from choroid plexi in the lateral ventricles[126,127] and the remainder from plexi in the 3rd and 4th ventricles. However, secretion of CSF directly into the subarachnoid spaces or ventricles from brain parenchyma appears to be functionally and therapeutically important in animal and possibly in man.[128]

In man CSF is secreted at a rate of 500 ml per 24 hours[129] or between 0.2% and 0.5% of the total volume per minute.[130] At CSF pressures below 200 mm water, production of CSF is independent of pressure.[131]

TABLE 4-4.

COMMON CAUSES OF MACROCEPHALY AND TIME OF CLINICAL PRESENTATION

EARLY INFANTILE (Birth to Six Months)

Hydrocephalus (progressive or arresting)
    Induction Disorders:
        Spina bifida cystica, cranium bifidum, Chiari malformations
        (types I, II and III), aqueductal stenosis, holoprosencephaly
    Mass Lesions:
        Neoplasms, A-V malformations, congenital cysts
    Intra-uterine Infections:
        Toxoplasmosis, cytomegalic inclusion disease, syphilis, rubella
    Peri- or Postnatal Infections:
        Bacterial, granulomatous, parasitic
    Peri- or Postnatal Hemorrhage:
        Hypoxia, vascular malformation, trauma
    Hydranencephaly
Subdural Effusion
    Hemorrhagic, infectious, cystic hygroma
Normal Variant (often familial)

LATE INFANTILE (Six months to two years)

Hydrocephalus (progressive or arresting)
    Space-occupying Lesions:
        Tumors, cysts, abcess
    Post-bacterial or Granulomatous Meningitis
    Dysraphism:
        Dandy-Walker syndrome, Chiari type I malformation
    Post-hemorrhagic:
        Trauma or vascular malformation

TABLE 4-4. (Continued)

COMMON CAUSES OF MACROCEPHALY AND TIME OF CLINICAL PRESENTATION

Subdural Effusion
Increased Intracranial Pressure Syndrome
  Pseudotumor Cerebri:
        Lead, tetracycline, hypoparathyroidism, steroids, excess or
        deficiency of Vitamin A, cyanotic congenital heart disease
Primary Skeletal Cranial Dysplasias (thickened or enlarged skull)
        Osteogenesis imperfecta, hyperphosphatemia, osteopetrosis,
        rickets
Megalencephaly (increase in brain substance)
  Metabolic CNS Diseases:
        Leukodystrophies (e.g., Canavan's, Alexander's),
        lipidoses (Tay-Sachs), histiocytosis, mucopolysaccharidoses
  Proliferative Neurocutaneous Syndromes:
        von Recklinghausen's, tuberose sclerosis, hemangiomatosis,
        Sturge-Weber
  Cerebral Gigantism:
        Sotos' syndrome
  Achondroplasia
  Primary Megalencephaly:
        May be familial and unassociated with abnormalities of cellular
        architecture, or associated with abnormalities of cellular archi-
        tecture

EARLY TO LATE CHILDHOOD (After Two Years)

Hydrocephalus ("arrested" or progressive)
  Space-occupying Lesions
  Pre-existing Induction Disorder:
        Aqueductal stenosis, Chiari type I malformation
  Post-infectious
  Hemorrhagic
Megalencephaly
  Proliferative neurocutaneous syndromes
  Familial
Pseudotumor Cerebri
Normal Variant

The biochemistry of CSF secretion is un-clear. In part CSF formation depends on glial carbonic anhydrase which facilitates the movement of sodium between blood and CSF. Water diffuses passively across the blood-CSF barrier to maintain the iso-osmotic state.[132] The administration of acetazolamide (Diamox) which inhibits car-bonic anhydrase and impairs sodium move-ment reduces CSF production by 60%.[133,134] In the experimental animal, a sodium-potas-sium-activated ATPase appears to provide energy for the active transport of sodium and potassium ions. An inhibitor of this enzyme,

the cardiac glycoside ouabain, reduces CSF production by 75%.[135] Metabolic or respira-tory alkalosis, cortisone, and hypervitaminosis A cause a decrease in CSF production in the experimental animal.[136,137]

The cells of the choroid plexus are rich in hydrolytic enzymes and ATP, and preside over oxidative phosphorylation within their mitochondria. The ependymal cells are like-wise rich in ATP and in acid and alkaline phosphatase. These enzymes provide the basis not only for a very active secretory role, but also for an absorptive one, and allow certain substances to be actively reabsorbed into the blood by choroid plexi and ependyma ("sink action").[129]

The arterial pulsations of the choroid plexi pump the CSF and begin its circulation throughout the neuraxis. This phenomenon, called the "third circulation" by Cushing,[137a] was originally formulated as early as the seventeenth century,[138] and conceptually modernized by Weed in 1913.[123] The fluid, beginning its ultimate sojourn, leaves the lateral ventricles via the foramina of Monro, enters the third ventricle from whence it moves via the aqueduct into the 4th ventricle. From there the fluid exits into the cisterns and spinal subarachnoid space via the foramina of Magendie and Luschka.

The cranial circulation proceeds posteriorly into the cisterna magna and over the cerebellum and posterior cerebral cortex. The cranial circulation also proceeds anteriorly into the basal cisterns (pontine and interpeduncular). From the basal cisterns CSF flows forward through the chiasmatic and lateral terminalis cisterns into the corpus callosum cistern. CSF also flows laterally from the basal cisterns into the ambient cisterns encircling the cerebral peduncles and emptying into the superior cistern. The superior cistern connects with the corpus callosum cistern and the cisternal circle of flow is completed, followed by widespread flow into the cerebral subarachnoid space. Eighty percent of CSF enters directly into the cisternal system with subsequent drainage from the cerebral subarachnoid space into the cortical venous system. Twenty percent circulates into the subarachnoid space of the spinal cord, but it too is eventually drained from cerebral subarachnoid space with negligible drainage from the spinal subarachnoid space into the spinal venous system.[129] CSF drainage occurs by way of the arachnoidal villi. These are single layer microtubular evaginations (up to 8 microns diameter) of the subarachnoid space into the lumen of large dural and venous sinuses. They are located principally in pacchionian granulations along the superior sagittal sinus posteriorly and at dural reflections over cranial nerves.

Three factors control CSF drainage: CSF pressure, pressure within the dural sinuses and cortical venous system, and resistance of the arachnoidal villi to CSF flow. Changes in any of these variables will significantly affect CSF flow. The normal CSF pressure is 150 mm of water in the laterally recumbent adult, and up to 180 mm in the child. The capacity for drainage is two to four times the normal rate of CSF production.[131,133]

When CSF pressure is 20–50 mm CSF, the arachnoid villi become distended with CSF and discharge their contents into the sinuses. This causes sinus pressure to rise, equalizing and then surpassing CSF pressure, causing the villi to collapse, and preventing back flow of sinus blood into the subarachnoid space. Therefore, it appears that the villi behave as "one-way valves," the critical opening pressure of which is 20–50 mm CSF,[139] and drainage is determined by hydrostatic pressure differences between CSF and sinuses. Furthermore, it appears that drainage does not depend upon colloid osmotic pressure difference between CSF and sinus blood, since the tubules are permeable to protein.[139]

Pathogenesis

It will be appreciated from the foregoing that any block in the CSF pathway from the foramina of Monro to the tubular arachnoid villi of the subarachnoid space will result in increased CSF fluid under increased pressure, and dilatation of ventricular and subarachnoid spaces. Therefore, with one possible exception, all hydrocephalic conditions are obstructive. Obstructive hydrocephalus by convention is divided into noncommunicating and communicating.

In the former the obstructive site is within the ventricular cavity, including the outlet foramina of the 4th ventricle. In the latter the obstruction occurs distally to the 4th ventricle foramina, in the cisterns or cerebral subarachnoid space itself. "Internal hydrocephalus" is used in the older literature and refers to obstructive hydrocephalus. "Hydrocephalus ex vacuo" refers to ventricular dilatation secondary to cerebral atrophy or hypoplasia. Although it is imprecise, it remains a venerable historical term. The same may be said for "external hydrocephalus," due to a developmental arachnoidal cyst and traditionally distinguished from communicating or noncommunicating obstructive hydrocephalus.

Regardless of the site of obstruction, it is the arterial pulse thrust of the choroid plexus that remains responsible for compressing the ventricular wall, enlarging the ventricular cavity,[140] and producing parenchymal disruption.[141] This pulse thrust increases with increasing mean CSF pressure and splits the ventricular ependymal lining, as demonstrated in the experimental animal.[141,142,143] This allows free and continuing transependymal flow of CSF into white matter producing spongy, atrophic, and edematous dissolution of nerve fibers and a significant degree of neuronal and astrocytic swelling in the deep areas of gray matter.[144] This is a major cause for a thin cerebral mantle. The problem of alternative avenues of CSF drainage in hydrocephalus has intrigued recent investigators.[145] To what extent normally nonfunctioning drainage routes, including the choroid plexi and the periventricular capillaries, become operative with increased CSF pressure and contribute to stabilization of pressure in the human hydrocephalic patient is unclear. However in hydrocephalic animals[133,146,147] and in man[148,149] normal ventricular pressure and the cessation of growth of the ventricular cavity appear to be due to these other drainage pathways. In hydrocephalic children, ventricular pressure varies greatly with respiration, cardiovascular changes, and activity.[150] CSF pressure is increased by sucking and crying and is normal during sleep. Therefore, normal pressure and high pressure hydrocephalus may be the same phenomenon, differing only in time and rate of development, degree of obstruction, and parenchymal integrity.[146]

Pathology

There are three general causes for hydrocephalus: 1) excess secretion due to choroid plexus papilloma; 2) obstruction within the ventricular cavity (noncommunicating); and 3) absorptive block within the subarachnoid space (communicating).

Excess Secretion-Choroid Plexus Papilloma.[151] The papilloma is a very large aggregate of choroidal fronds that are microscopically similar to normal choroid plexi and produce great quantities of CSF. They account for 1%–4% childhood intracranial tumors (see Chapter 10). They usually present after infancy and are associated with signs of increased intracranial pressure. However, some of the over 400 reported cases were found incidentally at postmortem examination. Since papillomas are prone to periodic bleeding, the CSF is proteinaceous and xanthochromic. This factor, together with the lack of proof that a normal absorptive system is unable to drain large excesses of CSF, has led to the argument that hydrocephalus in choroid plexus papillomas occurs as a consequence of arachnoidal adhesions, and obstruction of the subarachnoid space secondary to elevated CSF protein and frequent bleeding.[129,131,151,152]

Noncommunicating Hydrocephalus. Any obstruction from the foramina of Monroe or to the foramina of Magendie and Luschka will produce noncommunicating hydrocephalus. Space-occupying lesions in the cerebral hemispheres tend to compress the ventricular system, while tumors in the posterior fossa or arteriovenous malformations involving the vein of Galen may produce kinking or obstruction of the aqueduct or obstruction at the fourth ventricular outflow. These conditions are discussed in Chapter 10. At this point we will restrict ourselves to a review of the other more complex causes of aqueductal obstruction.

AQUEDUCTAL STENOSIS. This condition is responsible for 20% of hydrocephalus. Normally, the aqueduct, lined by ependyma, is 3 mm in length at birth and its mean cross section is 0.5 mm^2.[152a] with the cross sectional area ranging from 0.2 mm^2 to 1.8 mm^2.[160] In aqueductal stenosis the aqueduct is reduced in size but remains histologically normal. In particular, there is no gliosis. Constrictions of the aqueduct to less than 0.14 mm^2 may occur at two points. The first is beneath the midline of the superior quadrigeminal bodies, and the second at the intercollicular sulcus.[153]

The onset of symptoms is usually insidious and may occur at any time from birth to adulthood. In many instances aqueductal stenosis is accompanied by aqueductal forking, or marked branching of the channels. Associated malformations of neighboring structures are common.[66] These include fusion of the quadrigeminal bodies, fusion of the third nerve nuclei and more caudal defects of neural tube closure such as spina bifida cystica or occulta. These associated anomalies raise the possibility that aqueductal stenosis itself probably represents a mild expression of a neural tube defect. A small percentage is caused by a sex-linked recessive gene, representing the only known example in man of an isolated structural abnormality due to a single gene effect with autosomal recessive or sex-linked recessive transmission.[154,155]

AQUEDUCTAL GLIOSIS. This is a post-inflammatory process, usually secondary to a perinatal infection or hemorrhage.[153] With the increasing survival of newborns affected with bacterial meningitis or intracranial hemorrhage this condition has assumed increasing importance. The ependymal lining is permanently destroyed since it is highly vulnerable to insult and without regenerative power. There is marked fibrillary gliosis of adjacent tissue and granular ependymitis is seen below the obstruction. The occlusion is progressive and like aqueductal stenosis its onset is insidious. Aqueductal gliosis frequently accompanies von Recklinghausen's disease. A variant, also post-inflammatory in nature, appears as a septal obstruction at the caudal end of the aqueduct. This is due to a membrane of neuroglial overgrowth associated with a granular ependymitis.[66,153] Aqueductal stenosis and gliosis have been produced in experimental animals by viral infections, and a patient has been reported with aqueductal stenosis following mumps encephalitis.

Descending the ventricular system, the next major area of obstruction is at the fourth ventricle. This represents the site of obstruction in 50% of all hydrocephalic children.

Two major entities, both congenital malformations involving the fourth ventricle, deserve special attention:

CHIARI MALFORMATIONS. This defect alone or in combination with other anomalies accounts for 40% of all hydrocephalic children.[156] This entity is discussed elsewhere in detail. In essence it is a neural tube defect, presenting with malformations of the lower brain stem and cerebellum and herniation of these structures through the foramen magnum (Fig. 4–3). Whether the obstruction is due to fourth ventricle block secondary to atresia of the foramina, aqueductal stenosis,[153] or herniation with obliteration of subarachnoid pathways around the brainstem or higher, remains in dispute.[66]

DANDY-WALKER SYNDROME. This condition, described by Dandy in 1921,[157] and so named by Benda,[92] represents a hugely dilated fourth ventricle which behaves like a cyst and is roofed by a neuroglial-vascular membrane lined with ependyma. This "cyst" herniates caudally and separates the cerebellar hemispheres posteriorly (Fig. 4–11). The vermis and choroid plexi are rudimentary. The foramina of the fourth ventricle are often occluded by membranes or are atretic. Occasionally hydrocephalus fails to develop, either because the foramina are small but patent, or because CSF is absorbed through their membranes. The basic embryonic failure appears unrelated to occlusion of the foramina for two reasons. First, the foramina are occasionally open and secondly, the associated malformations of vermis and fourth ventricle occur prior to development of the foramina. Benda and others consider the Dandy-Walker syndrome to be a defect of neural tube closure at the cerebellar level.[92,157a] This entity must be distinguished from arachnoidal cysts of the 4th ventricular roof, which lie above the foramen of Magendie.[158] It is noteworthy that in Dandy-Walker syndrome hydrocephalus often does not herald itself until after infancy. The condition is characterized by a bulging occiput, nystagmus, ataxia and, cranial nerve deficits.

Other conditions which frequently obstruct 4th ventricular outflow are space-occupying lesions, particularly those involving the posterior fossa. Less often a retro-cerebellar subdural hematoma or bacterial or granulomatous meningitis will occlude the foramina of Magendie and Luschka.[159]

Communicating Hydrocephalus. This represents 30% of all childhood hydrocephalus. Once the CSF leaves the foramina of the

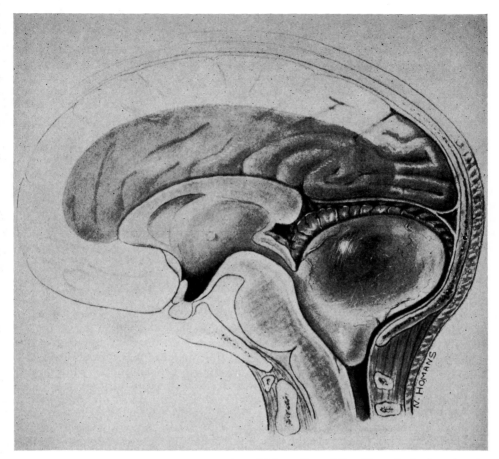

Fig. 4–11. Congenital obstruction of the foramina of Magendie and Luschka. Sagittal section showing dilatation of fourth ventricle to form a huge cyst within the posterior fossa. The tentorium is displaced upwards and the cerebellum is compressed. (From Matson, D. D.: *Neurosurgery of Infancy and Childhood*, 2nd ed., 1969, courtesy of Charles C Thomas Publisher, Springfield.)

4th ventricle and enters the cisterns it must progress into the cerebral and cerebellar subarachnoid space. Drainage is in jeopardy if the cisterns or the arachnoid villi over the cerebral cortex are obstructed by thickened arachnoid or meninges. This may be due to intracranial hemorrhage, or bacterial or granulomatous meningitis.

In premature infants intraventricular hemorrhage is secondary to neonatal hypoxia. Subarachnoid hemorrhage is usually seen in full-term infants and is due to trauma. The pathogenesis and pathology of these conditions are discussed more fully in Chapter 5.

Meningitis may produce communicating hydrocephalus during the acute phase by clumping of purulent fluid in the drainage channels, and in the chronic phase by organization of exudate and blood resulting in fibrosis of the subarachnoid spaces (see Chapter 6).[152] As a rule, bacterial meningitis tends to produce cerebral cortical arachnoiditis, while granulomatous or parasitic meningitis produces cisternal obstruction. Rarely, viral meningitis may result in obstruction at either point. Intra-uterine infections are discussed in Chapter 6.

Two causes of communicating hydrocephalus, though uncommon, deserve mention. The first of these is diffuse meningeal malignancy due to lymphoma or leukemia. The second is an extra-axial arachnoid cyst which may be located in the basal cistern or over the cerebral cortex. The cyst traps CSF without allowing full drainage into the sinuses. As it enlarges it eventually produces extrinsic compression of the ventricular system or of the subarachnoid channels.

Finally, obstruction within the veins and sinuses may rarely be responsible for communicating hydrocephalus.[161,162,163] Sinus pressure is independent of CSF pressure by virtue of the support given to the sinuses by their fibrous dura.[129] However an increase in pressure within the sinuses due to either their obstruction or increased venous pressure will result in a striking elevation of CSF pressure. Surprisingly, there is no experimental evidence supporting the clinical impression that chronic obstruction of any of the major sinuses or of the vein of Galen can produce permanent hydrocephalus.[164,165] It is interesting to note that occasionally large space-occupying lesions within the posterior fossa may cause hydrocephalus without impinging on the 4th ventricle, perhaps the result of venous obstruction.

Clinical Picture

Two major factors influence the clinical course in hydrocephalus. These are the time of onset and preexisting structural lesions. The time when hydrocephalus develops in relation to closure of the cranial sutures will determine whether enlargement of the head will be the presenting sign. Prior to two years of age progressive enlargement of the head is an almost invariable presenting complaint. When hydrocephalus develops after two years of age, any changes in head circumference are overshadowed by other neurologic manifestations. In older infants and in children the space-occupying lesions responsible for hydrocephalus often produce focal neurologic signs before causing CSF obstruction.

Neonatal Period Through Infancy (0–2 Years). Hydrocephalus causing an abnormally large head or abnormally accelerating head growth during this time is usually due to a major defect in embryogenesis. The Chiari malformations with or without spina bifida cystica,

aqueductal stenosis, and aqueductal gliosis account for 80% of all hydrocephalus in this period and represent 60% of all hydrocephalus regardless of age.[156] The remainder are a consequence of intra-uterine infection, anoxic or traumatic perinatal hemorrhage, and neonatal bacterial or viral meningoencephalitis. Rare causes include congenital midline tumor, choroid plexus papilloma, and arteriovenous malformation of the vein of Galen or straight sinus. Apart from the features unique to each disease entity, they all produce a stereotyped clinical picture.

The head grows at an abnormal rate (Fig. 4–8) and is macrocephalic within one to two months, if not at birth. The forehead is disproportionally large, lending an inverted triangular appearance to the head. The skull is thin and the sutures are excessively separated. This results in an accentuated "cracked pot" sound on percussion of the skull. The anterior fontanelle is tense and nonpulsatile. The scalp veins are dilated and strikingly so when the infant cries. A divergent strabismus with the eyeballs rotated downwards is often noted. This "setting sun sign" is a consequence of pressure upon a thinned orbital roof, or pressure of the suprapineal recess of the 3rd ventricle upon the mesencephalic tectum. Other ocular disturbances include unilateral or bilateral abducens nerve paresis, nystagmus, ptosis, and a diminished pupillary light response. Optic atrophy due to compression of the chiasm and optic nerves by a dilated anterior portion of the 3rd ventricle may occur. Papilledema is rare, however, perhaps because of the presence of open sutures.

Early infantile automatisms persist, indicating a failure in the development of normal cortical inhibition. Responses such as the parachute reflex, expected to appear later in infancy, fail to develop. Opisthotonus may be striking. A common finding is spasticity of the lower extremities. This results from proportionately more stretching and distortion of myelinated paracentral corticospinal fibers arising from the leg area of the motor cortex. These fibers have a longer distance to travel around the dilated ventricle than do the corticospinal and corticobulbar fibers supplying the upper extremities and face.[166] However, mild spasticity and weakness will occur in the upper limbs. Clinical signs are due more to myelin disruption than to cellular loss.[166b]

Of great importance is the development of deranged lower brain stem function due to bilateral corticobulbar disruption, so-called pseudobulbar palsy. This is manifested by difficulty in sucking, feeding, phonation, and results in regurgitation, drooling, and aspiration. Laryngeal stridor, although not common, is very distressing.[166a] It is related to vagal nerve traction or perhaps infarction of the vagal nuclei in the medulla. Corticobulbar deficits together with a change in acoustic properties of brain and calvarium account for the characteristic shrill, brief and high pitched cry.

Other features of early infantile hydrocephalus relate more to specific causes. The Dandy-Walker syndrome, although infrequent in early infancy, results in a large posterior fossa and a dolichocephalic appearance. The Chiari malformation type 2 is almost always associated with spina bifida cystica, and occasionally with short malformed necks due to basilar impression, platybasia, or the Klippel-Feil syndrome.

If hydrocephalus is rapidly progressive, as in acute bacterial meningitis or diffuse cortical thrombophlebitis, emesis, somnolence, irritability, seizures, and cardiopulmonary embarrassment will occur despite open sutures. Neonates with severe hydrocephalus associated with congenital anomalies usually do not survive the neonatal period.

Early to Late Childhood (2–10 Years). In this age group neurologic symptoms due to increased intracranial pressure, or focal deficits referable to the primary lesion, tend to appear prior to any significant changes in head size.

At this time the most common causes for hydrocephalus are posterior fossa neoplasms and obstructions at the aqueduct. The Chiari type 1 malformation, with abnormalities of the craniobasal bones and cervical vertebrae, while rare, is most likely to be encountered in this age group.

The clinical picture of the various space-occupying lesions is discussed in Chapter 10. A unique hydrocephalic syndrome is characterized by mental retardation, 3 per second head oscillations, and dysesthesias of the head especially to touch.[167,168] Between 2 and 10 years the infections most likely to cause hydrocephalus are tuberculosis and fungal or parasitic infections. Hydrocephalus resulting from any one of these agents has its special features. However, in almost all instances increased intracranial pressure produces headache upon awakening in the morning with improvement following emesis or upright posture, papilledema, and strabismus. On radiographic examination of the skull there is diastasis of the sutures with erosion of the clinoids and sella turcica. The "cracked pot" sound is prominent on skull percussion. Pyramidal tract signs are more marked in the lower limbs for reasons noted earlier.

Additional features seen in this late onset group are also encountered in the early onset group in whom hydrocephalus has become arrested or marginally compensated either spontaneously or due to surgical intervention. These features include endocrine changes resulting in small stature, obesity, gigantism, delayed or precocious puberty, primary amenorrhea or menstrual irregularities, absent secondary sexual characteristics, and diabetes insipidus.[169,169a] They are probably due to abnormal hypothalamic function, a consequence of increased intracranial pressure. Spastic diplegia is prominent and both upper limbs exhibit mild pyramidal tract signs resulting in fine motor incoordination. Perceptual motor deficits and visual spatial disorganization ensue as a consequence of stretched corticospinal fibers of parietal and occipital cortex due to dilated posterior horns of the lateral ventricles. Performance intelligence is considerably worse than verbal intelligence, and learning problems are common.[170] Children are sociable, cute, conversationally bright, and exhibit relatively good memory, but are often hyperkinetic, emotionally labile and unable to conceptualize.[171]

Diagnosis

In infancy the diagnosis of hydrocephalus is based on a head circumference that, regardless of absolute size, crosses one or more grid lines in the course of two to four weeks (Figs. 4–8, 4–12). Such an infant requires prompt

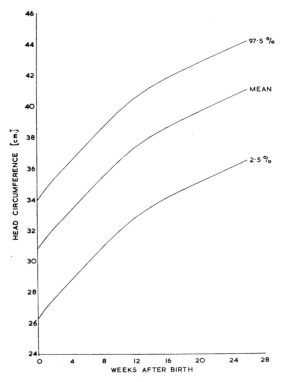

Fig. 4–12. Head circumference chart for premature infants. (Courtesy of O'Neill, E. M.: Archives of Disease in Childhood, 36:241, 1961).

diagnostic evaluation, particularly when neurologic signs are present and progressive. We should stress that in all instances it is necessary to localize the site of CSF obstruction and, if possible, its cause prior to the institution of surgical procedures. In evaluating a premature infant for hydrocephalus, the apparent abnormal acceleration of head growth must be considered, and special head circumference charts should be consulted (Fig. 4–12).[172]

Diagnostic studies, in order of their complexity, include the following: transillumination of the skull is performed in a totally darkened room after a three-minute dark adaptation by the examiner. A strong flashlight with a rubber adapter* that fits snugly against the infant's head is used. In the normal full-term infant a halo of light extends 1 to 2 cm from the rim of the light

* MacBick Co., Boston, Massachusetts.

source. The extent of transillumination may be greater in the premature infant. Transillumination is greatest over the frontal regions and normally fingerlike projections may extend up to 3 cm over the area of the anterior fontanelle.[173,173a] The extent of illumination is normal in full-term hydrocephalic infants, unless the cortical mantle is less than 1 cm in thickness. In hydranencephaly transillumination is striking. Transillumination of subdural effusions or porencephalic cysts is limited to the area of pathology, and is therefore often asymmetric. The presence of posterior fossa cysts, as in the Dandy-Walker syndrome, may also be suspected from an asymmetric transillumination.

In the Chiari type 2 malformation, 50% of neonates display craniolacuniae on radiographic examination of the skull (Fig. 4–13). In this condition, probably a defect in membranous bone formation, there is an irregular honeycomblike configuration of the skull with multiple, oval radiolucencies separated by dense bony ridges. X rays of the spine are indicated in any evaluation of infantile hydrocephalus. These may reveal spina bifida occulta or abnormalities of the cervical vertebrae.

A technetium 99 m brain scan is performed to detect neoplasms or A-V malformations greater than 1 cm diameter. Ultrasound A scanning for ventricular size may be employed

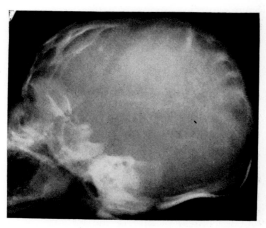

Fig. 4–13. Craniolacunae. Multiple radiolucencies are separated by bony ridges. (Courtesy of Dr. Gabriel Wilson, Department of Radiology, UCLA, Los Angeles.)

but in the absence of striking hydrocephalus lacks reliability.[174,174a]

Subdural taps are done through the open sutures with a ventricular needle. Ventricular taps and ventriculography are best reserved for the neurosurgeon. The needle is advanced into the lateral ventricle simultaneously measuring the thickness of the cortical mantle. A "bracketing" study is then done by introducing a lumbar needle and obtaining pressure measurements. With noncommunicating blocks at any level the CSF pressures in ventricular and lumbar spaces neither correlate with each other nor are they affected by jugular compression or postural changes. Furthermore, lumbar CSF protein is often strikingly elevated. Next, 60 to 100 cc of oxygen, exchanged for CSF, is injected into the ventricle and 20 to 30 cc of oxygen into the lumbar space. Proper positioning of the gas will bracket neatly the exact site of obstruction. Rare blocks at the foramina of Monro, and the more common obstructions at the 3rd ventricle, aqueduct and 4th ventricle exits can be appreciated. If the lateral ventricle chosen for initial exploration, itself appears blocked, then the other should be tapped and studied as well.

Absence of gas beyond the pontine or interpeduncular cisterns may represent a basal cistern block. In 90% of communicating hydrocephalus, no gas will progress beyond these basal cisterns.[175] However, failure to see gas over the cerebral convexities does not necessarily mean a block in the subarachnoid space. Up to 40% of nonhydrocephalic infants may have little or no gas over the cerebral cortex due to a shallow subarachnoid space or narrow channels connecting the subarachnoid space with the major cisterns.[175]

If better visualization of the intraventricular system is necessary, positive contrast ventriculography can be performed with Pantopaque. Dural sinography in infants with 50% Hypaque injected into the longitudinal sinus via the anterior fontanelle may be useful for complete study of outlet blocks at the foramina of Magendie and Luschka.[34]

The use of an inert dye marker such as phenolsulphonephthalein or indigo carmine, while of historical interest, is an unreliable method of distinguishing communicating from noncommunicating hydrocephalus.

Carotid and vertebral angiography is used to exclude the presence of a subdural hematoma and is an important diagnostic adjunct when the presence of an arteriovenous malformation is suspected. Its use to ascertain the site of CSF obstruction is still under investigation.[176,176a]

The child whose head circumference is greater than the 97th percentile, but whose head growth parallels the normal curve, presents an important diagnostic problem. This type of patient should not initially be subjected to air encephalography, with its attendant risks of reactivating hydrocephalus which has been partially or completely arrested. Rather, two relatively new and safe techniques may be employed in such a case. The first consists of the injection into the lumbar sac or cisterna of I^{131} labelled human serum albumin (RISA) or technetium (Tc 99m).[177] Gamma emission is measured by an external scanner. In communicating hydrocephalus I^{131} RISA collects entirely within the ventricular system and persists there for 24 to 48 hours. The ventricular persistence of RISA for this period of time correlates with shunt responsiveness in adults.[180] In noncommunicating hydrocephalus and in normal patients there is no retrograde ventricular filling. In the normal patient this is due to the high flow of CSF dynamics and by four hours, all the supratentorial cisterns (callosal and sylvian) are well-visualized. By 12 to 24 hours, RISA concentrates over the cerebral convexities, toward the parasagittal area. In 48 hours the CSF is clear. Thus, in such a patient, the main use of isotope ventriculography is to assess for communicating hydrocephalus and simultaneously to exclude hydrocephalus ex vacuo. This test is useful in the diagnosis of normal pressure hydrocephalus. This is a condition which is characterized by symptomatic hydrocephalus in the face of normal CSF pressure. Although usually limited to adult life, it has also been encountered in children as a complication of posterior fossa surgery.[179] It must be appreciated that in hydrocephalus RISA penetrates ventricular boundaries with ease and enters the surrounding brain.[178] This procedure can therefore not be used exclusively to demonstrate obstructive blocks.[178,181] In combined communicating and noncommunicating hydrocephalus results obtained on a RISA study may be uninterpretable.

Another diagnostic procedure which, however, is more liable to disturb CSF dynamics, is the recently devised constant infusion manometric study.[182,183] Artificial CSF is infused via the lumbar route and indirect measurements of reserve drainage capacity can be performed. Normally an infusion rate twice the CSF formation rate will produce slow and modest elevations in CSF pressure. In communicating hydrocephalus the CSF pressure rises abruptly and markedly with such an infusion rate. Increasingly better standardization of CSF pressure rises at given infusion rates will make this a valuable diagnostic tool, particularly in assessing children with "arrested" or "compensated" communicating hydrocephalus or hydrocephalus ex vacuo, and in evaluating suspected shunt obstructions.

When hydrocephalus develops after infancy, children present with symptoms and signs of increased intracranial pressure. Their diagnostic evaluation is similar to that suggested for tumor suspects (see Chapter 10).

Differential Diagnosis

The differential diagnosis of macrocephaly at various ages is presented in Table 4-4.

Treatment

The treatment of hydrocephalus is by surgery. With few exceptions, noted later, medical reduction of CSF formation has proved ineffective, and radiotherapy is limited to the rare radiosensitive tumor obstructing an outflow channel. The general principles of treatment are: 1) surgical correction of CSF obstruction; 2) reduction of CSF production by drugs or surgical therapy; 3) ventricular bypass into a normal intracranial channel in noncommunicating hydrocephalus; and 4) ventricular bypass into an extracranial compartment in either noncommunicating or communicating hydrocephalus.

In the child with rapidly progressive hydrocephalus of whatever cause, the need for therapy is obvious. However, the patient in whom hydrocephalus progresses slowly, or who is suspected to have arrested spontaneously, presents a difficult therapeutic problem. Matson has suggested that the child whose head circumference is greater than the 97th percentile, but whose head growth parallels the normal curve, does not have arrested hydrocephalus and therefore is a candidate for surgery.[34,184] We recommend a somewhat more conservative approach and believe that the decision on whether to operate should be based on the clinical condition of the patient and the results of the RISA studies. In the absence of intellectual or neurologic deficits, temporizing is indicated. The finding of communicating hydrocephalus, particularly postmeningitic hydrocephalus, or mild hydrocephalus associated with spina bifida cystica, which is likely to be arrested spontaneously,[185] argues for conservative therapy. On the other hand, needless procrastination or failure to treat may result in subtle compromise of both cognitive function and fine and gross motor coordination, recognized after infancy and too late to be reversed by shunting.[186]

Although the underlying cause[202] of hydrocephalus and serial developmental examinations may provide clues to the ultimate prognosis, they cannot be used as the basis for a decision on whether to submit the patient to surgery. Neither the width of the cortical mantle nor the head circumference correlate with the ultimate intellectual and neurologic status of the child.[203]

Surgical Treatment

Direct Attack. If the obstruction is surgically accessible a shunt may be avoided. Cystic or neoplastic obstruction of the foramina of Magendie or Luschka may be resected at suboccipital craniotomy and upper cervical laminectomy. Adhesions within the cisterna magna may be catheterized from the posterior fossa.[34] In hydrocephalus caused by these accessible lesions, shunting may be done prior to direct surgery to allow normalization of pressure and to insure a lower operative mortality and morbidity.

Indirect Attack. There are two techniques of great historical interest: endoscopic choroid plexus extirpation (plexectomy or electric coagulation) and third or fourth ventriculostomy. The former has been used successfully in communicating hydrocephalus[187] and reasons have been advanced for its continuing use.[188] Although complicated by intracerebral hemorrhage and potentially by cystic dilatations of the endoscopic tracts[189] and an operative mortality of 10%, the arrest rate is 65%. The elimination of the choroid plexus pulse effect, the main reason for ventricular dilatation, provides a pathophysiologic rationale for this approach. The procedure is often unsuitable for infants because of technical difficulties and frequently inadequate due to coexisting obstructions of the subarachnoid space.

Ventricular Bypass. The vast majority of progressive hydrocephalus must be shunted primarily and exclusively. Therapeutically the distinction between communicating (extraventricular) and noncommunicating (intraventricular) hydrocephalus has been rendered less important by modern shunt technology. In both types the lateral ventricle is utilized as the drained reservoir. The CSF is bypassed from the ventricle, the site of production, around the obstruction and into a freely draining compartment of the body.

Ventricular-cisterna magna shunts are utilized in older children with noncommunicating hydrocephalus or in hydrocephalus due to posterior fossa mass lesions obstructing outflow, with acceptable results in 75% of patients.[151] Technical difficulties preclude the use of this procedure in infants.[34]

Vascular Shunts. Currently, the treatment of choice for communicating hydrocephalus and for infantile noncommunicating hydrocephalus is to drain the CSF from the lateral ventricle into an extracranial compartment— the superior vena cava—via the one-way valved ventricular-venous shunt. The slit one-way valves used in this procedure open at a predetermined intraventricular pressure and close once the pressure falls below that level, thus preventing retrograde flow of venous blood into the ventricular cavity. With an operative mortality under 3% in the past 15 years and an arrest rate over 75%,[151]

this technique is generally preferred in both communicating and noncommunicating hydrocephalus. Two types of valves are widely used and newer ones are under investigation.[189a] The Holter valve consists of two stainless steel check valves connected by silicone tubing. The Pudenz-Heyer-Schulte is a plastic bubble pump placed under the scalp with its distal end connected to the slit valve. The latter apparatus can be "pumped" to check for patency and to clear partial obstructions. The Holter can be attached to a Rickham or Ommaya reservoir placed in the burr hole to measure ventricular pressure and instill antibiotics. Therefore, this reservoir is useful when hydrocephalus is due to infection or hemorrhage, or associated with high CSF protein and infected spina bifida cystica.

The venous end of the shunt is placed in the superior vena cava at the level of the sixth thoracic vertebrae. If it enters the auricle, endocardial contusions and clotting occur resulting in bacterial endocarditis, bacteremia, and ventriculitis. A 20%–30% incidence of these complications in ventricular venous shunts 10 years ago[191] currently has been reduced to 15%.[34,191a,192] *Staphylococcus albus* and diphtheroids are the usual offending organisms[34,193] and the infection is often inapparent. Long-term penicillin therapy often suffices but shunt replacement is usually necessary. If the venous end of the shunt is above the fifth thoracic vertebra, blood flow will not be sufficiently turbulent to prevent the tube clotting or jugular-superior vena cava thrombosis. Decreased platelet survival time may also contribute to thrombosis.[190] Shunt obstruction in communicating hydrocephalus is best evaluated by RISA cisternography and constant infusion studies.

In the experience of Matson, two-thirds of 162 ventricular-venous shunts required at least one revision for infection, shunt obstruction, or prophylaxis when the distal end rises to the fourth thoracic vertebra or higher because of body growth.[34] Logue in a similar group recommends routine shunt revision in the second year and again at four to six years of age to maintain a high functional level.[151] Recently, a ventricular-direct atriotomy shunt to replace obstructed ventricular-venous shunts has been reported with good results,[194] and has been used effectively as a primary procedure in the newborn period.[49]

The long-term complications are as yet unknown since routine shunting has been employed less than 20 years. The incidence of short-term complications is presented in Table 4–5. In children the success of ventricular-venous shunts, including revisions, has been over 70% in noncommunicating and over 90% in communicating hydrocephalus.[151,186] It remains unclear when the child may outgrow the need for CSF diversion. However it appears that the younger the child when shunted, the more likely shunt dependence will be permanent.[195]

Drainage into other body compartments from the lateral ventricle in noncommunicating hydrocephalus, and from the subarachnoid space in communicating hydrocephalus, has been employed as an alternative to ventricular-venous shunts with an arrest rate approaching 65%.[196] However, shunts drained into the peritoneal or pleural compartment have a 50% incidence of obstruction. Ureteral shunts entail the sacrifice of one kidney and are complicated by hyponatremic-hypochloremic dehydration.

The reader is referred to Matson[34] for a more detailed presentation of neurosurgical techniques.

Medical Treatment. Working on the same principle as choroid plexus extirpation, i.e., reduction of CSF formation, acetazolamide (Diamox), a carbonic anhydrase inhibitor, has been used with modest success in selected cases. A borderline or very slowly progressive hydrocephalus, growing at a rate of less than 1.5 cm per month in the first two years, in whom spontaneous arrest or compensation is anticipated, may benefit. A dose up to 50 mgm per kilo body weight per day in divided amounts is recommended.[198] Higher doses are complicated by metabolic acidosis. Acetazolamide is ineffective in hydrocephalus of any cause producing rapid increase in head size or unrelenting raised intracranial pressure.[198,199] Acetazolamide may be used as a temporizing or preoperative measure in acute hydrocephalus that is not brought to surgery promptly for whatever reasons. It may be used alone or together with urea,[200] glycerol,[133] or mannitol. The latter agents are hyperosmolal solutions and, as osmotic diuretics, cause a net flow of water out of brain cells into blood with a subsequent reduction in intraventricular pres-

TABLE 4-5.

RESULTS AND COMPLICATIONS OF VENTRICULAR BYPASS PROCEDURES

Operation	No. Cases	Operative Mortality (Percent)	Initial Success Rate (Percent)	Total Complications (Percent)	Complications Obstruction	Infection (Percent)	Other
Third ventriculostomy	529	15	70	2			
Cauterization of choroid plexus	91	15	60	3			
Torkildsen procedure	136	30	58	50	50		
Cardiac shunts	345	6	62	46	28	12	6*
Pleural shunts	108	8	53	100	100		
Peritoneal shunts	230	13	55	58	58		
Ureteral shunts	108	1	65	44	16	8	20**

* Thrombosis of superior vena cava
** Salt depletion
Pooled data from literature; Paine.[197]

sure. Another osmotic agent, isosorbide (Hydronal), acts as both an osmotic diuretic and an inhibitor of CSF production.[201,201a]

Prognosis. Based on studies of the natural course of untreated[195,204,205] and spontaneously arrested hydrocephalus,[171,206,207] it is clear that surgery represents a major advance in reducing mortality and limiting morbidity.[186,197] Untreated hydrocephalus has a 50% mortality. In one study 50% of the survivors were mentally retarded in the illiterate range or worse, and less than 10% intellectually normal. Over two-thirds of survivors had major physical handicaps.[205] Other studies of spontaneously arrested hydrocephalus revealed an IQ over 90 in one-third of survivors and disabling neurologic defects in two-thirds.[171] The latter included ataxia, spastic diplegia, compromised fine motor coordination, and perceptual deficits.

In surgically treated hydrocephalus the survival rate is about 80%[186] with two-thirds of deaths occurring within a year of the initiation of treatment. About one-third of survivors are both intellectually and neurologically normal, and one-half have neurologic deficits. Generally, noninfective hydrocephalus carries the best prognosis.

HYDRANENCEPHALY

Pathology

In this condition the greater portion of both the cerebral hemispheres and the corpus striatum are reduced to membranous sacs composed of glial tissue covered by intact meninges and encompassing a cavity filled with clear, protein-rich CSF. Basal portions of frontal, temporal, and occipital lobe are preserved, together with scattered islands of cortex elsewhere. The diencephalon, midbrain, and brain stem are usually normal except for rudimentary descending corticobulbar and corticospinal tracts. The cerebellum may be normal[208] or markedly hypoplastic or damaged.[209] In some cases the ependyma lining the covering membrane is intact, the choroid plexus is preserved, and the aqueduct stenotic. Other cases present as large bilateral schizencephalic clefts in which pia and ependyma are joined, and demonstrate other migration anomalies of fetal morphogenesis. In still other brains there are bilateral porencephalic cysts which replace the parenchyma normally perfused by the middle and anterior cerebral arteries. In the latter instances there is pathologic evidence of a destructive lesion.

Pathogenesis

The pathology suggests at least four different pathogenetic mechanisms. First, it has been argued that hydranencephaly is a type of hydrocephalus which has run its course in utero.[93] The presence of preserved ependyma and aqueductal stenosis in some cases supports this as one possible mechanism. In other instances hydranencephaly may be the consequence of intra-uterine infections or other gestational insults.[209,210] In other cases the condition may represent a genetically determined defect in vascular ontogenesis or the outcome of vascular occlusion of both internal carotid arteries or their main branches.[208,211,212,213] A few cases appear to be due to defects in embryogenesis and subsequent cellular migration resulting in schizencephaly and cortical agenesis.[14]

Clinical Picture

Infants appear normal at birth or present with a somewhat large head which enlarges progressively. Spontaneous and reflex activity is often normal. However, failure in the development of cerebrocortical inhibition results in the persistence and exaggeration of reflexes, which become apparent by the second or third postnatal week. Over the subsequent weeks hyperreflexia, hypertonia, quadriparesis, and decerebration develop, together with irritability, infantile spasms, and disconjugate extraocular movements. Generalized or minor motor seizures also become apparent. Electroencephalography may be normal at first but later becomes abnormal, varying from a diffusely slow to an isoelectric pattern.

Diagnosis

Transillumination (Fig. 4–14) suggests the presence of hydranencephaly. With an enlarged head or abnormally accelerating head growth, an air encephalogram is mandatory to exclude severe obstructive hydrocephalus,

TABLE 4-6.

**UNUSUAL CONGENITAL DEFECTS OF THE CRANIAL NERVES
AND RELATED STRUCTURES**

Condition	Effect	Reference
Marcus Gunn's syndrome	Eyelid lifts when jaw is opened and closes when jaw is closed, or vice versa	Falls, et al.[225]
Duane's syndrome	Fibrosis of one or both lateral rectus muscles results in retraction of the globe on adduction of the eye	Duane[226]
Congenital optic atrophy	Congenitally small and atrophic disks; poor vision, diminished pupillary light response	Walton and Robb[227]
Congenital nystagmus	Rapid and fine nystagmus, often pendular; head often turned so that eyes are in the position of least nystagmus; may be dominant or sex-linked recessive trait	Cox[228]
Congenital anomaly of facial nerve	Weakness associated with deformities of ipsilateral ear	Dickinson, et al.[229]

of normal proliferation of vessel media and elastica.

A review of the embryology of the cerebral vascular system is presented by Padget[230] and Arey.[6]

ANGIOMA

Angiomas are developmental malformations and not vascular neoplasms,[231] although some, through proliferation, may produce progressive destructive changes in surrounding parenchyma.[232] Malformations range from huge cavernous venous angiomas that often do not bleed to tiny subependymal "cryptic" angiomas that bleed massively and simultaneously obliterate themselves. They are the most common cause of nontraumatic intracranial hemorrhage in children.

ARTERIOVENOUS MALFORMATIONS

Arteriovenous malformations are the most common vascular lesion in the CNS and account for about 50% of all angiomas. The malformations may be located in any part of the neuraxis.[231,233,234,235,236,243] They result from the embryogenic failure of capillary development between artery and vein, producing enlargement of these vessels

and abnormal shunting of blood.[237] The "bag of worms" appearance is due to the tangled mass of dilated veins, to the frequently enlarged and tortuous arteries feeding these venous channels, and to interposed thickened, dilated, and hyalinized vessels. The malformation may extend from the cortical meningeal surface through the parenchyma to the ventricular cavity, and its size may vary from 1 mm to over 10 cm. Calcification within the walls of the vessel and the surrounding parenchyma is common, and there may even be some ossification. Hemosiderin may be found in the gliotic parenchyma, a reflection of extravasation of blood. The important though rare carotid-cavernous fistula is almost always traumatic in origin. However spontaneous fistulae have been reported with the Ehlers-Danlos syndrome.[243a]

Clinical Manifestations

Only about one-half of arteriovenous malformations are symptomatic during lifetime. In most large studies of symptomatic arteriovenous malformations, 10% become clinically manifest during the first decade[236] and up to 45% by the second or third decade.[236] The clinical picture of an arteriovenous malformation depends on its location, and as to whether it presents with an intracranial hemorrhage or as a space-occupying lesion.

An intracranial hemorrhage is the most common initial manifestation and occurs in 40%–80% of all symptomatic arteriovenous malformations. Depending on the location of the malformation, the hemorrhage may dissect into the subarachnoid space, the ventricles, or will be intracerebral and form a hematoma within the parenchyma. Life-threatening transtentorial or foramen magnum pressure cones may develop.[249] Any combination of the three courses may be observed.[236,236a] Sudden severe headache, nuchal rigidity, irritability, vomiting, neurologic deficits (particularly a progressive hemiparesis), focal or generalized seizures, and progressive deterioration of consciousness characterize the clinical course of a ruptured arteriovenous malformation.[236,238,239] An arteriovenous malformation occurring in an infant may rarely produce increased intracranial pressure as the initial symptom. This may be due to the mass effect of the lesion itself, an intracerebral hematoma, intraventricular hemorrhage, or dissection of a superficial cortical hemorrhage into the subdural space.

Depending on the location of the malformation a variety of focal neurologic signs may be encountered.

Subcortical Midline Syndrome. This syndrome is associated with an arteriovenous malformation of the vein of Galen, or the posterior or superior cerebellar arteries, and is generally encountered in infancy. The so-called "aneurysm of the vein of Galen" is actually an arteriovenous malformation. Signs appearing during the neonatal period are primarily those of congestive heart failure.[240,240b] Shunting of a large volume of blood results in decreased peripheral resistance and increased cardiac output. This produces a high output congestive heart failure with cardiomegaly and left axis deviation on EKG. A loud intracranial bruit, often heard without auscultation, a palpable thrill, and engorged scalp veins are other notable features.

Signs occurring during early infancy are due to hydrocephalus, hemorrhage, or both.[240a] Hydrocephalus is caused by aqueductal ob-struction by the vein of Galen, or is due to aqueductal ependymitis and subarachnoid adhesions associated with intracranial hemorrhage. The older child presents with signs of an acute subarachnoid hemorrhage.

Posterior Fossa Syndrome. Although common in the adult, malformations in the posterior fossa become manifest prior to 20 years of age in less than 10% of subjects.[233] Symptoms are those of a cerebellar or brain stem lesion and bruits are only rarely heard, since most arteriovenous malformations in this region are small, usually less than 2 cm in diameter. Hydrocephalus may complicate this type of arteriovenous malformation.[233]

Hemispheric Syndrome. While this is the most common of the clinical syndromes in the adult, it is relatively rare in childhood. Manifestations include a sudden massive intracranial hemorrhage, periodic headaches, focal seizures with Todd's paralysis,[238] and progressive hemiplegia or hemihypesthesia. Progressive behavioral abnormalities and dementia are frequent.[236]

Spinal Cord Syndrome. This syndrome is also quite rare in childhood. It is characterized by sudden and recurrent pain and paresthesias of girdle or root distribution which may present as fluctuating lower abdominal pain or sciatica, and may last several minutes to hours. Symptoms are produced by small hemorrhages, and stepwise progression of long tract signs below the lesion follows each attack.[234,241]

Diagnosis

The presence of an arteriovenous malformation is suggested by the sudden onset of an intracranial hemorrhage. In such cases the presence of an intracranial bruit should always be sought. Auscultation of the skull is performed with the child in the erect position using a bell stethoscope over six standard listening points: both globes, the temporal fossae, and the retroauricular or mastoid region. In all cases conduction of a cardiac murmur should be excluded. Spontaneous intracranial bruits are common in children. These are augmented by contralateral carotid compression and obliterated by homolateral carotid compression. Wadia and Monckton heard unilateral or bilateral bruits in 60% of four to five-year-olds, 10% of ten-year-olds, and 4% in fifteen to sixteen-year-olds.[242] Intracranial bruits are heard in over 80% of patients with angiomas. Unlike benign bruits they are accompanied by a thrill and have a much louder and harsher quality. Intracranial bruits are also heard in a variety of conditions characterized by increased cerebral blood flow. These include anemia, thyrotoxicosis, and meningitis. Bruits also accompany hydrocephalus and some, not necessarily vascular, intracranial tumors.

CSF examination in patients with intracranial hemorrhage will reveal blood, xanthochromia, and increased protein. In some instances there may be a pleocytosis and increased pressure. In the patient who is deteriorating acutely as a consequence of an expanding hematoma or intraventricular dissection of blood, and who presents with signs of tentorial or foramen magnum herniation, CSF examination through the lumbar route should be deferred.

Other diagnostic procedures include a brain scan, which can demonstrate arteriovenous malformations greater than 1 cm in diameter. Skull films rarely reveal intracranial calcifications in children. When angiography is elected as in children with persistent focal seizures and focal neurologic signs, bilateral carotid and vertebral studies are indicated, since other vascular malformations may coexist with the one responsible for neurologic symptoms. In addition, saccular aneurysms may coexist with angiomas in some 5%–10% of patients.[231,236] Angiography should be done four to six weeks after the acute stage unless an expanding hematoma threatens life.[34] Air encephalography is necessary in patients suspected of hydrocephalus.

Treatment

The decision whether to treat a given case surgically depends on the location and accessibility of the lesion. Indications for surgery include an intracerebral hematoma with mass effects, raised intracranial pressure, and focal seizures which are poorly controlled by medication.[34,243b] The younger the child the greater the indication for an attempted resection of an accessible lesion, in view of the longer vulnerable period for either rupture or gliosis and atrophy of the adjacent parenchyma. However, the decision for a surgical procedure which has a 2%–10% operative mortality in the absence of coma,[34] should be weighed against an almost 85% five-year survival rate in unoperated patients.[238]

VENOUS ANGIOMA

Pathologically, these deserve separate status although clinically they do not differ from arteriovenous malformations. The anomalous vein has a reduced amount of smooth muscle and elastic tissue. The lesion tends to be smaller than an arteriovenous malformation, although it may vary from 1 mm up to several centimeters in diameter. Fifteen to twenty percent will calcify and occasionally ossification and amyloid deposition may occur.[231] Because capillaries are interposed between artery and vein, bruits are seldom heard and jugular blood is venous in oxygen content. It is Ford's[106] impression that these angiomas are often associated with other defects of embryogenesis and that they manifest earlier in life than do most arteriovenous malformations. The spinal cord syndrome is most commonly due to venous angiomas, however they range throughout the neuraxis.

CAPILLARY ANGIOMA (TELANGIECTASIA)

Much smaller than either arteriovenous malformations or venous angioma, these are usually found in the posterior fossa, particularly in the pons, medulla, or occasionally in the cerebellum.[233] This lesion, admixed with a venous angioma, constitutes the basic abnormality in Sturge-Weber syndrome (see Chapter 10). They may also be found in the subependymal deep subcortical region. They are solitary and often discovered incidentally at post mortem. Because of their highly vulnerable location in the brain stem or subependymal region they may be responsible for a massive and catastrophic hemorrhage. The surrounding parenchyma becomes gliotic and calcified. The posterior fossa syndrome and intraventricular hemorrhage presents as it does in the arteriovenous malformation, but many other manifestations such as congestive heart failure, seizures, and noncommunicating hydrocephalus do not occur in capillary angiomas because of their size and location.

ANEURYSM

Approximately 7% of the population develop an aneurysm, 2 mm or more in size, by the time they die.[231] However, the condition is rare in children, and the percentage of cases developing symptoms prior to 15 years varies from 0% to 3%.[231] Only one-quarter of these are of the saccular type.[244] There is no sexual or racial predilection, and no relationship between systemic hypertension, or physical activity and their rupture.

Pathology and Etiology

The etiology is variable. The most common cause appears to be a congenital weakness of the vascular media inducing the formation of a saccular aneurysm. Less often, intracranial aneurysms are associated with coarctation of the aorta, polycystic kidneys, and collagen vascular disease. In all these instances there is intracranial hypertension with subsequent dilatation of an embryogenically predisposed vascular wall. On anatomic examination the aneurysm consists of an ovoid, smooth, thin-walled arterial sac, usually located at the bifurcation of one of the major vessels of the circle of Willis or less often in one of the distal branches. The media and elastica of the arterial wall are attenuated and thrombosis of the aneurysms is occasionally seen. Multiple aneurysms occur in 20% of all subjects but are uncommon in children.

Clinical Picture

The larger the aneurysm the more likely it is to rupture. This is particularly true for aneurysms greater than 5 mm—the size of those that become symptomatic during childhood.

Sudden massive intracranial hemorrhage is by far the most common clinical manifestation in children. The ruptured aneurysm evacuates blood into the subarachnoid space, producing sudden severe headache, vomiting, meningeal irritation, and increased intracranial pressure. With progressive bleeding there may be focal neurologic deficits, sei-

zures, and impaired consciousness. Retinal hemorrhages occur. These may be flame-shaped and localized near blood vessels, or ovoid and near or on the disc and may dissect between retinal layers (subhyaloid hemorrhage). Complicating intracerebral hematoma occurs in 50% of patients and may produce a sudden increase in intracranial pressure. Other clinical manifestations, such as cranial nerve palsies, are almost always confined to adults.

Diagnosis

Bruits are seldom heard in the unruptured aneurysm. If a ruptured aneurysm is suspected the spinal fluid should be examined. This is usually bloody during the acute phase. In infants the hemorrhage may enter the subdural space, and a subdural tap will be required. Angiography may be necessary during the acute phase, especially when an intracerebral hematoma is suspected. The angiographic complications of arterial spasm and subsequent cerebral infarction are more of a problem in adults than in children who have more resilient and relatively larger arteries.

Treatment

Unless there is a life-threatening intracerebral hematoma, surgery should be postponed until the patient has stabilized and arterial spasm and cerebral edema have subsided. It was Matson's experience that most aneurysms improve progressively and spontaneously, and that bleeding does not recur during the acute phase.[34] He therefore recommended deferring surgery for from one to six weeks.

OTHER VASCULAR MALFORMATIONS[245,246,247,248]

A variety of rare vascular malformations deserve brief comment. These include large communicating veins between the extracranial and intracranial circulation, and carotid-basilar anastomoses. The latter normally involute by the end of the fifth week. They are termed the trigeminal, acoustic, and hypoglossal arteries as they embrace the respective cranial nerves. The trigeminal artery is the most common of these. It may coexist with a saccular aneurysm or angioma and produce dysfunction of the fifth, third, fourth, or sixth cranial nerve or spontaneous subarachnoid hemorrhage.

Anomalies of the circle of Willis are extremely common, being encountered in nearly 50% of autopsy cases but in children are probably of no clinical significance.

REFERENCES

1. Dobbing, J.: In Davison, A. N. and Dobbing, J. (eds.): *Applied Neurochemistry*, Oxford: Blackwell Scientific Publications, 1968.
2. Dubos, R., Savage, D., and Schaedler, R.: Biological Freudianism. Lasting effects of early environmental influences, Pediatrics 38:789, 1966.
3. Adams, R. D. and Sidman, R. L.: *Introduction to Neuropathology*, New York: McGraw-Hill Book Co., 1968.
4. Kurtzke, J. F., et al.: The distribution of deaths from congenital malformations of the nervous system, Neurology (Minneap.) 23:483, 1973.
5. Fox, M. W.: Neuro-behavioral ontogeny, a synthesis of ethological and neurophysiological concepts, Brain Research 2:3, 1966.
6. Arey, L. B.: *Developmental Anatomy*, Philadelphia: W. B. Saunders Co., 1965.
7. Truex, R. C. and Carpenter, M. B.: *Human Neuroanatomy*, 6th ed., Baltimore: Williams & Wilkins Co., 1969.
8. Jacobson, M.: *Developmental Neurobiology*, New York: Holt, Rinehart & Winston, Inc., 1970.
9. Rugh, R.: Ionizing radiations and congenital anomalies of the nervous system, Milit. Med. 127:883, 1962.
10. Angevine, J. B., Jr.: Time of neuron origin in the hippocampal region, an autoradiographic study in the mouse, Exp. Neurol. Suppl. 2:1, 1965.
11. Kitchin, I. C.: The effects of notochordectomy in amblystoma mexicanum, J. Exper. Zool. 112:393, 1949.
12. Rakic, P. and Yakovlev, P. I.: Development of the corpus callosum and cavum septi in man, J. Comp. Neurol. 132:45, 1968.
13. Woodward, J. S.: Origin of the external granule layer of the cerebellar cortex, J. Comp. Neurol. 115:65, 1960.
14. Yakovlev, P. I. and Wadsworth, R. C.: Schizencephalies, J. Neuropath. Exp. Neurol. 5:116, 169, 1946.
15. Schadé, J. P., Meeter, K., and Van Groeningen, W. B.: Maturational aspects of the dendrites in the human cortex, Acta Morph. Neerl. Scand. 5:37, 1962.
16. Nance, W. E.: Anencephaly and spina bifida: An etiologic hypothesis, Birth Defects Original Article Series 7:97, 1971.

17. Johnson, R. T.: Viral infections and malformations of the nervous system, Birth Defects Original Article Series, 7:56, 1971.
18. Navarrete, V. N., et al.: Subsequent diabetes in mothers delivered of a malformed infant, Lancet 2:993, 1970.
19. Thiersch, J. B.: Therapeutic abortions with a folic acid antagonist, 4-aminopteroylglutamic acid (4-amino P.G.A.) administered by the oral route, Amer. J. Obstet. Gynec. 63:1298, 1952.
19a. Speidel, B.D.: Folic acid deficiency and congenital malformation, Develop. Med. Child Neurol. 15:81, 1973.
20. Cohlan, S. Q.: Congenital anomalies in the rat produced by excessive intake of vitamin A during pregnancy, Pediatrics 13:556, 1954.
21. Giroud, A.: "Causes and Morphogenesis of Anencephaly," in Wolstenholme, G. E. W. and O'Connor, C. M. (eds.): *CIBA Foundation Symposium on Congenital Malformations*, London: Churchill, 1960.
22. Russell, L. B.: X-ray induced developmental abnormalities in the mouse and their use in the analysis of embryological patterns, J. Exp. Zool. 114:545, 1950.
23. Dekaban, A. S.: Anencephaly in early human embryos, J. Neuropath. Exp. Neurol. 22:533, 1963.
24. Padget, D. H.: Development of so-called dysraphism; with embryologic evidence of clinical Arnold-Chiari and Dandy-Walker malformations, Johns Hopk. Med. J. 130:127, 1972.
25. Grabowski, C. T.: "Embryonic Oxygen Deficiency—A Physiological Approach to Analysis of Teratological Mechanisms," in Woollam, D. H. M. (ed.): *Advances in Teratology*, Vol. 4, New York: Academic Press Inc., 1970.
25a. Toop, J., et al.: Muscle differentiation in anencephaly, Develop. Med. Child Neurol. 15:164, 1973.
26. Macmahon, B. and Naggan, L.: Ethnic differences in the prevalence of anencephaly and spina bifida in Boston, Massachusetts, New Eng. J. Med. 277:1119, 1967.
26a. Richards, I. D. G., et al: A genetic study on anencephaly and spina bifida in Glasgow, Develop. Med. Child Neurol. 14:626, 1972.
26b. Elwood, J. H.: Major central nervous malformations notified in Northern Ireland 1964–1968, Develop. Med. Child Neurol. 14:731, 1972.
27. Macmahon, B. and Yen, S.: Unrecognized epidemic of anencephaly and spina bifida, Lancet 1:31, 1971.
28. Paulson, G. W. and Gottlieb, G.: Developmental reflexes: The reappearance of fetal and neonatal reflexes in aged patients, Brain 91:37, 1968.
29. Frandsen, V. A. and Stakemann, G.: The site of production of oestrogenic hormones in human pregnancy. III. Further observation on the hormone excretion in pregnancy with anencephalic foetus, Acta Endocr. 47:265, 1964.

30. Brocklehurst, G.: The pathogenesis of spina bifida: A study of the relationship between observation, hypothesis, and surgical incentive, Develop. Med. Child Neurol. 13:147, 1971.

31. Dryden, R.: The fine structure of spina bifida in an untreated three-day chick embryo, Develop. Med. Child Neurol. Suppl. 25:116, 1971.

32. Dekaban, A. S.: Effects of x-radiation on mouse fetus during gestation: Emphasis on distribution of cerebral lesions, Part II, J. Nucl. Med. 10:68, 1969.

33. Warkany, J., Monroe, B. B., and Sutherland, B. S.: Intrauterine growth retardation, Amer. J. Dis. Child. 102:249, 1961.

34. Matson, D. D.: *Neurosurgery of Infancy and Childhood*, 2nd ed., Springfield: Charles C Thomas Publisher, 1969.

35. Mackenzie, N. G. and Emery, J. L.: Deformities of the cervical cord in children with neurospinal dysraphism, Develop. Med. Child Neurol. Suppl. 25:58, 1971.

36. Emery, J. L. and Lendon, R. G.: Clinical implications of cord lesions in neurospinal dysraphism, Develop. Med. Child Neurol., Suppl. 27:45, 1972.

37. Blaauw, G.: Defect in posterior arch of atlas in myelomeningocele, Develop. Med. Child Neurol. Suppl. 25:113, 1971.

38. Gardner, W. J.: Hydrodynamic mechanism of syringomyelia: its relationship to myelocele, J. Neurol. Neurosurg. Psychiat. 28:247, 1965.

39. Hankinson, J.: "Syringomyelia and the Surgeon," in Williams, D. (ed.): *Modern Trends in Neurology*, vol. 5, London: Butterworth, 1970.

40. Penfield, W. and Coburn, D. F.: Arnold-Chiari malformation and its operative treatment, Arch. Neurol. Psychiat.: 40:328, 1938.

41. Russell, D. S. and Donald, C.: The mechanism of internal hydrocephalus in spina bifida, Brain 58:203, 1935.

42. Margolis, G. and Kilham, L.: Experimental virus-induced hydrocephalus, J. Neurosurg. 31:1, 1969.

43. Lemire, R. J., et al.: Skin covered sacrococcygeal masses in infants and children, J. Pediat. 79:948, 1971.

44. Ingraham, F. D. and Swan, H.: Spina bifida and cranium bifidum, New Eng. J. Med. 228:599, 1943.

44a. Suwanwela, C. and Suwanwela, N.: A morphological classification of sincipital encephalomeningoceles, J. Neurosurg. 36:201, 1972.

44b. Naggan, L.: The recent decline in prevalence of anencephaly and spina bifida, Amer. J. Epidem. 89:154, 1969.

45. Neel, J. V.: A study of major congenital defects in Japanese infants, Amer. J. Hum. Genet. 10:398, 1958.

46. Stark, G. D.: Neonatal assessment of the child with meningomyelocele, Arch. Dis. Child. 46:539, 1971.

47. Mortier, W. and von Bernuth, H.: The neural influence on muscle development in myelomeningocele: Histochemical and electrodiagnostic studies, Develop. Med. Child Neurol. Suppl. 25:82, 1971.

48. Laurence, K. M.: Natural history of spina bifida cystica: Detailed analysis of 407 cases, Arch. Dis. Child. 39:41, 1964.

49. Lorber, J.: Ventriculo-cardiac shunts in the first week of life, Develop. Med. Child Neurol. Suppl. 20:13, 1969.

50. Naik, D. R. and Emery, J. L.: The position of the spinal cord segments related to the vertebral bodies in children with meningomyelocele and hydrocephalus, Develop. Med. Child Neurol. Suppl. 16:16, 1968.

50a. Stark, G.: Prediction of urinary continence in myelomeningocele, Develop. Med. Child Neurol. 13:388, 1971.

51. Stark, G.: The pathophysiology of the bladder in myelomeningocele and its correlation with the neurological picture, Develop. Med. Child Neurol. Suppl. 16:76, 1968.

52. Thomas, M. and Hopkins, J. M.: A study of the renal tract from birth in children with myelomeningocele, Develop. Med. Child Neurol. Suppl. 25:96, 1971.

53. Smith, E. D.: *Spina Bifida and the Total Care of Spinal Meningomyelocele*, Springfield: Charles C Thomas Publisher, 1965.

54. Sharrard, W. J. W., Zachary, R. B., and Lorber, J.: Survival and paralysis in open myelomeningocele with special reference to the time of repair of the spinal lesion, Develop. Med. Child Neurol. Suppl. 13:35, 1967.

55. Sharrard, W. J. W., et al.: Controlled trial of immediate and delayed closure of spina bifida cystica, Arch. Dis. Child. 38:18, 1963.

56. Buisson, J. and Formby, D.: Antibiotic spray during and after closure of myelomingoceles, Aust. Ped. J. 5:3, 1969.

57. Rickham, P. P. and Mawdsley, T.: The effect of early operation on the survival of spina bifida cystica, Develop. Med. Child Neurol. Suppl. 11:20, 1966.

58. Farmer, T. W.: *Pediatric Neurology*, New York: Harper & Row Publishers, 1964.

58a. Lorber, J.: Results of treatment of myelomeningocele, Develop. Med. Child Neurol. 13:279, 1971.

59. Gellis, S.: Commentary in *Yearbook of Pediatrics, 1967-1968*, Chicago: Yearbook Medical Publishers, pp. 407–408.

60. Laurence, K. M. and Tew, B. J.: Follow-up of 65 survivors from the 425 cases of spina bifida born in south Wales between 1956 and 1962, Develop. Med. Child Neurol. Suppl. 13:1, 1967.

61. Retik, A., Perlmutter, A. D., and Gross, R. E.: Cutaneous ureteroileostomy in children, New Eng. J. Med. 277:217, 1967.

61a. Eckstein, H. B.: Urinary control and children with myelomeningocele, Brit. J. Urol. 40:191, 1968.

62. Campbell, J. B.: Congenital anomalies of the neural axis, Amer. J. Surg. 75:231, 1948.

63. Laurence, K. M.: The survival of untreated spina bifida cystica, Develop. Med. Child Neurol. 11:10, 1966.

64. Mawdsley, T. and Rickham, P. P.: Further follow-up study of early operation for open myelomeningocele, Develop. Med. Child Neurol. Suppl. 20:8, 1969.

65. Chiari, H.: Ueber Veranderungen des Klein-hirns infolge von Hydrocephalie des Grosshirns, Deutsch. Med. Wschr. 17:1172, 1891.

66. Norman, R. M.: "Malformations of the Nervous System, Birth Injury and Diseases of Early Life," in Greenfield, J. G. (ed.): *Neuropathology*, London: Edward Arnold, Ltd., 1967.

67. Von Hoytema, G. J. and Von den Berg, R.: Embryological studies of the posterior fossa in connection with Arnold-Chiari malformation, Develop. Med. Child Neurol. Suppl. 11:61, 1966.

68. Davies, H. W.: Radiological changes associated with Arnold-Chiari malformation, Brit. J. Radiol. 40:262, 1967.

68a.Sieben, R. L., Hamida, M. B., and Shulman, K.: Multiple cranial nerve deficits associated with the Arnold-Chiari malformation, Neurology (Minneap.) 21:673, 1971.

69. Gardner, W. J.: Anatomic features common to the Arnold-Chiari and the Dandy-Walker malformations suggest a common origin, Cleveland Clin. Quart. 26:206, 1959.

69a.Peach, B.: Arnold-Chiari malformation. Anatomic features of 20 cases, Arch. Neurol. 12:613, 1965.

69b.Emery, J. L. and MacKenzie, N. G.: Medullocervical dislocation deformity (Chiari II deformity) related to neurospinal dysraphism (meningomyelocele), Brain 96:155, 1973.

70. Moes, C. A. F. and Hendrick, E. B.: Diastematomyelia, J. Pediat. 63:238, 1963.

71. Bremer, J. L.: Dorsal intestinal fistula; accessory neurenteric canal; diastematomyelia, Arch. Path. 54:132, 1952.

72. Sheptak, P. E. and Susen, A. F.: Diastematomyelia, Amer. J. Dis. Child. 113:210, 1967.

73. Poser, C. M.: *The Relationship Between Syringomyelia and Neoplasm*, Springfield: Charles C Thomas Publisher, 1956.

74. Walshe, F. M. R.: Syringomyelia, Proc. Roy. Soc. Med. 20: 1246, 1927.

75. Balocco, A.: Agenesia del segmento lombosacrale della colonna vertebrale con situs viscerum inversus, Minerva Pediat. 15:1482, 1963.

76. Matson, D. D. and Jerva, M. J.: Recurrent meningitis associated with congenital lumbosacral dermal sinus tract, J. Neurosurg. 25:288, 1966.

77. Bull, J. S., Nixon, W. L., and Pratt, R. T.: Radiological criteria and familial occurrence of primary basilar impression, Brain 78:229, 1955.

78. DeLong, W. B. and Schneider, R. C.: Surgical management of congenital spinal lesions associated with abnormalities of the cranio-spinal junction, J. Neurol. Neurosurg. Psychiat. 29:319, 1966.

79. Klippel, M. and Feil, A.: Un cas d'absence des vertebres cervicales, Soc. Anat. Paris Bull. et Mem. 14:185, 1912.

80. Gunderson, C. H. and Solitare, G. B.: Mirror movements in patients with Klippel-Feil syndrome, Arch. Neurol. 18:675, 1968.

81. Morrison, S. G., Perry, L. W., and Scott, L. P.: Congenital brevicollis (Klippel-Feil syndrome), Amer. J. Dis. Child. 115:614, 1968.

82. Foster, J. B., Hudgson, P., and Pearce, G. W.: The association of syringomyelia and congenital cervico-medullary anomalies: Pathological evidence, Brain 92:25, 1969.

83. Bach, C., et al.: La dysostose cleido-cranienne. Etude de six observations. Association a des manifestations neurologiques, Ann. Pediat. (Paris) 42:67, 1966.

84. Millen, J. W.: Timing of human congenital malformations, Develop. Med. Child Neurol. 5:343:, 1963.

85. Arakaki, D. T. and Waxman, S. H : Trisomy D in a cyclops, J. Pediat. 74:620, 1969.

86. De Myer, W., Zeman, W;, and Palmer, C. G.: Familial alobar holoprosencephaly (arhinencephaly) with median cleft lip and palate, Neurology 13:913, 1963.

87. Yakovlev, P. I.: Pathoarchitectonic studies of cerebral malformations, J. Neuropath. Exp. Neurol. 18:22, 1959.

88. De Myer, W.: The median cleft face syndrome, Neurology 17:961, 1967.

89. De Myer, W.: Classification of cerebral malformations, Birth Defects Original Article Series 7:78, 1971.

90. Dekaban, A. S.: Arhinencephaly, Amer. J. Ment. Defic. 63:428, 1948.

91. Dekaban, A.: Large defects in cerebral hemispheres associated with cortical dysgenesis, J. Neuropath. Exp. Neurol. 24:512, 1965.

92. Benda, C. E.: *Developmental Disorders of Mentation and Cerebral Palsies*, New York: Grune & Stratton, Inc., 1952.

93. Druckman, R., Chao, D., and Alvord, E. C., Jr.: A case of atonic cerebral diplegia with lissencephaly, Neurology (Minneap.) 9:806, 1959.

94. Rice, E. C. and Dekaban, A. S.: Congenital hemiplegia resulting from cerebral malformation, AMA Arch. Path. 68:348, 1959.

94a.Ettlinger, G., et al.: Agenesis of the corpus callosum: A behavioural investigation, Brain 95:327, 1972.

95. Menkes, J. H., Philippart, M., and Clark, D. B.: Hereditary partial agenesis of the corpus callosum, Arch. Neurol. 11:198, 1964.

96. Rakic, P. and Yakovlev, P.: Development of the corpus callosum and cavum septi in man, J. Comp. Neurol. 132:45, 1968.

97. Dooling, E. C., et al.: Cyst of the cavum septi pellucidi, Arch. Neurol. 27:79, 1972.

98. Nellhaus, G.: Head circumference from birth to eighteen years, Pediatrics 41:106, 1968.

99. Book, J. A., Schut, J. W., and Reed, A. C.: A clinical and genetical study of microcephaly, Amer. J. Ment. Defic. 57:637, 1953.

100. Connolly, C. J.: The fissural pattern of the primate brain, Amer. J. Phys. Anthrop. 21:301, 1936.

101. McKusick, V. A., et al.: Chorioretinopathy with hereditary microcephaly, Arch. Ophthal. 75:597, 1966.

102. Smith, D. W.: *Recognizable Patterns of Human Malformations*, Philadelphia: W. B. Saunders Co., 1970.

103. Dekaban, A.: Abnormalities in children exposed to x-radiation during various stages of gestation: Tentative timetable of radiation injury to the human fetus, Part I, J. Nucl. Med. 9:471, 1968.

104. Hicks, S. P.: Developmental malformations produced by radiation, Amer. J. Roentgen. 69:272, 1953.

105. Wood, J. W., Johnson, K. G., and Omori, Y.: In utero exposure to the Hiroshima atomic bomb: An evaluation of head size and mental retardation twenty years later, Pediatrics 39:385, 1967.

106. Ford, F. R.: *Diseases of the Nervous System in Infancy, Childhood and Adolescence*, 5th ed., Springfield: Charles C Thomas Publisher, 1966.

107. Ashby, W. R. and Stewart, R. M.: Size in mental deficiency, J. Neurol. Psychopath. 13:303, 1932.

108. O'Connell, E. J., Feldt, R. H., and Stickler, G. B.: Head circumference, mental retardation, and growth failure, Pediatrics 36:62, 1965.

109. Pryor, H. B. and Thelander, H.: Abnormally small head size and intellect in children, J. Pediat. 73:593, 1968.

110. Martin, H. P.: Microcephaly and mental retardation, Amer. J. Dis. Child. 119:128, 1970.

111. Virchow, R.: Ueber den Cretinismus, namentlich in Franken, und uber pathologische Schadelformen, Verh. Phys.-Med. Ges. Wurzburg 2:230, 1851.

112. Park, E. A. and Powers, G. F.: Acrocephaly and scaphocephaly with symmetrically distributed malformations of the extremities, Amer. J. Dis. Child. 20:235, 1920.

113. Cross, H. E. and Opitz, J. M.: Craniosynostosis in the Amish, J. Pediat. 75:1037, 1969.

114. Reilly, B. J., Leeming, J. M., and Fraser, D.: Craniosynostosis in the rachitic spectrum, J. Pediat. 64:396, 1964.

115. Comings, D. E., Papazian, C., and Schoene, H. R.: Conradi's disease: Chondrodystrophia calcificans congenita, stippled epiphyses, J. Pediat. 72:63, 1968.

116. Menking, M., et al.: Premature craniosynostosis associated with hyperthyroidism in 4 children with reference to 5 further cases in the literature, Mschr. Kinderheilk. 120:106, 1972.

116a. Fishman, M. A., et al.: Concurrence of hydrocephalus and craniosynostosis, J. Neurosurg. 34:621, 1971.

117. Dodge, H. W., Jr., Wood, M. W., and Kennedy, R. L. J.: Craniofacial dysostosis: Crouzon's disease, Pediatrics 23:98, 1959.

117a. Dohn, D. F.: Surgical treatment of unilateral coronal craniostenosis (plagiocephaly), Cleveland Clin. Quart. 30:47, 1963.

118. Freeman, J. M. and Berkowf, S.: Craniostenosis, review of the literature and report of thirty-four cases, Pediatrics 30:57, 1962.

119. Anderson, F. M. and Geiger, L.: Craniosynostosis: A survey of 204 cases, J. Neurosurg. 22:229, 1965.

120. Watts, J. W., and Miller, M. H.: The surgical treatment of craniosynostosis, Clin. Proc. Child. Hosp. (Wash.) 23:83, 1967.

120a. Pawl, R. P. and Sugar, O. P.: Zenker's solution in the surgical treatment of craniosynostosis, J. Neurosurg. 36:604, 1972.

121. Shillito, J. and Matson, D. D.: Craniosynostosis: A review of 519 surgical patients, Pediatrics 41:829, 1968.

122. Wilson, S.A.K.: Megalencephaly, J. Neurol. Psychopath. 14:193, 1934.

122a. Popich, G. A. and Smith, D. W.: Fontanels: Range of normal size, J. Pediat. 80:749, 1972.

123. Weed, L. H.: The development of the cerebrospinal spaces in pig and man, Carnegie Inst. Wash., Contribs. Embryol. 5:1, 1917.

124. Shuangshoti, S. and Netsky, M. G.: Histogenesis of choroid plexus in man, Amer. J. Anat. 118:283, 1966.

125. Brocklehurst, G.: The development of the human cerebrospinal fluid pathway with particular reference to the roof of the fourth ventricle, J. Anat. 105:467, 1969.

126. Lorenzo, A. V., Page, L. K., and Watters, G. V.: Relationship between cerebrospinal fluid formation, absorption and pressure in human hydrocephalus, Brain 93:679, 1970.

127. Bering, E. A. and Sato, O.: Hydrocephalus: Changes in formation and absorption of cerebrospinal fluid within the cerebral ventricles, J. Neurosurg. 20:1050, 1963.

128. Milhorat, T. H.: Choroid plexus and CSF production, Science 166:1514, 1969.

129. Davson, H.: *Physiology of the Cerebrospinal Fluid*, Boston: Little, Brown & Co., 1967.

130. Masserman, J. H.: Cerebrospinal hydrodynamics, Arch. Neurol. Psychiat. 32:523, 1934.

131. Cutler, R. W. P., et al.: Formation and absorption of cerebrospinal fluid in man, Brain 91:707, 1968.

132. Shaywitz, B. A., Katzman, R., and Escriva, A.: CSF formation and ^{24}Na clearance in normal and hydrocephalic kittens during ventriculocisternal perfusion, Neurology 19:1159, 1969.

133. Davson, H.: "The Cerebrospinal Fluid Pressure," in Cumings, J. N. and Kremer, M. (eds.): *Biochemical Aspects of Neurological Disorders*, Oxford: Blackwell Scientific Publications, 1968.

134. Davson, H.: Dynamic aspects of CSF, Develop. Med. Child Neurol., Suppl. 27:1, 1972.

135. Vates, T. S., Jr., Bonting, S. L., and Oppelt, W. W.: Na-K activated adenosine triphosphatase formation of cerebrospinal fluid in the cat, Amer. J. Physiol. 206:1165, 1964.

136. Garcia-Bengochea, F.: The effect of cortisone on cerebrospinal fluid production in castrated adult cats, Neurology 16:512, 1966.

137. Hurt, H. D., et al.: Rates of formation and absorption of cerebrospinal fluid in chronic bovine hypervitaminosis A, J. Dairy Sci. 50:1941, 1967.

137a. Cushing, H. W.: *Studies in Intracranial Physiology and Surgery; the Third Circulation, the Hypophysis, the Gliomas,* London: Oxford University Press, 1926.

138. Brisman, R.: Pioneer studies in the circulation of the cerebrospinal fluid with particular reference to studies by Richard Lower in 1669, J. Neurosurg. 32:1, 1970.

139. Welch, K. and Friedman, V.: The cerebrospinal fluid valves, Brain 83:454, 1960.

140. Bering, E. A.: Circulation of the cerebrospinal fluid, J. Neurosurg. 19:405, 1962.

141. Weller, R. O. and Wisniewski, H.: Histological and ultrastructural changes with experimental hydrocephalus in adult rabbits, Brain 92:819, 1969.

142. Sahar, A., et al.: Cerebrospinal fluid absorption in animals with experimental obstructive hydrocephalus, Arch. Neurol. 21:638, 1969.

143. Milhorat, T. H., et al.: Structural, ultrastructural and permeability changes in the ependyma and surrounding brain favoring equilibration in progressive hydrocephalus, Arch. Neurol. 22: 397, 1970.

144. Weller, R. O. and Shulman, K.: Infantile hydrocephalus, clinical, histological, and ultrastructural study of brain damage, J. Neurosurg. 36:255, 1972.

145. Milhorat, T. H., et al.: Evidence for choroidplexus absorption in hydrocephalus, New Eng. J. Med. 283:286, 1970.

146. Levin, V. A., et al.: Physiological studies on the development of obstructive hydrocephalus in the monkey, Neurology (Minneap.) 21:238, 1971.

147. Hochwald, G. M., et al.: Experimental hydrocephalus: changes in cerebrospinal fluid dynamics as a function of time, Arch. Neurol. 26:120, 1972.

148. Shulman, K. and Marmarou, A.: Pressure-volume considerations in infantile hydrocephalus, Develop. Med. Child Neurol. Suppl. 25:90, 1971.

149. Cutler, R. W. P., et al.: Overproduction of CSF in communicating hydrocephalus, Neurology (Minneap.) 23:1, 1973.

150. Hayden, P. W., Shurtleff, D. B., and Foltz, E. L.: Ventricular fluid pressure recordings in hydrocephalic patients, Arch. Neurol. 23:147, 1970.

151. Logue, V.: "Hydrocephalus," in *Biochemical Aspects of Neurological Disorders,* Cumings, J. N. and Kremer, M. (eds.), Oxford: Blackwell Scientific Publications, 1968.

152. Voris, H. C.: Postmeningitic hydrocephalus, Neurology (Minneap.) 5:72, 1955.

152a. Emery, J. L. and Staschak, M. C.: The size and form of the cerebral aquaeduct in children, Brain 95:591, 1972.

153. Russell, D. S.: Observations on the pathology of hydrocephalus, Med. Res. Counc. Spec. Rep. (London) 265:1, 1949.

154. Bickers, D. S. and Adams, R. D.: Hereditary stenosis of the aqueduct of Sylvius as a cause of congenital hydrocephalus, Brain 72:245, 1949.

155. Edwards, J. H., Norman, R. M., and Roberts, J. M.: Sex-linked hydrocephalus—report of a family with 15 active members, Arch. Dis. Child. 36:481, 1961.

156. Laurence, K. M.: The pathology of hydrocephalus, Ann. Roy. Coll. Surg. Eng. 24:388, 1959.

157. Dandy, W. E.: Diagnosis and treatment of hydrocephalus due to occlusion of the foramina of Magendie and Luschka, Surg. Gynec. Obstet. 32:112, 1921.

157a. Hart, N. M.: The Dandy-Walker syndrome: A clinicopathological study based on 28 cases, Neurology (Minneap.) 22:771, 1972.

158. Gardner, W. J., Abdullah, A. F., and McCormack, L. J.: The varying expressions of embryonal atresia of the fourth ventricle in adults, J. Neurosurg. 14:591, 1957.

159. Gilles, F. H. and Shillito, J.: Infantile hydrocephalus: Retrocerebellar subdural hematoma, J. Pediat. 76:529, 1970.

160. Woollam, D.H.M. and Millen, J. W.: Anatomical considerations in the pathology of stenosis of the cerebral aqueduct, Brain 76:104, 1953.

161. Byers, R. K. and Hass, G. M.: Thrombosis of the dural venous sinuses in infancy and in childhood, Amer. J. Dis. Child. 45:1161, 1933.

162. Yang, D. C., Sohn, D., and Anand, H. K.: Thrombosis of the superior longitudinal sinus during infancy, J. Pediat. 74:570, 1969.

163. Hooper, R.: Hydrocephalus and obstruction of the superior vena cava in infancy, Pediatrics 28:792, 1961.

164. Schlessinger, B.: The tolerance of the blocked galenic system against artificially increased intravenous pressure, Brain 63:178, 1940.

165. Russell, D. S. and Beck, D. J. K.: Experiments on thrombosis of the superior longitudinal sinus, J. Neurosurg. 3:337, 1946.

166. Yakovlev, P. I.: Paraplegias of hydrocephalics, Amer J. Ment. Defic. 51:561, 1947.

166a. Adeloye, A., et al.: Stridor, myelomeningocele and hydrocephalus in a child, Arch. Neurol. 23:271, 1970.

166b. Rubin, R. C.: The effect of severe hydrocephalus on size and number of brain cells, Develop. Med. Child Neurol., Suppl. 27, 117, 1972.

167. Benton, J. W., et al.: The Bobble-head doll syndrome. Report of a unique truncal tremor associated with third ventricular cyst and hydrocephalus in children, Neurology (Minneap.) 16:725, 1966.

168. Mayher, W. E. and Gindin, R. A.: Head bobbing associated with third ventricular cyst, Arch. Neurol. 23:274, 1970.

169. Kim, C. S., Bennett, D. R., and Roberts, T. S.: Primary amenorrhea secondary to non-communicating hydrocephalus, Neurology (Minneap.) 19:533, 1969.

170. Miller, E. and Sethi, L.: The effect of hydrocephalus on perception, Develop. Med. Child Neurol. Suppl. 25:77, 1971.

171. Hagberg, B. and Sjogren, I.: The chronic brain syndrome of infantile hydrocephalus, Amer. J. Dis. Child. 112:189, 1966.

172. O'Neill, E. M.: Normal head growth and prediction of head size in infantile hydrocephalus, Arch. Dis. Child. 36:241, 1961.

173. Dodge, P. R. and Porter, P.: Demonstration of intracranial pathology by transillumination, Arch. Neurol. 5:594, 1961.

173a.Mazur, R.: Transillumination of the skull in the diagnosis of intracranial disease in children up to 3 years, Develop. Med. Child Neurol. 7:634, 1965.

174. Kazner, E., Kunze, S., and Schiefer, W.: Echoencephalography as an aid to the diagnosis of space-occupying lesions of the posterior fossa by measuring the size of the third and lateral ventricles, J. Neurosurg. 26:511, 1967.

174a.Schlagenhauff, R. E. and Mazurowski, J.: Ultrasonic measurement of cerebral ventricular system: Critical and comparative study of echoencephalographic and pneumoencephalographic determinations in 100 patients, Neurology (Minneap.) 21:1134, 1971.

175. Granholm, L. and Rådberg, C.: Congenital communicating hydrocephalus, J. Neurosurg. 20:338, 1963.

176. Raimondi, A. J.: Angiographic diagnosis of hydrocephalus in the newborn, J. Neurosurg. 31:550, 1969.

176a.Raimondi, A. J.: *Pediatric Neuroradiology*, Philadelphia: W. B. Saunders Co., 1972.

177. DiChiro, G., Ashburn, W. L., and Briner, W. H.: Technetium Tc 99m serum albumin for cisternography, Arch. Neurol. 19:218, 1968.

178. Milhorat, T. H. and Hammock, M. K.: Isotope ventriculography. Interpretation of ventricular size and configuration in hydrocephalus, Arch. Neurol. 25:1, 1971.

179. Stein, B.M., Fraser, R. A. R., and Tenner, M. S.: Normal pressure hydrocephalus: Complication of posterior fossa surgery in children, Pediatrics 49:50, 1972.

180. McCullough, D. C., et al.: Prognostic criteria for the CSF shunting from cisternography in communicating hydrocephalus, Neurology (Minneap.) 20:594, 1970.

181. Brocklehurst, G.: Use of radio-iodinated serum albumin in the study of cerebrospinal fluid flow, J. Neurol. Neurosurg. Psychiat. 31:162, 1968.

182. Katzman, R. and Hussey, F.: A simple constant infusion manometric test for measurement of CSF absorption, Neurology (Minneap.) 20:534, 665, 1970.

183. Nelson, J. R. and Goodman, S. J.: An evaluation of the cerebrospinal fluid infusion test for hydrocephalus, Neurology (Minneap.) 21:1037, 1971.

184. Schick, R. M. and Matson, D. D.: What is arrested hydrocephalus? J. Pediat. 58:791, 1961.

185. Laurence, K. M. and Coates, S.: Further thoughts on the natural history of hydrocephalus, Develop. Med. Child Neurol. 4:263, 1962.

186. Lorber, J. and Zachary, R. B.: Primary congenital hydrocephalus: Long-term results of controlled therapeutic trial, Arch. Dis. Child. 43:516, 1968.

187. Putnam, T. J.: Treatment of hydrocephalus by endoscopic coagulation of choroid plexuses. Description of new instrument, New Eng. J. Med. 210:1373, 1934.

188. Scarff, J. E.: Treatment of nonobstructive (communicating) hydrocephalus by endoscopic cauterization of the choroid plexuses, J. Neurosurg. 33:1, 1970.

189. Lorber, J. and Emery, J. L.: Intracerebral cysts complicating ventricular needling in hydrocephalic infants. A clinico-pathologic study, Develop. Med. Child Neurol. 6:125, 1964.

189a.Hakim, S.: A critical analysis of valve shunts used in the treatment of hydrocephalus, Develop. Med. Child Neurol. 15:230, 1973.

190. Stuart, M., et al.: Shortened platelet lifespan in patients with hydrocephalus and ventriculo-jugular shunts, J. Pediat. 80:21, 1972.

191. Matson, D. D.: Hydrocephalus, New Eng. J. Med. 271:1360, 1964.

191a.Shurtleff, D. B.: Ventriculoauriculostomy-associated infection: A 12 year study, J. Neurosurg. 35:686, 1971.

192. McLaurin, R. L. and Dodson, D.: Infected ventriculo-atrial shunts: Some principles of treatment, Develop. Med. Child Neurol. Suppl. 25:71, 1971.

193. Fokes, E. C.: Occult infections of ventriculo-atrial shunts, J. Neurosurg. 33:517, 1970.

194. Blaze, J. B., Forrest, D. M., and Tsingoglou, S.: Atriotomy using the Holter shunt in hydrocephalus, Develop. Med. Child Neurol. Suppl. 25:27, 1971.

195. Foltz, E. L., and Shurtleff, D. B.: Five-year comparative study of hydrocephalus with and without operation (113 cases), J. Neurosurg. 20:1064, 1963.

196. Scarff, J. E.: Treatment of hydrocephalus: an historical and critical review of methods and results, J. Neurol. Neurosurg. Psychiat. 12:1, 1963.

197. Paine R. S.: Hydrocephalus, Pediat. Clin. N. Amer. 14:779, 1967.

198. Huttenlocher, P. R.: Treatment of hydrocephalus with acetazolamide: Results in 15 cases, J. Pediat. 66:1023, 1965.

199. Mealey, J. and Barker, D. T.: Failure of oral acetazolamide to avert hydrocephalus in infants with myelomeningocele, J. Pediat. 72:257, 1968.

200. Reed, D. J. and Woodbury, D. M.: Effect of urea and acetazolamide on brain volume and cerebrospinal fluid pressure, J. Physiol. 164:265, 1962.

201. Hayden, P. W., Foltz, E. L., and Shurtleff, D. B.: Effect of an oral osmotic agent on ventricular fluid pressure of hydrocephalic children, Pediatrics 41:955, 1968.

201a.Hayden, P. W. and Shurtleff, D. B.: The medical management of hydrocephalus, Develop. Med. Child Neurol., Suppl. 27:52, 1972.

202. Guthkelch, A. N. and Riley, N. A.: Influence of aetiology on prognosis in surgically treated infantile hydrocephalus, Arch. Dis. Child. 44:29, 1969.

203. Yashon, D., Jane, J. A., and Sugar, O.: Course of severe untreated infantile hydrocephalus: Prognostic significance of cerebral mantle, J. Neurosurg. 23:509, 1965.

204. Laurence, K. M.: Natural history of hydrocephalus, Lancet 2:1152, 1958.

205. Laurence, K. M. and Coates, S.: Natural history of hydrocephalus: Detailed analysis of 182 unoperated cases, Arch. Dis. Child. 37:345, 1962.

206. Laurence, K. M.: Neurologic and intellectual sequelae of hydrocephalus, Arch. Neurol. 20:73, 1969.

207. Hagberg, B.: The sequelae of spontaneously arrested infantile hydrocephalus, Develop. Med. Child Neurol. 4:583, 1962.

208. Lindenberg, R. and Swanson, P. D.: Infantile hydrancephaly, report of five cases of infarction of both cerebral hemispheres in infancy, Brain 90:839, 1967.

209. Fowler, M., et al.: Congenital hydrocephalus-hydrancephaly in five siblings with autopsy studies: a new disease, Develop. Med. Child Neurol. 14:173, 1972.

210. McElfresh, A. E. and Arey, J. B.: Generalized cytomegalic inclusion disease, J. Pediat. 51:146, 1957.

211. Becker, H.: Uber Hirngefaszausschaltungen II. Intrakranielle Gefaszverschlusse. Ueber experimentelle Hydrancephalie (Blasenhirn),- Deutsch. Z. Nervenheilk. 161:446, 1949.

212. Vogel, F. S. and McClenahan, J. L.: Anomalies of major cerebral arteries associated with congenital malformations of the brain, Amer. J. Path. 28:701, 1942.

213. Myers, R. E.: Brain pathology following fetal vascular occlusion: An experimental study, Invest. Ophthal. 8:41, 1969.

214. Hoffman, J. and Liss, L.: Hydranencephaly, Acta Paediat. Scand. 58:297, 1969.

215. Bergstrom, K., Laurent, U., and Lundberg, P. O.: Neurological symptoms in achondroplasia, Acta Neurol. Scand. 47:59, 1971.

216. Dandy, W. E.: Hydrocephalus in chondrodystrophy, Bull. Hopkins Hosp. 52:5, 1921.

217. James, A. E., Jr., et al.: Hydrocephalus in achondroplasia studied by cisternography, Pediatrics 49:46, 1971.

218. Cohen, M. E., Rosenthal, A. D., and Matson, D. D.: Neurological abnormalities in achondroplastic children, J. Pediat. 71:367, 1967.

219. Möbius, P. D.: Uber angeborene doppelseitige Abducens-Facialis-Lahmung, München. Med. Wschr. 35:91, 1888.

220. Van Allen, M. W. and Blodi, F. C.: Neurologic aspects of the Möbius syndrome, Neurology (Minneap.) 10:249, 1960.

221. Richter, R. B.: Congenital hypoplasia of the facial nucleus, J. Neuropath. Exp. Neurol., 17:520, 1958.

222. Pitner, S. E., Edwards, J. E., and McCormick, W. F.: Observations of pathology of Möbius syndrome, J. Neurol. Neurosurg. Psychiat. 28:362, 1965.

223. Henderson, J. L.: The congenital facial diplegia syndrome: Clinical features, pathology and etiology, Brain 62:381, 1939.

224. Hanson, P. A. and Rowland, L. P.: Möbius syndrome and facioscapulohumeral muscular dystrophy, Arch. Neurol. 24:31, 1971.

224a.Konigsmark, B. W.: Hereditary deafness in man, New Eng. J. Med. 281:713, 774, 827, 1969.

224b.Konigsmark, B. W., Mengel, M. C., and Haskins, H.: Familial congenital moderate neural hearing loss, J. Laryng. 84:495, 1970.

224c.Parker, N.: Congenital deafness due to a sex-linked recessive gene, Ann. Hum. Genet. 10:196, 1958.

224d.Waardenburg, P. J.: A new syndrome combining developmental anomalies of the eyelids, eyebrows and nose root with pigmentary defects of the iris and head hair and with congenital deafness, Amer. J. Hum. Genet. 3:195, 1951.

225. Falls, H. F., Kruse, W. T., and Cotterman, C. W.: Three cases of Marcus Gunn phenomenon in two generations, Amer. J. Ophthal. 32:53, 1949.

226. Duane, A.: Congenital deficiency of abduction, associated with impairment of abduction, retraction movements, contractions of the palpebral fissure and oblique movements of the eye, Arch. Ophthal. 34:133, 1905.

227. Walton, D. S. and Robb, R. M.: Optic nerve hypoplasia, Arch. Ophthal. 84:572, 1970.

228. Cox, R. A.: Congenital head nodding and nystagmus: Report of a case, Arch. Ophthal. 15:1032, 1936.

229. Dickinson, J. T., Srisomboon, P., and Kamerer, D. B.: Congenital anomaly of the facial nerve, Arch. Otolaryng. (Chicago) 88:357, 1968.

230. Padget, D. H.: The development of the cranial arteries in the human embryo, Carnegie Institution of Washington Contributions to Embryology 32:205, 1948.

231. McCormick, W. F.: "Vascular Disorders of Nervous Tissue: Anomalies, Malformations, and Aneurysms," in Bourne, G. H. (ed.): *The Structure and Function of Nervous Tissue*, New York: Academic Press Inc., 1969.

232. Russell, D. S. and Rubinstein, L. J.: *The Pathology of Tumours of the Nervous System*, 3rd ed., Baltimore: Williams & Wilkins Co., 1970.

233. McCormick, W. F., Hardman, J. M., and Boulter, T.R.: Vascular malformations ("angiomas") of the brain with special reference to those occurring in the posterior fossa, J. Neurosurg. 28:241, 1968.

234. Bergstrand, A., Hook, O., and Lidvall, H.: Vascular malformations of spinal cord, Acta Neurol. Scand. 40:169, 1964.

235. Logue, V. and Monckton, G.: Posterior fossa angiomas—a clinical presentation of nine cases, Brain 77:252, 1954.

236. Paterson, J. H. and McKissock, W. A.: A clinical survey of intracranial angiomas with special reference to their mode of progression and surgical treatment: A report of 110 cases, Brain 79:233, 1956.

236a.Tay, C. H., et al: Intracranial arteriovenous maformations in Asians, Brain 94:61, 1971.

237. Kalplan, H. A., Aronson, S. M., and Browder, E. J.: Vascular malformations of the brain, J. Neurosurg. 18:630, 1961.

238. Henderson, W. R. and Gomez, R. deR. L.: Natural history of cerebral angiomas, Brit. Med. J. 4:571, 1967.

239. Pool, J. L. and Potts, D. G.: *Aneurysms and Arteriovenous Anomalies of the Brain*, New York: Hoeber Medical Division, Harper & Row Publishers, 1965.

240. Carroll, C. P. H. and Jakoby, R. K.: Neonatal congestive heart failure as the presenting symptom of cerebral arteriovenous malformation, J. Neurosurg. 25:159, 1966.

240a.Montoya, G., et al.: Arteriovenous malformation of the vein of Galen as a cause of heart failure and hydrocephalus in infants, Neurology (Minneap.) 21:1054, 1971.

240b.Holden, A. M., et al.: Congestive heart failure from intracranial arterio-venous fistula in infancy: Clinical and physiological considerations in 8 patients, Pediatrics 49:30, 1972.

241. Buchanan, D. N. and Walker, A. E.: Vascular anomalies of the spinal cord in children, Amer. J. Dis. Child. 61:928, 1941.

242. Wadia, N. H. and Monckton, G.: Intracranial bruits in health and disease, Brain 80:492, 1957.

243. McCormick, W. F. and Boulter, T. R.: Vascular malformations ("angiomas") of the dura mater, J. Neurosurg. 25:309, 1966.

243a.Schoolman, A. and Kepes, J. J.: Bilateral spontaneous carotid-cavernous fistulae in Ehlers-Danlos syndrome, J. Neurosurg. 26:82, 1967.

243b.Moyes, P. D.: Intracranial and intraspinal vascular anomalies in children, J. Neurosurg. 31:271, 1969.

244. Laitinen, L.: Arteriella aneurysm med subarachnoidalblodnigg hos barn, Nord. Med. 71:329, 1964.

245. Madonick, M. J. and Ruskin, A. P.: Recurrent oculomotor paresis, Arch. Neurol. 6:353, 1962.

246. Wise, B. L. and Palubinskas, A. J.: Persistent trigeminal artery (carotid-basilar anastomosis), J. Neurosurg. 21:199, 1964.

247. Wolpert, S. M.: The trigeminal artery associated aneurysms, Neurology (Minneap.) 16:610, 1966.

248. Gerlach, J., et al.: Traumatic caroticocavernous fistula combined with persisting primitive hypoglossal artery, J. Neurosurg. 20:885, 1963.

249. Plum, F. and Posner, J. B.: *Diagnosis of Stupor and Coma*, 2nd ed., Philadelphia: F. A. Davis Co., 1972.

Perinatal Trauma

CHAPTER 5

CEREBRAL BIRTH INJURIES

Although more than 100 years have elapsed since Little's classic paper linking abnormal parturition, difficult labor, premature birth, and asphyxia neonatorum with a "spastic rigidity of the limbs,"[1] the pathogenesis of cerebral birth injuries is far from being completely understood. This is not due to a lack of clinical studies. The evolution and ultimate neurologic picture of the various syndromes of disordered movement and posture resulting from nonprogressive brain disease—collectively termed cerebral palsy—have been recorded in innumerable papers. These include Little's paper on spastic diplegia, and Cazauvielh's 1827 monograph on congenital hemiplegia,[2] both also containing descriptions of childhood dyskinesia. Prospective and retrospective studies have attempted to link the various neurologic abnormalities to specific disorders of gestation or the perinatal period.

Pathologic studies, on the other hand, have resulted in the careful description of various cerebral abnormalities in patients with nonprogressive neurologic disorders and have led to attempts, often highly speculative, at formulating their etiology. A combined clinical and pathologic approach has demonstrated, however, that a given neurologic deficit can result from a cerebral malformation of prenatal origin, a destructive process of perinatal or early postnatal onset, or malformation and perinatal trauma acting in concert.

A third line of investigation has been to induce perinatal injury in experimental animals and to correlate the subsequent pathologic and clinical picture with that observed in patients.

From all these investigations a complex picture of the pathogenesis of perinatal brain trauma is beginning to emerge, which is summarized in the subsequent section.

Cerebral palsy occurs in two people of every thousand,[3] there being about one-half million affected persons in the United States, males slightly in excess of females.[4] In an area of 100,000 population, seven infants destined to have cerebral palsy are born each year. Of these, one will die, one will be overwhelmingly incapacitated by neuromotor difficulties, two will be incapacitated by coincident severe mental retardation, and one will have so mild a deficit as not to require special treatment. It is in relation to the remaining two, whose disabilities need treatment but are not devastating, and who have sufficient intelligence to cooperate in therapy, that skilled rehabilitative measures are essential.

Pathogenesis and Pathology

Several factors acting solely or conjointly may produce brain damage during the perinatal period. Physical trauma to the central or peripheral nervous system is probably the one insult which is best understood. A disorder of cerebral circulation, caused by shock or arterial or venous insufficiency and acting as a sole factor, is probably an uncommon cause of brain damage. More often metabolic disorders—notably hypoxia, acidosis, and hypoglycemia—may damage the brain directly or result in edema and various secondary circulatory disturbances.

Physical trauma to the fetal head may produce extracranial lesions, notably caput succedaneum and cephalhematoma. The former represents an area of edema of the scalp, associated with hyperemia and microscopic hemorrhages. Cephalhematoma denotes a subperiosteal hemorrhage produced by the differential between intra- and extrauterine pressure. A variety of skull fractures may be seen in the newborn. Linear fractures are commonly associated with a cephalhematoma and are found in the underlying parietal bone in about 25% of affected infants.[5] A depressed skull fracture may result from pressure of the head against the pelvis or may be induced by an incorrect application of the obstetrical forceps. The latter is often responsible for the small, "Ping-Pong ball" depression.

When molding of the fetal head becomes extreme, hemorrhages and tears of the tentorium or cerebral falx may ensue. These are more common in term than in premature infants. Compression of the head along its occipitofrontal diameter, resulting in vertical molding, may occur with vertex presentations, while compression of the skull between the vault and the base, resulting in an anterior-posterior elongation, is likely to be the outcome of face and brow presentations. Tears of the falx and of the tentorium can be caused by both forms of overstretch. The damage is usually located in the region where the falx joins the anterior edge of the tentorium. Tears and thromboses of the dural sinuses and of the larger cerebral veins, including the vein of Galen, are commonly accompanied by subdural hemorrhages. These may be major and potentially fatal, or minor and clinically unrecognizable. The hemorrhages are mainly localized to the base of the brain or, when the tears extend to involve the straight sinus and the vein of Galen, expand into the posterior fossa. The latter tend to be poorly tolerated and are rapidly fatal.

Overriding of the parietal bones rarely produces a laceration of the superior sagittal sinus and a major fatal hemorrhage. Tearing of the superficial cerebral veins is probably a relatively common phenomenon. The subsequent hemorrhage results in a thin layer of blood over the cerebral convexity. As the superficial cerebral veins of the premature infant are still underdeveloped, this type of hemorrhage is limited to full-term infants.[6] Minor neonatal hemorrhages of this type are probably not uncommon, if the presence of blood in the cerebrospinal fluid can be deemed to be a criterion. Up to 14% of newborn infants have a significant amount of blood in their spinal fluid. Only a few of these show clinical evidence of neurologic abnormalities.[7]

Traumatic lesions to the brain stem and spinal cord are found in 10%–33% of newborn autopsies.[8] Traction of the fetal neck during labor or delivery is accompanied by flexion, hyperextension, and torsion of the spine, and may produce a variety of injuries to the brain stem and spinal cord. This form of birth trauma is particularly common in breech deliveries.[9] Laceration of the cerebellar peduncles accompanied by local brain stem hemorrhage is a sequel of stretch injuries to the brain stem.

Physical damage to the brain, while contributing significantly to mortality during the neonatal period, is a rare cause for persistent major neurologic deficits. These far more commonly are the outcome of hypoxia and other complex metabolic alterations.[10]

When the primate fetus is subjected to acute total asphyxia, a reproducible pattern of brain pathology is observed.[11] This includes bilaterally symmetric lesions in the thalamus, and in a number of brain stem nuclei—notably those of the inferior colliculi, the superior olive, and the lateral lemniscus. These pathologic changes, observed soon after the initial insult, are followed by the gradual appearance of widespread transneuronal degeneration. With progressively longer periods of total asphyxia, the destructive changes in the thalamus become more extensive, and damage begins to appear in the putamen, and in the deeper layers of the cortex. In its extreme form, asphyxiated animals show an extensive cystic degeneration of both cortex and white matter with connective tissue replacement of the damaged areas in the forebrain but a relative lack of cellular reaction in the central nuclear areas.[12]

This experimentally produced picture resembles central porencephaly or cystic degeneration of the human brain, a condition characterized by the formation of cystic cavities in white matter (Fig. 5–1). When small, the cysts are trabeculated and do not communicate with the ventricular system. In their most extensive form they may involve both hemispheres, leaving only small remnants of cortical tissue. The relationship of cystic degeneration to neonatal asphyxia was already established by Little.[1] The cavities are felt to be due to an insufficient glial reaction, perhaps the result of cerebral immaturity, or they may reflect the sudden and massive tissue damage.[13] The pathologic differentiation between this condition and hydranencephaly is discussed in Chapter 4.

It is still unclear whether these gross and microscopic changes are the end result of acute oxygen deprivation acting alone, or whether cell destruction also requires a failure of capillary circulation and an accumulation of various intermediary metabolites which alter intracellular pH and osmotic pressure.

The biochemical and electrical changes attending acute anoxia have been well-studied. Within seconds after the induction of cerebral anoxia, there is a conversion of NAD to NADH, and an increase in the ion permeability of the neuronal membranes. This results in depolarization of neurons and loss of spontaneous electrical activity. Entrance of sodium, chloride, and water into dendrites parallels a marked reduction in the concentration of gray matter triphosphoinositide, a phospholipid known to have a close affinity for calcium and magnesium ions.[14] Accompanying these shifts in electrolyte concentration, lactate accumulates, and the amount of high energy phosphates falls. Glucose and glycogen also drop rapidly, and within 10 minutes become undetectable. The water content increases, and some brain swelling may already be evident within 15 minutes.[15] On electron microscopy there is swelling and disruption of the internal mitochondrial structure, and an increase in the density of the cytoplasmic matrix.[16] After an as yet undetermined period, a point of

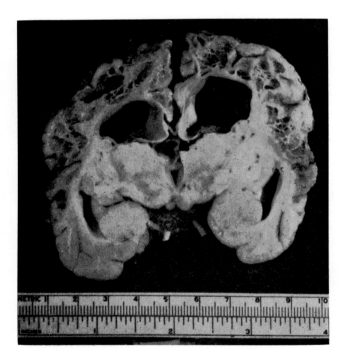

Fig. 5–1. Cystic degeneration of dorsal parts of the hemispheres. Coronal section of brain. (Courtesy of Dr. Nathan Malamud, Langley Porter Neuropsychiatric Institute, San Francisco and the editors of the Journal of Neuropathology and Experimental Neurology.)

irreversibility is reached. Subsequent histochemical changes consist of a widespread accumulation of glycogen within glial cells and a disturbance of the blood-brain barrier.[17]

The relative resistance of the newborn brain to oxygen lack has been known for a long time.[18] Although it has been ascribed to a greater dependence on glycolytic metabolism, it is more likely that it reflects a reduction in overall cerebral metabolism, and decreased energy demands by the newborn brain in comparison with that of the adult organ. Total metabolism of the newborn mouse brain is about one-tenth of the adult, and glycolysis also proceeds at a much slower rate.[19]

While these studies have been limited to acute total asphyxia, the distribution of cerebral lesions induced by these conditions only rarely reproduces those found in infants subjected to perinatal trauma and anoxia. Rather, experimentally induced partial but prolonged asphyxia approximates more closely the pathophysiology of human perinatal anoxia. When primates are subjected to prolonged partial asphyxia, they develop high pCO_2 levels, and a mixed metabolic and respiratory acidosis.[20] This is usually accompanied by marked brain swelling. The relative significance of each of the three variables: hypoxia, hypercarbia, and acidosis in the induction of cerebral edema is still unclear. Two other factors, neonatal hypoglycemia, which hastens the depletion of energy stores under anoxic conditions,[21] and the ability of the newborn brain to utilize ketone bodies as a source of energy by induction of beta-hydroxybutyric acid dehydrogenase, have not been studied sufficiently to assess their contribution to the induction or prevention of anoxic cerebral damage.

Brain swelling compresses the small blood vessels of the cerebral parenchyma. The resultant increase in vascular resistance is often associated with shock and a drop in the systemic blood pressure. These factors combine to lead to failure in cerebral perfusion, and in turn to a number of cerebral circulatory lesions the location of which is governed in part by vascular patterns, and in part by the gestational age of the fetus at the time of the hypoxic insult.[8,22] For many years

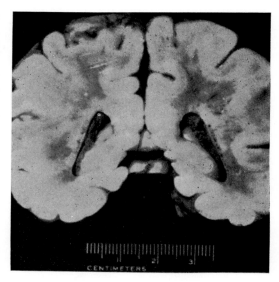

Fig. 5–2. Periventricular encephalomalacia. Note the semicircular areas of malacia surrounding both lateral ventricles. (Courtesy of Dr. Betty Q. Banker, Western Reserve University, Cleveland. From Cooke, R. E.: *The Biologic Basis of Pediatric Practice,* 1968, courtesy of McGraw-Hill Book Co., New York.)

several distinct pathologic lesions have been known to occur singly or conjointly.

One form of brain damage which occurs with particular frequency in the premature infant is periventricular encephalomalacia[23] (Fig. 5–2). Essentially this condition consists of a bilateral but not necessarily symmetric necrosis having a periventricular distribution. Tissue destruction is accompanied by proliferation of astrocytes and microglia, a loss of ependyma, and areas of subcortical degeneration.

Towbin[8] has postulated that the location of the primary lesion in this condition is influenced by the high metabolic activity of the periventricular region, the persistence in the brain of the premature infant of a highly cellular and richly vascularized germinal matrix in the tissue surrounding the lateral ventricles, and the relative prominence of the deep venous system, which becomes prone to thromboses during the last trimester of gestation. Inadequate circulatory perfusion of this area through the deep penetrating arteries may contribute to the evolution of this condition.[23a]

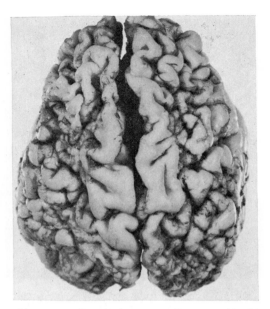

Fig. 5–3. Watershed pattern. Ten-year-old with history of prolonged labor, spastic quadriparesis. Symmetric atrophy in border zones of anterior, middle and posterior cerebral arteries. (Courtesy of Dr. Richard Lindenberg, Baltimore, and the editors of the Journal of Neuropathology and Experimental Neurology.)

In the full-term infant the most common site of brain damage is in the cortex. In this area infarctional lesions are secondary to arterial or venous stasis and thromboses. One common pattern for the distribution of lesions ("arterial border zone" or "watershed") is usually the direct result of a sudden fall in systolic blood pressure. The lesions characteristically involve the territory supplied by the most peripheral branches of the three large cerebral arteries[24] (Fig. 5–3). Damage is maximal in the posterior parietal occipital region, becoming less marked in the more anterior portions of the cortex. Towbin[8,22] has emphasized that in the full-term infant the localization of the infarctional damage to the cerebral cortex not only reflects the "watershed" pattern stressed by Lindenberg, but also the increased metabolic activity of this region during the last few weeks of pregnancy. The lesions in the affected area may be located preferentially in the cortex or in the white matter. Lindenberg[25] has postulated that when right heart

failure is predominant, the white matter is injured preferentially, while the cortex tends to remain intact. When the gray matter is affected, damage usually involves the portions around the depth of the sulci, reflecting the effect of cerebral edema on the drainage of the cortical veins. The subsequent lesion has been termed ulegyria (mantle sclerosis, nodular cortical sclerosis). This is a common abnormality, and accounts for about one-third of clinical defects caused by circulatory disorders during the neonatal period.[24] Its characteristic feature is the localized destruction of the lower parts of the wall of the convolution with relative sparing of the crown. This produces a "mushroom" gyrus (Fig. 5–4). The margins of affected gray matter often contain abnormally dense aggregates of myelinated fibers, while the adjacent white matter shows a considerable amount of myelin loss and compensatory gliosis.[26] Ulegyria may be extensive, or so restricted that the appearance of the brain is grossly normal.[10,27] When ulegyria is widespread, there is often an associated cystic defect in the subcortical white matter (porencephalic cyst) and dilatation of the lateral ventricles. The meninges overlying the affected area are thickened and the small arteries may occasionally show calcifications in the elastica. Less often, ulegyria involves the cerebellum.

Abnormalities within the basal ganglia are seen in the majority of patients subjected to perinatal trauma (84% in the series of Christensen and Melchior).[28] One common lesion seen in this area has been termed status marmoratus. This picture was first described by Anton[29] in 1885 and later by the Vogts,[30] and is characterized by a gross shrinkage of the striatum, particularly the globus pallidus, associated with defects in myelination. While in some cases myelinated nerve fibers may be found in coarse networks resembling the veining of marble—hence the name of the condition (Fig. 5–5)—in other cases the principal pattern is one of a symmetric demyelination (status dysmyelinisatus). It is clear that both hypermyelination and demyelination represent different responses to the same insult. Nerve cells in the affected areas are usually conspicuously reduced in number, with the smaller neurons in the putamen and

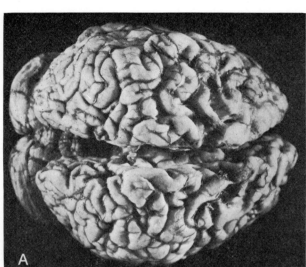
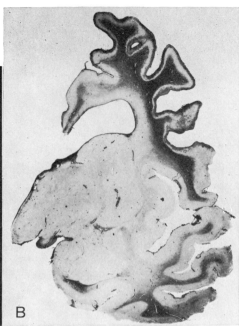

Fig. 5–4. **A.** Lobar sclerosis (ulegyria) in a five-year-old mentally retarded and spastic since infancy. There is sclerosis and distortion of the frontoparietal convolutions of the cerebrum. **B.** Coronal section of same brain showing shrunken and gliotic convolutions. The sulci are deepened and widened (Holzer stain for myelin fibers). (From Towbin, A.: *The Pathology of Cerebral Palsy*, 1960, courtesy of Charles C Thomas, Publisher, Springfield.)

caudate nucleus appearing to be more vulnerable. Cystic changes within the basal ganglia are stressed by Denny-Brown[31] but are rarely extensive.[8] While in many cases the abnormalities within the basal ganglia are the most striking, a variety of associated cortical lesions can be detected in most instances.

The etiology of this condition is still under some dispute. Fundamentally, the pathologic picture is one of glial scarring corresponding to the areas of tissue destruction.[32] It seems clear that selective demyelination of the globus pallidus is one of the most consistent sequelae of kernicterus with or without severe perinatal anoxia.[28,33] Schwartz[34,35,36] has postulated that this pathologic picture is a response to venous hemorrhage secondary to an obstruction of the galenic venous system, and has produced some experimental evidence in support of his theory. Such a mechanism would account for the majority of cases in which there are destructive lesions both within the basal ganglia and the cortex.[13] Although Towbin[8] believes that premature infants are more prone to an infarction of the galenic venous system, the pathologic picture of altered myelination within the basal ganglia can be observed in both full-term and premature infants.[28]

Rarely, the major structural alterations resulting from perinatal injury are localized to the cerebellum. In the majority of instances the involvement is diffuse with widespread disappearance of the cellular elements of the cerebellar cortex and dentate nucleus.[37]

Circulatory lesions of the brain stem secondary to perinatal trauma have received relatively little attention. It is likely, however, that transient compression of the vertebral arteries in the course of rotation or hyperextension of the infant's head during delivery may be a relatively common cause for circulatory lesions of the brain stem.[38]

Intracranial hemorrhages can result not only from direct trauma to the brain but also

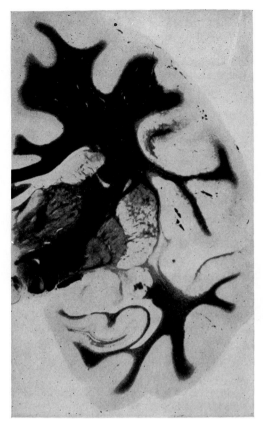

Fig. 5–5. Status marmoratus. This coronal section is stained for myelin fibers and demonstrates aggregations of myelinated fibers throughout the basal ganglia. (Courtesy of Dr. E. P. Richardson, Harvard Medical School, Boston. From Cooke, R. E.: *The Biologic Basis of Pediatric Practice*, 1968, courtesy of McGraw-Hill Book Co., New York.)

from anoxia. Towbin[8] distinguishes two major types of lesions. In premature infants intraventricular hemorrhage is relatively common and is found in 15% of premature babies subjected to autopsy.[39] The condition is often associated with chorioamnionitis and congenital pneumonia, and affected infants tend to be growth retarded for their gestational age. Harcke and associates have found abnormalities in the structure of small arteries which predispose them to hypoxic insults.[39a] Bleeding originates from the choroid plexus or the terminal subependymal veins in the walls of the lateral ventricles The extent of the hemorrhage varies from slight oozing to a massive intraventricular bleed with extension

to the subarachnoid space of the posterior fossa. Circumscribed intraventricular clots detectable by air contrast studies have been reported.[40] The hemorrhage is probably the result of hypoxic systemic circulatory failure, and infarction of the subependymal germinal matrix.[8,41] Blood usually clears rapidly from the subarachnoid spaces. In a few instances, however, it induces a fibrotic reaction which obliterates the subarachnoid spaces and produces hydrocephalus (see Chapter 4).

The second variety of intracranial bleeding is a subarachnoid hemorrhage. It is seen in both premature and full-term infants and is due to hypoxia and stasis within the superficial venous circulation. It accounts for approximately 30% of intracranial hemorrhages of the newborn.[42] Bleeding is usually circumscribed and relatively minor.

A hemorrhage into the brain substance secondary to anoxia is relatively rare and in the experience of Craig[42] accounted for only some 5% of all intracranial hemorrhages of the newborn.

In addition to direct trauma, anoxia, and circulatory disturbances, malformations of the central nervous system play an important part in the genesis of the lesions of perinatal trauma. There is little doubt that in the premature infant, for instance, both faulty maturation of the nervous system and a

TABLE 5-1.
NEUROPATHOLOGY IN
PREMATURE AND FULL-TERM INFANTS
WITH CEREBRAL PALSY*

	Pathology	
Birth Weight (gm)	Birth Injury Number of Cases	CNS Malformation Number of Cases
Less than 2000	3	3
0020–2500	2	1
2501–3000	0	6
3001–3500	10	4
Greater than 3500	7	7
Total known	22	21

* From Malamud et al.[33]

greater vulnerability to perinatal trauma and anoxia are responsible for the high incidence of neurologic deficits.

In any given patient, an evaluation of the pre- and perinatal history may give an indication as to the predominant etiology of the neurologic handicap.[33] A prolonged second stage of labor, the use of a combination of different anesthetics or drugs at delivery, and clinical signs of maternal and infant distress suggest perinatal trauma. In the experience of Malamud and his coworkers[33] parameters of infant distress correlating significantly with neuropathologic lesions of perinatal trauma were impaired respiration, abnormal color, the need for resuscitative measures, seizures, and excessive weight loss during the neonatal period.

Mothers of infants whose neurologic handicap was secondary to cerebral malformations had a statistically higher incidence of vaginal bleeding during pregnancy, and a suggestively higher incidence of prenatal infections. In premature infants with residual neurologic deficits (cerebral palsy) both types of neuropathology were observed (Table 5–1).

Clinical Manifestations

The clinical findings in the child who has been subjected to perinatal trauma are initially fluctuating and limited in their expression by the immaturity of the nervous system. With maturation the neurologic picture evolves and becomes more manifold so that a number of categories can be delineated, with the classification of a given patient usually based on his major clinical involvement.

In this section we will describe the clinical appearance of the neonate who has been subjected to perinatal trauma, trace the evolution of the spastic and extrapyramidal deficits, and conclude with a discussion of the various syndromes of cerebral palsy, acknowledging that in many instances cerebral malformations may play an etiologic role equaling that of birth trauma.

NEONATAL PERIOD. The neonate who has sustained perinatal trauma does not present a consistent appearance. In some, the existence of brain injury is readily apparent, while in others, neurologic abnormalities

may be absent or may only be detected with a careful examination. In describing the neurologic picture we assume that the reader is somewhat familiar with the essentials of a neurologic examination of the small child. A description of techniques is given by Paine and Oppe,[43] and Paine, et al.[44] As a considerable portion of the neurologic examination is devoted to the elicitation and evaluation of postural and segmental reflexes, these are summarized in Table 5–2.

It should be stressed that many of the reflexes exhibited by the newborn infant are also observed in a "spinal animal," one in which the spinal cord has been permanently transected. With progressive maturation, some of these reflexes disappear. This should not be construed to mean that they are actually lost—a reflex once acquired in the course of development is retained permanently—but rather that they are suppressed by the higher centers as they become functional.

A number of segmental medullary reflexes become functional during the last trimester of gestation. They include the following: 1) respiratory activity; 2) cardiovascular reflexes; 3) coughing reflex mediated by the vagus nerve; 4) sneezing reflex evoked by afferent fibers of the trigeminal nerve; 5) swallowing reflex mediated by the trigeminal and glossopharyngeal nerves; and 6) sucking reflex evoked by the afferent fibers of the trigeminal and glossopharyngeal nerves and executed by the efferent fibers of the facial, glossopharyngeal, and hypoglossal nerves.

Another reflex demonstrable in the isolated spinal cord is the flexion reflex. This response is elicited by the noxious stimulation of the skin of the lower extremity and consists of dorsiflexion of the great toe and flexion of the ankle, knee, and hip. This reflex has been elicited in very immature fetuses, and may persist as a fragment, the extensor plantar response, for the first two years of life. Reflex stepping, which, in part at least, is a function of the flexion response, is present in the normal newborn when he is supported in the standing position, and disappears in the fourth or fifth month of life. The normal muscle tone of newborn infants is one of flexion of both upper and lower extremities.

TABLE 5-2.
POSTURAL REACTIONS*

Postural Reflex	Stimulus	Origin of Afferent Impulses	Age Reflex Appears	Age Reflex Disappears
Local static reactions	Gravitation	Muscles		
Stretch reflex			Any age	
Positive supporting action			Well-developed in 50% of the newborn	Indistinguishable from normal standing
Placing reaction			Newborn	Covered up by voluntary action
Segmental static reactions	Movement	Contralateral muscles		
Crossed extensor reflex			Newborn	7–12 months
Crossed adductor reflex to quadriceps jerk			3 months	8 months
General static reactions	Position of head in space	Otolith Neck muscles Trunk muscles		
Tonic neck reflex			Never sustained and complete	
Neck-righting reflex			4–8 months	Covered up by voluntary action
Grasp reflex:				
Palmar			5th intra-uterine month	4–5 months
Plantar			Newborn	9–12 months
Moro reflex			3rd intra-uterine month	4–5 months
Labyrinthine accelerating reactions	Change in rate of movement	Semicircular canals		
Linear acceleration: Parachute reaction			7–9 months	Covered up by voluntary action
Angular acceleration: Postrotational nystagmus			Any age	

* Menkes, J. H.: "The Neuromotor Mechanism" in Cooke, R. E. (ed.): *The Biological Basis of Pediatric Practice,* New York: McGraw-Hill Book Co., 1968.

The flexion tone is generally lost in the upper extremities by four months of age, and in the lower extremities shortly thereafter. Up to then the posture assumed by the infant resembles that seen in paraplegia-in-flexion after spinal cord transection.

The newborn who has sustained perinatal anoxia may demonstrate abnormalities of respiration and muscular tone, evidence of cerebral irritation, and increased intracranial pressure.

Respiratory abnormalities may include a failure to initiate breathing after birth. This suggests a hypoxic depression of the respira-

tory reflex within the brain stem. Tachypnea or dyspnea in the absence of pulmonary or cardiac disease also suggests a neurologic abnormality. Periodic bouts of apnea, while normal in the smaller premature infant, may result from a depression of the respiratory reflex, but in the newborn can also be indicative of a convulsive disorder (see Chapter 11).

The infant who has sustained serious perinatal brain injury is often hypotonic. The sucking and swallowing reflexes are weak or absent, producing difficulties in feeding; palmar and plantar grasps are weak and the placing and stepping reactions are impossible to elicit. Mild degrees of hypotonia can be documented by a head lag and a lack of the normal biceps flexor tone in the traction response from the supine position. The Landau reflex is often abnormal. To elicit this response the infant is lifted with one hand under its trunk, face downward. Normally, there is a reflex extension of the vertebral column, causing the newborn infant to lift its head to slightly below the horizontal, resulting in a slightly convex upward curvature of the spine.[44] With hypotonia the infant's body tends to collapse into an inverted-U shape. Van Harreveld has postulated an electrophysiologic mechanism for hypotonia due to asphyxia.[45]

Less often, an infant who has sustained perinatal hypoxia exhibits hypertonia and rigidity during the neonatal period. The clinical picture of spasticity in the neonate is modified by the immaturity of some of the higher centers. In the spastic infant the deep tendon reflexes are not exaggerated but may even be depressed as a result of muscular rigidity. Hyperreflexia becomes evident only during the second half of the first year of life. More reliable physical signs indicating spasticity include the presence of a sustained tonic neck response. This indicates a tonic neck pattern which can be imposed on the infant for an almost indefinite time and which

he cannot break down. Such a response is never normal (Fig. 5–6). The presence of spastic hemiparesis is manifest during the period in only some 10% of infants[46] usually by a reduction of spontaneous movements, or excessive fisting in the upper extremity. Obvious paralyses during the neonatal period are rarely due to cerebral damage; rather they should suggest a peripheral nerve or spinal cord lesion.

Evidence of cerebral irritation is common in infants who have sustained brain injury, particularly when this is associated with major intracranial hemorrhages. The cry is shrill and monotonous, the face assumes a staring or "worried" appearance, and the infants are irritable and jittery.[47] Often there is an exaggeration of the Moro response, or of the startle reaction to sound.

Convulsions secondary to birth trauma

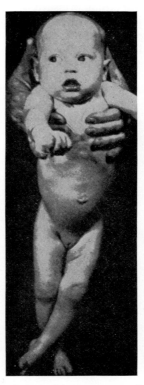

Fig. 5–7. Infant with upper motor lesion demonstrating scissoring of the lower extremities when held in vertical suspension. (Courtesy of the late Dr. Richmond S. Paine, Washington, D.C. From Cooke, R. E.: *The Biologic Basis of Pediatric Practice*, 1968, courtesy of McGraw-Hill Book Co., New York.

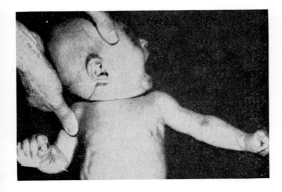

Fig. 5–6. Tonic neck response in a two-month-old infant with mild spasticity. Note the excessive fisting in both hands which is also present. (Courtesy of the late Dr. Richmond S. Paine, Washington, D.C. From Cooke, R. E.: *The Biologic Basis of Pediatric Practice*, 1968, courtesy of McGraw-Hill Book Co., New York.)

usually occur during the second day of life. Generalized tonic-clonic convulsions are rare in the newborn. More often, tonic and clonic movements are observed on separate occasions. Clonic movements are usually focal and tend to move from one part of the body to another. Tonic seizures are manifested by transient opisthotonos, and rotation of the head and eyes. Unusual forms of seizure activity are not rare during the neonatal period. They include paroxysmal blinking, changes in vasomotor tone, nystagmus, chewing, swallowing, pedaling or swimming movements, and periods of apnea or paroxysmal hyperpnea (see Chapter 11). Seizures due to birth trauma often cease spontaneously within a few days or weeks, or are relatively easy to control with anticonvulsant medication.

A full or tense fontanelle is indicative of increased intracranial pressure. This may be a consequence of a massive intracranial hemorrhage, an acute subdural hemorrhage,[47] or cerebral edema.

EVOLUTION OF MOTOR PATTERNS. Infants who have suffered perinatal trauma experience various sequential changes of muscle tone and an abnormal evolution of postural reflexes.

Most often there is a gradual change from the generalized hypotonia of the newborn period to spasticity of later life. In these subjects the earliest sign of spasticity is the presence of increased resistance on passive supination of the forearm, or on flexion and extension of ankle or knee. In spastic diplegia, this abnormal stretch reflex is first evident in the lower extremities and is often accompanied by the appearance of extension and scissoring in vertical suspension (Fig. 5–7), the late appearance or asymmetry of the placing response, a crossed adductor reflex that persists beyond eight months of age, and the increased mobilization of extensor tone in the supporting reaction.[48] In spastic hemiplegia, abnormalities first become apparent in the upper extremity. They include inequalities of muscle tone and asymmetry of fisting, and inequalities of the "parachute" reaction (Fig. 5–8). In many instances,

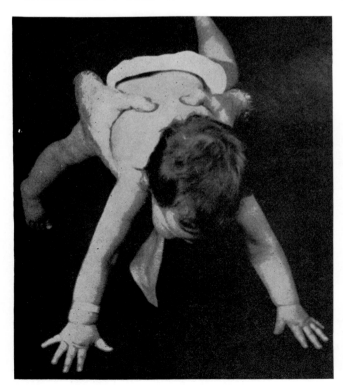

Fig. 5–8. Normal infant demonstrating the "parachute" reaction. Note the extended arms and spreading of fingers. (Courtesy of the late Dr. Richmond S. Paine, Washington, D.C. From Cooke, R. E.: *The Biologic Basis of Pediatric Practice*, 1968, courtesy of McGraw-Hill Book Co., New York.)

parents note poor feeding and frequent re-gurgitation.

Ingram[49] has observed a remarkably con-stant sequence of neurologic manifestations in the progression from hypotonia to spas-ticity. The hypotonic stage may last from 6 weeks to 17 months or even longer. In general, the longer its duration, the more severely handicapped the child.

In a significant percentage of children— 1.3% in the series of Skatvedt,[50] but 20% of the cerebral palsied group at the Southbury Training School[51]—the hypotonic state per-sists for a sufficiently long time, to be desig-nated as atonic cerebral palsy, a term first proposed by Förster in 1910.[52] The condi-tion is characterized by marked generalized hypotonia. In contrast to hypotonia resulting from disorders of muscles or peripheral nerves, the deep tendon reflexes are normal or even hyperactive, but never absent, and the elec-trical reactions of muscle and nerve are normal. Mental deficiency is striking, and in a large percentage there are major cerebral malformations. Muscle biopsy has revealed an abnormal persistence of type II fibers in some children. Type II fibers are rich in glycolytic enzymes and are predominant at 25 weeks gestation but not at term. This abnormality may be a consequence of dis-ordered cerebral influence on muscular de-velopment.[53] The differential diagnosis be-tween atonic cerebral palsy and abnormalities in muscle function is covered more fully in Chapter 12.

A stage of intermittent dystonia often be-comes apparent when the infant is first able to hold up his head. At that time abrupt changes in position, particularly extension of the head, will elicit a response which is similar to extensor decerebrate rigidity. It is likely that the frequency with which this inter-mediate dystonic stage is observed is a func-tion of the care with which neurologic obser-vations are performed. In the majority of children, dystonic episodes are present for between 2 and 12 months; ultimately, as rigidity appears, they become less frequent and more difficult to elicit.

In a smaller number of cerebral palsied children there is a transition from the diffuse hypotonia seen in the neonatal period to an

TABLE 5-3.
EVOLUTION OF ATHETOSIS IN INFANTS WITH EXTRAPYRAMIDAL CEREBRAL PALSY*

Age (in Months)	Cumulative Percentage of Patients Showing Athetosis in Reaching for Objects
6	0
9	12
12	36
15	56
18	64
21	64
24	72
27	76
30	84
33	88
36	92

* From Paine.[48]

extrapyramidal form of cerebral palsy. While a characteristic feature of the motor activity of the normal premature and full-term infant is the presence of choreo-athetoid movements of hands and feet, the fully developed clinical picture of dyskinesia is not usually apparent until the second year of life[48] (Table 5–3). Up until then the neurologic picture is marked by persistent hypotonia accompanied by a retention of the immature postural reflexes. In particular the tonic neck reflex, the righting response, and the Moro reflex are retained for longer periods in infants with extrapyramidal cerebral palsy, than in those in whom a spastic picture predominates.[48] In general, the earliest evidence of extra-pyramidal disease is observed in the posturing of the fingers when the infant reaches for an object (Fig. 5–9). This may be noted as early as nine months of age and, as a rule, the early appearance of extrapyramidal movements in-dicates that the ultimate disability will be mild. In the child with dyskinesia, dystonic posturing can be elicited by sudden changes in the position of the trunk or limbs, particu-larly by extension of the head. Characteris-tically, when an infant is placed with support in the sitting position, he will resist passive flexion of the neck and tend to retroflex his back and shoulders.

Every physician examining infants sus-

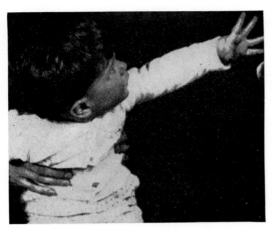

Fig. 5–9. Athetotic posture of the hand in an infant. The child is attempting to reach a proffered object. (Courtesy of the late Dr. Richmond S. Paine, Washington, D.C. From Cooke, R. E.: *The Biologic Basis of Pediatric Practice*, 1968, courtesy of McGraw-Hill Book Co., New York.)

pected of having sustained a cerebral birth injury has encountered a group of patients who appear to have clear-cut neurologic signs in early infancy but who, on subsequent examinations, have lost all of their motor dysfunctions. Some of these infants may show delayed milestones and ultimately are found to be grossly retarded, while others may only demonstrate mild perceptual handicaps, or a hyperkinetic behavior pattern. It is therefore obvious that in a minority of infants abnormalities in motor function are potentially reversible.[48]

CLINICAL FINDINGS IN CHILDHOOD. In older children, the manifestations of cerebral birth injuries are so varied that it becomes difficult to devise an adequate scheme of classification. Yet the differences in etiology, clinical picture, and prognosis require that patients with cerebral palsy be subdivided into various entities based on their clinical picture. In this chapter the following system will be used:
Spastic cerebral palsy
   1. Spastic quadriplegia
   2. Spastic diplegia
   3. Spastic hemiplegia
Extrapyramidal cerebral palsy
Mixed forms

The incidence of each of these forms is presented in Table 5–4. It should be emphasized that as many as one-quarter of children show a mixture of pyramidal and extrapyramidal signs, and that almost every child with spastic diplegia will be found to have spastic quadriplegia upon careful examination. A number of authors have distinguished an ataxic form of cerebral palsy.[49,50] In Skatvedt's series this condition accounts for about 7% of cerebral palsied children. In most instances neuropathologic studies on patients with cerebellar signs have revealed malformations of the cerebellum, often accompanied by even more conspicuous malformations of the cerebral hemispheres.[37] Conversely, most patients with histologically verified lesions of the cerebellum attributable to birth injury did not show cerebellar signs during their lifetime.[28] While both Woods[54] and Crothers and Paine[46] distinguish a condition termed spastic monoplegia (Table 5–4), this entity is probably quite rare. Most children fitting this designation turn out to have spastic hemiplegia on subsequent examinations.[46]

SPASTIC QUADRIPLEGIA (spastic rigidity, bilateral hemiplegia). Under this heading we designate a group of children whose appearance corresponds to the description of "spastic rigidity" as given by Little in his classic paper on cerebral palsy.[1] This

TABLE 5-4.
INCIDENCE OF VARIOUS FORMS OF CEREBRAL PALSY

Classification	Crothers and Paine* (1959)	Woods† (1957)
Cerebral Palsy		
Spastic	**64.6%**	**69.5%**
Quadriplegia	19.0	19.4
Diplegia	2.8	7.9
Hemiplegia	40.5	36.6
Monoplegia	0.4	5.6
Triplegia	1.9	
Extrapyramidal	**22.0**	**11.1**
Mixed Types	**13.1**	**21.1**

* Crothers and Paine.[46]
† Woods.[54]

category includes some of the most severely damaged patients.

While there is a mixed etiology for this as well as for the other forms of cerebral palsy, abnormalities in delivery, particularly a prolonged second stage of labor, precipitate delivery, or fetal distress, are common. On pathologic examination, Benda has frequently noted an extensive cystic degeneration of the brain (polyporencephaly) (Fig. 5–1).[13]

Subjects demonstrate a generalized increase in muscular tone, and rigidity of the limbs on both flexion and extension. In its most extreme form, the child is stiff and assumes a posture of decerebrate rigidity. As a rule, impairment of motor function is more severe in the upper extremities. There are few voluntary movements, and vasomotor changes in the extremities are common. Most children have pseudobulbar signs with difficulties in swallowing, and recurrent aspiration of food material. Optic atrophy and grand mal seizures are noted in about one-half of patients.[49]

Intellectual impairment is severe in all instances, and no child in Ingram's series was considered to be educable.[49]

SPASTIC DIPLEGIA. As defined by Freud,[55] who coined the term "diplegia," this condition is characterized by bilateral spasticity, with greater involvement of the legs than arms. The incidence of spastic diplegia is difficult to ascertain. In the experience of Ford[56] this was the most common form of cerebral palsy encountered at Johns Hopkins Hospital. On the other hand, Woods[54] does not use this designation, while Crothers and Paine[46] group most diplegic patients with those having spastic quadriplegia. For reasons as yet unclarified, a number of centers have observed that the incidence of spastic diplegia in low birth weight infants born since 1969 is significantly lower than in infants born prior to that date.[56a]

A high proportion of diplegic children have a history of an abnormal gestation, labor, or delivery. The frequency of prematurity is particularly striking.[57] In the series of Ingram,[49] 44% of patients suffering from spastic diplegia had a birth weight of $5\frac{1}{2}$

pounds or less. Of the full-term patients, 18% had only abnormal gestation, 23% had only abnormal delivery, and 25% had both abnormal gestation and delivery. Conversely, 81% of premature infants developing the cerebral palsy syndrome have spastic diplegia.[57] As a rule, those patients in whom a history of birth injury is readily apparent, have a higher intelligence than those having an uneventful perinatal period. It is likely that the latter group includes patients with cerebral malformations.[58]

A variety of pathologic abnormalities can be found on autopsy. One particularly common entity is periventricular encephalomalacia[23] (Fig. 5–2). The location of the white matter lesions produces an interruption of the downward course of the pyramidal fibers from the cortical leg area as they traverse the internal capsule, explaining the predominant involvement of the lower extremities. Cortical abnormalities, porencephaly, and congenital malformations of the gyri (micropolygyria) have also been seen in children who were diplegic during their lifetime.[28]

The most striking physical finding in children with spastic diplegia is the increased muscular tone in the lower extremities. The severity of the diplegia varies from case to case. In the most involved patients Ingram[49] is able to distinguish a state when rigidity predominates, and limbs tend to be maintained in extension. Thus when a child is held vertically, the rigidity of the lower extremities becomes most evident, while the adductor spasm of the hips maintains them in a scissored position (Fig. 5–7). This stage is succeeded by the spastic phase, when flexion of the hips, knees, and to a lesser extent of the elbows becomes predominant. When the diplegia is less severe, patients will only show impaired dorsiflexion of the feet, with increased tone at the ankles, causing them to walk with the feet in the equinus position ("toe-walking"). In such instances the tone in the upper extremities is often normal to passive movement, but the child will maintain his elbows flexed when walking. In others, spasticity of the lower extremities is accompanied by impaired coordination of fine and rapid finger movements, and a slight weakness of the wrist extensors. Sensory impairment is rare. The deep tendon reflexes are hyperactive in all extremities, unless muscular rigidity makes them difficult to elicit. An ankle clonus and an extensor plantar response can usually be obtained. Dystonia, athetosis, and mixed types of involuntary movements are occasionally seen in the more severely involved patients and may interfere considerably with muscular control. After a variable period, usually more than two years, contractures appear. These tend to be most severe in the distal musculature, particularly at the ankles. As a consequence, feet tend to become fixed in plantar flexion, knees in flexion, and hips in flexion and adduction. Vasomotor changes and dwarfing of the pelvis and lower extremities are often striking and, in general, parallel the severity of the paresis. Optic atrophy, field defects, and involvement of the cranial nerves are relatively rare. A convergent strabismus is common, however, and was seen in 43% of Ingram's diplegic patients.[49] Forty-four percent of Ingram's children had a speech defect; most often this was a matter of retarded speech development and an inability to pronounce consonants.

Seizures are a common accompaniment of spastic diplegia and were seen in 27% of Ingram's series.[49] These are most often grand mal in type, and their incidence is unrelated to the severity of the motor handicap, although the presence of minor motor seizures is usually limited to patients with significant involvement of the upper extremities.

The extent of mental retardation in diplegic patients is difficult to ascertain. As expected, the more severe the motor deficit, the more retarded the patient. Six out of 29 children with little impairment of the upper extremities (spastic paraplegia) had IQs above 100, but all of 27 children with major involvement of the upper extremities had an IQ below 100.[49]

SPASTIC HEMIPLEGIA. This condition is characterized by a unilateral paresis, which nearly always affects the upper extremity to a greater extent than the lower, and which is ultimately associated with some spasticity and flexion contracture of the affected limbs.

In about half of those afflicted, the hemiparesis is evident at birth or during the first two years of life. In the remainder the hemiparesis develops as an acute episode during infancy or childhood. While technically the latter condition, termed acute infantile hemiplegia, is not a birth injury, it is discussed in this chapter under a separate heading.

The correlation of congenital hemiplegia with cerebral abnormalities was established by Cazauvielh[2] in 1827, while an antecedent history of abnormalities of labor and delivery was established by McNutt,[59] Freud and Rie,[60] and Ford.[61] As in the other forms of cerebral palsy the pathologic picture in congenital hemiplegia is varied. Benda has emphasized the frequency with which mantle sclerosis (ulegyria) can be found[13] (Fig. 5–4), but malformations of the cerebral hemispheres are encountered with an almost equal frequency.[33] The high incidence of abnormalities of pregnancy and delivery is striking (Table 5–5).

Children with congenital hemiplegia are only rarely recognized at birth. Usually, the age at which the hemiparesis becomes apparent is a function of the care of parental observation. Most commonly, parents note the early establishment of handedness. Dominance will become apparent prior to 18 months of age, as contrasted with a normal of two to four years. This is associated with disuse and abnormal posturing of the affected arm. Less often, a disturbance of gait or

TABLE 5-5.
INCIDENCE OF ABNORMALITIES OF PREGNANCY AND DELIVERY IN PATIENTS WITH CONGENITAL HEMIPLEGIA*

Abnormality	Number of Patients
Pregnancy	6
Delivery	7
Pregnancy and delivery	16
Neither	1
TOTAL	30

* From Ingram.[49]

developmental retardation are the presenting complaints.

In most series the right side is more commonly affected, the incidence of right-sided involvement in three major series being 55%,[62] 59%,[49] and 66%.[46]

The evolution of hemiplegia from the flaccid stage seen in the neonatal period to the spasticity of the older child has been traced by Byers.[63]

In the older child the extent of impaired voluntary function varies considerably from one patient to another.

As a rule, the most affected are fine movements of the hand, notably the pincer grasp of thumb and forefinger, extension of the wrist, and supination of the forearm. In the lower extremity, dorsiflexion and eversion of the foot are most frequently impaired. Increased flexor tone is invariably present, leading to a hemiparetic posture, with flexion at the elbow, wrist, and knees, and an equinus position of the foot. The deep tendon reflexes are increased, and the Babinski and, less often, the Hoffmann responses can be elicited. In most children there is a persistence of the palmar grasp reflex.

A large proportion of hemiplegic children have involuntary movements of the affected limbs. These are most clearly seen in the hand. Here one observes an avoidance response, and athetotic posturing of the hand, producing overextension of the fingers and occasionally the wrist, as the hand makes an attempt at holding an object.[64] This type of posture has a marked similarity to that of patients with parietal lobe lesions. The affected side will also participate in overflow movements, which are involuntary changes in position associated with voluntary movements of the unaffected side.

Sensory abnormalities of the affected limbs are common and could be documented by Tizard and associates[65] in 68% of patients with congenital hemiplegia. Stereognosis is impaired most frequently; less often two-point discrimination and position sense are defective. In addition to sensory impairment there is frequently a neglect and unawareness of the affected side, deficits which aggravate considerably the handicap induced by the hemi-paresis. In general, the severity of the sensory defect does not correlate with that of the hemiparesis.

Growth disturbances of the affected limbs are extremely common and, like the sensory defects, probably reflect damage to the parietal lobes. Failure of growth is most evident in the upper extremities, particularly in the terminal phalanges and in the size of the nail beds, and is a result of underdevelopment of muscle and bone. The presence of growth arrest is not always accompanied by sensory changes.

Between 17%–27% of patients with congenital hemiplegia have homonymous hemianopsia. When adequate testing of the visual fields is possible, sparing of the macula can often be demonstrated.[46] The anatomic basis for the hemianopsia has been studied by Walsh and Lindenberg;[66] they call attention to the vulnerability of the visual pathways to perinatal cerebral edema on the basis of compression of the posterior cerebral arteries and their branches, thus compromising the vascular supply to the occipital lobes.

Abnormalities in cranial nerve function are common and usually due to a supranuclear involvement of the muscles enervated by the lower cranial nerves. Facial weakness is probably the most common abnormality, being noted in about three-quarters of the patients.[49,63] Deviation of the tongue and convergent strabismus are seen less often.

About one-half of patients with congenital hemiplegia develop seizures. In the majority, convulsions first appear between one and four years. They continue for several years, ceasing spontaneously in about half of the patients. Seizures are usually in the nature of grand mal or focal attacks, but a considerable proportion of patients who for months or even years have focal seizures only, may later go on to develop generalized convulsions.[61] As a rule, anticonvulsant therapy is effective in reducing the frequency of attacks. There exists, however, a sizeable group of seizure patients in whom attacks persist despite medication, and who may require surgical removal of the portion of the cerebral cortex from which the seizure focus originates, or even a hemispherectomy, should there be more than one focus.

In congenital hemiplegia, neither the IQ nor the incidence of speech defects depends on which of the hemispheres has sustained the major damage. About one-third of children have average IQs or better, and nearly all of these are educationally competitive. In general, there is little relationship between IQ level and the severity of the hemiparesis.[49]

EXTRAPYRAMIDAL CEREBRAL PALSIES. These conditions are characterized by the predominant presence of a variety of involuntary movements, generally considered to be the result of damage to the extrapyramidal motor system.

Varieties of etiologies are responsible for the extrapyramidal deficits. A number of patients have a history suggestive of birth injury with an abnormal delivery and distress during the immediate neonatal period. Only about 15% of these are premature infants.[49] In a second group no abnormalities of delivery can be elicited, and cerebral malformations are often evident on pathologic examination. In a third group there is a history of significant jaundice, often the result of blood group incompatibility, appearing during the first 24 hours of life. The neuropathology in these patients indicates that the extrapyramidal disorder is a result of kernicterus. This group of patients is discussed more fully in Chapter 9.

The clinical picture of extrapyramidal cerebral palsy evolves gradually from diffuse hypotonia with lively reflexes in infancy to choreo-athetosis during childhood.[67]

The onset of choreo-athetosis is usually between the second and third year of life (Table 5–3)[48] but may be as late as the eighth year. This delay in the clinical expression of a static cerebral lesion has been attributed to a disparity between the maturation of injured and uninjured areas of the central nervous system.[68] As a rule the most severely affected children continue to manifest hypotonia for the longest.

In the final stage of dyskinesia, a number of involuntary movements are recognized. Collectively these have been termed choreo-athetosis, but actually the clinical picture is more complex. In most patients, a variety of involuntary movements appearing discretely or in transition forms can be recognized.

Athetosis indicates an instability of posture, with slow swings of movement most marked in the distal portions of the limbs. The movements fluctuate between two extremes of posture in the hand, one of hyperextension of the fingers with pronation and flexion of the wrist, and supination of the forearm, the other one of intense flexion and adduction of the fingers and wrist, and pronation of the forearm.

Choreiform movements refer to more rapid and jerky movements similar in their range to the athetoid movements but so rapid and continuous that the two extremes of posture are no longer evident.[31] Commonly they involve the muscles of the face, tongue, and proximal portions of the limbs. Athetosis and choreiform movements occur far more frequently as associated than as isolated phenomena.[49]

In dystonia, there is fixation or relative fixation in one of the athetotic postures. Dystonia is always accompanied by other involuntary movements. The other manifestations of basal ganglia disorder, tremors, and myoclonus, are usually less apparent. Tremors are rhythmic alterations in movement, while myoclonus is a relatively unpredictable contraction of one or more muscle groups. It may be precipitated by a variety of stimuli, particularly sudden changes in position, or by the start of voluntary movements. In addition to these movement disorders, children with dystonic cerebral palsy also exhibit sudden increases in muscle tone, often precipitated by attempts at voluntary movement ("tension").

These various dyskinesias combine with spasticity, which is seen in a large porportion of children, to interfere markedly with all types of voluntary movements.

Development of motor function is usually far more retarded than would be expected from the intelligence level of the child. About one-half will walk prior to the fourth year; in Ingram's series, the average age at which unsupported walking was achieved was two years and five months.[49] The delay in gait correlates well with delays in the other motor milestones. Crothers and Paine[46] have shown that persistence of the obligatory tonic neck reflex (Fig. 5–6) suggests a bad prognosis in terms of the ability to walk without assistance and, to a lesser extent, of the severity of athetosis. In their experience, walking is highly improbable as long as an obligatory tonic neck response is elicitable. Correlation of obligatory tonic neck response with intelligence was not uniform, and the persistence of the reflex should not indicate intellectual incompetence.

Skilled hand movements, such as those which are required for feeding, dressing, and writing, are equally impaired, and the disability in hand function may be so severe as to render a child virtually helpless. An occasional patient may learn to perform these skilled movements with his mouth or feet.

Speech defects occur frequently in children with extrapyramidal cerebral palsy. In many, development of speech is retarded due to the incoordinated movements of lips, tongue, palate, and respiratory muscles. In about two-thirds of children, incoordination of the muscles of respiration and speech is responsible for delayed speech.[50] Yet, about

half of patients begin to say intelligible words before 2½ years of age,[46] and all children who are not severely retarded are able to speak by four years of age.

A number of patients with moderately severe dyskinesia have impaired swallowing and control of saliva. As a result, drooling may persist for as long as five to six years of age. Cranial nerve involvement is less common than in the other forms of cerebral palsy. However, strabismus is seen in about one-third of patients, and one-third have nystagmus.[49] Optic atrophy is rare, and seizures are no more frequent than in the general population.[46]

As a rule, children with extrapyramidal involvement have less intellectual deficit than any other group of cerebral palsied. In the experience of Crothers and Paine,[46] some 65% had IQs over 70, and 45% had IQs of 90 or better. In a considerable number, the delay in developing language skills, and the gross motor handicap result in an erroneous underestimation of intelligence (Table 5–6).[46] However, a large proportion

TABLE 5-6.
VALIDITY OF EARLY ESTIMATE OF INTELLIGENCE
IN TWO TYPES OF CEREBRAL PALSY

Type of Cerebral Palsy	Original Estimate		Estimate at Follow-up		
	Range	No. of Patients	Same	Higher	Lower
Hemiplegia	Superior	4	2	—	2
	Average	17	13	1	3
	Below average	19	11	1	7
	Inadequate or defective	27	25	2	—
Extrapyramidal	Superior	5	5	—	0
	Average	13	10	0	3
	Below average	6	6	0	0
	Inadequate or defective	27	16	11	—

* From Crothers and Paine.[46]

of children with normal or near normal intelligence have sufficiently severe educational disability to require their attendance at special schools.

MIXED FORMS OF CEREBRAL PALSY. In the experience of most physicians a considerable proportion of cerebral palsied exhibit a mixture of spasticity and extrapyramidal movements (Table 5–4). This may manifest itself by minor amounts of athetotic posturing, as observed in a high percentage of children with spastic hemiplegia, or by the presence of extensor plantar responses in patients with predominantly extrapyramidal disease. When the mixed form is most obvious, the clinical picture is one of marked hyperreflexia, spasticity, and contractures in a child with frank dystonia or other extrapyramidal movements.

Diagnosis

The diagnosis of a neurologic disorder which has resulted from perinatal injury rests upon the following factors:

1. A history of perinatal distress. In particular, a second stage of labor lasting more than 30 minutes, often accompanied by sufficient maternal distress to require blood transfusion or administration of oxygen. Breech presentation and the application of mid-forceps are both significantly associated with perinatal trauma.

2. A history of an abnormal neonatal course. This would include delayed or impaired respiration, requiring resuscitative measures or stimulative drugs in the delivery room, abnormal muscle tone, color or cry, seizures, or a bulging fontanelle. Intracranial hemorrhage during the neonatal period may also be caused by blood dyscrasias, such as thrombocytopenic purpura, hemophilia, or—in a rare instance—hemorrhagic disease of the newborn.[69]

3. Evidence for a nonprogressive neurologic disorder. Nonprogression of neurologic symptoms is not easy to demonstrate, for in the course of development, particularly during the first two years of life, new motor patterns evolve, which may suggest a progressive disease, such as a lipoidosis, or one of the leukodystrophies. Furthermore, severely handicapped children may transiently or permanently lose ground as a consequence of intercurrent infections, or in association with the onset of seizures.

4. During the neonatal period, laboratory studies may assist in arriving at a diagnosis of cerebral trauma. Examination of the cerebrospinal fluid can provide evidence for a recent intracranial hemorrhage. Fluid which contains more than 500 red cells/mm^3 will appear grossly bloody. When this is the case, it becomes important to exclude the possibility of a traumatic tap by performing cell counts on three sequential samples of fluid. In the presence of an intracranial hemorrhage there is little difference in the count obtained on the first and last specimens. However, erythrocyte counts up to about 600 cells/mm^3 have been recorded in asymptomatic infants after an uncomplicated delivery.[70] Performing sequential cell counts constitutes a more reliable method for demonstrating intracranial bleeding than observing the presence of xanthochromic fluid or crenated red cells.[71] Crenation of red cells in cerebrospinal fluid occurs promptly,[72] while xanthochromia may be noted whenever contamination by red cells is heavy. Spectrophotometric analysis of the pigment will be of assistance when the tap is performed after sufficient time has elapsed, usually several days, to allow the conversion of oxyhemoglobin to bilirubin.[73] The conversion of hemoglobin to bilirubin is catalyzed by a microsomal oxidase localized to the arachnoid, the choroid plexus, and the cerebral cortex. Enzyme induction occurs within 12 hours after blood enters the CSF.[73a] In jaundiced infants, CSF bilirubin must be corrected for the amount present as a consequence of the elevated concentrations in the serum. A formula for calculating CSF bilirubin from serum levels is:

$$\text{CSF bilirubin} = \text{Serum bilirubin} \times \frac{\text{CSF protein}}{\text{Serum protein}}$$

If the CSF bilirubin is 30% or more than the amount calculated from serum levels by means of this equation, a recent intracranial hemorrhage is likely.[74]

In the presence of perinatal trauma, the concentration of cerebrospinal fluid protein may be above the normal range, which in the newborn extends to about 150 mg%.[70] The presence of blood from any source raises the total protein by 1.5 mg per 100 ml of fluid for every 1000 fresh red blood cells per cu mm.[73] An elevation in the activity of cerebrospinal fluid creatine phosphokinase has been found in infants who have sustained recent perinatal trauma. Since the presence of blood in the spinal fluid does not influence the value of creatine phosphokinase, enzyme levels may parallel the extent of cerebral parenchymal damage.[75]

It should, however, be stressed that a normal cerebrospinal fluid does not exclude the possibility of perinatal brain trauma. Other studies that can be utilized in confirming recent perinatal trauma include radiographs of the skull. These may reveal the presence of linear or depressed fractures. One common variety of the latter is the "Ping-Pong ball" fracture, which is characterized by an absence of an actual break in the continuity of the bone, which has simply been bent inward. It is produced by extreme molding of the head during passage through the birth canal, or by a difficult forceps delivery. In most instances it is not associated with damage to the underlying brain.[76]

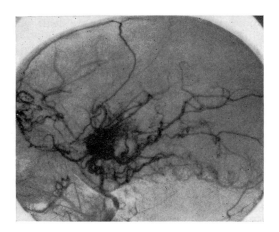

Fig. 5–10. Moyamoya disease. The left cerebral angiogram demonstrates an obstruction of the internal carotid artery probably at the origin of the posterior communicating artery. There is a netlike cluster of blood vessels in the area of the basal ganglia probably arising from the lenticulo-striate arteries. Three-year-old boy with acute right hemiplegia. (Courtesy of Dr. Gabriel Wilson, Department of Radiology, UCLA.)

Diagnostic studies applicable to older children with a history of perinatal trauma are usually less helpful. The cerebrospinal fluid is normal, skull films may show microcephaly, or in cases of hemiplegia, thickening of the ipsilateral cranial vault, hypertrophy of the frontal and paranasal sinuses, and an elevation of the slope of the petrous ridge—a radiographic picture first described by Dyke, Davidoff, and Masson.[77] Atrophy of the cerebral substance is demonstrable by contrast studies. Abnormalities of the cerebral circulation are minor and are limited to a shortened circulation time and impaired vascularization of the affected side.[78]

Treatment

The treatment of the cerebral palsied has been the subject of innumerable publications, most of them surprisingly uncritical and devoid of controls. In the main, treatment consists of physical therapy, with or without bracing and orthopedic surgery. From the studies of Crothers and Paine,[46] and Paine,[79] it seems clear that to be most effective, the choice of program is determined by the nature of the handicap.

Intensive physical therapy appears to be helpful for children with spastic hemiplegia. Most of these require regular physiotherapy as soon as they begin to walk, with special attention being paid to the presence of contractures in the lower extremity. Bracing may often be necessary. Despite physical therapy about one-half of the patients will ultimately require some form of orthopedic surgery, most commonly lengthening of the heel cords or hamstrings. There is much controversy as to the management of the hemiplegic hand. Ultimate hand function is usually not improved by physical therapy or surgery, and there is little doubt that when the hemiplegia is complicated by a hemisensory deficit, the affected hand will never be more than an assist to the good hand. Growth of the affected side is not improved by any mode of treatment. When the hemiplegia is mild, children will achieve a good gait whether treated or not.

A similar program is advisable for children with spastic diplegia. Here too, the treatment is directed to prevention of contractures

heterogeneous and that children who develop hemiplegia following a prolonged seizure have a clinical picture that differs somewhat from those who develop hemiplegia without antecedent seizures. By means of arteriography, occlusive vascular disease can be demonstrated in a considerable proportion. Solomon, et al.[92] have distinguished five categories on the basis of the angiographic picture. One common entity is characterized by marked stenosis or complete occlusion of the supraclinoid segment of the internal carotid, and the proximal portions of the middle and anterior cerebral arteries. Associated with this there is a prominent telangiectasis of the vessels in the basal ganglia (Fig. 5–10). These abnormalities are usually bilateral. This radiographic picture has been recognized by Japanese physicians for over a decade and has been termed "Moyamoya" disease. Moyamoya refers to something hazy, "just like a puff of cigarette smoke drifting in the air."[93] It is thought that the moyamoya vessels represent collaterals resulting from the occlusion of the carotid arteries. This vascular pattern is usually transient and disappears as the cerebral circulation is maintained by collaterals from the external carotid or vertebral arteries. The basis for the occlusion of the carotid arteries is still obscure.

Another common arteriographic pattern in acute hemiplegia is a unilateral occlusion of the carotid artery in its supraclinoid portion, but unaccompanied by a telangiectatic pattern. The occlusion is believed to be due to an arteritis, possibly as an aftermath of ear, throat, or sinus infection.[94]

Less often, Solomon, et al. encountered a stenosis at the origin of the internal carotid artery, or occlusion of one or more branches of the distal portion of the middle cerebral artery.[92] As a rule, children who demonstrate occlusive vascular disease do not have convulsions at the onset of their hemiparesis.[95]

In the remainder of children, arteriography is normal. In the majority of this group the hemiparesis follows multiple generalized or focal seizures.[92,95] Norman[91] has postulated that neuronal destruction resulting from the seizures and occurring in a laminar distribution within the cerebral cortex may be responsible for the hemiparesis. While in most cases of status epilepticus the neuronal loss is bilateral, in a number of instances cortical damage can be almost exclusively unilateral, particularly when seizures are superimposed on a pre-existing but clinically inapparent malformation or birth injury.[91]

The mechanism by which seizures induce brain damage is not completely understood but is discussed in Chapter 11.

Clinical Manifestations

Little can be added to the clinical description of acute hemiparesis as given by Freud:[88]

The Clinical Course of a Typical Case:

A child who has hitherto been well, and without hereditary predisposition is suddenly taken ill at an age between a few months to three years. The etiology of the disease either remains unexplained or is attributed to a concurrent infection. The presenting symptoms may be either stormy, with fever, convulsions, and vomiting, or insignificant; they may last one day or up to several weeks. The disease cannot be diagnosed with certainty in this initial stage. A hemiparesis may appear at this point, or not until later. It spreads in the usual manner: first face, then arm, then leg. At first it is a flaccid paresis, but very soon it becomes spastic, with increased reflexes and contractures. Partial or complete aphasia appear commonly, but are usually transient; hemianopsia or paralyses of the ocular muscles are rare. The paresis may vanish, or else recur in bouts with increasing severity; most commonly it is permanent. Improvement is more likely in the leg than the arm; in such a case the child walks with circumduction of the affected hip. Improvement of the paresis is very commonly associated with post-hemiplegic chorea together with a greater or lesser degree of residual spasticity. Growth atrophy of the affected limbs, which is often extensive, becomes apparent during the pubertal growth spurt. Impaired intelligence of varying degree is seldom absent. Epileptic seizures may make their appearance at a variable interval following the initial illness. These are at first unilateral, later they become generalized and severe. There is no time limit to the appearance of epileptic seizures.

As indicated by Freud's description, acute hemiplegia usually occurs prior to three years of age. This is borne out by our experience, and by the series of Ingram,[49] who encountered nearly 90 percent of his cases prior to the age of three. About 60% of patients have unilateral or generalized seizures at the onset of their hemiplegia.[49] The duration of the convulsion is variable, and may be as long as 24 hours. Following this there is loss or severe impairment of neurologic function. In a few instances the onset of the hemiplegia is subacute and develops over the course of several months, apparently unassociated with any illness. As Freud indicated, involvement of the arm is almost always more extensive than of the leg. Contrary to his experience, Crothers and Paine, and Aicardi, et al. found disturbances in sensation and hemianopsia to be relatively common.[46,95]

Although Freud considered children who develop acute hemiplegia as being "hitherto well," it is likely that in some cases a minor degree of hemiplegia may have preexisted. About one-third or children have a history of an abnormal birth or pregnancy,[49] and some 20% have a history of previous convulsions.[95] In most of these patients, single or multiple seizures initiate the hemiparesis (postconvulsive hemiparesis).

In the acutely hemiparetic child the cerebrospinal fluid is usually normal. In a few cases there is a mild pleocytosis (less than 50 cells per mm^3), and an elevated protein. The electroencephalogram may reveal unilateral or predominantly unilateral slowing, and decreased voltage over the affected side. Pneumoencephalography may initially demonstrate edema of the affected hemisphere with a shift of the midline to the unaffected side. Subsequent studies will usually show unilateral cerebral atrophy, as evidenced by dilatation of the lateral ventricles. In long-standing hemiplegias, particularly those having their onset before three years of age, alterations of the bony structure of the vault, referred to as the Dyke-Davidoff-Masson syndrome[77] may become evident as early as nine months after the onset of the hemiparesis.[92] The results of cerebral angiography have already been referred to. Complications from this procedure are rare, even when carried out shortly after the onset of the hemiparesis. This study is therefore indicated for every child with an acute onset of hemiparesis in order that an anatomic diagnosis can be established.

Differential Diagnosis

Various conditions may produce a sudden onset of hemiplegia in a child. In addition to the causes already enumerated, lupus erythematosus, periarteritis nodosa, bacterial or viral infections, trauma, cardiac abnormalities, sickle cell disease and other hemoglobinopathies, arteriovenous malformations, and homocystinuria may all be responsible for hemiplegia of acute onset.[95a] Todd's paralysis must also be considered in the differential diagnosis of acute hemiplegia. This is a transient paresis that follows a generalized, focal, or Jacksonian seizure. While in most cases the weakness clears within a few hours, apparently uncomplicated Todd's paralysis may not clear completely for up to several days (see Chapter 11). The sudden onset of hemiparesis is characteristic of hemiplegic migraine. This is a relatively common condition, often familial, characterized by the association of migraine and hemiplegia, with the latter usually occurring as an aura to the attack.[96] Cerebral angiography during the prodrome shows a decrease in the caliber of the internal carotid artery system. The condition is more common in older children, particularly teenagers, and is referred to in Chapter 11.

Treatment and Prognosis

There is no evidence that the use of anticoagulants or fibrinolytic agents reduces the severity of the hemiplegia. Hypothermia and inhalations of carbon dioxide or oxygen have also been ineffective for most children.

Seizures persist in about three-quarters of the postconvulsive hemiplegias, particularly in those whose illness began with multiple seizures.[92,95] In this group, complete recovery both with respect to the motor deficit and residual intellectual and behavioral abnormalities, is less likely than in patients whose hemiparesis is unaccompanied by seizures.

In many children, seizures continue for years, and prove to be intractable to anti-

convulsant medications. Under these circumstances hemispherectomy should be considered. Positive criteria for surgery include
a relatively good intelligence and radiographic evidence that the contralateral
hemisphere is normal. Bilateral electroencephalographic abnormalities do not con-
traindicate surgery. In the experience of
Wilson[97] surgery completely or substantially
reduced seizures in 82% of subjects, with concurrent improvement of behavior in most.
About one-third of patients subjected to
hemispherectomy have a prolonged morbidity
in the form of persistent and recurrent subdural hemorrhages, obstructive hydrocephalus, and recurrent episodes of aseptic meningitis. The latter may produce siderosis of the
central nervous system.[97,98]

PERINATAL TRAUMA TO THE SPINAL CORD

Although first described during the nineteenth century, much of our understanding
of spinal birth injuries can be attributed to the
classic papers of Crothers,[99] Ford,[9] and
Crothers and Putnam.[100] While relatively
common several decades ago, the incidence
of this type of birth injury has diminished with
improved obstetric practice, and it comprised
only 0.6% of the series of cerebral palsied encountered by Crothers and Paine.[46] However the apparent rarity of this condition may
in part reflect the fact that few infants with
major spinal cord damage survive the neonatal period.[100a]

Pathogenesis and Pathology

Perinatal traumatic lesions of the spinal
cord more commonly result from stretching
of the cord than compression or transection.[101]
Traction to the infant's neck, particularly in
the course of a difficult breech delivery, will
stretch the cord, its covering meninges, the
surface vessels, and the nerve roots. Lesions
are most frequent in the lower cervical and
thoracic regions. The most common gross
pathologic findings are epidural hemorrhage,
dural laceration with subdural hemorrhage,
tears of the nerve roots, laceration and distortion of the cord, and focal hemorrhage and
malacia within the cord.[101] Ischemic lesions
of the cord are less common.[102] Gross or

petechial hemorrhages may also be seen
within the substance of the cord.

Clinical Manifestations

Most infants who have suffered a spinal
birth injury have a history of a difficult
breech delivery, with arrest of the after-
coming head. When damage to the cord is
severe, death of the neonate occurs during
labor or soon after. When injury is less extensive, infants show respiratory depression
and generalized hypotonia, or flaccid paraplegia. There is an associated urinary retention, and abdominal distention with
paradoxical respirations.[103] In addition to
impaired motor function, sensation and perspiration are absent below the level of injury.
The deep tendon reflexes are usually unelicitable during the neonatal period, and
mass reflex movements do not become apparent until later.

In about 20% of cases, damage to the
brachial plexus can also be documented. In
others the lower brain stem is involved as
well, with consequent bulbar signs.

The evolution of the clinical picture following complete transection of the spinal cord
is covered in Chapter 8. A high percentage
of survivors have normal intelligence.

Diagnosis

The presence of poor muscle tone and
flaccid weakness involving all extremities or
only the legs following a breech extraction
should suggest a cord injury. Although not
easy to demonstrate, loss of sensory function
should always be sought for.

Neuromuscular disorders, notably infantile
muscular atrophy (Werdnig-Hoffmann disease), are not associated with loss of sensory
function or sphincter control. Of the other
neuromuscular disorders, congenital myasthenia gravis is diagnosed by reversibility
of symptoms following injection of anticholinesterase drugs (see Chapter 12).

Occasionally an infant with a congenital
tumor of the cervical or lumbar cord may
present a clinical picture akin to that of a
spinal cord injury. Abnormalities of the
skin along the posterior lumbosacral midline,
including dimpling, hemangiomata, or tufts
of hair are commonly seen in the latter.[104]

Treatment and Prognosis

In most infants, fractures or fracture dislocations of the spine are absent and there is no specific treatment for spinal cord injuries. While the majority of clinically apparent spinal birth injuries are severe and irreversible, milder degrees of injury are potentially reversible.

BIRTH INJURIES OF THE CRANIAL NERVES

FACIAL NERVE

The most common cranial nerve to be involved in birth trauma is the facial nerve. According to Hepner,[105] some facial nerve injury is evident in 6% of neonates. The injury is the result of pressure of the sacral prominence of the maternal pelvis against the facial nerve distal to its emergence from the stylomastoid foramen (pes anserinus). Less often, compression results from forceps application. These insults are more likely to produce swelling of tissue around the nerve rather than complete or partial anatomic interruption of the fibers.

The degree of facial paresis ranges from complete loss of function in all three main branches to weakness limited to a small group of muscles. One common picture is a mild paresis of the lower portion of the face, particularly the depressor muscle of the lower lip and the depressor muscle of the angle of the mouth which manifests itself most clearly when the infant cries by a failure in downward movement of the affected corner of the mouth. Since the mentalis muscle, enervated by the same nerve fibers as the depressor anguli oris, is usually unaffected, the condition may reflect a maldevelopment rather than perinatal trauma.[105a]

In most instances the facial nerve palsy is mild, and some improvement becomes evident within a week. In the more severe cases, the start of recovery may be delayed for several months. Electric studies can be used to detect the presence of voluntary muscle potentials. The ability to produce contraction of the muscle by stimulating the nerve implies that the conductivity of the nerve is only partially interrupted, and suggests a favorable prognosis. However, good recovery is possible even when electric reactions are completely absent.[106] It is important to wait three to four days before undertaking these studies to allow any injured fibers to degenerate (see Bell's palsy, Chapter 7). Less often, facial nerve palsy present at birth is the result of a basilar skull fracture. Möbius syndrome (see Chapter 4) generally involves a bilateral facial palsy, often accompanied by weakness of one or both abducens nerves or of other cranial nerves. Occasionally, Möbius syndrome will be limited to one side of the face, or even one part of the face.

Treatment of the facial nerve palsy is limited to protection of the eye by application of methyl cellulose drops, and taping of the paralytic lid. Electric stimulation of the nerve does not hasten recovery. Neurosurgical repair of the nerve should only be considered when there is evidence that the nerve is severed.

OTHER CRANIAL NERVES

While conjunctival and retinal hemorrhages are common in the newborn infant, birth injury involving the optic nerve exclusively is relatively rare. Unilateral and bilateral optic atrophy have been reported, and result from direct injury to the nerve through fracture of the orbit or, less often, the base of the skull.[107,108]

A transient postnatal paralysis of the abducens and oculomotor nerves is occasionally encountered, the latter may take the form of a transient postnatal ptosis.[109]

While impaired hearing is seen in about one-quarter of children with cerebral palsy, direct unilateral or bilateral damage to the acoustic nerves in the course of delivery rarely has been documented.

BIRTH INJURIES TO THE PERIPHERAL NERVES

INJURIES OF THE BRACHIAL PLEXUS

Although first described by Smellie,[110] we owe our present-day understanding of the interrelationship between palsies of the upper extremity and injuries of the brachial plexus to a group of nineteenth-century French neurologists. This includes Danyau[111] and Duchenne,[112] who were the first to describe obstetric injuries to the fifth and sixth cervical roots (Erb-Duchenne palsy), and Klumpke,[113] who described the lesion of the lower trunk of the cervical plexus which now bears her name.

Pathogenesis and Pathology

The most common form of brachial plexus injury is one involving the fifth and sixth cervical roots. In most instances this is the consequence of stretching of the plexus due to traction of the shoulder in the course of delivering the after-coming head in a breech presentation, or of turning the head away from the shoulder in a difficult cephalic presentation of a large infant.[114,115] In most cases the brachial plexus is compressed by hemorrhage and edema within the nerve sheath. Less often there is an actual tear of the nerves or avulsion of the roots from the spinal cord with segmental damage to the gray matter of the spinal cord.[114] With traction, the fifth cervical root gives way first, then the sixth, and so on down the plexus. Thus the mildest plexus injuries only involve C_5 and C_6, and the more severe the entire plexus.[115]

Clinical Manifestations

Erb-Duchenne Paralysis. In the majority of infants the paralysis is confined to the upper brachial plexus.[116] In about 93%, involvement is unilateral. The weakness is recognized soon after delivery. The affected arm assumes a characteristic posture. The shoulder is adducted and internally rotated, the elbow extended, the forearm pronated and the wrist occasionally flexed. This position results from paralysis of the deltoid, supra- and infraspinatus, biceps, and brachioradial muscles. The Moro reflex is absent or markedly diminished on the affected side, but the grasp reflex remains intact. The biceps reflex is abolished, or is less active than the triceps reflex, a picture which is the converse of normal. In most infants, one is unable to demonstrate a sensory loss, although occasionally there is loss of cutaneous sensation over the deltoid region, and the adjacent radial surface of the upper arm. Fractures of the clavicle or of the humerus often accompany an Erb-Duchenne paralysis. When there is a significant degree of injury to the fourth cervical root, phrenic nerve paralysis may accompany injury to the upper brachial plexus.[117] Such an infant may present with signs of respiratory distress, including tachypnea, cyanosis, and decreased movement of the affected hemithorax. When the phrenic nerve palsy is unaccompanied by injury to the brachial plexus, as occurs occasionally, the condition may mimic congenital pulmonary or heart disease.[118,119]

Klumpke Paralysis. This injury is relatively uncommon, and constituted only 2.5% of brachial plexus birth palsies in the experience of Ford.[56] In this type of lesion, the paralysis involves the intrinsic muscles of the hand with weakness of the flexors of the wrist and fingers. The grasp reflex is absent, and there is often a unilateral Horner's syndrome due to involvement of the cervical sympathetic nerves. Loss of sensation and sudomotor function over the hand may also be found. Interference with the sympathetic innervation of the eye results in a delay or failure in pigmentation of the iris, and is one of several causes for heterochromia iridis.[120] In some instances there is complete paralysis of the arm. The limb is flaccid, the Moro and grasp reflexes are unelicitable, deep tendon reflexes are absent, and there is sensory loss over most of the extremity.

Diagnosis

The diagnosis of brachial plexus injury is usually readily apparent from the posture of the affected arm, and from the absence of voluntary and reflex movements. Congenital Horner's syndrome may occur in the absence of trauma and may be associated with anomalies of the cervical vertebra, enterogenous cysts, or congenital nerve deafness.[121] The association of heterochromia iridis, congenital nerve deafness, white forelock, broad root of the nose, and lateral displacement of the medial canthi of the eyes and inferior lacrimal puncta is well recognized under the term Waardenburg's syndrome.[121] (See Chapter 4.)

Radiographic examinations to detect associated fractures and fluoroscopy to ascertain any limitation of diaphragmatic movement are indicated. In severe injuries causing avulsion of the spinal roots and bleeding into the subarachnoid space, the cerebrospinal fluid may be bloody. Myelography may be used to indicate root avulsion.[122] Electromyography may confirm the extent of denervation.

Therapy and Prognosis

Gentle passive exercises of the affected arm should be begun after about one week of birth. The infant's sleeve should be pinned in a natural position, rather than in abduction and external rotation as is suggested in many texts.[56] Follow-up studies indicate that over-immobilization of the affected arm is conducive to contractures and deformities which can persist despite spontaneous recovery of nerve function.[123]

If no improvement is noted within three to six months, surgical exploration of the brachial plexus should be considered, although it must be remembered that in most instances where recovery is poor, nerve damage is due to avulsion of the spinal roots, and surgical repair therefore is impossible.

Although a number of authors state that the prognosis for brachial plexus injuries is far from good, this has not been our experience. In the Erb-Duchenne palsy, recovery may be complete within a few weeks, and in the remaining children, maximum recovery is achieved within 1–18 months.[124] In the complete brachial plexus injury, and in Klumpke's paralysis, the outlook is less good. In Gjørup's follow-up of what probably were the more serious brachial plexus injuries,[116] results were good in about 40% of children, and definitely poor in about one-third. Permanent lesions are accompanied by muscle atrophy, contractures, and impaired limb growth.

OTHER PERIPHERAL NERVES

Birth injuries to the other peripheral nerves are relatively uncommon. Sciatic nerve palsy has been observed following injection of hypertonic glucose into the umbilical artery. It is due to thrombosis of the inferior gluteal artery and is accompanied by circulatory changes in the buttock.[124,125]

Palsies of the radial nerve,[126] and obturator nerve,[127] have also been recorded.

REFERENCES

1. Little, W. J.: On the influence of abnormal parturition, difficult labor, premature birth, and asphyxia neonatorum on the mental and physical conditions of the child, especially in relation to deformities, Trans. Lond. Obstet. Soc. 3:293, 1862.
2. Cazauvielh, J. B.: Recherches sur l'agenese cerebrale et la paralysie congenitale, Arch. Gen. Med. 14:1, 347, 1827.
3. Hansen, E.: Cerebral palsy in Denmark, Acta Psychiat. Scand. 35: suppl. 136, 1960.
4. Courville, C. B.: *Cerebral Palsy*, Los Angeles: San Lucas Press, 1954.
5. Kendall, N. and Woloshin, H.: Cephalhematoma associated with fracture of skull, J. Pediat. 41:125, 1952.
6. Gröntoft, O.: Intracranial hemorrhage and blood-brain barrier problems in the newborn, Acta Path. Microbiol. Scand., suppl. C, 1954.
7. Roberts, M. H.: Spinal fluid in newborn with special reference to intracranial hemorrhage, JAMA 85:500, 1925.
8. Towbin, A.: Central nervous system damage in the human fetus and newborn infant, Amer. J. Dis. Child. 119:529, 1970.
9. Ford, F. R.: Breech delivery in its possible relations to injury of the spinal cord, Arch. Neurol. Psychiat. 14:742. 1925.
10. Courville, C. B.: *Birth and Brain Damage*, Pasadena: M. F. Courville, 1971.
11. Ranck, J. B. and Windle, W. F.: Brain damage in the monkey, macaca mulatta, by asphyxia neonatorum, Exp. Neurol. 1:130, 1959.
12. Myers, R. E.: Cystic brain alteration after incomplete placental abruption in monkey, Arch. Neurol. 21:133, 1969.
13. Benda, C. E.: *Developmental Disorders of Mentation and Cerebral Palsies*, New York: Grune & Stratton, Inc., 1952.
14. Birnberger, A. C. and Eliasson, S. G.: Experimental ischemia and polyphosphoinositide metabolism, Neurology (Minneap.) 20:356, 1970.
15. Clendenon, N. R., et al.: Biochemical alterations in the anoxic-ischemic lesion of rat brain, Arch. Neurol. 25:432, 1971.
16. Brown, A. W. and Brierley, J. B.: The nature and time course of anoxic-ischaemic cell change in the rat brain. An optical and electron microscope study, in "Brain Hypoxia" ed. by Brierley, J. B. and Meldrum, B. S., Clin. Dev. Med. 39/40:49, 1971.
17. Mossakowski, M. J., et al.: Early histochemical changes in neonatal asphyxia, J. Neuropath. Exp. Neurol. 27:500, 1968.
18. Fazekas, J. F., Alexander, F. A. D., and Himwich, H. E.: Tolerance of the newborn to anoxia, Amer. J Physiol. 139:281, 1941.
19. Thurston, J. H. and McDougal, D. B.: Effect of ischemia on metabolism of the brain of the newborn mouse, Amer. J. Physiol. 216:348, 1969.

20. Myers, R. E., Beard, R., and Adamsons, K.: Brain swelling in the newborn rhesus monkey following prolonged partial asphyxia, Neurology (Minneap.) 19:1012, 1969.

21. Jones, E. L. and Smith, W. T.: Hypoglycaemic brain damage in the neonatal rat, in "Brain Hypoxia" ed. Brierley, J. B. and Meldrum, B. S., Clin. Devel. Med. 39/40: 231, 1971.

22. Towbin, A.: Cerebral hypoxic damage in fetus and newborn, Arch. Neurol. 20:35, 1969.

23. Banker, B. Q. and Larroche, J. C.: Periventricular leukomalacia of infancy, Arch. Neurol. 7:386, 1962.

23a. deReuck, J., Chattha, A. S., and Richardson, E. P.: Pathogenesis and evolution of periventricular leukomalacia in infancy, Arch. Neurol. 27:229, 1972.

24. Freytag, E. and Lindenberg, R.: Neuropathological findings in patients of a hospital for the mentally deficient: A survey of 359 cases, Johns Hopkins Med. Journ. 121:379, 1967.

25. Lindenberg, R. in James, L. S., Myers, R. E., and Gaull, A. E. (eds.): Brain Damage in the Fetus and Newborn from Hypoxia or Asphyxia, Report of the 57th Ross Conference on Pediatric Research, Columbus: Ross Laboratories, 1967.

26. Norman, R. M., Urich, H., and McMenemey, W. H.: Vascular mechanisms of birth injury, Brain 80:49, 1957.

27. Towbin, A.: Organic causes of minimal brain dysfunction, JAMA 217:1207, 1971.

28. Christensen, E. and Melchior, J.: Cerebral palsy—A clinical and neuropathological study, Clin. Dev. Med. 25:1, 1967.

29. Anton, G.: Ueber die Betheiligung der grossen basalen Gehirnganglien bei Bewegungsstorungen und insbesondere bei Chorea, Jahrb. Psych. Neurol. 14:141, 1896.

30. Vogt., C. and Vogt, O.: Zur Lehre der Erkrankungen des striaren Systems, J. Psychol. Neurol. 25:631, 1919–1920.

31. Denny-Brown, D.: The Basal Ganglia, Oxford: Oxford University Press, 1962.

32. Malamud, N.: Sequelae of perinatal trauma, J. Neuropath. Exp. Neurol. 18:141, 1959.

33. Malamud, N., et al.: An etiologic and diagnostic study of cerebral palsy, J. Pediat. 65:270, 1964.

34. Schwartz, P.: Birth Injuries of the Newborn, New York: Hafner Publishing Company, 1961.

35. Schwartz, P.: Erkrankungen des Zentralnervensystems nach traumatischer Geburtsschadigung, Z. Neurol. Psychiat. 90:263, 1924.

36. Schwartz, P.: Die traumatischen Schadigungen des Zentralnervensystems durch die Geburt, Ergebn. Inn. Med. Kinderheilk. 31:165, 1927.

37. Courville, C. B.: Structural alterations in the cerebellum in cases of cerebral palsy, Bull. Los Angeles Neurol. Soc. 24:148, 1959.

38. Yates, P. O.: Birth trauma to vertebral arteries, Arch. Dis. Child. 34:436, 1959.

39. Schaffer, A. J. and Avery, M. E.: Diseases of the Newborn, Philadelphia: W. B. Saunders Co., 1971.

39a. Harcke, H. T., et al.: Perinatal intraventricular hemorrhage, J. Pediat. 80:37, 1972.

40. Murtagh, F. and Baird, R. M.: Circumscribed intraventricular hematoma in infants: Associated with craniosynostosis and secondary hydrocephalus, J. Pediat. 59:351, 1961.

41. Ross, J. J. and Dimette, R. M.: Subependymal cerebral hemorrhage in infancy, Amer. J. Dis. Child. 110:531, 1965.

42. Craig, W. S.: Intracranial haemorrhage in the newborn. A study of diagnosis and differential diagnosis based on pathological and clinical findings in 126 cases, Arch. Dis. Child. 13:89, 1938.

43. Paine, R. S. and Oppe, T. E.: Neurological examination of children, Clin. Dev. Med. 20/21:1–279, 1966.

44. Paine, R. S., et al.: Evolution of postural reflexes in normal infants and in the presence of chronic brain syndromes, Neurology (Minneap.) 14:1036, 1964.

45. van Harreveld, A.: "Acute and Chronic Effects of Asphyxiation of Central Nervous System," in James, L. S., Myers, R. E., and Gaull, A. E. (eds.): Brain Damage in the Fetus and Newborn from Hypoxia or Asphyxia, Report of the 57th Ross Conference on Pediatric Research, Columbus: Ross Laboratories, 1967.

46. Crothers, B. and Paine, R. S.: The Natural History of Cerebral Palsy, Cambridge: Harvard University Press, 1959.

47. Schipke, R., Riege, D., and Scoville, W. B.: Acute subdural hemorrhage at birth, Pediatrics 14:468, 1954.

48. Paine, R. S.: The evolution of infantile postural reflexes in the presence of chronic brain syndromes, Develop. Med. Child Neurol. 6:345, 1964.

49. Ingram, T. T. S.: Paediatric Aspects of Cerebral Palsy, Edinburgh: E. and S. Livingstone, Ltd., 1964.

50. Skatvedt, M.: Cerebral palsy. A clinical study of 370 cases, Acta Paediat. 46, suppl. 3, 1958.

51. Yannet, H. and Horton, F.: Hypotonic cerebral palsy in mental defectives, Pediatrics 9:204, 1952.

52. Förster, O.: Der atonische-astatische Typus der infantilen Cerebrallahmung, Deutsch. Arch. Klin. Med. 98:216, 1910.

53. Fenichel, G.: Cerebral influence on muscle fiber typing, Arch. Neurol. 20:644, 1969.

54. Woods, G.: Cerebral Palsy in Childhood. Bristol, England: Wright, 1957.

55. Freud, S.: Zur Kenntnis der cerebralen Diplegien des Kindesalters, Leipzig: Deuticke, 1893.

56. Ford, F. R.: Diseases of the Nervous System in Infancy, Childhood and Adolescence, 5th ed., Springfield: Charles C Thomas Publisher, 1966.

56a.Teberg, A. J., Wu, P. Y. K., and Hodgman, J. E.: Developmental and neurological outcome of infants with birth weight under 1500 grams, Clin. Res. 21:322, 1973.

57. McDonald, A. D.: Cerebral palsy in children of very low birth weight, Arch. Dis. Child. 38:579, 1963.

58. Drillien, C. M., Ingram, T. T. S., and Russell, E. M.: Further studies of the causes of diplegia in children, Develop. Med. Child Neurol. 6:241, 1964.

59. McNutt, S. J.: Apoplexie neonatorum, Amer. J. Obstet. 1:73, 1885.

60. Freud, S. and Rie, O.: *Klinische Studie ueber die halbseitige Cerebrallahmung der Kinder*, Vienna: M. Perles, 1891.

61. Ford, F. R.: Cerebral birth injuries and their results, Medicine (Baltimore) 5:122, 1926.

62. Perlstein, M. A. and Hood, P. N.: Infantile hemiplegia, Pediatrics, 14:436, 1954.

63. Byers, R. K.: Evolution of hemiplegias in infancy, Amer. J. Dis. Child. 61:915, 1941.

64. Twitchell, T. E.: The grasping deficit in infantile hemiparesis, Neurology (Minneap.) 8:13, 1958.

65. Tizard, J. P. M., Paine, R. S., and Crothers, B.: Disturbances of sensation in children with hemiplegia, JAMA 155:628, 1954.

66. Walsh, F. B. and Lindenberg, R.: Hypoxia in infants and children. A clinical-pathological study concerning the primary visual pathways, Bull. Hopkins Hosp. 108:100, 1961.

67. Polani, P. E.: The natural history of choreoathetoid cerebral palsy, Guy. Hosp. Rep. 108:32, 1959.

68. Hanson, R. A., Berenberg, W., and Byers, R. K.: Changing motor patterns in cerebral palsy, Develop. Med. Child Neurol. 12:309, 1970.

69. Alagille, D. and Charles, J.: Les hemorragies intra craniennes chez l'enfant hemophile, Arch. Franc. Pediat. 23:795, 1966.

70. Naidoo, B. T.: Cerebrospinal fluid in healthy newborn infants, S. Afr. Med. J. 42:933, 1968.

71. McMenemy, W. H.: The significance of subarachnoid bleeding, Proc. Roy. Soc. Med. 47:701, 1954.

72. Mauer, A. M.: Crenated red cells in spinal fluid, Amer. J. Dis. Child. 108:451, 1964.

73. Tourtellotte, W. W., et al.: A study on traumatic lumbar punctures, Neurology (Minneap.) 8:129, 1958.

73a.Roost, K. T., et al.: The formation of cerebrospinal fluid xanthochromia after subarachnoid hemorrhage, Neurology (Minneap.) 22:973, 1972.

74. Hellström, B. and Kjellin, K. G.: The diagnostic value of spectrophotometry of the CSF in the newborn period, Develop. Med. Child Neurol. 13:789, 1971.

75. Belton, N. R.: Creatine phosphokinase, blood and CSF levels in newborn infants and children, Arch. Dis. Child. 45:600, 1970.

76. Matson, D. D.: *Neurosurgery of Infancy and Childhood*, 2nd ed., Springfield: Charles C Thomas Publisher, 1969.

77. Dyke, C. G., Davidoff, L., and Masson, C.: Cerebral atrophy with homolateral hypertrophy of the skull and sinuses, Arch. Neurol. Psychiat. 29:412, 1933.

78. Walter, W. and Brandt., P.: Die Angiographie bei den fruehkindlichen Hirnschaeden, Acta Neurochir. (Wien) 6:310, 1958.

79. Paine, R. S.: On the treatment of cerebral palsy, Pediatrics 29:605, 1962.

80. Marsh, H. O.: Diazepam in incapacitated cerebral-palsied children, JAMA 191:797, 1965.

81. Rosenthal, R. K., McDowell, F. H., and Cooper, W.: Levodopa therapy in athetoid cerebral palsy, Neurology (Minneap.) 22:1, 1972.

81a.Cooper, I. S.: Effect of stimulation of posterior cerebellum on neurological disease, Lancet 1: 1321, 1973.

82. Douglas, A. A.: Ophthalmological aspects of cerebral plasy, Spastics' Quart. 11:37, 1962.

83. Guibir, G. B.: Eye defects in cerebral palsy, Amer. J. Ophthal. 36:1719, 1953.

84. Keats, W. M.: *Operative Orthopedics in Cerebral Palsy*, Springfield: Charles C Thomas Publisher, 1970.

85. Denhoff, E. and Robinault, I. P.: *Cerebral Palsy and Related Disorders*, New York: McGraw-Hill Book Co., 1960.

86. Cruickshank, W. M. and Raus, G. M.: *Cerebral Palsy. Its Individual and Community Problems*, Syracuse: Syracuse University Press, 1955.

87. Finnie, N. R.: *Handling the Young Cerebral Palsied Child at Home*, London: Wm. Heinemann, 1968.

88. Freud, S.: "Die Infantile Cerebrallahmung," in Nothnagel, H.: *Specielle Pathologie und Therapie*, vol. 9, part 3, Vienna: Hölder, 1897.

89. Ford, F. R. and Schaffer, A. J.: The etiology of infantile (acquired) hemiplegia, Arch. Neurol. Psychiat. 18:323, 1927.

90. Dekaban, A. S. and Norman, R. M.: Hemiplegia in early life associated with the thrombosis of the sagittal sinus and its tributary veins in one hemisphere, J. Neuropath. Exp. Neurol. 17:461, 1958.

91. Norman, R. M.: Neuropathological findings in acute hemiplegia in childhood, Clin. Dev. Med. 6:37, 1962.

92. Solomon, G. E., et al.: Natural history of acute hemiplegia of childhood, Brain 93:107, 1970.

93. Suzuki, J. and Takaku, A.: Cerebrovascular "Moyamoya" disease, Arch. Neurol. 20:288, 1969.

94. Bickerstaff, E. R.: Aetiology of acute hemiplegia in childhood, Brit. Med. J. 2:82, 1964.

95. Aicardi, J., Amsili, J., and Chevrie, J. J.: Acute hemiplegia in infancy and childhood, Develop. Med. Child Neurol. 11:162, 1969.

95a.Scheffner, D. and Wille, L.: Acute infantile hemiplegia due to obstruction of intracranial arterial vessels, Neuropaediatrie 4:7, 1973.

96. Ohta, M. S., Araki, S., and Kuroiwa, Y.: Familial occurrence of migraine with a hemiplegic syndrome and cerebellar manifestations, Neurology (Minneap.) 17:813, 1967.

97. Wilson P. J. E.: Cerebral hemispherectomy for infantile hemiplegia, Brain 93:147, 1970.

98. Hughes, J. T. and Oppenheimer, D. R.: Superficial siderosis of the central nervous system. A report on nine cases with autopsy, Acta Neuropath. 13:56, 1969.

99. Crothers, B.: Injuries of the spinal cord in breech extractions as an important cause of foetal death and paraplegia in childhood, Amer. J. Med. Sci. 165:94, 1923.

100. Crothers, B. and Putnam, M. C.: Obstetrical injuries of the spinal cord, Medicine (Baltimore) 6:41, 1927.

100a.Jellinger, K. and Schwingshackl, A.: Birth injury of the spinal cord, Neuropaediatrie 4:111, 1973.

101. Towbin, A.: Latent spinal cord and brain stem injury in newborn infants, Develop. Med. Child Neurol. 11:54, 1969.

102. Adams, J. H. and Cameron, H. M.: Obstetrical paralysis due to ischemia of the spinal cord, Arch. Dis. Child. 40:93, 1965.

103. Melchior, J. C. and Tygstrup, I.: Development of paraplegia after breech delivery, Acta Paediat. Scand. 52:171, 1963.

104. Schwartz, H. G.: Congenital tumors of spinal cord, Ann. Surg. 136:183, 1952.

105. Hepner, W. R., Jr.: Some observations on facial paresis in the newborn infant: Etiology and incidence, Pediatrics 8:494, 1951.

105a.Nelson, K. B. and Eng, G. D.: Congenital hypoplasia of the depressor anguli oris muscle: Differentiation from congenital facial palsy, J. Pediat. 81:16, 1972.

106. Douglas, D. B. and Kessler, R. E.: Significance of electrical reactions in facial palsy of newborn, Behav. Neuropsychiat. 2:6, 1971.

107. Vannas, M.: Zur Sehnervenatrophie nach Geburtsverletzung, Acta Ophthal. (Kobenhavn) 11:514, 1933.

108. Gifford, H.: Congenital defects of abduction and other ocular movements and their relation to birth injuries, Amer. J Ophthal. 9:3, 1926.

109. Cogan, D. G.: Neurology of the Ocular Muscles, Springfield: Charles C Thomas Publisher, 1956.

110. Smellie, L.: "A Collection of Preternatural Cases and Observations in Midwifery," London, 1768.

111. Danyau, N.: Paralysie du membre superieur, chez le nouveau-ne, Bull. Soc. Chir. Paris 2:148, 1851.

112. Duchenne, G. B. A.: De L'Electrisation Localisee, Paris: Bailliere et fils, 1872.

113. Klumpke, A.: Contribution a l'etude des paralysies radiculaires du plexus brachial, Rev. Med. (Paris) 5:739, 1885.

114. Schoemaker, J.: Ueber die Aetiologie der Entbindungslahmungen, speziell der Oberarmparalysen, Z. Geburtsch. Gynaek. 41:33, 1899.

115. Clark, L. P., Taylor, A. S., and Trout, T. P.: A study on brachial birth palsy, Amer. J. Med. Sci. 130:670, 1905.

116. Gjørup, L.: Obstetrical lesion of the brachial plexus, Acta Neurol. Scand. Suppl. 18, 42:9, 1966.

117. Schifrin, N.: Unilateral paralysis of the diaphragm in the newborn infant due to phrenic nerve injury, with and without associated brachial palsy, Pediatrics 9:69, 1952.

118. Adams, F. H. and Gyepes, M. T.: Diaphragmatic paralysis in the newborn infant simulating cyanotic heart disease, J. Pediat. 78:119, 1971.

119. Smith, B. T.: Isolated phrenic nerve palsy in the newborn, Pediatrics 49:449, 1972.

120. Robinson, G. C., Dikranian, D. A., and Roseborough, G. F.: Congenital Horner's syndrome and heterochromia iridium, Pediatrics 35:103, 1965.

121. DiGeorge, A. M., Olmsted, R. W., and Harley, R. D.: Waardenburg's syndrome: Syndrome of heterochromia of irides, lateral displacement of medial canthi and lacrimal puncta, congenital deafness and other characteristic associated defects, J. Pediat. 57:649, 1960.

122. Tarlov, I. M. and Day, R.: Myelography to help localize traction lesions of the brachial plexus, Amer. J. Surg. 88:266, 1954.

123. Adler, J. B. and Patterson, R. L.: Erb's palsy: Long-term results of treatment in 88 cases, J. Bone Joint Surg. (USA) 49A:1052, 1967.

124. Penn, A. and Ross, W. T.: Sciatic nerve palsy in newborn infants, S. Afr. Med. J. 29:553, 1955.

125. San Agustin, M., Nitowsky, H. M., and Borden, J. N.: Neonatal sciatic nerve palsy after umbilical vessel injection, J. Pediat. 60:408, 1962.

126. Lightwood, R.: Radial nerve palsy associated with subcutaneous fat necrosis in the newborn, Arch. Dis. Child. 26:436, 1951.

127. Craig, W. S. and Clark, J. M. P.: Obturator palsy in the newly born, Arch. Dis. Child. 37:661, 1962.

Infections of the Nervous System

CHAPTER 6

Marvin L. Weil

INTRODUCTION

The central nervous system responds to injury in a limited number of ways. Regardless of the nature of the invading organism, infectious diseases share a number of clinical and pathologic features, with various unique symptom complexes being due to the tropism or virulence of the particular invading organism. Generally, it is difficult to distinguish between bacterial and fungal infections, or between chronic granulomatous disease and viral, spirochetal, or protozoan infections solely from the physical examination of the patient. The diagnosis requires laboratory studies including the isolation and propagation of the suspected organism.

MENINGITIS

ACUTE PURULENT MENINGITIS

Pathology and Pathophysiology

The most common sequel to bacterial assault on the nervous system is meningitis. Organisms reach the meningeal region along four routes: direct hematogenous spread, passage through the choroid plexus, rupture of superficial cortical abscesses, and contiguous spread of an adjacent infection. Direct hematogenous spread may be accomplished through passive transfer as organisms are carried by diapedetic leukocytes, or by spread from damaged or malformed blood vessels.

Infection of the pia-arachnoid from foci in the underlying cerebral or choroid parenchyma has been postulated in tuberculosis of the nervous system.[1] Other sites of infection prone to direct spread to the meninges include the skull and the spine in the course of osteomyelitis, or thrombophlebitis of the bridging and penetrating vessels. The latter mode of bacterial spread is particularly common in otitis media and sinusitis. The subarachnoid space resists infection in normal animals; seeding of the meninges by induced bacteremia is difficult to produce in laboratory animals but occurs more readily if the spinal fluid pressure is altered while there are bacteria in the blood stream.[2] Bacterial infection of the meninges also may be introduced as the result of developmental anomalies[3] or penetrating injuries of the skull, which establish continuity between the central nervous system and the external environment.

Almost any of the pathogenic bacteria may induce meningitis. Table 6–1 presents the frequency of the most common forms. Pathologic changes have been summarized by Adams et al.[4] The fundamental process is an inflammation of the leptomeninges, with the first stage being hyperemia of the meningeal vessels followed by migration of neutrophils into the subarachnoid space (Fig. 6–1). The subarachnoid exudate rapidly increases and extends into the sheaths of blood vessels and

In one-third of the patients meningitis is associated with ventriculitis; involvement of the ependyma, choroid plexus, and subependymal tissues may result. Ependyma and subependymal tissues change little early in meningitis, but cellular infiltration of the subependymal perivascular spaces and glial proliferation may occur in severe or prolonged meningitis, resulting in overgrowth of the ependymal lining and obliteration of the aqueduct of Sylvius.

Obstructive hydrocephalus may result from ependymal or glial proliferation with aqueductal obstruction, or block of the fourth ventricular foramina may result from creamy or gelatinous pus at the base of the brain (Fig. 6–1). Communicating hydrocephalus may result from involvement of the basilar meninges, the absorptive surfaces, the arachnoid villi, or the dural sinuses.

Disorder of cortical neurons with change in mental state or seizures occurs as much as several days before microscopic alterations are demonstrated. This is not due to bacteria within the substance of the brain and must be a metabolic or toxic encephalopathy.

The leptomeningeal inflammation increases vascular permeability for fluid and at the same time reduces bulk absorption. This results in an increase in intracranial pressure which progressively impedes cerebral perfusion and produces further tissue hypoxia. The pathophysiology of increased intracranial pressure accompanying meningitis is similar to that with brain tumor and is discussed in Chapter 10.

Clinical Manifestations

Signs and symptoms associated with the fully developed picture of acute purulent meningitis include fever, headache, nausea and vomiting, nuchal and spinal rigidity, alterations of sensorium, convulsions, cranial nerve palsies, disturbances in vision, and occasionally papilledema.[6,7]

Headache results from inflammation of the meningeal vessels and from increased intracranial pressure. It is often accompanied by photophobia and hyperesthesia. Head retraction, neck stiffness, and spinal rigidity are due to irritation of the meninges and spinal roots which elicits protective flexor reflexes intended to shorten the spinal axis and immobilize the irritated tissue.[8] On lengthening the spine, nerve roots are stretched, and the resulting pain and reflex spasm is the basis of Kernig's sign, as well as the neck and leg Brudzinski signs.

Alterations in sensorium are related to a toxic and metabolic encephalopathy or may be postictal.[8a]

Seizures may be both generalized and focal. They occur in 44% of patients with *H. influenzae* meningitis, in 25% of *D. pneumonia* infections, in 10% of meningococcal infection, and in 78% of patients with streptococcal meningitis. Focal seizures can be the result of localized involvement of the cerebral hemispheres. In a study by Samson et al.,[9] 18% of patients had their first febrile convulsion in the course of meningitis. Significantly, 40% of these, all under 16 months of age, had no clinical evidence of meningitis. A lumbar puncture is therefore advised at the time of the first febrile convulsion.

Cranial nerve involvement is due to local inflammation of the perineurium, as well as impaired vascular supply to the nerves; VI, III, and IV are most commonly affected. Since the decreased use of ototoxic chemotherapeutic agents, cochlear and vestibular deficits have become rare.

Sustained increased intracranial pressure only rarely results in papilledema, unless the acute meningitis is associated with mass lesions such as abscesses or subdural collections.

Focal cerebral signs are usually secondary to cortical necrosis or occlusive vasculitis, most commonly thrombosis of the cortical veins. Focal signs may occur with cerebral vasculitis, cerebritis, or abscess formation. Hemiparesis or seizures that appear after the tenth day of the infection may signify delayed vascular thrombosis.

Cranial bruits over the anterior fontanelle and the posterior temporal areas are more common in children with purulent meningitis than in both febrile and afebrile controls.[10] The tache cerebrale is a common but not pathognomonic finding in meningitis.

Complications of bacterial meningitis include subdural effusion, electrolyte disturbances, and recurrent infections.

Subdural Effusions

This complication has become more apparent since the advent of effective antibiotic therapy, although it was already noted in the last century. Almost all subdural effusions occur over the frontoparietal region, although localized occipital collections have been reported. The mechanism of this complication is not clear.[11] It may be related to thrombophlebitis of the veins bridging the subdural space, small tears in these vessels secondary to shifting of the brain, reduction in pressure by lumbar puncture, or spread of the infection from an arachnoiditis. Compared to serum, subdural fluid has a disproportionately high albumin to globulin ratio. The effusion is almost invariably bilateral and the incidence has varied considerably from one series to another and is probably proportional to the vigor with which this complication is sought.[12] Subdural effusions are seen with all organisms; they are most common following meningitis due to *Haemophilus influenzae* (45% of all effusions), pneumococcus (30% of all effusions) and meningococcus (9%). Most cases are in children less than two years of age. This, in part, is undoubtedly related to the ease with which subdural taps can be performed through the open fontanelle, and there is evidence that subdural effusions occur in older individuals as well.

Indications for suspecting a subdural effusion in the presence of meningitis are presented in Table 6–2. The condition can best be diagnosed by subdural taps, although the presence of the effusion may be suggested by transillumination of the skull, or by a progressive enlargement of the head circumference. Dodge and Porter[13] discuss the use of transillumination in demonstrating a variety of intracranial pathology, including hydrocephalus, hydranencephaly, and porencephaly. The EEG may reveal focal slowing or voltage depression but is too often normal to be a reliable diagnostic tool. Calcified subdural membranes are detected by x rays of the skull;[14] cerebral angiography and pneumoencephalography may be of assistance when the diagnosis is in doubt. Initially, the fluid is xanthochromic or blood-tinged, and may become less yellow with repeated taps. The protein content ranges between 50 and 1000

TABLE 6-2.
INDICATIONS FOR SUSPECTING A SUBDURAL EFFUSION IN INFANTS WITH PURULENT MENINGITIS*

1. Failure of temperature curve to show progressive decline after 72 hours of adequate antibiotic and supportive treatment.
2. Persistent positive spinal cultures after 72 hours appropriate antibiotic therapy.
3. Occurrence of focal or persistent convulsions.
4. Persistence or recurrence of vomiting.
5. Development of focal neurologic signs.
6. An unsatisfactory clinical course, particularly evidence for increased intracranial pressure after 72 hours of antibiotic therapy.

* From Matson.[15]

mg/100 cc and is always higher than the CSF protein obtained simultaneously. In about 10% of patients, cultures of the fluid are positive.

The treatment of subdural effusions is controversial. The technique for a subdural tap is described by Matson.[15] In most instances, repeated aspiration of the subdural space results in complete disappearance of the fluid collections, and sequelae are more frequent than in patients who did not develop effusions.[15] When the fluid collection fails to respond to repeated aspiration, craniotomy and stripping of the subdural membrane has been recommended. Others have used a subdural-peritoneal shunt.[16] We treat the effusions conservatively, with repeated taps, removing no more than 15 to 30 cc fluid at each occasion, to relieve increased intracranial pressure. The persistence of subdural effusions reflects underlying cortical damage, for normal cerebrum would sooner or later obliterate the subdural space.[17]

Electrolyte Disturbances

Disturbance in sodium metabolism, usually with hyponatremia, is seen in about 6% of patients with meningitis. Hyponatremia may be due to an intracellular shift of sodium with an extracellular shift of potassium as a consequence of the inflammation, inappropriately high secretion of antidiuretic hormone (ADH), or both. Inappropriate ADH release leads to hypervolemia, oliguria, and increased urinary osmolality. The symptoms are those of water intoxication, and include restlessness, irritability, and convulsions, all of which may be ascribed to meningitis. The condition is treated by restricting water intake, and administering small amounts of additional sodium. In some of the chronic meningitides inappropriate ADH secretion may induce a secondary diminution in aldosterone or third factor secretion and increased urinary sodium loss.

Recurrent Meningitides

Recurrent bacterial meningitis may be due to acquired or congenital gross anatomic defects, foci of infection, or disorders in immune mechanism.

Anatomic defects which allow continuity between the nervous system and the exterior may be gross with frank leakage of CSF, or minute and difficult to find. Skull fractures, especially those affecting the base of the brain and extending to the sinuses and petrous pyramids, are the most common cause of recurrent meningitis. They are discussed in Chapter 8. Congenital defects include myelomeningoceles, neurenteric cysts, and midline or spinal dermal sinuses.[3,18,19] Neuroschisis may also occur in the anterior portion of the pharynx as an anterior encephalocele, or as a fine defect in the cribriform or orbital plate.

Recurrent meningeal infections secondary to defects in the immune response may occur after splenectomy,[20] or in the various immunopathies. Children with leukemia and lymphoma have a particularly high incidence of recurrent purulent and fungal meningitis. Recurrences due to the same organism may be seen after inadequate therapy or relative resistance of the organism to treatment.[21]

The incidence of chronic complications of meningitis are listed in Table 6–3.

Diagnosis

The diagnosis of meningitis requires prompt examination and culture of the spinal fluid. Characteristically, the fluid is under increased pressure and cloudy. During the acute stage the cells are predominantly polymorpho-

TABLE 6-3.
MAJOR COMPLICATIONS SEEN IN 71 CHILDREN AFTER RECOVERY FROM MENINGITIS

Complication	Number of Cases
Mental retardation	3
Seizures	3
Hemi- or quadriparesis	1
Bilateral deafness	4
Vestibular disturbance	1
Hydrocephalus	1
TOTAL	13 (18%)

* After Dodge and Swartz.[7]

nuclear while a monocytic response appears in the later stages. The cell counts range between 1000 and 10,000 per mm^3 but may be normal during the earliest stage of the infection. Much higher counts suggest a meningitis secondary to rupture of a brain abscess. Organisms may be seen intra- and extracellularly in smears, and occasionally may be visualized or cultured in the absence of pleocytosis.

Characteristic in bacterial and tuberculous meningitis is a decrease in the CSF glucose content. This was first observed by Lichtheim,[22] and initially attributed to use of glucose by bacteria growing in the fluid. This explanation, as many subsequent ones, has been abandoned in view of conflicting experimental evidence, and the mechanism of the low CSF sugar remains uncertain. Prockop and Fishman[23] have found the facilitated diffusion of glucose both from blood to CSF and from CSF to blood to be impaired. There is also some evidence for a significant decrease in cerebral glucose oxidation, and an increase in glycolysis, so that a combination of these metabolic alterations may be responsible.[24] Low CSF sugars are also seen in sarcoidosis, mumps leptomeningitis, CNS leukemia, and meningeal carcinomatosis.

CSF protein is elevated in 80% to 92% of patients.[6] Lactic dehydrogenase[25] and glutamic oxalacetic transaminase[26] and creatine phosphokinase[26a] may be increased. In general, the more striking elevations are seen with severe cerebral involvement and indicate a poor prognosis. The chloride level, once thought to differentiate between bacterial and tuberculous meningitis, is of little value. Low CSF chloride levels, common in chronic meningitis, reflect the low systemic levels seen with persistent fever and vomiting.

Blood cultures are positive in about 40% of patients. Nose and throat cultures are generally less informative.

Treatment

Treatment of purulent meningitis falls into two categories: antibacterial chemotherapy, and specific measures designed to reverse systemic and neurologic complications.

The principal aim of antibiotic therapy is to use the proper antibiotic in a sufficiently high dosage to maintain effective CSF concentrations. The choice of the antibiotic depends on the causative organism, and currently recommended schedules for antibiotics in the treatment of the more common forms of bacterial meningitis are presented in Table 6–4.

We believe that patients should be continued on parenteral therapy for at least five days after fever has subsided, and preferably for the full 14 days. The intravenous route of administration is recommended, since reconstitution of the blood-brain barrier as healing progresses makes optimum blood levels of antibiotics imperative. The oral route allows for considerable uncertainty with respect to blood levels, while the subcutaneous or intramuscular routes may incite severe local reaction.

Treatment should be continued for at least one week after spinal fluid cultures have become sterile. While experimental data suggest that certain combinations of antibiotics are antagonistic, clinical evidence does not offer much support for this. However, increasing the number of antibiotics will increase the incidence of toxic reaction.

Corticosteroids have been advocated in the control of endotoxin shock, but their effectiveness has not been verified by controlled studies. Increased intracranial pressure is reduced by osmotic agents, such as mannitol, slow repeated removal of CSF, or treatment with steroids. Ventricular taps in the course of an acute meningitis may promote brain abscess by intracerebral seeding of bacteria.

TABLE 6-4.
CURRENT RECOMMENDATIONS FOR ANTIBIOTIC THERAPY

Organism	Drug of Choice
Aerobacter	Gentamicin or kanamycin
Bacteroides	Gentamicin
Clostridium	Penicillin G
Corynebacterium	Penicillin G
Diplococcus pneumoniae	Penicillin G
Escherichia coli	Gentamicin or kanamycin
Haemophilus influenzae	Ampicillin or chloromycetin
Klebsiella	Gentamicin or kanamycin
Listeria monocytogenes	Penicillin G
Neisseria meningitidis	Penicillin G
Neisseria gonorrhoeae	Penicillin G
Proteus mirabilis (indole negative)	Ampicillin
Proteus morganii (indole positive)	Gentamicin or kanamycin
Pseudomonas	Gentamicin, colistin, or polymyxin
Salmonella	Ampicillin, gentamicin, or chloromycetin
Staphylococci-penicillinase negative	Penicillin G
Staphylococci-penicillinase positive	Methicillin
Streptococci	Penicillin G
Unknown	Ampicillin, gentamicin, or kanamycin, methicillin if question of staphylococcal infection

Indications for lumbar punctures depend upon the clinical course of the patient. In a patient with uncomplicated purulent meningitis who responds well to treatment, a second lumbar puncture should be performed at the termination of therapy.

In general, the amount of intravenous fluid to be given to a patient with meningitis should be on the low side of the daily maintenance and replacement requirements, so as to avoid the complications of hypervolemia and hyponatremia induced by an inappropriate antidiuretic hormone output.

A secondary rise in fever after four days of antibiotic therapy may be due to phlebitis at the site of intravenous therapy or be drug fever.[27] Prolonged fever may be due to persistence of the organism, the consequence of an inappropriate antibiotic, subdural effusions or empyema, brain abscess, purulent arthritis, otitis media, mastoiditis or ophthalmitis. A second infection such as pulmonary tuberculosis or tuberculous meningitis may also be encountered.

Recurrent infections with the same organism may be seen after inadequate therapy or when relative resistance to antibiotics permits the organism to be dormant in a cryptic focus.

Prognosis

The outcome of meningitis depends primarily on four factors: 1) Nature of the infectious agent and severity of the initial process.

2) Age of the patient. 3) Duration of symptoms before diagnosis and institution of intensive antibiotic therapy. The incidence of residua is higher in children whose diagnosis and treatment is delayed. Kresky et al.[28] observed residua in 12% of children whose treatment was started less than 24 hours after the onset of symptoms, in contrast to 59% in those treated after three or more days of symptoms. 4) Type and amount of antibiotic used. Bacteriocidal drugs seem to act somewhat more rapidly than bacteriostatic ones.

While the mortality rate for all forms of bacterial meningitis has decreased over the past few years, a high incidence of residua is still encountered (Table 6–5).[29] These range from transient minimal subjective complaints and electroencephalographic abnormalities which are seen in as many as 25% of survivors,[32] to severe incapacitating deficits. The frequency with which minimal residua are encountered depends upon the care with which reevaluation of survivors is performed.

In long-term follow-up studies on survivors from *H. influenzae* meningitis 29% were found to have significant handicaps, and 48% were apparently free of sequelae. However, children in the latter group functioned at a significantly lower level than their peers.[33]

Several forms of purulent meningitis present sufficiently distinctive clinical pictures to warrant new discussion under a separate heading.

TABLE 6-5.
INCIDENCE OF MORTALITY AND RESIDUA AFTER VARIOUS FORMS OF MENINGITIS

Infection	Number of Cases	Deaths	Mental Retardation or Major Neurologic Residua	Minor Neurologic Residua
Haemophilus influenzae (1951–1964)	40	7	4	11
Diplococcus pneumoniae (1960–1964)	10	2	0	1
Neisseria meningitidis (1960–1964)	12	0	1	3
Mixed infections (1948–1963)	20	7	6	—

* From Sproles et al.,[29] Herweg et al.,[30] and de Lemos and Haggarty.[31]

MENINGOCOCCAL MENINGITIS

Infections with *N. meningitidis* may assume three distinct clinical courses:[34] 1) meningitis; 2) septicemia which may precede invasion of the nervous system or may appear in an isolated, but fulminant form (Waterhouse-Friderichsen syndrome) accompanied by a variety of skin lesions; 3) chronic meningococcemia, in which an equilibrium between bacteria and host appears to have become established.

The epidemiology of meningococci has changed in recent years. Until 1962 group A organisms which are very susceptible to sulfonamide therapy were predominant. Since then group B organisms have become the dominant type in the United States, and group C organisms have become more frequent. Neither group responds to sulfonamide therapy.

The meningococcus produces distinctive skin lesions in approximately 75% of cases. The rash may be petechial, maculopapular, or morbilliform. Petechiae are also seen in occasional patients with *H. influenzae*, pneumonococcal, or streptococcal meningitis.

Meningococcal septicemia may cause a fulminant, rapidly progressive, potentially fatal condition which often represents a medical emergency. The severe septicemia may result in embolic formation of fine bacterial petechiae, or in local tissue sensitization which leads to large ecchymotic areas as a consequence of intravascular coagulation similar to the Shwartzman phenomenon.[35] In about two-thirds of fatal cases there are bilateral adrenal hemorrhages.

Gram-negative endotoxin shock in meningococcemia is similar to that due to *E. coli* and other gram-negative organisms. This has been extensively reviewed by Lillehei et al.,[36] who point out the harmful role of splanchnic pooling of blood, increased peripheral vascular resistance, and decreased visceral perfusion.

Chronic meningococcemia is associated with intermittent and relatively mild episodes of chills, fleeting rashes, joint pain or swelling, or joint effusions. Symptoms may regress without specific therapy or cause recurrent episodes over several days or weeks. The rash may be in the form of petechiae, erythema nodosum, papulonecrotic tuberculids, macules, or maculopapules. The accompanying fever is of variable severity.

Complications of meningococcal bacteremia may be seen with or without meningitis. Pericarditis has been reported in 0%–1.6%, arthritis in 2.7%–5.8%, and eye involvement in 0.4%–3.1% of cases.[37] Eye lesions include hypopyon and panophthalmitis. Autopsy study of 200 fatal cases of meningococcal infection revealed acute interstitial myocarditis with focal necrosis and hemorrhage in 78%.[38]

Specific therapy for meningococcal meningitis is outlined in Table 6–4. Supportive therapy becomes of prime importance in meningococcemia. It includes the use of colloids, alpha-adrenergic blocking agents (phenoxybenzamine) or beta-adrenergic drugs (isoproterenol)[36,38] and hypothermia (artificial hibernation).[39] The use of adrenal cortical hormones such as hydrocortisone has been under dispute. The hemorrhagic adrenal glands found in many of the fatal cases of meningococcemia suggest adrenal insufficiency, and studies by Migeon et al.[40] have demonstrated a diminished adrenal stress response in severe meningococcal meningitis. However, adrenal insufficiency may only contribute to the circulatory collapse. Nevertheless, pharmacologic doses of cortisol in combination with administration of plasma reduce mortality in experimental endotoxin shock.

There is a close correlation between the prognosis and the presence of a consumption coagulopathy. Unfavorable prognostic features include: 1) presence of petechiae for more than 12 hours prior to admission to a hospital; 2) presence of shock; 3) absence of meningitis; 4) a normal or low blood leukocyte count; and 5) a normal or low erythrocyte sedimentation rate. In the experience of Stiehm and Damrosch[41] patients with only two of the above features had a mortality rate of about 7% or less, while patients with three or more had a mortality of 85% or greater. The use of heparin to interrupt coagulation and fibrinogen to restore minimal coagulation has also been recommended to stop intravascular coagulation which leads to multiple capillary thrombi.

HEMOPHILUS MENINGITIS

This is almost limited to children and is most commonly due to *Haemophilus influenzae* type B. Less often hemophilus meningitis may be caused by types A through F, *Haemophilus parainfluenzae* or *Haemophilus aphrophilus*.[42]

Meningitis due to *Haemophilus influenzae* occurs almost exclusively in children under six[6] and is at present the most common form of bacterial meningitis in this age group (see Table 6–1). After the age of six the incidence is so low that one should suspect defects in resistance or parameningeal infection when it occurs.

Symptoms of influenzal meningitis in the older child are those associated with any acute meningitic infection. Pericarditis, influenzal epiglottitis, myocarditis, and septic arthritis may accompany influenzal meningitis. Residua include convulsions, bilateral nerve deafness, visual and speech deficits, awkwardness, incoordination, and facial paresis. Delay in motor maturation may be directly related to vestibular or cerebellar dysfunction. Residual electroencephalographic abnormalities may be present in as many as one quarter of patients who recover, and psychologic interview and testing may disclose residual anxiety related specifically to the hospital experience in as many as 50% of older children.

PNEUMOCOCCAL MENINGITIS

The most common cause of meningitis for all age groups is *Diplococcus pneumoniae*; it is third in rank for children under 10 years of age. Predisposing factors for pneumococcal meningitis of the pediatric age group include an upper respiratory infection, acute or chronic otitis media, purulent conjunctivitis, and cerebrospinal fluid rhinorrhea secondary to developmental abnormalities or trauma.[6]

The pathogenesis of pneumococcal meningitis may differ from that of meningitis due to other organisms in that pneumococci elaborate neuraminidase and N-acetyl neuraminic acid (NANA) aldolase whereas *H. influenzae* and *N. meningitidis* do not.[43] As a consequence, elevated concentrations of free cerebrospinal fluid N-acetyl neuraminic acid are detected only in patients with pneumococcal meningitis. In general, these correlate positively with a more florid infection and residual neurologic signs.

Pneumococcal meningitis is seen more often in children with sickle cell disease than in control populations. This is due to the decrease in heat-labile opsonins[44] and functional asplenia[45] of these children.

The general clinical signs and symptoms of pneumococcal meningitis are similar to the other bacterial meningitides. The diagnosis is made by culturing the organism from the CSF or the blood. While blood cultures are positive in 50% of patients, nasopharyngeal and ear cultures are positive in only 24% and are therefore less reliable for diagnosis.[6] Penicillin given by constant intravenous infusion is preferred as this produces sustained CSF concentrations within four to six hours after the start of the infusion (see Table 6–4). By contrast, single intravenous injections produce higher CSF levels but these are much less sustained. Therapy with penicillin is much more effective early in the infection. In vitro and in vivo experiments have demonstrated rapid killing of bacteria when the drug is added four hours after the beginning of an experimental infection, but little effect when treatment was withheld for 12 hours.

Erythromycin has been suggested for the recently described strains of pneumococci which are significantly resistant to penicillin.

STAPHYLOCOCCAL MENINGITIS

Staphylococcal meningitis may be due to secondary invasion of the nervous system as the result of traumatic wounds or nearby infections; it is prone to occur with cavernous sinus thrombosis or epidural abscesses. Metastatic embolic lesions from acute bacterial endocarditis may result in bacterial meningitis but more commonly result in an embolic lesion followed by cerebritis and brain abscess.[46]

Staphylococcus albus infections have been a frequent indolent meningitic complication of ventriculoatrial and ventriculoperitoneal shunts.[47,47a] In the latter the location of the distal end of the shunt is an important factor in the frequency of shunt infections and meningitis; placement below T_7 often results in bacteremia while placement at a level of

T_4 or higher is less likely to be associated with an infection but often results in block.[48] In some cases more than one staphylococcal subgroup may colonize the shunt at a time, each having a different antibiotic spectrum. This is important in selecting an antibiotic since single colony antibiotic sensitivities may not be sufficient. Sequential shunt infections may be due to the same or different subgroups.

ACUTE PURULENT MENINGITIS IN THE NEONATE

Neonatal meningitis differs from that in older infants and children in its clinical manifestations, in the high incidence of gram-negative organisms, and the generally poor prognosis.

About 30% of infections are due to *E. coli* and 10% to paracolon strains. This spectrum of invaders is due to an alteration in the immune state during the neonatal period. Neonates are deficient in gram-negative bacteriocidins because there is no transplacental transfer of IgM. The human infant is capable of responding to an antigenic stimulus within the initial weeks of life but there is a delay in the first appearance of antibody and in the transition from the initially appearing IgM to the IgG antibody which is more efficient in

neutralizing soluble toxins. The transition from a granulocytic response to a mononuclear preponderance is also slower and less striking in the newborn, and plasma cells appear more slowly and are less abundant.[49]

Complications during pregnancy, labor, and delivery, especially if associated with fetal distress, are associated with an increased incidence of neonatal meningitis. Maternal infections, particularly of the uterus and urinary tract, predispose to infection. The same agent may be isolated from the site of infection in the mother and from the spinal fluid of her infant. Premature rupture of the membranes, when associated with peripartum infection and chorioamnionitis, may contribute to meningitis.[49]

Initial infections of the fetus, particularly those of the respiratory tract and skin, predispose to meningitis. Septicemia with positive blood cultures occurs in 55% to 61% of patients with meningitis.

The paucity of clinical signs in neonatal meningitis makes the diagnosis extremely difficult. The major signs and symptoms are presented in Table 6–6. Classic signs of meningitis are rare. A bulging fontanelle was observed in 30%, and nuchal rigidity in only 18%. Rather, the most common abnormalities are fever, poor activity and poor feeding, a gray appearance, and seizures.[50]

TABLE 6-6.
SIGNS AND SYMPTOMS IN 39 INFANTS
WITH NEONATAL MENINGITIS*

	Premature Infants		Full-Term Infants	
	Initial	Overall	Initial	Overall
Anorexia or vomiting	4	10	4	15
Lethargy	3	12	1	13
Irritability	0	0	4	15
Jaundice	3	10	2	3
Respiratory distress	5	11	1	5
Diarrhea	1	3	1	4
Bulging fontanelle	0	0	0	13
Convulsions	0	2	1	9
Nuchal rigidity	0	1	0	6
Fever	0	2	8	19
Pyoderma	0	0	1	6
TOTAL PATIENTS	16		23	

* From Groover et al.[50]

The diagnosis can only be made by lumbar puncture; even in the CSF the response to infection may be atypical, and there may be only a minimal pleocytosis. Blood cultures are positive in about 75% of infants and usually yield the same organism as the spinal fluid. Culture of the nasopharynx yields the same organism as the CSF in 40% of cases.

The prognosis is poor. In Overall's fairly typical series, the mortality was about 60%, and 50% of the survivors had neurologic sequelae.[49]

Therapy should be specific for the invading organism and instituted as early as possible. Choice of antibiotic is as for older children (see Table 6–4 and pp. 219–220 and 226–229).

Intrathecal polymyxin B has been utilized to treat some of the more refractory forms of gram-negative meningitis. Infections of the central nervous system have been successfully treated with intrathecal polymyxin B with or without other antibiotics.[51]

CHRONIC AND GRANULOMATOUS INFECTIONS OF THE MENINGES

TUBERCULOUS MENINGITIS

Despite recent advances in chemotherapy, tuberculous meningitis due to *Mycobacterium tuberculosis* remains a serious pediatric problem, particularly in some of the under-developed nations. In the United States it currently causes more deaths than any other form of tuberculosis.

Pathology and Pathogenesis

In children tuberculous meningitis almost always accompanies generalized miliary tuberculosis. In some of the older clinical series[52] 68% of children with meningitis had miliary tuberculosis, and conversely 81% of children with miliary disease developed tuberculous meningitis.

In the majority of cases in the United States, infection is due to the human type of mycobacteria. Bovine tuberculosis has become uncommon due to the widespread pasteurization of milk. In tropical countries, the human form is also more common due to the relative inaccessibility of nonhuman milk and milk products.

Involvement of the meninges is probably secondary to a small tuberculoma in the cor-tex or the leptomeninges,[1] and most brains of patients who succumb to tuberculous meningitis will demonstrate superficial foci of an older date. Tuberculomas of the choroid plexus may be a less common site for the infection.

At autopsy the meninges look gray and opaque and a gelatinous exudate fills the basal cisterns, particularly the anterior portion of the pons. Small tubercles may appear over the convexity of the brain or the periventricular area.

On microscopic examination the exudate consists of lymphocytes, plasma cells, and large histiocytes with typical caseation. Langhans giant cells are rare. The meningeal arteries are inflamed and thrombosed, and secondary infarctions of the superficial cortex are common.

Tuberculomas are now relatively rare but at one time were one of the most common causes for a posterior fossa mass in children.[53] They occurred most commonly in the cerebellum, and less often within the brain stem.

Clinical Manifestations

The most common form of tuberculous meningitis, comprising about 70% of all cases, is a caseous meningitis due to direct invasion of the meninges. In about 75% of children this occurs while the primary focus is fresh, less than six months old. The illness is often precipitated by an acute infectious disease, not uncommonly measles. Prior to 1955 its incidence in the United States was highest in the spring. When tuberculous meningitis is part of the initial attack its incidence is highest among infants aged one to two years. When it is a complication of systemic tuberculosis, it is more likely to affect older children.

Untreated, tuberculous meningitis is rapidly fatal, with an average duration of only three weeks. Lincoln[54] has distinguished three stages of the illness, each lasting about a week.

In the initial stage, gastrointestinal symptoms predominate. The child is apathetic or irritable, but the neurologic examination is negative. In about 10% of patients, commonly in infants, a febrile convulsion may be the most significant symptom of this stage.

During the second stage of the illness the child enters into progressive stupor, Kernig's and Brudzinski's signs become positive, the deep tendon reflexes are hyperactive, abdominal reflexes disappear, and there may be ankle and patellar clonus. Cranial nerve signs most commonly include involvement of III, IV, VI, and VII. Ten percent of patients have choroid tubercles.

During the third stage the patient is comatose, although there still may be periods of intermittent wakefulness. The pupils are fixed and recurrent clonic spasm of the extremities, irregular respiration, and a rising fever are present. Hydrocephalus develops in about two-thirds of patients whose illness lasts longer than three weeks. It is particularly common when treatment is delayed or inadequate.

A serous form of tuberculous meningitis is encountered less commonly. It presents with meningeal irritation in children known to have active primary tuberculosis. In contrast to tuberculous meningitis, the CSF is normal.

A third form of tuberculous meningitis, seen in 17% of instances, comprises cases with primary spinal cord infection. These children may present major problems with blockage of the spinal canal which may or may not be associated with Pott's disease. Spinal tuberculosis may be differentiated from the other types by its history and laboratory findings. The duration of symptoms is usually longer, often up to six months before meningitis is considered. A fall often produces back pain and staggering or clumsy gait. Abdominal pain, presumably of root origin, is common. Nuchal or spinal rigidity may develop while the sensorium remains clear. Spinal fluid may be scant and show marked elevation in protein.

Diagnosis

Anergy to tuberculosis is relatively uncommon. In the Bellevue Hospital experience, 85% of patients reacted positively, while another 10% were inadequately tested or died before tuberculin tests could be completed.[54,55]

The spinal fluid findings are quite characteristic. The fluid has a ground glass appearance and when spun down forms a pellicle wherein the organisms may occasionally be visualized. The total counts range between 10 and 350. Eighty-seven percent of patients have more than 50% lymphocytes and 96% show a sugar of 38 mg% or less. CSF protein is invariably increased.

The diagnosis of tuberculous meningitis rests upon the spinal fluid changes, a history of exposure to the disease, often from an otherwise asymptomatic older relative, a positive skin test, and the clinical picture of a subacute meningitis.

Treatment

Therapy for tuberculous meningitis[56] must be prompt and adequate. It includes appropriate chemotherapy, correction of fluid and electrolyte disturbances, and relief of increased intracranial pressure. All patients should receive isoniazid (20 mg/kilo up to a maximum of 500 mg/day). If the patient is vomiting intravenous or intramuscular preparations should be used. Streptomycin is given as a single daily injection of 20 mg/kilogram not to exceed 1 gm/day. This may be reduced to two or three times per week as the clinical condition improves and is discontinued as soon as warranted by the clinical condition and the cerebrospinal fluid. Paraaminosalicylic acid may be used as a companion drug when combined therapy is employed.[56] This is given in doses of 200 mg/kilo/day in one to three doses per day. Experience with this drug indicates a high incidence of gastrointestinal disturbances which interfere with other oral medication and adequate nutrition. The optimum duration of treatment with isoniazid is not known but it should be continued for at least two years. Corticosteroids, such as prednisone 1 to 2 mg per kg per day, have been recommended for seriously ill patients for one to three months, followed by gradual withdrawal.[56] Evidence for benefit from intrathecal or oral prednisone is unclear.[57] Steroids may reduce intracranial pressure and cerebral edema without altering morbidity or mortality[58] and relieve pulmonary symptoms in miliary tuberculosis.[56] Complications from steroid therapy such as hypothermia and gastrointestinal hemorrhage limit its usefulness.[58]

Patients who have consistent severe elevations of intracranial pressure (CSF pressure over 400 mm water) may require short courses of dexamethasone (6 mg/m^2 every 4–6 hours) to reduce edema, or neurosurgical intervention with ventriculoexternal or ventriculoperitoneal shunts to relieve acute hydrocephalus.[58a] Intracranial pressures above 400 mm of CSF significantly impair perfusion of cerebral tissue. This becomes more marked at pressures up to 600 mm CSF, by which point perfusion has fallen to about 40% of normal.

Recent reports indicate that 6% of strains in the United States are resistant to isoniazid and another 3% to streptomycin and/or PAS. This percentage is much higher in other regions of the world and makes a laboratory evaluation of drug susceptibility imperative. Ethambutol, ethionamide, and pyrazinamide or cycloserine should be used whenever drug resistance to standard chemotherapeutic agents is known.[59,60]

Peripheral neuritis may complicate the use of isoniazid in some patients. This can be prevented or relieved by pyridoxine (25–50 mg daily). Added pyridoxine is probably not necessary for infants or children unless they are malnourished, but is recommended for adolescents.[56]

Metabolic disturbances during tuberculous meningitis include metabolic alkalosis, hyponatremia, hypochloremia, and hypotonic expansion of extracellular fluid. Intracellular potassium concentration is normal or decreased while sodium concentration within red cells and skeletal muscle generally increases. An increase in antidiuretic hormone levels may occur. Vomiting often tends to aggravate electrolyte disturbances. There is no evidence for a "salt losing" renal lesion in tuberculous meningitis although hypervolemia may result in secondary hypoaldosteronism.

Prognosis

Untreated tuberculous meningitis is invariably fatal. Even with treatment, many survivors have major sequelae.[61] About 9% require custodial care and only 57% become able to support themselves Major neurologic sequelae were seen in 21% of patients, including spastic pareses and seizures. Para-

plegia and sensory disturbances of the extremity may occur. Late ophthalmologic complications include optic atrophy. Hearing and vestibular residua occur as a consequence of streptomycin therapy as well as of the disease process itself. Minor neurologic sequelae include cranial nerve palsies, nystagmus, ataxia, mild disturbances of coordination, and spasticity. Intellectual defects occur in about one-half of survivors; these patients have a high incidence of encephalographic abnormalities, which correlate with the persistence of sequelae such as convulsions and mental subnormality. Intracranial calcifications develop in about one third of children who recover from tuberculous meningitis.[62] Panhypopituitarism has been reported after cured tuberculous meningitis[63] as well as selective pituitary disturbances such as deficiencies in antidiuretic hormone, growth hormone, and gonadotropin, or endocrinopathies such as sexual precocity.[62]

The most important prognostic factor is the stage of disease when therapy is started. Children under three years of age have a poorer prognosis for survival than do older children, a fact which in part may be due to easier recognition of the disorder in older children.[64]

MENINGITIS DUE TO UNUSUAL ORGANISMS

The essential clinical features of the various meningeal infections produced by some of the less common organisms, and the currently recommended forms of treatment are summarized in Table 6–7.

ANTIBIOTIC THERAPY

Current recommendations for antibiotic therapy based upon recent experience with bacterial meningitis are summarized in Table 6–4.

Penicillin G is recommended for infections by Group A beta-hemolytic and other susceptible streptococcal infections, susceptible staphylococci, pneumococci, meningococci, gonococci, and clostridia.

Resistant organisms are penicillinase secreting gram-positive organisms and gram-negative bacilli.

Dosage for infants is 60,000 units/kilo/day; older children and adults should receive

TABLE 6-7.
SOME RARER ORGANISMS RESPONSIBLE FOR MENINGITIS

Organism	Clinical Features	Antibiotics of Choice
Listeria monocyto-genes[65]	Primary meningitis in newborn infants, or later in first month of life.	Ampicillin (150-250 mg/kg/day) i.v., alone or in combination with kanamycin or gentamicin
B. proteus[66]	Neonatal meningitis or secondary to otitis media, genitourinary tract infection. Hydrocephalus, hemorrhagic necrosis of brain common complications. CSF cultures may be negative with ventricular cultures positive.	Variable sensitivities: usually penicillin, kanamycin, ampicillin, chloramphenicol
Mima polymorpha[67]	Neonatal meningitis	Variable: sensitivities necessary (usually sensitive to ampicillin or gentamicin)
Salmonella[68]	Neonatal meningitis	Chloramphenicol, ampicillin
Klebsiella pneumoniae[69]	Secondary to middle ear or respiratory tract, wound infections. Usually under age one, high mortality.	Variable: sensitivities necessary. Usually kanamycin, gentamicin, polymyxin (may have to be given intrathecally)

16,000,000 units/m²/day (approximately 500,-000 units/kilo/day) up to 24,000,000 units per day. Patients will receive 1.68 mEq of potassium with each million units of potassium penicillin or 1.68 mEq of sodium with each million units of sodium penicillin, amounts which may be significant in the electrolyte management of sick children. CNS toxicity to high doses of intravenous penicillin has been reported.

Ampicillin is recommended for organisms such as *Haemophilus influenzae, Streptococcus viridans,* enterococci, and penicillin-susceptible organisms. Resistant organisms include indole-positive *Proteus, Pseudomonas,* and an increasing number of strains of *Aerobacter, E. coli, Salmonella,* and *Shigella.*

Parenterally 200–400 mg/kilo per day are given in four equal divided doses. Solutions should be freshly prepared and given within one hour of constitution, preferably as an intravenous bolus over five minutes every six hours. Ten percent loss of activity may occur during a four-hour intravenous drip. Therapy should last 10–14 days or longer. The child should be afebrile and free of signs of active infection for at least five days before the parenteral route is discontinued. Oral administration may result in capricious absorption.

Methicillin is recommended for penicillin-susceptible penicillinase-producing organisms and is used for staphylococcal infections. Dosage is 7 gm/m² per day (200–300 mg/kilo per day) given in four to six equal divided doses.

Patients with allergy to methicillin may demonstrate skin rash, urticaria, or pruritus. Transient neutropenia, bone marrow depression, or renal impairment have been reported.

Gentamicin is recommended for infections with *Aerobacter, Bacteroides, D. pneumoniae, E. coli, E. freundii, H. influenzae, Klebsiella, Mima (Moraxella, Herellea), Mycobacterium tuberculosis, Mycoplasma, Pasteurella multocida,* indole-negative *Proteus, Pseudomonas, Serratia,* all penicillin-sensitive and some methicillin-resistant strains of *Staphylococcus aureus,* and Group A streptococci. Variably sensitive organisms include *Brucella, Listeria, Paracolobactrum, Proteus inconstans, Salmonella, Shigella,* and some strains of streptococci. Resistant organisms include *Clostridium, Corynebacterium, N. gonorrhoeae* and *N. meningitidis,* and *Pseudomonas pseudomallei.* Resistance develops very slowly in susceptible organisms.

Dosage for patients with normal renal function is 0.8–1.2 mg/kilo per day in two to four equally divided doses. This may be increased to 5 mg/kilo per day in life-threatening disease. Intrathecal dosage is recommended for selected cases of bacterial meningitis caused by gram-negative organisms in neonates and *Pseudomonas aeruginosa* infections of all age groups. The dose for older children, which in some instances may be given intraventricularly, is 0.5–1.0 mg daily; adults may receive 5 mg/day for as long as nine days.

Ototoxicity usually causes greater vestibular than auditory impairment. Both vestibular and auditory function should be checked regularly while on this drug.

Kanamycin is recommended for infections by *Klebsiella, Aerobacter, Proteus* species (indole-positive), and *E. coli.* Other organisms sensitive to the drug include *Vibrio, Neisseria, Brucella, M. tuberculosis,* and atypical mycobacteria. An increasing number of resistant strains of organisms makes successful therapy less certain for *Aerobacter, Proteus* species (indole-positive), *E. coli* and other usually sensitive forms such as *Salmonella, Shigella, S. aureus,* and the paracolon group.

Resistance to kanamycin is common for pneumococci, *Alcaligenes, Streptococcus pyogenes, Pseudomonas,* enterococci, *Bacteroides,* clostridia and other anaerobes, *Streptococcus viridans,* and mycotic infections.

Dosage for neonatal infections during the first three days of life is 7.5 mg/kilo per day divided into two to four doses; older infants should receive 5–15 mg/kilo per day intramuscularly. Older children and adults should receive 15 mg/kilo per day in two to three equally divided doses. The maximum daily dose should not exceed 1.5 gm, total dose should not exceed 15 gm.

Evolution of resistant staphylococci and *E. coli* occurs with serial subcultures on increasing concentrations of antibiotics in media. Mycobacteria become rapidly resistant in vitro. Conjugation transfer of resistance occurs. Cross resistance between kanamycin, neomycin, and paramycin is complete.

Ototoxicity with cochlear and vestibular damage is usually bilateral. The drug is neurotoxic with curarelike effects on the neuromuscular junction. Nephrotoxicity has been reported.

Polymyxin B is recommended for many strains of *Pseudomonas* and for organisms resistant to more conventional antibiotics. These include *Aerobacter, Eberthella, Escherichia, Haemophilus, Klebsiella, Pasteurella, Salmonella, Shigella,* and *Vibrio.*

Resistance to polymyxin is common for gram-positive organisms, and cross resistance with colistin is complete. The development of new resistant strains is rare.

Dosage for all ages is 1.5–2.5 mg/kilo per day, not to exceed 200 mg/day given in four equally divided doses. As the drug does not gain access to the cerebrospinal fluid through inflamed meninges, intrathecal therapy is necessary. Intrathecal dose for children under two years of age is 2 mg daily for three to four days, then 2.5 mg every other day; older children and adults should receive 5 mg daily for three to four days, then 5 mg every other day. Adults may receive up to 10 mg daily. Duration of therapy should be three weeks. Intrathecal solutions should be prepared to yield 5 mg of drug per 1.0 ml of 0.9% saline or artificial spinal fluid. Injections of more than 5 mg of polymyxin B may produce signs of meningeal irritation, headache, fever, and an increase in cells and protein in the cerebrospinal fluid.

Toxicity is primarily neuromuscular and renal. Ophthalmoplegia, decreased reflexes, dysphagia, and increased weakness resulting in a myasthenic picture may occur. Nephritis with impaired renal function has been reported.

Colistin is recommended for susceptible strains of *Pseudomonas.* The dosage for children and adults is 2.5–5.0 mg/kilo per day. The intrathecal dose for children is 2–5 mg; for adults it is 20 mg repeated as indicated.

Toxicity is primarily neuromuscular or renal. Paresthesias, visual and speech disturbances, partial deafness, dizziness, severe ataxia, and respiratory paralysis similar to those observed from polymyxin as well as adverse renal effects have been reported.

Streptomycin is recommended for infections with *Mycobacterium tuberculosis.* Dosage for children is 20–30 mg/kilo per day for three to six months, then two or three times a week for two or three years. Dosages for older children and adults is 1.0 gm daily for two to three months, then 1.0 gm two or three times per week. Ototoxicity may result in disturbances of auditory or vestibular function.

Because of its toxicity, *chloramphenicol* is not recommended in the treatment of meningitis unless no other effective drug is available. The drug has been recommended for *H. influenzae* meningitis when, as is rarely the case, ampicillin is ineffective.[69a] Sensitive organisms include a number of gram-negative and gram-positive organisms, *Mycoplasma*, rickettsiae, and large viruses of the psittacosis-lymphogranuloma venereum group.

Dosage in children under one month is 25 mg/kilo per day; older children should receive 75–100 mg/kilo per day for the first two to three days, followed by 50 mg/kg/day for the subsequent seven to ten days.

A number of gram-negative organisms may acquire resistance by bacterial conjugation and acquisition of an acetyl transferase.

Serious toxicity is primarily due to bone marrow depression. Symptoms occur with an incidence of 1 in 20,000 to 1 in 100,000 patients. Two types of syndromes have been described: 1) a temporary depression of the erythroid series resulting in anemia, occasionally accompanied by thrombocytopenia and leukopenia; and 2) a severe and usually irreversible pancytopenia. In infants the "gray syndrome," manifested by cardio-respiratory collapse and respiratory distress, is unassociated with bone marrow depression.

BRAIN ABSCESSES

A brain abscess consists of localized free or encapsulated pus within the brain substance. Although the condition has been known for more than 200 years, and its association with cyanotic congenital heart disease described over 100 years ago, the absence of classic signs and symptoms hinder its early diagnosis and treatment.

Etiology and Pathogenesis

The pyogenic organisms gain access to the brain substance by one of four routes: 1) the blood stream from a distant infection, or as a consequence of sepsis; 2) extension of contiguous infections such as in the middle ear, and the paranasal sinuses either directly, or as a result of septic thrombophlebitis of bridging veins; 3) as a complication of a penetrating wound; and 4) in association with a cardio-pulmonary malfunction, most commonly, cyanotic congenital heart disease, in which there may be a real or a potential right-to-left shunt.

The most common causative organisms in

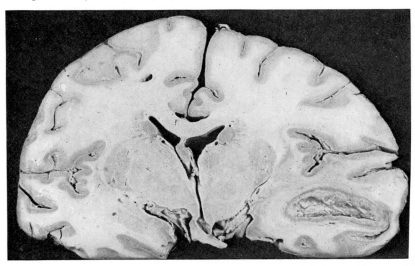

Fig. 6–3. Temporal lobe abscess in child with cyanotic congenital heart disease. The brain is edematous with flattening of the gyri. There is an abscess in the right temporal lobe. (Courtesy of Dr. P. Cancilla, Department of Pathology, UCLA, Los Angeles.)

order of frequency are *Staphylococcus aureus*, anaerobic streptococci, beta-hemolytic streptococci, alpha-hemolytic streptococci, pneumococci, *Bacteroides* and other gram-negative rods—particularly *Haemophilus aphrophilus*.[70] Infections caused by fungi such as *Aspergillus*, *Nocardia*, *Actinomyces*, *Leptothrix*, and cryptococci occur less often; abscesses due to *Corynebacterium*, *Mycobacterium* as well as protozoans such as *Entamoeba histolytica* are even rarer.[71] Approximately 6%–20% of abscesses are due to mixed flora.[72]

Abscesses resulting from hematogenous spread may be localized within any part of the brain but most commonly at the junction of gray and white matter of the cerebral hemispheres. By contrast, abscesses derived from contiguous sources tend to be superficial and close to the infected bone or dura. Multiple abscesses occur in 6% of patients, usually when sepsis or congenital heart disease are the predisposing causes.

Pathology

The earliest stage of an abscess is cerebritis (septic encephalitis). This is usually localized in the white matter even when infection has to pass through the cortex. It is an edematous area with softening and congestion of brain tissue often with numerous petechial hemorrhages. The center becomes liquefied, thus forming the abscess cavity (Fig. 6–3). Initially, its wall is poorly defined and irregular. Gradually, a firmer, thicker wall develops which ultimately may become a thick firm concentric capsule of fibrous tissue.

The adjacent brain tissue is infiltrated with polymorphonuclear leukocytes and plasma cells near the abscess, with lymphocytes in the more peripheral zones and heavy lymphocytic cuffing of vessels in the area. In more chronic abscesses, a border of granulation tissue merges gradually into a collagenous capsule. Abscesses enlarge within the softer and less vascular white matter, and extend toward the ventricles, rupturing into this space rather than into the subarachnoid fluid. Seeding of the leptomeninges and subsequent meningitis results from local thrombophlebitis more often than from actual rupture.

TABLE 6-8.
INCIDENCE OF SYMPTOMS AND NEUROLOGIC FINDINGS IN 19 CASES OF BRAIN ABSCESS WITH CONGENITAL HEART DISEASE*

Symptoms:	Number of Patients
Headache and/or vomiting	15
Seizures	7
Fever (101° F or more)	6
Listlessness	4
Disorientation	4
Neck pain	4
Neurologic Signs:	
Lateralizing signs	15
Papilledema	13
Hemiparesis	12
Increased deep tendon reflexes	12
Extensor plantar responses	9
Pupillary changes	7
Stupor	6
Neck stiffness	5
Aphasia	5
Homonymous hemianopsia	4
Localized percussion tenderness of skull	**

* Adapted from Raimondi et al.[82]
** Although not cited, this is a common neurologic sign and is valuable in localizing the abscess.

Clinical Manifestations

During initial stages of the brain abscess, the clinical picture may be nonspecific. The patient, who may have cyanotic congenital heart disease or a primary infection, develops the complex of headache, vomiting, and convulsions, either partially or in its entirety. With progression of the abscess the neurologic signs, which initially were minimal or completely absent, become readily apparent. As indicated in Table 6–8 they include papilledema, lateralizing signs—particularly a hemiparesis or homonymous hemianopsia— and more obvious indications of increased intracranial pressure. Untreated, the condition is usually fatal, either as a consequence of decompensated increased intracranial pressure, or from sudden rupture of the abscess into the ventricular system. The latter event is marked by a sudden high fever, meningeal signs, and deterioration of consciousness.

Cerebellar abscesses are most commonly seen in association with mastoid infections and occur most frequently during the second and third decade. Symptoms and neurologic signs are those associated with any posterior fossa mass lesion.

Peripheral blood counts are usually of little value in establishing the diagnosis of brain abscess in children. However, the cerebrospinal fluid is usually abnormal. There is increased pressure, pleocytosis, and later on, protein concentrations become elevated. Cultures are generally negative unless the abscess is leaking into the ventricular system. As a rule, the more striking the pleocytosis, the closer the abscess to the ventricular lining.

The electroencephalogram almost always shows a focal slowing, which corresponds closely to the location of the abscess. A ventriculogram, often done if increased intracranial pressure precludes a pneumoencephalogram, usually reveals a mass lesion. The danger of abscess rupture or marked increase in brain swelling after an air study makes cerebral arteriography the method of choice for all suspect cases except those markedly polycythemic patients with cyanotic congenital heart disease who have an increased risk of procedural complications including seizures and vascular thromboses. Focal arterial displacement or the presence of the "ripple sign," a concentric, curvilinear displacement of opacified sulci in the late arterial phase due to perifocal edema, are helpful radiographic findings.[74] Conventional brain scan techniques or use of carotid perfusion with I^{131} microaggregate may also help delineate the lesion.[75] The echoencephalogram may disclose a midline shift. In patients with cyanotic congenital heart disease, a brain abscess must primarily be differentiated from intracranial vascular accidents and hypoxic attacks.

Thromboses of arteries, veins, and dural sinuses are particularly common in severely cyanotic infants. While dehydration and stasis play a minor role in the evolution of cerebral vascular thromboses, virtually every infant who experiences a thrombosis has an arterial oxygen saturation of 10 volumes percent or less.[75a] Except for a more abrupt onset of symptoms, the clinical picture may mimic that of an abscess. However, the age of the patient is of considerable importance in the differential diagnosis. Brain abscesses are rare under the age of two, while vascular thromboses are rare in patients over two.[75a] Emboli in patients with congenital heart disease are highly unusual, and when present are precipitated by cardiac or other surgery.

Hypoxic attacks, often accompanied by headaches, are seen in 12–15% of patients with cyanotic congenital heart disease. Attacks are more common during the first two years of life, occur many times a day, and are related to activity, such as exercise, feeding, or bowel movement.

A partially treated meningitis should also be considered. The latter lacks the neurologic and electroencephalographic evidence of focal central involvement.

Clark[72] has pointed out that old focal neurologic signs, which are often present in the patient with cyanotic congenital heart disease, are aggravated by stress, including a recent infection. The ensuing picture simulates a progressive lesion.

Treatment

During the stage of its formation, antibiotic therapy will heal an abscess. When it is fully established, surgical treatment is required. Therapy for brain abscess suspects should be instituted only when focal lesions have been established either by the presence of advancing neurologic signs, percussion tenderness on tapping the skull, a slow wave focus on EEG, focal brain scan or x-ray contrast studies. The area in question is surgically tapped and any abscess aspirated. Only then is a massive antibiotic regimen instituted, usually with intravenous methicillin and ampicillin. Intravenous fluid is usually limited to 1500 ml/m² in order to minimize cerebral edema.

Micropaque barium may be instilled into the abscess region.[76] This will disperse through the area of the abscess as well as be phagocytized by scavenger cells to provide a readily localizable lesion at the time of surgery when local cerebritis has been controlled. This procedure is recommended to verify the location and size of the abscess.

Open surgical drainage may be required or excision may be necessary. Wright and Ballantine[77] recommend total excision of brain abscesses since they had no deaths with this approach whereas drainage or medical treatment alone was associated with significant mortality. A short course of steroids to reduce life-threatening edema may safely be administered.

Patients with marked increase in intracranial pressure and danger of brain stem herniation should have a careful selection of anesthetic agents since halothane, trichlorethylene, and methoxyflurane may cause a considerable rise in intracranial pressure in patients with space-occupying lesions.[78]

Occasionally a patient with a cyanotic heart disease has equivocal signs of brain abscess. It then becomes advisable to obtain bacteriologic cultures, to stop all antibiotic therapy and follow the patient with repeated neurologic examinations, EEGs and brain scans. If after about two weeks neurologic signs have failed to advance and no definite focus is seen on brain scan or EEG, the patient is discharged.

Sequelae

Residual defects include: 1) seizure activity; 2) localized neurologic abnormalities; 3) mental retardation, and 4) hydrocephalus. Mortality rate for untreated cases is high

and remains in the range of 27–38%[73] for treated cases.

EPIDURAL ABSCESSES

Epidural abscesses may develop from contiguous infection of structures which surround the brain and spinal cord. They may arise from local infection or secondary to congenital anomalies such as dermal sinuses.[79,80,81] Subdural empyema may result from direct extension of infection or by bacterial contamination of a subdural effusion in meningitis, subdural hematoma, or as a result of sepsis. Rarely intramedullary abscesses, often in the dorsal region, may produce symptoms of cord compression.

Infection of the spinal epidural space is extremely rare in childhood, but when it does occur, it produces a devastating neurologic picture. The infection is limited to the dorsal surface of the cord except in its lower sacral portion where the space completely surrounds the cord. The anatomy of the space limits extension to vertical spread and produces extradural compression.

The clinical course may be acute and rapidly progressive or chronic. The former, more common in children, is usually the result of a metastatic infection while chronic lesions are most commonly due to a direct extension of a spinal osteomyelitis.

The classic case of spinal epidural abscess follows a fairly typical pattern of development. Within one to two weeks of an infection, there is a backache, enhanced by jarring or straining, and accompanied by local spinal tenderness; this progresses within a few days to radicular pain followed by symptoms of cord involvement, including weakness of voluntary movements and impaired sphincter control. Paraplegia may be complete within a few hours or days.

In many patients, the history or neurologic signs are impossible to differentiate from those of acute transverse myelitis. A similar clinical picture may be produced by intradural extramedullary tumors.

Lumbar puncture aids early diagnosis of the condition. This is done carefully with a large gauge needle and frequent aspiration of the spinal needle so as not to miss any pus in the extradural space which might be carried subdurally. Generally, there is a marked CSF pleocytosis and elevated protein levels. A myelogram will confirm the block and show the presence of an extradural mass.

An epidural abscess which has produced neurologic deficit is treated by laminectomy with decompression and drainage. Antibiotic therapy is secondary, and in view of the rapid progression of potentially irreversible symptoms, this condition is a surgical emergency.

CONGENITAL INFECTIONS OF THE NERVOUS SYSTEM

Infections of the fetal nervous system differ from those of older children and adults in that they may cause significant damage to development and to the elaboration of neural relationships, and thus produce multiple defects. The induction of congenital anomalies in the infected developing embryo depends on the time of action of the teratogen. Prior to the blastula stage, the embryo is very resistant to the action of teratogens, and damage will result either in death or in recovery without malfunction. When the primary germ layers have become established, and during organogenesis, the embryo becomes vulnerable to infectious agents. Occasional instances of congenital malformations have resulted from infections incurred during the second trimester.[83] After the second trimester, congenital malformations become increasingly uncommon. For these reasons the fetal brain is highly susceptible to some infectious agents which are of little consequence to older children.

Another feature of prenatal infections is the altered biologic response to injury. The immature fetal brain is able to repair damage, remove abnormal cells, and compensate for missing tissue. The inflammatory response, which often contributes to the damage produced by viruses at a later age, is absent or less marked in the fetus.[84]

The two main pathways for transmission of infection to the fetus are the ascending cervical-amniotic route, and the transplacental route. Bacteria usually invade by the ascending route, while toxoplasmosis, syphilis, rubella, cytomegalovirus, and other viruses

generally assume the transplacental route.[85] Placental changes have been demonstrated in most of these conditions.[86] The pathogenesis of prenatal viral infections has been reviewed by Mims[87] who states that while maternal viremia is relatively common, the fetus will only become infected and damaged when the virus breaches the placental barrier.

Viral spread through the human embryo during the first three weeks of gestation must be by cell contiguity since there is no established circulation. In the older fetus, virus spread may be similar to that seen in adults.

The invading virus may be cytopathic for fetal cells or cause reduction and cessation of cell growth and division. Thus, a fetus infected with rubella and cytomegalovirus has a subnormal number of cells, but a normal cytoplasmic mass. Certain viruses, notably rubella, produce lesions in the endothelium of chorionic and fetal blood vessels, which by themselves may result in maldevelopment secondary to ischemia, and faulty tissue proliferation.

The course of fetal infection may be influenced by the specific immune response. IgG antibodies, mainly of maternal origin, have been demonstrated in the blood of three to four-month-old fetuses. Specific fetal IgM and IgG antibodies may be produced from the twentieth week on, so that inordinately high IgM levels at birth may be diagnostic of a prenatal infection. Some 34% of newborns with IgM levels above 19.5 mg % can be shown to have infections as compared with 0.8% of infants with IgM values below this level.[88,89]

The production of interferon has not been demonstrated in the rubella-infected fetus.[90]

Four conditions that affect the fetal brain will be further discussed. They are rubella, cytomegalic inclusion disease, toxoplasmosis, and herpes simplex.

RUBELLA

Rubella was first noted to produce congenital malformations by Gregg some 30 years ago.[91] It is now known that severe central nervous system involvement may accompany congenital rubella, the incidence and severity of the malformations depending on the time of maternal infection. Infection during the first trimester will result in an abnormal fetus with a frequency ranging from 10%–70%. In general, the earlier in pregnancy the infection is incurred, the greater the risk to the fetus, and the discrepancy in the incidence is in part due to the lack of appearance of some of the induced anomalies. Congenital rubella following maternal disease during the second trimester results in more subtle abnormalities in some two-thirds of infants, notably disorders in communication and delayed mental development.[83]

Pathology

The histopathologic abnormalities of rubella infection of the nervous system are of two types: those due to retardation or inhibition of cell growth, and those resulting from cellular necrosis. The parenchyma of the brain demonstrates multiple small areas of liquefactive necrosis and gliosis with vasculitis and perivascular calcification. The lesions may be in the periventricular white matter, the basal ganglia, and less frequently in midbrain, pons, and spinal cord.[93] In addition, there is usually a chronic leptomeningitis with round cell infiltration.

Clinical Manifestations

The clinical picture of the congenital rubella syndrome is summarized in Table 6–9. Cataracts, glaucoma, and cardiac malfunctions occur when the infant is infected during the first two months of gestation; hearing loss and psychomotor retardation may follow infection any time in the first trimester and rarely as late as 16 weeks' gestation.[92,95] In about 80% of rubella-infected infants, symptoms referable to the nervous system can be observed during the first year of life.[92]

The neurologic picture tends to follow one of three clinical patterns.[92,94,95] In 72% of the cases, the clinical picture at birth is marked by lethargy, hypotonia, and a large, full, or bulging fontanelle. Later on, between one and four months of age, irritability, restlessness, constant movements, vasomotor instability, and photophobia become the most prominent clinical features. Opisthotonic posturing, and a marked developmental

TABLE 6-9.
CLINICAL MANIFESTATIONS OF CONGENITAL RUBELLA INFECTIONS*

Findings	Percent of Patients	
Deafness	67.0	
Heart disease	48.5	
Bilateral cataracts	15.4	
Unilateral cataract	13.4	
Glaucoma	3.2	
Chorioretinitis	39.1	
Psychomotor retardation	45.2	
Mild		22.4
Moderate		10.6
Severe		12.2
Thrombocytopenia	22.5	
Spasticity	12.2	

* From Cooper et al.[92]

delay is common. Between 6 and 12 months, about half of these infants improve and begin to develop.

Sixteen percent of infants are small, hypotonic, and unreactive, with little evidence of irritability. In 11% convulsions start shortly after birth or there are symptoms of meningitis.

Seizures occur in one-quarter of children. Minor motor attacks or abrupt vasomotor changes are the most common forms.[92]

When the central nervous system is involved during prenatal life, congenital malformations including microcephaly, hydrocephalus, and spina bifida may develop,[96] but may not be recognized until developmental or speech retardation become obvious. Retarded language development may be due to a peripheral hearing loss (44%), or central auditory imperception (42%) as well as due to mental retardation.[97]

The most common ocular abnormality in congenital rubella is chorioretinitis. It is characterized by areas of discrete, patchy, black pigmentation interspersed with similar patchy depigmentation; the so-called "salt and pepper" appearance. There is no evidence that this defect of retinal pigmentation interferes with vision. Microphthalmia, nuclear cataracts, glaucoma, and severe myopia are also common.

In about one-third of children, a variety of abnormal electroencephalographic tracings can be obtained.

In the majority of patients, the CSF protein is abnormally high at birth, diminishing to normal levels by three months of age. Rubella virus may be isolated from the spinal fluid for as long as 18 months after birth.[95]

Diagnosis

The diagnosis of congenital rubella can be made by finding an elevated IgM level at birth and identifying this IgM as specific rubella antibody. The virus may be isolated from nasopharynx, urine, stool, or cerebrospinal fluid. In older children the diagnosis of congenital rubella may be established by administering rubella vaccine. By age five, hemagglutination inhibition antibody is seronegative in 18.5% of patients. In the seronegative children with congenital rubella, only 10% respond with a rise in the titer of hemagglutination inhibition antibodies in contrast to 99% of nonimmune normal children.[98]

Treatment

There is no specific treatment for rubella. The control of congenital rubella infections rests on the prevention of maternal viremia by vaccination with attenuated viral strains. Rubella vaccine given to a pregnant woman has resulted in intra-uterine infection by vaccine virus.[99] Infants with congenital rubella are a potential source of virus for nursing personnel.

Prognosis

Nearly all long-term survivors of congenital rubella are left with deafness.[96] Cataracts and chorioretinopathy are commonly seen.[100] Severe mental retardation (24%) and spasticity (20%) occur, but most patients who have sustained severe neurologic damage die during the early years of life.[95,100]

CYTOMEGALOVIRUS

Cytomegalovirus is ubiquitous and may be isolated from the urine of approximately 1.0%–1.4% of asymptomatic newborn infants.[101] The factors responsible for a clinically apparent infection are unclear, but Hanshaw has pointed out that in these patients the infection occurs during the second and third trimester of pregnancy.[101]

The virus has an affinity for the rapidly growing subependymal cells lining the cerebral ventricles. Multiplication of virus, and subsequent deposition of calcium in this area result in characteristic periventricular or diffuse calcifications and subsequent failure of brain growth. Intranuclear inclusion bodies appear within endothelial cells, neurons, and in cells surrounding the cerebral vasculature.

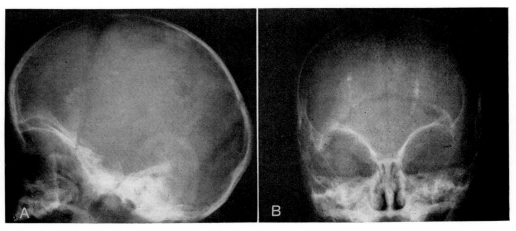

Fig. 6–4. Cytomegalic inclusion disease. There are extensive periventricular calcifications. A. Lateral view of the skull. B. Anterior-posterior view of the skull. (Courtesy of Dr. G. Wilson, Department of Radiology, UCLA, Los Angeles.)

TABLE 6-10.
CLINICAL AND LABORATORY MANIFESTATIONS
IN 19 CHILDREN WITH CONGENITAL
CYTOMEGALOVIRUS INFECTIONS*

Finding	Number of Patients
Hepatomegaly	17
Splenomegaly	16
Jaundice	13
Low birth weight (less than 2500 gm)	12
Thrombocytopenia	11
Petechiae	10
Cerebral calcifications	5
Microcephaly	5
Hemolytic anemia	4
Chorioretinitis	2
Hydrocephalus	1

* From Shinefield and Eichenwald.[106]

Clinical Manifestations

The clinical manifestations are most often seen during the early neonatal period or early infancy, in infants who are premature or small for gestational age. They are summarized in Table 6–10.

The classic picture of congenital cytomegalic inclusion disease is one of persistent jaundice, hepatosplenomegaly, thrombocytopenia, and severe anemia. Neurologic abnormalities include microcephaly and, on rare occasions, hydrocephalus. Microgyria and other cortical malformations, cerebellar aplasia, porencephaly, and calcifications of the cerebral arteries may also be encountered (Fig. 6–4).[102] About 10%–35% of children with congenital microcephaly have cytomegalovirus infections, contrasted with a 4%–7% incidence in controls.[101] There is also some evidence that congenital cytomegalovirus infections may produce milder neurologic manifestations including mental retardation.[103] Ocular abnormalities include chorioretinitis, anomalies of the optic disc, microphthalmia, cataracts, optic atrophy, retinal calcifications, and other malformations.[102]

Whether congenital or acquired, the cytomegalovirus infection may persist for months despite high antibody levels and viruria may be demonstrated after two years of age.[104] The virus can also be found in saliva and leukocytes, and infant-to-infant transmission resulting in inapparent infections may occur in nurseries.[105]

The diagnosis of the condition rests upon the demonstration of inclusion bodies in cells from the urinary sediment, a characteristic pattern of periventricular calcification and isolation of the virus.

Both 5-fluoro-2′-deoxyuridine (floxuridine) and 5-iodo-2′-deoxyuridine (idoxuridine) have been used in the treatment of cytomegalovirus infections.[107] The effectiveness of these drugs is still uncertain.

VARICELLA

Multiple neurologic defects, including mental retardation, abnormalities of the ocular fundus, seizures, and dilated ventricles are associated with congenital varicella.[107a]

TOXOPLASMOSIS

Toxoplasmosis is caused by the protozoan *Toxoplasma gondii*, a parasite first found in the gondi, a North African rodent. It infects a wide range of birds and mammals, and is an obligatory intracellular parasite lacking host and tissue specificity.[108]

Toxoplasma infection in the human infant was first described by Wolf et al. in 1939.[109] The incidence of congenital infections in the human has been estimated at 1 per 1000 to 3500 live births, and when still births are included, about 1% of all pregnancies.[108]

It involves fetal transmission of an infection incurred during the last seven months of pregnancy. Infection of the placenta occurs before fetal infestation.[108] Maternal antibodies may develop and modify the course of the fetal infection. Eighty-five percent of mothers who give birth to children with toxoplasmosis have no history of respiratory illness. Only an infection newly acquired by the mother during her pregnancy seems to endanger the fetus; chronic infection does not seem to be of importance. The most dangerous period is the second trimester of pregnancy; maternal infection prior to the third month and during the third trimester may result in congenital toxoplasmosis that is initially relatively benign with the infection

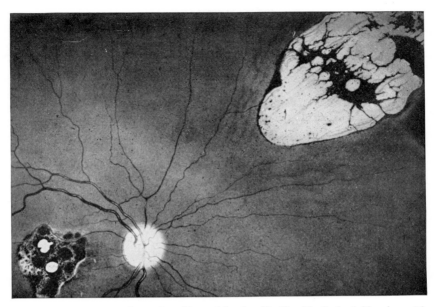

Fig. 6–5. Chorioretinitis in toxoplasmosis. (From Merritt, H. H.: *Textbook of Neurology*, 4th ed., 1970, courtesy of Lea & Febiger, Philadelphia.)

being latent for at least the first few years of life.[110]

Postnatally acquired toxoplasmosis is a common inapparent infection. When clinical manifestations become obvious, patients may develop hepatomegaly, lymphadenopathy, pneumonia, and occasionally a mild encephalitis.[111] Less often one encounters isolated facial palsy,[112] generalized seizures,[113] or a picture mimicking a space-occupying lesion.[114] The spinal fluid in acquired toxoplasmosis usually shows an elevated protein and a variable degree of mononuclear pleocytosis.

Pathology

Cerebral lesions are of three types: large granulomatous areas with a necrotic center, diffuse inflammation and small miliary granulomas. The last are most common in the cerebral cortex, and consist of large epithelioid and round cells. Adherent overlying meninges are congested and densely infiltrated. Organisms may be found free in the most recent lesions and in the subarachnoid space. They are mainly extracellular but may also be within large epithelioid cells. With progression of the infec-tion, areas of necrosis develop and calcium salts become deposited in amorphous masses, with predilection for the ventricular walls.

Hydrocephalus is frequent, most often due to ependymitis occluding the aqueduct.[115] Hydranencephaly may also occur.[115a]

Classic Features

The severest forms of congenital toxoplasmosis are the most familiar, but cases with few symptoms are common.[116]

The severe form may be apparent at birth or may remain asymptomatic for a few days or weeks. The clinical picture is either generalized or primarily affects the nervous system. In both types, the principal findings are a chorioretinitis (Fig. 6–5), which in 85% of patients is bilateral,[117] an abnormal CSF, anemia and seizures (Table 6–11). When the nervous system bears the major impact of toxoplasmosis, there is, in addition, a higher incidence of cerebral calcifications and hydrocephalus (Table 6–11).

The prognosis for both groups is quite poor; overall mortality for patients with apparent early neurologic disease was 11.1% while that for the group with generalized disease was 13.6%. Major sequelae were found in a

TABLE 6-11.
CLINICAL AND LABORATORY MANIFESTATIONS IN
INFANTS WITH CONGENITAL TOXOPLASMOSIS*

	Generalized Form	Neurologic Form
Chorioretinitis	66	94
CSF pleocytosis, elevated protein	84	55
Anemia	77	51
Convulsions	—	50
Intracranial calcifications	—	50
Jaundice	79	29
Hydrocephalus	—	28
Fever	77	25
Splenomegaly	90	21
Lymphadenopathy	68	17
Hepatomegaly	77	17
Vomiting	48	17
Microcephaly	—	13
Cataracts	—	4.6
Optic atrophy	—	1.9
Pneumonitis	41	—

* After Eichenwald.[116]

large majority of survivors.[116] A four-year follow-up of the group with apparent neurologic disease in infancy disclosed mental retardation (89%), convulsions (83%), spasticity and palsies (69%), severely impaired sight (42%), hydro- and microcephalus (44%), deafness (17%); only 9% were normal. The group with generalized involvement had only a slightly better long-term picture with mental retardation (81%), convulsions (77%), spasticity (58%), hydro- and microcephalus (10%); 16.1% were normal.

With the widespread use of serologic tests for toxoplasmosis, incomplete forms of the disease have been recognized. The frequency of positive serologic reactions is higher in patients with isolated chorioretinitis than in controls.[110] The incidence of toxoplasmosis is about 50% in patients with isolated cerebral calcifications.[117] Rarely, toxoplasmosis may be responsible for seizures or psychomotor retardation.[118]

Diagnosis

The most widely used tests for the diagnosis of toxoplasmosis are the Sabin-Feldman dye test, the complement fixation test, the hemagglutination test, and the fluorescent antibody

test utilizing the IgM or mixed globulin antibody of human serum.[108,119]

The isolation of the parasite by inoculation of mice may be extremely difficult as well as hazardous to laboratory workers.

The dye test is probably the most sensitive test. Titers appear within two weeks of the infection, persist until age two years at levels of 1 to 1000, and gradually decline to around 1 to 50 or less by age five years.[110]

The complement fixation test does not become positive until several weeks after the dye test, and remains positive for a shorter period of time.

Antibody levels on the fluorescent antibody test generally parallel those obtained by the dye test.

Cerebral calcifications, while suggestive of toxoplasmosis, are not pathognomonic. The radiologic features of the intracranial calcifications have been reviewed by Mussbichler.[120] The deposits are scattered irregularly throughout the brain, tending to cluster in the caudate nucleus, meninges, choroid plexus, and subependymal region. None were found in the subtentorial region or spinal cord. The shape of the lesion varies considerably.

The clinical picture of congenital toxoplasmosis may be identical to that seen in cytomegalic inclusion disease, syphilis, prenatal sepsis, and hemolytic disease of the newborn.

Treatment

Of the many drugs that demonstrate activity against toxoplasmosis, only the sulfonamides and pyrimethamine (Daraprim) are of potential value. The combination of pyrimethamine with triple sulfa or sulfadiazine[108] has been reported as beneficial in the acute illness. This treatment eliminates trophozoites but not encysted forms. The progressive nature of congenital toxoplasma infections suggests that treatment be considered in hope of arresting progress; in a small series, such benefits could not be demonstrated, although the spinal fluid and the antibody titers reverted to normal more rapidly than without therapy. Therapy for small children is sulfadiazine (100 mg per kilo body weight per day in divided doses); pyrimethamine (1 mg per kilo per day—a double dose is used for the first three days); leukovorin (1 mg per day), and fresh bakers' yeast (100 mg daily). Older children and adults receive the usual dosage of sulfadiazine with 25 mg in children and 50 mg in adults of pyrimethamine for the first three days and half of that dose thereafter. Five to 15 mg of leukovorin and two fresh yeast cakes per day are also given. Duration of therapy is four weeks for both congenital and acquired toxoplasmosis. As pyrimethamine is a folic acid antagonist, platelet and leukocyte counts are done twice weekly during therapy, and the drug is discontinued if one or both are significantly reduced.[119]

HERPES SIMPLEX

Infection of the fetus with herpes simplex virus may result in a fatal generalized disease. In most instances of congenital herpes, the infection is recognized between one and three weeks of age and is usually due to type II strains. Most cases result from exposure to herpetic lesions of the mother's genitalia, but transplacental infection has also been demonstrated.[120a]

The clinical picture may be that of a visceral form with cyanosis, jaundice, fever, and respiratory distress, or of encephalitis. In the latter type, the infection is almost always due to type II virus.

Although a number of chemotherapeutic agents (including idoxuridine, or cytosine arabinoside)[121] have been used in the treatment of herpes encephalitis in older children, their effectiveness in congenital infections remains unproven..

POSTINFECTIOUS AND POSTVACCINAL ENCEPHALOMYELITIS

The neurologic complications encountered in the course of the various exanthemata, notably measles, chickenpox, and rubella as well as in mumps, are considered in Chapter 7.

The complications of prophylactic immunization, particularly those associated with vaccination and rabies prophylaxis, are also discussed in Chapter 7.

PROTOZOAN AND PARASITIC INFECTIONS OF THE NERVOUS SYSTEM

Aside from toxoplasmosis, discussed elsewhere in this chapter, none of these organisms commonly invade the nervous system of American or Western European children.[121a] Consequently, our experience with these diseases is limited, and the reader is referred to references appended to Table 6–12.

Generally speaking, parasitic infestations of the CNS may produce symptoms of meningoencephalitis or of a space-occupying lesion. Because of their relative frequency in Latin American countries, trichinosis and cysticercosis are singled out for a fuller discussion.

TRICHINOSIS

This condition is due to a nematode *Trichinella spiralis*, which infests hogs and is eaten as raw or poorly cooked pork. The encysted larvae escape to all parts of the body by the blood stream but survive and grow only in skeletal muscle.

On microscopy, parasites are seen within the muscle fibers, where they set up a focal inflammation and ultimately become calcified. Within the central nervous system filiform larvae are found in the capillaries and in parenchyma, where they engender a focal inflammatory response.[122]

TABLE 6-12.
PROTOZOAN AND PARASITIC INFECTIONS OF THE NERVOUS SYSTEM

Condition (Organism)	Major Clinical Features	Treatment	Reference
Malaria (Plasmodium falciparum)	Sudden high fever, convulsions, focal cerebral signs	Chloroquine	Chalgren and Baker,[128] Thomas[129]
African trypanosomiasis (T. gambiense or T. rhodesiense)	Fever, lymphadenopathy, hepatosplenomegaly. Months or years later: apathy, meningeal signs, somnolence, seizures	Often fatal once CNS signs appear. Tryparsamide	Van Bogaert and Janssen[130]
American trypanosomiasis (T. cruzi)	In acute type seen in infants: convulsions, nuchal rigidity. In chronic type: spastic diplegia, choreoathetosis, with or without bulbar palsy	No adequate treatment. Nitrofurfurylidene (Bay 2502) has been tried.	Jorg and Orlando[131]
Amebiasis ((Naegleria)	Meningoencephalitis	Amphotericin B	Duma et al.[132,133]
Amebiasis (Entamoeba histolytica)	Meningoencephalitis, brain abscess secondary to hepatic or pulmonary involvement	Emetine, chloroquine ?metronidazole	Orbison et al.[134]
Gnathostoma spinigerum	Encephalomyelitis	None effective	Chitanondh and Rosen[135]
Dracunculus medinensis	Extradural abscesses	Niridazole	
Visceral larva migrans (Toxocara canis or T. cati)	Encephalitis, optic neuritis	None effective	Schochet,[136] Bird et al.[137]
Schistosomiasis (S. japonicum, S. mansoni, S. haematobium)	Transverse myelitis, granulomatous tumor of the spinal cord, radiculitis, meningeal signs, encephalitis	S. haematobium-niridazole S. japonicum-stibophen S. mansoni-stibophen	Carroll,[38] Zilberg[139]
Paragonimiasis	Meningoencephalitis, granulomata, ultimately calcification, seizures, headaches, visual disturbances, focal neurologic signs, mental deterioration	Bithionol	Oh,[140,141] Shim and Park,[142] Higashi et al.[142a]
Hydatidosis (Echinococcus)	Location of cysts in children: 77% in brain, 8% in skull, 18% in spine. CNS cysts give symptoms of space-occupying lesion	Surgery	Arana-Iniguez and Lopez-Fernand[143]

The clinical picture is highlighted by fever, myalgia, and abdominal pain. Muscles innervated by the cranial nerves, including the extraocular and masticatory muscles may be involved. In 10%–20% of infestations the nervous system is also invaded within the first weeks of the onset of infection. An encephalitis or meningeal signs may be present, and there may be papilledema and focal neurologic abnormalities.[123,124,125]

The most striking laboratory findings include an eosinophilia and, occasionally, electrocardiographic abnormalities compatible with a myocarditis. The diagnosis rests on a history of potential exposure, persistent eosinophilia, rising serum antibody titer, and a positive muscle biopsy. In about one-quarter of patients larvae may be seen in the cerebrospinal fluid.[125]

Several investigators have reported symptomatic benefit from corticosteroid therapy, but improvement is generally not dramatic. When the infection has not been extensive, the prognosis for life is good, but weakness and electrocardiographic abnormalities may persist for long periods after apparent clinical recovery. In chronic infections, x rays of the muscles, particularly those of the calves, will reveal the calcified filarial cysts.

CYSTICERCOSIS

Cysticercosis of the central nervous system is rare in the United States and in other countries that have adequate sanitation. It is not unusual in Chile, Mexico, Peru, India, and in the Middle East. In Mexico, for instance, cysticercosis accounts for about 25% of intracranial tumors. The condition is almost always due to the encysted form of *Taenia solium*. The organisms may encyst within the parenchyma or the basilar cisterns producing chronic inflammation of the leptomeninges and ependyma.[126]

The most common symptoms are increased intracranial pressure, found in about 75% of cases, focal or generalized seizures, and cranial nerve palsies. Tumor and encephalitic and basilar meningitic forms of infestation have also been described. In about one- to two-thirds of cases there is a CSF eosinophilia. About one-half of patients show intracranial calcifications on x ray.[127]

Surgical removal of the cysticercus, and correction of the CSF obstruction, when present, are necessary.

VIRUS INFECTIONS

INTRODUCTION

In a naturally acquired infection, the major pathway for spread of virus to the central nervous system is hematogenous. Viral growth generally begins in extraneural tissue such as the gut or regional lymphatics (poliomyelitis), respiratory tract (herpes simplex), vascular epithelium (arbovirus), and brown fat (coxsackie, poliomyelitis, reovirus, rabies, variola). The viremia is maintained by shedding of the virus, by absorption onto red blood cells, or by growth within leukocytes. Virus in blood may enter the cerebrospinal fluid by either passing or growing through the choroid plexus. Growth of virus in the choroid plexus may explain the ease with which ECHO and coxsackie virus can be isolated from the cerebrospinal fluid. Migration of infected phagocytes through cerebral vessels and replication of virus in the endothelial cells with growth or passive transfer through the blood brain barrier may also occur. Once within the nervous system the virus may spread by direct continuity or through the limited extracellular space.

Less commonly, the virus may enter the nervous system tissue by centripetal spread along the endoneurium and perineural Schwann cells and fibrocytes of peripheral nerves. Once the virus has gained access to the spinal cord by this route, it may spread randomly along the endoneurium or the interstitial space within the nerve. The latter method of spread is significant for rabies, and for some herpes simplex infections.

A third route of invasion, utilizing the olfactory system, has been demonstrated in herpes simplex, poliomyelitis, and arbovirus infections. These viruses spread along the interstitial spaces, endoneurium and perineurium of the olfactory nerves to the parenchymal cells of the olfactory bulb, and thence along the subarachnoid cuffs to the meninges.

Cells of the central nervous system vary in their susceptibility to infection. Herpes simplex seems to infect all cell types while polio has a predilection for the larger motor cells, Purkinje cells, and reticular formation. Susceptibility is determined by cell receptor sites and by the route of entry.

The reactions of brain tissue to viral invasion are similar in all forms of encephalitis. The most obvious histologic lesion is a cellular infiltration. Initially, this consists largely of polymorphoneutrophils; later, round cells predominate.

Proliferation of microglial cells may be diffuse or focal. In the latter case, the cells accumulate around degenerated or dying nerve cells, a phenomenon associated with neuronophagia. Alterations may be seen within the nerve cells, commonly a loss of Nissl granules and eosinophilia of the cytoplasm. Inclusion bodies within neurons and glial cells such as the Negri bodies seen in rabies may be typical of the disease or may represent nonspecific degeneration products.

An arteritis and other alterations of the vessel walls are observed in a number of conditions, notably in equine encephalitis. Demyelination, when present, may result from the loss of cortical nerve cells, or may occur independently as in subacute sclerosing panencephalitis or other slow virus infections.

Immune response to infection may contribute to the disease picture. For instance, in experimental lymphocytic choriomeningitis, the virus causes severe meningeal infiltrates only in immunologically mature and competent animals.

ENTEROVIRUS INFECTIONS

This group of RNA viruses includes poliomyelitis (3 types), coxsackie—group A (24 types) and B (6 types), and the ECHO virus group (34 types).[144] The organisms enter the body via the gastrointestinal tract, replicate there and in adjacent lymphoid tissue, induce a viremia and subsequently may invade the nervous system.[145] The clinical picture presented by these agents depends on viral factors such as type and virulence of the virus, the site of central nervous system invasion and, in the case of poliomyelitis, host factors such as degree of susceptibility and recent inoculations or trauma.[146]

Transmission of enterovirus infection occurs principally by means of direct or indirect contamination through infected fecal material. Organisms may be isolated from oropharynx, stool, blood, or spinal fluid. Isolation of virus from cerebrospinal fluid confirms the etiology of a specific episode.[145] Diagnosis by isolation of an enterovirus from stool may be misleading since virus may be excreted for 12–17 weeks after infection. In such a situation, only a definite rise in antibody titer to the agent isolated can confirm a recent significant infection.

POLIOMYELITIS

Poliomyelitis is an acute infectious disease first described by Heine in 1840.[147] It is characterized by preferential involvement of the motor neurons of the spinal cord and brain, and results in an asymmetric flaccid paralysis of the voluntary muscles. The severity of the illness varies; asymptomatic or mild cases are more common than the classic paralytic disease. The illness occurs throughout the world; in areas that have adequate sanitation, it is contracted later in life and is more likely to be symptomatic than in regions where poor sanitation is conducive to exposure at an age when transferred maternal immunity may attenuate the clinical picture.

With widespread immunization, poliomyelitis has become a preventable disease, and the recurrent major epidemics are no

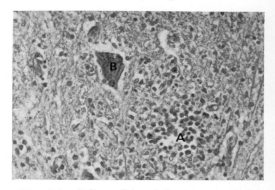

Fig. 6–6. Poliomyelitis. Inflammatory reaction in the anterior horn. One anterior horn cell (A) has disappeared and only the neuronophagia is evident. The other anterior horn cell is still evident, although it already has undergone degenerative changes (B). H and E stain × 80. (Courtesy of Dr. P. Cancilla, Department of Pathology, UCLA, Los Angeles.)

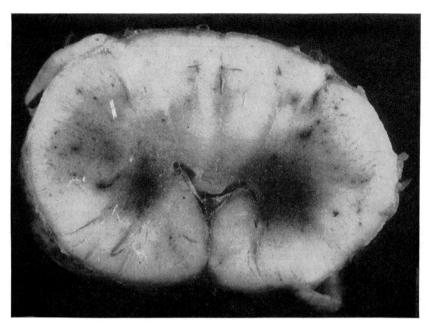

Fig. 6–7. Poliomyelitis. Congestion and inflammation in gray and white matter of cervical cord. (From Merritt, H. H., *Textbook of Neurology*, 4th ed., 1970, courtesy of Lea & Febiger, Philadelphia.)

longer encountered. Recent cases have been sporadic, and in some instances have been associated with vaccine strains.[148]

Pathology

Alterations within the central nervous system depend on the stage of the disease at the time of death. In the early days of the illness, neurons undergo a variety of nonspecific microscopic changes which vary in severity and result directly from viral invasion. These are accompanied by an initially polymorphonuclear reaction, which later becomes mononuclear. With progression of the illness, motor neurons degenerate, become surrounded by inflammatory cells, and undergo neuronophagia (Fig. 6–6). The distribution of lesions is characteristic of poliomyelitis. In the forebrain, lesions are usually mild and restricted to layers three and five in the precentral gyrus and adjacent cortex,[149] the thalamus, and the globus pallidus.[145] Cerebellar vermis and deep cerebellar nuclei are often severely involved,[150] whereas the cerebellar hemispheres are usually free of lesions. There is also marked involvement

of motor and sensory cranial nuclei of the medulla, especially the vestibular and ambiguus nuclei, and throughout the reticular formation.[145]

In the spinal cord, lesions are usually restricted to the anterior horn cells although some cases also show spotty involvement of the neurons in the intermediate, intermediolateral and posterior gray columns. Extension of lesions to the sensory spinal ganglia is the rule in more extensive cord involvement. Cervical and lumbar cord tend to be more affected than the thoracic region (Fig. 6–7).

Clinical Manifestations

The clinical picture of poliomyelitis ranges from a nonspecific mild febrile illness to a severe and potentially fatal paralytic disease. An inapparent infection is estimated to occur in 90%–95%, a minor nonparalytic illness in 4%–8% and paralytic poliomyelitis in 1%–2% of infected individuals (Fig. 6–8). The incubation period ranges between 5 and 35 days, with an average of 17 days.[151]

The minor illness coincides with the period of viremia and the presence of virus in the

but muscles totally paralyzed one month after the onset of the illness become completely normal only 1.4% of the time. Muscles severely paralyzed at the end of the acute period regain functional strength in 50% of instances, becoming normal in 20%. Moderately paralyzed muscles recover in 90% of instances. Half the affected muscles continue to improve after one year. Three-quarters of functional recoveries occur in the first year, slightly less than one-quarter during the second year and 5% during the third year. In general, prognosis is best for the proximal muscles in the lower extremities; it is poorest for the opponens pollicis and abdominal muscles.[161]

Relapses and second attacks are extremely rare.

Differential Diagnosis

Currently, poliomyelitis only occurs sporadically, and the diagnosis has become relatively difficult. A number of other enteroviruses, notably coxsackie and ECHO viruses, may produce a flaccid paralysis. When these conditions are unassociated with exanthem, their diagnosis rests on serologic studies or viral isolation.

Infectious polyneuritis presents with a symmetric paralysis, usually progressing for more than three to four days and unaccompanied by fever. When sensory deficits can be documented, they confirm the diagnosis of polyneuritis. The absence of pleocytosis in presence of a progressive paralysis also argues for polyneuritis.

Treatment

Control of poliomyelitis has been achieved by the use of orally administered live attenuated virus vaccine (Sabin). This has largely replaced the formalin-inactivated preparation (Salk). For a detailed discussion of the response to vaccination, the characteristics of immunity, and the complications of vaccination, the reader is referred to Bodian and Horstmann.[145]

During the acute phase of the illness, treatment is symptomatic.

Involvement of the spinal cord between C_3 and T_{12} may result in impaired respiratory motor function. Respiratory assistance is generally given when vital capacity drops below 50% of normal, when arterial oxygen saturation is 94% or less, or in the presence of respiratory acidosis. The normal adult or older child can often count to 40 with one breath; respiratory assistance may be required if he can only count to 10 or less. Cyanosis may not appear until O_2 saturation is 80%–85%, a level which may have already contributed to the damage of virus infected cells. Respiratory assistance can be rendered by means of mechanical respirators or phrenic nerve stimulators. In most instances, tracheostomy will be required.

For a full discussion of the various techniques of handling respiratory complication, the reader is referred to Russell.[162]

Other complications of the acute stage of poliomyelitis include infections of the respiratory tract and atelectasis. Urinary retention is treated with furfuryl trimethylammonium iodide (Furmethide) or may require drainage. Paralytic ileus with gastric atony may result from viral damage to the vegetative centers or altered serum potassium concentrations.

Urinary calculi result from the mobilization of bone calcium due to immobilization. Hemorrhagic diathesis may occur secondary to hypoxia with increased capillary permeability or nutritional hypoprothrombinemia.

Treatment of the chronic stage involves physiotherapy and orthopedic measures.[162]

COXSACKIE VIRUSES

An increasing number of coxsackie virus strains have been reported as causing infections of the human nervous system. The clinical picture produced by the various strains is indistinguishable. Neurologic manifestations include encephalitis, paralysis, acute meningitis, and epidemic pleurodynia. These occur with both type A and B infections.

Group A virus may cause acute lymphonodular pharyngitis, acute parotitis, hand-foot-and-mouth disease, and respiratory infections. Group B viruses have been associated with pleurodynia (Bornholm disease or epidemic myalgia), diarrhea, and both types have been associated with pericarditis and myocarditis. Anatomic alterations within the central nervous system are slight and nonspecific. They include meningeal inflammation and focal glial infiltration of gray and white matter of cerebrum, brain stem, and cerebellum.[163,164]

The clinical picture of aseptic meningitis due to infection with coxsackie virus is nonspecific. The illness is preceded by a prodromal phase manifested by malaise and gastrointestinal disturbances, during which viremia can be demonstrated. Neurologic symptoms may occur in association with pleurodynia, particularly in older children infected with B_1 and B_3 viruses. Exanthemata are rare.

A mild paralytic disease has been reported[165,166] as well as acute cerebellar ataxia,[167] unilateral paralysis of the oculomotor nerve,[168] and a postencephalitic Parkinson's picture.[166]

The diagnosis of coxsackie infection is made by recovering the virus from blood or cerebrospinal fluid, feces, and oropharyngeal swabbings, and by demonstrating a concurrent increase in neutralizing antibodies against the isolated virus.

The prognosis for recovery is usually excellent, and treatment is purely symptomatic.

ECHO VIRUS INFECTIONS

This group of viruses is the most frequent cause of enterovirus infection of the nervous system. Sporadic infections have been described for 25 members of the group while outbreaks usually occur with types 4, 6, 9, 11, 16, 18, and 30.

The clinical manifestations are variable. Most common is an aseptic meningitis.[169] This illness is biphasic, and generally self-limited. It presents a nonspecific picture of fever, headache, signs of meningeal irritation, sore throat, neck and back pain, and occasionally myalgia. The illness usually terminates in seven to ten days. While in most cases there are no paralytic residua, a few patients have been left with impaired strength in the anterior neck muscles.

A paralytic disease indistinguishable from poliomyelitis may occur with ECHO infections. Paralysis may be mild and transient or so severe as to be permanent or fatal. In the latter type of case, the virus has been isolated from central nervous tissue.

Encephalitis manifested by focal or generalized seizures, disorders of sensorium, tremor, cranial nerve deficits, disorders of ocular movement, choreiform movements, paresthesias, and other signs of cerebral dysfunction has been associated with ECHO virus infections.[170] Cerebellar ataxia of short duration as well as acute ascending polyradiculomyelitis have also been described.[171]

The diagnosis of ECHO virus usually rests on laboratory tests. Certain viral strains may produce an illness associated with exanthematous or petechial rashes which may antecede or associate with the period of central nervous involvement.

The association of lymphadenopathy, pericarditis, myocarditis, conjunctivitis, and photophobia distinguishes ECHO virus from poliomyelitis but is not sufficiently characteristic for a diagnosis.

ADENOVIRUSES

Adenovirus infection usually causes an acute respiratory disease associated with conjunctivitis or keratoconjunctivitis. In a small percentage of cases, these symptoms are associated with involvement of the nervous system, notably a severe encephalitis or meningoencephalitis.[172]

ROSEOLA

Roseola, the most common exanthem of infancy, is characterized by the relative absence of prodromata, a rapid rise in temperature, and conspicuously little listlessness or irritability. The temperature remains elevated for three to five days, subsiding with the appearance of a maculopapular rash.

Seizures are a common concomitant to the disease, their incidence varying considerably from one series of cases to another. While these are by and large benign, persistent neurologic complications have been reported.[173] These include hemiparesis, recurrent seizures, and mental retardation. The etiology of the residual encephalopathy is unknown.

ARBOVIRUSES

INTRODUCTION

Arthropod-borne (Arbo) viruses are RNA viral agents transmitted between susceptible vertebrate hosts by means of bloodsucking arthropods.[174,175] About 200 viruses have been tentatively classified into this group, and about 150 of these are assigned to 21 groups which share common antigens. At least 51 have been associated with disease in man. The epidemiology of this disease is largely determined by the nature and life-style of the vector. Most of the infections are sustained in sylvan hosts, with transmission through man and domestic animals usually incidental and insignificant in the natural history of virus. Of greatest significance in this country are California encephalitis (CE), St. Louis encephalitis (SLE), western equine encephalomyelitis (WE), eastern equine encephalomyelitis (EEE), Venezuelan equine encephalomyelitis (VE), and Colorado tick fever.

In man, these viruses may fail to elicit any manifestation or may produce a mild generalized illness. The full-blown diseases, which are discussed in this section, are the least common manifestations of infection.

The nonspecific symptomatology requires diagnosis by means of laboratory studies. A significant antibody rise is usual within three weeks of onset, but may require as long as eight weeks. Neutralizing titers usually remain elevated for longer periods than hemagglutination inhibition or complement fixation titers.[174,175] The virus may be isolated from blood or nervous tissue, but not from spinal fluid.

CALIFORNIA ENCEPHALITIS

This condition is more prevalent in the midwestern and southern United States than in California. Since the first isolation of virus in 1943 and 1944 from naturally infected mosquitoes in the San Joaquin Valley of California, increasing numbers of human cases have been recognized and currently it is the most common arbovirus encephalitis in the United States.[176] The vectors for this virus are *Culex* and *Aedes* mosquitoes.

Pathology

The alterations within the brain are largely microscopic and are those of an acute encephalitis[177] without distinctive findings.

Clinical Manifestations

The peak incidence is between July and October. There is a strong association between rural outdoor exposure, and the presence of antibodies and clinical illness. Thus, the incidence of antibodies is 26.8% in rural populations and 15.3% in urban areas. Large increments in antibody occur between ages five and nine among rural and between 10 and 19 years among urban populations in endemic areas.[176]

The peak incidence of California encephalitis is between four and nine years of age; males are three times more commonly affected than females.

The clinical picture is that of a meningo-encephalitis with fever, changes in consciousness, headache, and meningeal irritation.[178,179,180,181]

The cerebrospinal fluid shows a pleocytosis, which in 85% is mainly mononuclear. The protein content is mildly elevated. The EEG is always abnormal, with abnormalities persisting for months or years.

Diagnosis

In contrast to infections caused by enteroviruses, the illness is not bi-phasic, is not associated with upper respiratory or gastroenteric signs or symptoms, and familial outbreaks are extremely rare.

Prognosis

California virus encephalitis is a relatively mild illness, with a low mortality. Initially, older patients tend to show emotional lability, difficulty in learning and personality problems.[180] Later on, difficulties in processing visual and auditory information become apparent and many children develop a personality resembling that of the "organic hyperkinetic syndrome."[181a]

ST. LOUIS ENCEPHALITIS

This encephalitis was first recognized in St. Louis in the summer of 1932 during an epidemic of encephalitis that originated in Paris, Illinois. Since then, sporadic outbreaks have occurred in the St. Louis area, as well as in California, the Rio Grande valley, in Florida, and in the central river valleys and western coastal regions of the United States.

The vector for this virus is the *Culex* mosquito.

Pathology

There is diffuse vascular congestion and edema, with meningeal and perivascular infiltration, petechiae, and glial nodules. Lesions predominate in the thalamus and substantia nigra. The cortex, the anterior horns of the spinal cord, the molecular and Purkinje cell layers and the dentate nucleus of the cerebellum are also involved.[185]

Clinical Manifestations

Most commonly, this virus produces a clinically inapparent infection. The attack rate, studied during the Houston epidemic of 1964, was 4.3 per 100,000 for children under the age of nine. Most cases occur in late summer and early fall; boys are three times more commonly affected than girls.

About 58% of children contract a benign disease with symptoms of viral meningitis. The remainder of children with clinically apparent infections develop a severe encephalitis. Its onset may be sudden, or it may follow a mild prodromal stage of 24–72 hours duration.[186] In the 1964 Houston epidemic, most children had fever, headache, and meningeal irritation. Ataxia was noted in 27% and fine tremors of the upper extremity in 19%. Cranial nerve palsies were encountered in 12%.[187]

The abnormalities in the cerebrospinal fluid are those expected for a viral encephalitis, namely a pleocytosis, which initially is predominantly polymorphonuclear, but later becomes monocytic,[186] a mild elevation of protein levels, and a normal sugar content. The EEG is often abnormal. Electromyographic studies have shown fasciculations (59%), fibrillations (8%), and excessive insertional potentials (54%). In some cases, these abnormalities have persisted for over one month.[187]

Prognosis

St. Louis encephalitis is intermediate in severity between California encephalitis and the equine encephalitides. The mortality in the 1964 St. Louis epidemic was 8% in children under 10. In more recent epidemics, it has ranged from 0%–22%. Major sequelae occur less often than following Eastern or Western equine encephalitis. They have been noted in 1.0%–7.7% of survivors. Most commonly, they involve disturbances of gait and equilibrium,[188,189,190] difficulties in speech and vision, and changes in personality.

Treatment

No vaccine is currently available, and control must be directed against the mosquito vector.

WESTERN EQUINE ENCEPHALITIS

Western equine encephalomyelitis is caused by a group A arbovirus which occurs in the western United States and in the central states west of the Mississippi Valley. The organism was first isolated in 1930 in California from horses with encephalitis. The chief vectors are several *Culex* mosquitoes although *Aedes* species have also been found to carry the virus.[174]

Pathology

The alterations within the nervous system are similar to those seen in the other encephalitides due to arboviruses. The greatest damage is usually in the basal ganglia and cerebral white matter, with foci of demyelination and necrosis. There may be extensive cystic degeneration of white matter in infants.

A striking finding, noted as late as five years after onset of the acute illness, is the presence of both chronic inactive areas of destruction, as well as the active foci glial proliferation and perivascular cuffing. This suggests that a slow progressive form of the disease may continue for years.[182]

In chronic cases, there may be significant endothelial proliferation with a vasculitis producing almost complete occlusion of small vessels. Scattered areas of focal necrosis often contain phagocytic elements. In some cases extensive cavities may replace brain tissue.[190,191]

Clinical Manifestations

Clinically inapparent infections far outnumber overt cases, although in infants under one year, there is an equal incidence of apparent and inapparent infections.[192]

In infants under one year of age, the clinical picture is one of sudden onset of high fever (92%), accompanied by focal or generalized seizures (77%).[193] In older children, the picture is one of a severe encephalitis with fever, headache, vomiting, changes in consciousness, and meningeal signs. Convulsions are less common in older children. They develop in about 50% of children aged one to four years, and in 9% of children in the 5 to 14-year-old group.

Symptoms usually persist for about 10 days, then gradually subside. In fatal cases, the course is rapidly downhill. The CSF findings resemble those encountered in the other arbovirus infections.[193]

The mortality rate in different epidemics has ranged from 9% to 23%. Sequelae are frequent and are most severe in very young infants. Of infants who contracted the illness when they were less than one month of age 56% had major sequelae.[190] These include microcephaly,[182] pyramidal or extrapyramidal motor impairment, seizures, and developmental retardation. From follow-up studies conducted on survivors it is apparent that the younger the patient at the time of his illness, the greater the incidence and severity of sequelae.[182,183] In older infants and in children the sequelae become less severe. In Finley's series, no patient contracting the illness between one and two years of age developed motor or behavior problems; 25%, however, developed seizures.[182] Such seizures represent persistence of convulsions which first appeared during the acute illness.

There is no vaccine or specific treatment.

EASTERN EQUINE ENCEPHALITIS

This group A arbovirus was first isolated in 1933 from brain tissue of infected horses. It is distributed along the Atlantic coast from the northeastern United States to Argentina. Small epidemics have been encountered in Massachusetts, New Jersey, and more recently in Jamaica. The virus is transmitted by a variety of mosquitoes.[174]

Pathology

The outstanding feature of eastern equine encephalitis is the predominance of neutrophilic leukocytes in the infiltrates. This undoubtedly reflects the rapid demise of most fatally infected patients. Focal or diffuse accumulations of neutrophils and histiocytes are prominent in the leptomeninges and in the cerebral cortex, particularly the occipital and frontal lobes and hippocampus.[194]

Foci of tissue damage with rarefaction necrosis permeated by neutrophilic leukocytes and pleomorphic ameboid cells are often found. Neuronolysis, often with adjacent neutrophilic leukocytes and microglial cells, is very common in fulminant cases.

Large perivascular collections of neutrophils, histiocytes, and other ameboid cells are detected in the white matter in regions of cortical involvement. Other sites of predilection are the basal ganglia and brain stem, in particular the thalamus, putamen, substantia nigra, and the basilar portion of the pons.

Edema and congestion are prevalent early. Vascular lesions characterized by numerous small thrombi in arterioles and venules may occur. Many vessels show complete involvement of their walls with neutrophilic infiltration and fibrin deposition.

As the disease progresses, the dominant cell type changes to mononuclear lymphocytes and macrophages.[190,195]

Clinical Manifestations

Infection with the virus of eastern equine encephalitis has the most serious prognosis of all virus infections prevalent in the United States.

The illness is particularly common in infants, two-thirds of the patients being less than two years old. It is usually fulminant with an abrupt onset, high fever, stupor or coma, convulsions, and signs of meningeal irritation. Patients may succumb within 48 hours of their initial symptoms or may survive for a few days, succumbing to damage of the vital medullary centers, dural sinus thrombosis, or subarachnoid hemorrhage. Survivors may remain comatose for several days or weeks before becoming responsive.

Laboratory studies are not diagnostic. The

TABLE 6-14.
CLINICAL CHARACTERISTICS OF NEUROTROPIC
ARBOVIRUSES

Name	Distribution	Vector	Reference
Japanese B	Eastern Siberia, China, Korea, Taiwan	Mosquito	190, 196, 197
Murray Valley encephalitis	Eastern Australia (valleys of Murray and Darling Rivers, Victoria, New South Wales), New Guinea	Mosquito	184
Tick-borne group B encephalitis (Russian spring-summer, far eastern tick-borne encephalitis)	Siberia, Czechoslovakia	Tick	175, 190, 198
Kyasanur forest disease	India	Tick	195
Powassan virus	Ontario, Canada	Tick	195, 199
Colorado tick fever	Western U.S.A.	Wood tick	190, 200, 201

peripheral blood may show a prominent leukocytosis.

The cerebrospinal fluid may be under a striking increase in pressure. Initial spinal fluid cell counts range between 250 and 2000 WBC per mm³, often with 60% to almost 100% polymorphonuclear cells. The pleocytosis diminishes rapidly, and mononuclear cells predominate after three days in patients who survive.[195]

Prognosis

The mortality rate in eastern equine encephalitis in patients under 10 years is approximately 68%.[190] Severe sequelae are noted, including mental retardation, motor dysfunction, deafness, and seizures. Complete neurologic recovery was only seen in a small proportion of survivors.

VENEZUELAN EQUINE ENCEPHALOMYELITIS

Although this group A arbovirus is indigenous to Colombia, Venezuela, and Panama, it was responsible for the 1971 Texas encephalitis epidemic. The organism has been isolated from many wild rodents as well as from *Aedes* and *Culex* mosquitoes.[174,196]

This disease is much more benign than the California, St. Louis, eastern, or western equine encephalomyelitides. There is sudden onset of malaise, chills and fever, nausea and vomiting, headache, myalgia, and bone pain. The fever lasts from 24 to 96 hours, then abruptly drops. A period of 2–3 weeks of marked asthenia may follow. The CSF findings are as in the other arbovirus infections.

Prognosis is good and, with good care, fatalities are rare.

The distribution of encephalitides due to other arboviruses is summarized in Table 6–14.

HERPES SIMPLEX

Herpes simplex virus is a widespread organism which commonly infects man. It produces a protean picture that only rarely results in neurologic manifestations.

Prenatal herpes infection, referred to elsewhere in this chapter, may result in various congenital malformations including microcephaly, intracranial calcifications, and retinal dysplasia.

Etiology

Herpes virus occurs in two distinct serologic and biologic types.[202] Type I strains are isolated mainly from the oropharynx and upper body, while type II is associated with the genital area. Newborn infants usually contract type II virus which may produce encephalitis, while older children and adults have herpes simplex type I isolated from the cerebrospinal fluid or brain tissue.[203]

Experimental virus invasion of the nervous system has been demonstrated following intranasal inoculation. The virus spreads through infection of mucosal and submucosal cells, ultimately crossing the cribriform plate or by infection of endoneural and perineural cells of the olfactory fibers to involve the parenchymal cells of the olfactory bulb.[204] This mode of entry is relevant to the tendency for herpes encephalitis to be associated with anosmia and to cause focal and rhinencephalic lesions.

Herpes virus spread may occur during primary exposure, or after prolonged infection.[205] Encephalitis has developed following long-term steroid therapy, and experimentally, after injection of adrenalin or induction of anaphylactic shock.[206]

Pathology

Central nervous system infection by herpes simplex virus shows the usual microscopic picture of viral encephalitis, i.e., lymphocytic infiltration of the meninges, perivascular aggregates of lymphocytes and histiocytes in the cortex and subadjacent white matter, and proliferation of microglia with formation of glial nodules. Several pathologic features are, however, distinctive:

1. Severity of the process. Necrosis is unusually severe in the areas of greatest involvement, with gross softening, destruction of architecture, hemorrhage, and, in severe cases, loss of all nervous and glial elements.

2. Topography of lesions. While lesions are generally widespread with many foci of hemorrhage and necrosis, the medial temporal and orbital regions are the most severely damaged.

3. Inclusion bodies. Intranuclear Cowdry type A inclusion bodies are recognized in neurons, oligodendroglia, and astrocytes.[207]

Clinical Manifestations

The incidence of central nervous system involvement in herpes simplex infections is uncertain, but the condition probably accounts for about 10% of all viral infections of the CNS. In general, its incidence is least between the ages of 5 and 15.[208]

Prodromal symptoms unrelated to central nervous system disease occur in about 60% of patients. Fever and malaise are most common; symptoms of respiratory infection were present in one-third of patients. When seen, this prodromal period usually lasts one to seven days.

Neurologic involvement includes aseptic meningitis and encephalitis of a diffuse or focal nature.[208] Aseptic meningitis is seen in about 20% of cases. Patients experience an acute febrile illness with headache, stiff neck, occasionally with orchitis or pneumonitis. Cerebrospinal fluid pleocytosis is common, ranging from 300 to 1000 cells with a protein concentration from 50 to about 200 mg%. In 12% of cases, the initial CSF examination may be normal.[208a] Though asymptomatic, spinal fluid changes may persist for months. Encephalitis may or may not accompany herpes elsewhere on the body.

Aseptic meningitis is relatively benign and patients recover uneventfully after four to seven days.

More commonly herpes is associated with encephalitis. The clinical findings are of two types: nonspecific changes of encephalitis including fever, papilledema, meningeal irritation, global confusion, and changes referable to focal necrosis, usually of the orbital or temporal regions of the brain, including anosmia, memory loss, disordered behavior, and olfactory or gustatory hallucinations.[207]

Initial signs of herpes encephalitis are frequently referable to the central nervous system. The most common early signs are fever, headache, and a sudden onset of major motor convulsions, often unilateral. The last are seen in about 40% of patients. In 10%–20%, the disease appears more subtly; expressive aphasia or paresthesias precede the more severe central nervous system signs. Generally the disease pursues an unremitting course. High fever, resistant to antipyretics, is common. Five-sixths of the patients become comatose, the remainder have other disturbances of consciousness.

Localizing signs are found in about three-fourths of patients, mostly focal seizures and paralyses. Patients with localized findings may also show focal EEG abnormalities.[210] Angiography suggests the presence of a mass lesion, often localized to the temporal lobe. When encephalitis is accompanied by seizures and coma, a fatal outcome can be expected in about three-fourths of instances.[209] Surviving patients usually improve after 10–25 days; they do not suffer from persistent chronic encephalitis.

Residua may include severe disturbances in mental function, either isolated damage to memory or speech areas or diffuse cerebral damage. Selective cognitive deficits, mental retardation, personality changes, incoordination, seizures, or hemiparesis may also remain.

The mortality from herpes encephalitis ranges from 20%[205] to 70%.[208] Approximately half of the survivors aged 5 to 11 had major residual deficits.[205]

The cerebrospinal fluid is normal in about one-quarter of patients. In the remainder it is under increased pressure, shows a pleocytosis and an elevation in protein concentration which may persist for months. In other cases, the fluid may be hemorrhagic or xanthochromic due to acute hemorrhagic encephalitis.

The electroencephalogram is usually diffusely abnormal. It may suggest a focal temporal or frontal lesion, or there may be focal centrotemporal spike complexes, recurring every one to two seconds against a slow wave background.[210] The brain scan may show diffuse or focal abnormalities.

Diagnosis

The clinical picture of herpes encephalitis or aseptic meningitis may be indistinguishable from that produced by other viral organisms. When present, focal temporal lobe or limbic symptoms suggest the diagnosis, as may the presence of a bloody or xanthochromic spinal fluid. A history of preceding herpetic infection, or the presence of mucocutaneous herpes is present in fewer than 50% of patients.

Serologic diagnosis has not been satisfactory for herpes encephalitis. Fourfold rises in titer may occur from herpes infection at other sites. Antecedent herpes virus infection may give elevations in titer which do not change significantly during neurologic involvement. A rise in IgM herpes antibody correlates best with an active herpetic process. Some acute cases of herpes encephalitis may represent reactivation of latent infection or reinfection rather than new infection.

Histologic confirmation or virus isolation may require early brain biopsy which must be taken from the involved area either by needle aspiration or direct surgical approach.[211] Histopathologic changes may be missed if the wrong site is biopsied or may be misinterpreted since Cowdry type A inclusion bodies occur in other diseases such as subacute sclerosing panencephalitis. Even in proven cases attempts at viral isolation may be unsuccessful.

The differentiation of herpes encephalitis from a rapidly evolving cerebral tumor is often difficult. Diffuse sclerosis may also present with focal neurologic signs and evidence of cerebral swelling. The presence of a bloody cerebrospinal fluid may suggest an intracranial hemorrhage from a variety of other causes.

Therapy

Recent experience with idoxuridine suggests that the drug may be effective when started early in the course of herpes encephalitis.[212,213] Cytosine arabinoside has also been used with apparent benefit.[214]

The combination of 5'-iodo-2'-deoxyuridine and surgical decompression has also been recommended.[215] Dexamethasone has been recommended to reduce cerebral edema but its role in therapy for this condition is not well-established.[216]

No treatment is required for herpetic aseptic meningitis.

HERPES ZOSTER

Herpes zoster is due to varicella virus localized to dorsal root ganglia and its connections, and to the skin area corresponding to the distribution of the involved sensory nerves.

Clinical, epidemiologic, and virologic evidence have established that the varicella virus also causes herpes zoster.[217] The localized nature of zoster infection, the age-group distribution and past history of varicella in many cases of herpes zoster indicate it to be an infection with varicella virus in a partially immune host. Zoster vesicle fluid can produce typical varicella lesions in susceptible children. Serologic and viral studies do not distinguish between the two agents though zoster patients carry a higher immune titer. It is believed that the initial varicella exposure results in viral infection of neuronal tissue; any subsequent reversion to generalized infection is suppressed by persistent immunity. Gradual attenuation of the resistance, or immune suppression for extrinsic or intrinsic reasons, may lower antibody to a level which permits the virus to activate. Once established, this exacerbation of infection elicits an anamnestic immune response too late to abort the process.[218]

The age-related incidence of herpes zoster is about 0.74 per 1000 for children 0–9 years of age, 1.38 for those 10–19 years, and remains about 2.5 per 1000 through age 49 when it rises steadily to 5.09 per 1000 in age 50–59

years and to 10.1 per 1000 in the group 80–89 years of age.[218] Neonatal cases have been described. As a rule children over two years old have had a previous attack of varicella; those under two years may have been exposed in utero or during infancy without clinical disease. Incidence of second attacks is 3–5 per 1000.[218] Rarely children may develop segmental symptoms of herpes zoster during an attack of varicella.

Pathology

The pathologic changes in herpes zoster are usually limited to one dorsal root or sensory ganglion, and the corresponding nerve.[219] Around a central area of congestion and hemorrhage due to intense inflammation and hemorrhagic necrosis there is infiltration with lymphocytes, plasma cells, and polymorphonuclear cells. Nerve cells in the area demonstrate degeneration and neuronophagia. Involvement often extends to the spinal cord where microglial cells abound in the dorsal horns and in Clarke's column, as well as in the lateral and ventral horns. Anterior horn cells may show chromatolysis and neuronophagy. Similar involvement in the brain

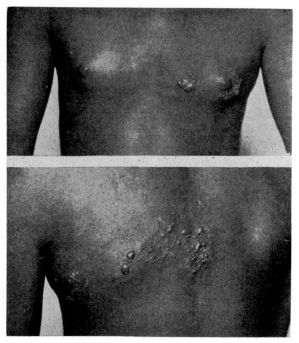

Fig. 6–9. Herpes zoster showing the skin eruption over the fifth thoracic dermatome. (From Ford, F. R.: *Diseases of the Nervous System in Infancy, Childhood and Adolescence*, 5th ed., 1966, courtesy of Charles C Thomas Publisher, Springfield.)

stem accompanies infection of the trigeminal or glossopharyngeal nerve.

Clinical Manifestations

Essential to herpes zoster are grouped vesicular lesions distributed over one or more dermatomes. Systemic reactions, usually fever, nuchal rigidity, headache, and enlargement of the regional lymph nodes, are common in children. In 89% of patients under 12 years the lesion is localized to the thoracolumbar area (Fig. 6–9). Cervical herpes is seen in 8% and maxillary lesions in 3% of children. Ophthalmic herpes and geniculate herpes are extremely rare.

The skin lesions first appear as erythematous papules, which progress to vesicles within 12–24 hours, and to pustules in 72 hours. Lesions often appear in the proximal area of the dermatome and spread peripherally. When pustulation appears, the surrounding erythema begins to subside, and in seven to eight days pustules begin to dry up. Crusts form in 10–12 days, which fall off in two or three weeks. Unilateral involvement is the rule, with bilateral involvement in only 0.5% of cases.

About two-thirds of children complain of pain. This may be a prodrome, occur during the acute infection, or develop after the skin inflammation has subsided. The pain is evanescent in some, persistent in others; it bears no relationship to the severity of cutaneous lesions. Patients describe it as pruritic, aching, stabbing, or burning in nature.

The most common adult complication of herpes zoster—postherpetic neuralgia—is uncommon in children.

Localized paralyses and atrophy of muscles are not unusual, and in some instances are permanent.

Ascending myelitis and a diffuse encephalomyelitis have been reported.[220]

The association of herpes zoster with leukemia and Hodgkins' disease has been well-documented. Treatment of the underlying malignancy with corticosteroids, antimetabolites and alkylating agents did not appear to have an untoward effect on the course of herpes.[221]

Disseminated herpes zoster occurs in 2%–

5% of cases. Widespread lesions involving the skin, mucous membranes, and lungs, and a clinical syndrome with many characteristics of varicella may develop within 2–12 days, usually by six days after the onset of herpes zoster.[222]

Diagnosis

The herpetic eruption has a characteristic appearance and distribution. In the differential diagnosis of facial palsy, herpetic lesions of the tympanic membrane and the external auditory canal should be looked for.

Treatment

Treatment is limited to the prevention of secondary infections of the skin lesion.

RABIES

Rabies is an acute infection of the nervous system, caused by an RNA virus with predilection for exocrine glands and kidneys as well as for the nervous system. The virus is in the saliva of infected mammals and is transmitted by bite. The disease was well described by Greek and Roman clinicians. Pasteur's study of the disease led to his development of a modified virus vaccine in 1885[223] which is still the basis for immunization.

Etiology and Pathology

The domestic dog is the principal cause of human infection. The virus carried in saliva is transmitted through a bite or skin abrasion. Other mammals responsible for human infections include a variety of bats, such as the vampire bat, various fruit-eating and insectivorous bats, and wolves. The skunk, bat, cat, fox, coyote, and raccoon are major reservoirs for the virus.[224] The disease has also been contracted by indirect exposure, probably by inhalation of virus particles in a bat-infested cave.[225] Depending on the site of the wound and the character of the bite, humans bitten by rabid dogs contract the disease in 10%–20% of instances.[226] A heavy inoculum accompanying considerable tissue damage (e.g., wolf bite) is much more likely to cause fatality than a lesser bite (e.g., dog). Bites about the face and neck are most dangerous. A fatal clinical illness is 10 times more

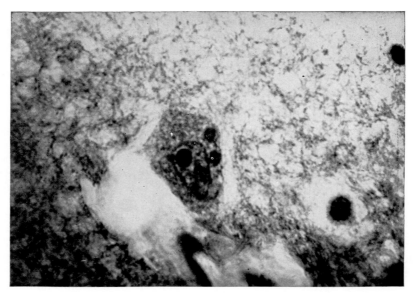

Fig. 6–10. Rabies. Inclusion bodies (Negri bodies) in cytoplasm of ganglion cell of cerebral cortex. (From Merritt, H. H.: *Textbook of Neurology*, 4th ed., 1970, courtesy of Lea & Febiger, Phialdelphia.)

likely following a face bite than a bite on the upper extremity and 28 times more likely than following a lower extremity bite.[227]

The virus reaches the central nervous system along peripheral nerves.[228] The essential pathology of rabies is that of a generalized encephalomyelitis. When the site of exposure is on the extremities, the corresponding posterior horn of the spinal cord will show marked hyperemia, neuronophagia, and cellular infiltration. Intracytoplasmic eosinophilic inclusions (Negri bodies) (Fig. 6–10) can be demonstrated in the neurons in most cases. These consist of many aggregated viral particles, and are pathognomonic of the disease.[229] They are most numerous in the forebrain; usually they abound in the pyramidal layer of the hippocampus but are also common in the cerebral cortex and in the cerebellar Purkinje cells. These inclusions are only seen after infection with street or "wild" virus, not with fixed or adapted virus. Another eosinophilic cytoplasmic body, the Lyssa body, is seen not only in rabies but also in a variety of other degenerative conditions not related to virus infection.

Distribution of microscopic lesions differs with the two clinical types of disease. In the classic form following a dog bite and charac-

terized clinically by restlessness and dysphagia, the chief lesions are in the brain stem, notably in the jugular, Gasserian, and dorsal root ganglia, and in the lower two-thirds of the medulla. Infiltrations may also be seen in the substantia nigra, the hypothalamic nuclei, the peripheral nerves, the spinal cord, and the cerebral and cerebellar hemispheres.

The paralytic form following bat bites results in congestion of the cord and striking softening of the lower cord. Neuronal degeneration is marked in both anterior and posterior horns and extends up into the medulla. Microglial infiltration is marked, but Negri bodies are often sparse.

Clinical Manifestations

The highest incidence of rabies in man occurs in children under 15. The incubation period usually ranges from one to three months but may be as short as 10 days or as long as eight months.[226]

There are three phases. The *initial* or *premonitory phase*, of two to four days' duration, is characterized by fever, headache, anorexia, malaise, and sore throat. The temperature may be mildly elevated but is seldom higher than 102° F. The most striking symptom during this period is numbness or paresthesia in the region of the bite. This occurs in about 80% of cases and has been ascribed to the direct action of the virus on sensory neurons. Decreased sensitivity to local pain can be demonstrated, yet paradoxically patients complain bitterly of drafts and bedclothes which cause general stimulation of the skin.

Symptoms of the second or *excitement phase* usually have a gradual onset. Hyperacusis and photophobia may occur. Objective signs include hyperactive deep tendon reflexes, increased muscle tone, and tics; facial expression becomes overactive. Symptoms referable to the autonomic system may be prominent; they include pupillary dilatation, lacrimation, excessive salivation, and increased perspiration.

As the excitement phase progresses, the patient is increasingly nervous, sleepless, anxious, and apprehensive. The outstanding clinical symptom of rabies is related to the act of swallowing. When fluid comes in contact with the fauces it is expelled with considerable violence; there are painful spasmodic contractions of the muscles of deglutition and of the accessory muscles of respiration. Subsequently, the sight, smell, or sound of liquids may precipitate spasm. Drooling of bloody saliva may be prominent at this time.[230] Choking with attempts at swallowing may result in such severe spasm of the respiratory muscles that prolonged apnea develops with cyanosis and anoxia. The term "hydrophobia" has derived from this phenomenon.

Convulsions are common, as is maniacal behavior, such as tearing of clothes and bedding. Periods of intense excitement are interspersed with relative quiet, during which the patient is oriented and responds intelligently.

Most patients die in the acute excitement stage during a convulsion, often before the *paralytic phase* becomes evident. Depressive or paralytic symptoms may dominate the disease picture from its onset or may supervene at any time. Weakness of muscle groups in the vicinity of the bite may become apparent early in the disease. If the patient survives the acute excitement stage, in one to three days muscle spasm often ceases and the patient becomes quiet. Ability to swallow with difficulty may be retained. The face becomes expressionless; anxiety and excitement are replaced by apathy, stupor, and coma. Bowel and bladder control may be lost. Then for a few hours the patient may seem to improve, but this apparent remission is rapidly followed by progressive paralysis.

In rare instances, ascending paralysis begins in the muscles of the legs and progresses without relationship to the original site of infection. Rabies in man, following the bite of the vampire bat as described in Trinidad, is uniformly of the paralytic type.[226]

Death may be due to heart failure as well as hypoxia; myocarditis has been reported.[231] The disease is uniformly fatal. One child has recovered after developing the disease in spite of immunization with duck embryo vaccine.[231a]

The white blood count is increased and may range from 20,000 to 30,000 WBC/mm^3 with a polymorphonuclear preponderance. There is frequently minimal proteinuria, glycosuria, and acetonuria. Cerebrospinal fluid cell count usually is within normal limits but a mononuclear pleocytosis of more than 100 cells has been encountered.[226]

Diagnosis

The diagnosis of rabies in man is based on the history, the clinical features, and laboratory procedures. Often the long incubation periods make the history of a bite unreliable, and laboratory tests, including serum antibodies, may be negative—possibly due to an inhibiting substance which neutralizes the rabies virus. Fluorescent antibody tests on saliva may be equally disappointing.[232]

Prevention and Treatment

Once symptoms are present, rabies progresses inexorably and is generally fatal; only one symptomatic person has been known to survive. The recommended procedure for prevention of the disease in the exposed child has been summarized recently.[226] Among infectious diseases, rabies is unique in that the long incubation period allows the induction of active as well as passive immunity prior to the onset of illness. The former is achieved by use of one of two types of rabies vaccines. The Pasteur-brain-fixed virus vaccine is a

severity. Motor and sensory functions are usually impaired, and cerebrospinal fluid changes similar to those in acute infectious polyneuritis (Guillain-Barré) have been reported.

Encephalomyelitis is a rare complication of infectious mononucleosis. It may present with cerebral, cerebellar, brain stem, or spinal cord signs, singly or in combination. Generalized or myoclonic seizures may be evident. A mononeuritis of a variety of nerves has also been reported. These have included an olfactory and an optic neuritis, the latter with papillitis,[245,246] as well as palsies of the third, fourth, and sixth cranial nerves,[247] one or both facial nerves, and the nerve to the serratus anterior muscle.[246]

Approximately 30% of patients with infectious mononucleosis upon examination of the cerebrospinal fluid have had five or more cells/mm^3.[248] These alterations may persist for months, often after complete clinical recovery.

Electroencephalographic abnormalities have been noted in 35% of children.[248]

The diagnosis of infectious mononucleosis is best established by serologic studies. Davidsohn[249] has suggested that a positive heterophile titer of over 1:224 before absorption, or 1:64 after absorption with guinea pig kidney as the criterion for diagnosis. Heterophile antibodies are occasionally demonstrated in the cerebrospinal fluid. A rise in serum antibody to EB virus may be diagnostic.

Recovery from the neurologic sequelae usually occurs rapidly,[250] and is complete in 85% of patients within a few days to several months. In some cases there is a poor correlation between the severity of the neurologic disorder and the clinical course, prognosis and laboratory findings.

No specific therapy or vaccine is available.

CAT SCRATCH DISEASE

This infectious illness, first described by Debré in 1950,[251] is in man caused by the scratch of a cat. It is characterized by fever, a primary cutaneous lesion with regional lymphadenitis, and occasional neurologic complications which form the principal topic of this section.

Etiology

The isolation of a hemagglutinating virus, and the demonstration of herpeslike particles under the electron microscope[252,253] suggest that a viral agent is responsible. Complement fixation tests with psittacosis-ornithosis-lymphogranuloma venereum-trachoma group of antigens show significant antibody titers in about 50% of adult patients as compared with 3%–6% of controls.[254]

Clinical Manifestations

Neurologic manifestations usually follow the initial symptoms of the illness by one to five weeks.[251] The most frequently observed complication is encephalitis, which accounts for 90% of neurologic cases, but encephalomyelitis (5%), and encephalomyeloradiculitis (5%) have also been reported.[255,256]

The onset of the encephalitic phase is usually precipitous, with convulsions, confusion, lethargy, stupor, and coma. Despite the apparent severity of the picture, improvement is rapid, and restoration of consciousness generally occurs within 2–10 days. Varieties of transient neurologic sequelae have been encountered, and an occasional patient has succumbed to the encephalitis.[255]

The cerebrospinal fluid is usually normal. Rarely, there is a mild to moderate mononuclear pleocytosis.[255] The electroencephalogram is almost uniformly abnormal during the acute phase of the illness; focal or generalized abnormalities may persist for several years even after an apparently complete clinical recovery.[255]

Diagnosis

The diagnosis is suggested by a positive intradermal skin test employing antigen prepared from suppurative human lesions and confirmed by positive lymphogranuloma venereum complement fixation titers. The Frei skin test antigen, which is also positive in some cases, may induce elevations in the complement fixation titer and is therefore not recommended for diagnostic purposes.

Treatment

No treatment or immunization has been successful.

SLOW VIRUS INFECTIONS AND RELATED DISORDERS

Although a chronic encephalopathy of sheep (scrapie) was first described by Sigurdsson in 1954,[257] the concept that a virus may continue to multiply within the host over the course of several months to years, ultimately producing a progressive debilitative disease of the nervous system, is relatively new. Such an infection has been termed a slow virus infection.[257,258]

Characteristically, slow viruses multiply in the host for prolonged periods without producing clinical symptoms. As these viruses are not recognized as "foreign" by the host, his immune response is either very late or absent. Therefore the disease produced by a slow virus may either be the result of a gradual destruction of affected cells, or an auto-immune response caused by termination of tolerance.

Of the various conditions believed to result from slow virus infections only three—kuru, subacute sclerosing panencephalitis (SSPE), and Creutzfeldt-Jakob disease—have been proven to have a viral etiology. The first two of these occur in children.

KURU

Kuru, first described by Berndt in 1954,[259] is a progressive degenerative disease of the central nervous system with predominantly cerebellar features. The disease is limited to the Fore tribe of the eastern highlands of central New Guinea, in a population that until recently practiced cannibalism.

Pathologic changes are only seen on microscopy.[260] They include widespread neuronal degeneration, most marked within the cerebellum, proliferation of astroglia and microglia, and minimal demyelination. The disease has been transmitted experimentally to the chimpanzee, in whom it develops after incubation periods ranging from 18 to 30 months.[261] It is now believed to have passed from human to human by the cannibalistic ingestion of infected human brain.

The clinical course is remarkably uniform. In boys, the mean age of onset is about 14 years. In females, the age of onset has a bimodal distribution, with one mode occurring at about eight years, the other at 33 years. The initial symptom is ataxia, which is progressive and accompanied by a fine tremor of the trunk, extremities, and head. During the second to third month of illness the tremor becomes more coarse and severe, and choreiform movements may appear. Intelligence is preserved, although alterations in mood are common. In most children the disease is fatal within six to nine months of onset.

Laboratory studies have been unremarkable; in particular, there have been no abnormalities of the cerebrospinal fluid.

Although no therapy has been effective once symptoms have become apparent, abolition of cannibalism among the Fore tribe has led to disappearance of the illness among children.

SUBACUTE SCLEROSING PANENCEPHALITIS (SSPE)

This slow virus infection, first described in Tennessee children by Dawson in 1933,[262] presents a clinical picture of a central nervous system degeneration characterized by myoclonic seizures, involuntary movements, and mental deterioration. An infection with a measleslike virus has been demonstrated by electron microscopy,[263] fluorescence microscopy,[264] rise in measles antibody titer,[265] and isolation of virus from brain and lymph nodes.[264,265,266,267]

Pathology and Etiology

The alterations within the brain are usually evident on both gross and microscopic examination. In essence, these consist of a subacute encephalitis, which is accompanied by demyelination.

Lesions generally involve the cerebral cortex, hippocampus, thalamus, brain stem, and cerebellar cortex. In the cerebral cortex the histologic picture is a nonspecific one of a subacute encephalitis, with cell loss, sometimes accompanied by neuronophagia, and meningeal and perivascular infiltration. Inclusions are seen within both the nucleus and the cytoplasm of neurons and glial cells. Most characteristically, they consist of homogeneous eosinophilic material (Cowdry, type A); less often the inclusions are small and multiple (Cowdry, type B).

The demyelination is particulately evident in the more chronic cases. It is sudanophilic with astrocytic and fibrillary gliosis, and is independent of the loss of cortical neurons. Electron microscopic studies indicate an evolution of type B to type A inclusions, which in turn become cytoplasmic inclusions, from which viral particles bud. Their structure is indistinguishable from those of the large myxoviruses such as measles or canine distemper.[268]

While these studies are highly suggestive of latent measles virus infection, recent virologic and epidemiologic evidence implicates a second virus in the activation of the disease process.[269,270]

Clinical Manifestations

Between 1965 and 1970 over 200 cases of SSPE were recorded. The age of onset ranged from five to fifteen years; boys were more frequently affected than girls by a factor of 5:1. In 75% the antecedent measles infection was contracted before age four; in 25% before age one.[271] In another 25% there was no history of measles infection. In the presence of elevated serum and CSF measles antibodies, this implies an early infection occurring during a period of partial immunity.

The regional distribution of SSPE is striking, with 50% of the cases being reported from the southeastern United States. Initial symptoms are those of personality changes and an insidious intellectual deterioration. Soon, usually within two months, seizures appear. Characteristically, these are myoclonic jerks initially of the head and subsequently the trunk and limbs. Muscular contraction is followed by one to two seconds of relaxation associated with a marked decrease in muscle action potentials, or complete electric silence. The myoclonic jerks do not interfere with consciousness. They are exaggerated by excitement and disappear during sleep. Initially, they are infrequent and may be regarded as stumbling, clumsiness, or possibly ataxia, but later in the course of the illness they occur every 5–15 seconds. Spontaneous speech and movements decrease, although comprehension seems to remain relatively well-preserved.

With further progression of the illness extrapyramidal dyskinesia and spasticity become more prominent. The former includes athetosis, chorea, ballismus, and dystonic movements with transient periods of opisthotonus. Swallowing difficulties may develop at this stage. A progressive visual loss, associated with focal chorioretinitis, cortical blindness, and occasionally optic atrophy has also been noted.[272]

In the terminal stages of the disease a progressive unresponsiveness is associated with increasing extensor hypertonus and decerebrate rigidity; respirations become irregular and stertorous, and there are a variety of signs of hypothalamic dysfunction, including vasomotor instability, hyperthermia, profuse sweating, and disturbances of pulse and blood pressure.

The entire course of the illness may be characterized by slow progressive deterioration or variable periods of remission.[273] The usual duration of the disease is about nine months; patients have lived for as short a period as six weeks following the onset of symptoms, or for as long as 10 years. Patients with periods of remission lasting up to three years have been described, but these too have ultimately succumbed.[273]

Typically, the cerebrospinal fluid contains a normal or slightly elevated protein concentration but the concentration of gamma globulin, predominantly IgG, is always increased, varying from amounts which are slightly above normal to 60% of the total protein concentration. The increase in gamma globulins produces a first zone colloidal gold curve, which is characteristic for the early stages of SSPE.[274] Antibodies against measles virus can be demonstrated in both serum and CSF by a variety of techniques. Generally the level of antibodies in the CSF is disproportionately low when compared to that in serum. This may be due to partial neutralization of antibody by liberated viral antigen.[275] CSF pleocytosis may be absent or minimal, with a variable proportion of mononuclear cells.

Characteristic electroencephalographic abnormalities may be seen early in the disease, sometimes even before the clinical appearance of myoclonus. Paroxysmal bursts of

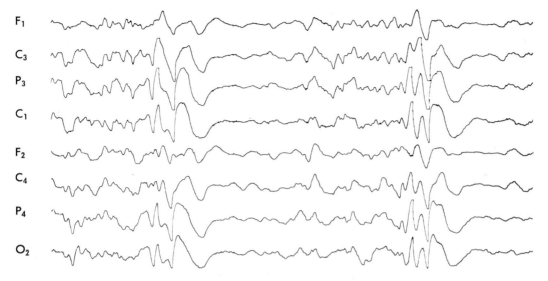

Fig. 6–11. Subacute sclerosing panencephalitis. Electroencephalogram in a five-year-old boy, showing characteristic suppression bursts. (Unipolar leads, F_1, C_3, P_3, O_1—left frontal, central, parietal and occipital leads. F_2, C_4, P_4, O_2, right frontal, central, parietal and occipital leads.)

2–3/second high voltage diphasic activity occur synchronously throughout the EEG and are often associated with spike discharges; they may be followed by a short period of flattened activity, the entire pattern being termed a suppression burst (Fig. 6–11). These discharges are believed to arise from the mesencephalic activating system.[276] Initially the background activity may be normal, later it becomes disorganized. Terminally, paroxysmal activity may decrease, and may disappear completely with periods of hyperpyrexia. The myoclonic contractions may coincide with paroxysmal bursts observed by means of the EEG, or may be disassociated from them. When associated with a burst, the muscular contraction commences prior to the large slow wave discharge, and disappears during the course of the latter. During sleep the myoclonic discharges disappear, but the paroxysmal EEG bursts continue.

Diagnosis

The clinical picture of intellectual deterioration associated with myoclonic seizures is always strongly suggestive of SSPE. The diagnosis is confirmed by the presence of suppression bursts on electroencephalographic examination, and the strikingly elevated levels of measles antibodies in the serum and CSF. Microscopic examination of a brain biopsy, and viral isolation from this tissue provides a final diagnostic proof.

SSPE should be differentiated from the group of late infantile or juvenile lipidoses (Chapter 1), or the various degenerations of white matter. Children frequently present with a history of recent falls which may suggest cerebral trauma or akinetic seizures. Occasionally patients may demonstrate lateralizing neurologic signs or, less commonly, papilledema, findings that may lead to an erroneous diagnosis of an intracranial space-occupying lesion.

Therapy

No adequate therapy is presently available. Immune suppression by means of steroids has not proved beneficial. Interferon induction by pyran copolymers, or the use of antiviral agents such as 5-bromo-2'-deoxyuridine or adamantadine, has not been shown to alter the course of the disease.[267,277]

LEPROSY

Though it still is a major health problem

elsewhere, the disease is rare in the continental United States. It is most prevalent in India, China, Nigeria, the Congo, and in the western hemisphere in Brazil, Colombia, Samoa, and Hawaii. Leprosy is essentially a systemic disease with a marked predilection for skin and nerves. The infection with *Mycobacterium leprae* has an incubation period of a few months to many years, most often between two and four years. Depending on the resistance of the host, two distinct types of infection may develop. With high resistance infection it is maculoanaesthetic or tuberculoid, with low resistance it is lepromatous or nodular. In the latter there are numerous bacilli, little tissue reaction, and T-lymphocyte populations deficient in number and function.[277a]

Initially, the infection is confined to sheaths of small nerves in the dermis where there are foci of lymphocytes, histiocytes, and epithelioid cells. From this lesion, the disease may progress to form subcutaneous granulomata (lepromatous form) or spread up nerves (tuberculoid or neural form). In the lepromatous form clusters of numerous bacilli in the Schwann cell cytoplasm and axonal space may burst out into surrounding tissue and produce a pronounced granulomatous reaction. Subcutaneous nodules and ulcerations of skin and mucosa may occur. In the neural form of infection cellular infiltration of the peri- and endoneural sheaths results in fusiform swelling along the nerves. The lesions bear some resemblance to tuberculosis; bacilli may be scanty. Infection gradually spreads up the nerve to involve some motor as well as sensory fibers and eventually reaches the dorsal root ganglia or less often the motor neurons of the spinal cord.

The neurologic lesions of leprosy are of three types.[278,279] Purely sensory polyneuritis results in loss of light touch, pain, and temperature in a "glove-stocking" distribution while deep pressure and pain, vibration, and joint sense are preserved. This may occur without characteristic skin lesions. Less common is a mixed sensory polyneuritis and mononeuritis with paralysis in a peripheral nerve distribution and sensory loss more widely distributed than in the first group of patients.[280] Rarely there is a pure mono-

neuritis, resulting in motor deficit in a peripheral nerve distribution or even a myositis.[281,282]

Symptoms may begin abruptly or develop insidiously. In addition to the sensory loss, sudomotor dysfunction with anhidrosis is commonly seen in the absence of evidence of vasomotor abnormality.

Sulfones, derivatives of 4, 4'-diamino diphenyl sulfone, have been used in the treatment of leprosy since 1941. In some instances steroids and thalidomide are also beneficial. Sulfones have been recommended for chemoprophylaxis in children.[283] BCG vaccination is reported to reduce the incidence of leprosy from 11 to 2.2 per 1000.[284]

LEPTOSPIROSIS

Leptospirosis, due to *L. icterohaemorrhagiae*, is an uncommon cause of meningitis. There is sudden onset of fever, muscle pain, epigastric pain, and headache. Obstructive jaundice and hepatosplenomegaly are common. Single or multiple relapses occur but almost all patients recover. Signs of meningeal irritation occur in about 10% of patients.[285,286,287]

Rarely encephalitis is demonstrated by diplopia, nystagmus, paralysis of cranial nerves, paraplegia, myoclonus, disturbances of sleep or psychic changes.

Of 41 patients 1–10 years after leptospirosis, 25 had neurologic deficits. Pyramidal symptoms were common and there were polyneuritis, cranial nerve deficits, and neurasthenic symptoms. EEG was abnormal in 16 of 34 and the EMG revealed lower motor neuron deficit in 42%.[286]

SYPHILIS

The resurgence of syphilis throughout the world gives added importance to congenital and acquired cases of neurosyphilis seen in infancy or childhood.

Pathology and Pathogenesis

The pathology of congenital neurosyphilis resembles that of the acquired forms.[288] Syphilitic infection may be transmitted to the fetus any time during gestation, but most often during the fourth through seventh months. Of the children of syphilitic parents 25%–

80% develop syphilis; clinical signs of congenital neurosyphilis occur in 2%–16% of these.

Neurosyphilis takes either the meningovascular or the parenchymatous form. In both, the infectious process begins in the meninges as a widespread diffuse arachnoiditis with inflammation concentrated around the meningeal vessels and the branches that penetrate into the cortex. Small meningeal vessels may show thickening and infiltration of the adventitia as well as intimal proliferation; syphilitic phlebitis is less common though both may result in infarction with localized lesions of the brain or spinal cord.

Obstructive or communicating hydrocephalus may result from meningeal fibrosis and obliteration of the subarachnoid spaces.

Diffuse meningeal inflammation of the secondary stage may be carried over into the tertiary stage with increased fibrosis of the meninges and the formation of small, often miliary gummata.

In parenchymatous congenital syphilis, as in juvenile paresis, there is diffuse degeneration with cerebral and cerebellar atrophy. Microscopic changes include a round cell meningeal and perivascular infiltration; loss and degenerative changes in the nerve cells, with an increase in microglia and astroglia, a disturbance of normal cytoarchitecture, deposition of iron pigment, and presence of spirochetes.

Clinical Manifestations

The central nervous system becomes involved during the first few months or years of life. In 50%–80% of cases of congenital neurosyphilis one or more of the stigmata of congenital syphilis are present. These include interstitial keratitis, chorioretinitis, defective teeth, malformed or "saddle" nose, frontal bossing of the skull, saber shins, Clutton's joints, and rhagades, either singly or in combination. Nerve deafness, which together with dental deformities and interstitial keratitis form the classic Hutchinson's triad, however, is infrequent. During the first few months of postnatal life, syphilitic meningitis is most common while vascular syndromes are prevalent during the first two years of life.

Syphilitic meningitis usually appears between 3–12 months of age with a sudden onset of convulsions, listlessness, apathy, vomiting, feeding difficulties, or progressive enlargement of the head. Nuchal rigidity, a full fontanelle, head retraction, various cranial nerve palsies with optic atrophy, or strabismus may develop in the course of the illness.

Chronic syphilitic meningitis may give rise to hydrocephalus. It is rarely present at birth but usually develops at 9–12 months with progressive enlargement of the head sometimes accompanied by cranial nerve deficits. Congenital cerebrovascular syphilis may result in diverse vascular syndromes because of arteritis and thrombosis of cerebral vessels.[288]

Mental deficiency, mental subnormality, and behavior disorders are more common in subjects with congenital syphilis than in the general population. This is not due to the infection itself, but to other hereditary and environmental factors.[289]

Tertiary congenital syphilis begins after an interval about as long as is in acquired syphilis.

Juvenile paresis is the most common form of congenital tertiary neurosyphilis. Its usual onset is between 6 and 21 years, with an average of 13 years. Males and females are affected equally often. It may appear in children with marked mental retardation in whom the onset is vague and impossible to date. When the children are moderately retarded or of normal intelligence onset is marked by loss of previously learned accomplishments.

In juvenile paresis there is most commonly simple mental deterioration characterized by regression, confusion, flattened affect, and restless purposive behavior.

The neurologic syndromes of juvenile paresis are more diverse and advanced than those in acquired paresis and in 25% of cases cerebellar deficits are conspicuous. In 50% of children one or more limbs are spastic. Seizures occur in 30%–40%. Spinal cord involvement indicating taboparesis is present in from 10%–15% of cases. Optic atrophy with or without chorioretinitis is present in

with two volumes of fluid and administered slowly. Lumbar sites of administration should be altered over about three vertebral levels in order to minimize drug induced arachnoiditis, revealed by a slight elevation in CSF cell count and protein concentrations. Cisternal antibiotic may result in headaches or nausea, both treated symptomatically by frequent changes in position and ambulation if possible. The use of a subcutaneous reservoir for intraventricular administration of the drug has been suggested.[301a]

Concomitant therapy with intravenous amphotericin B is started on a daily basis with 0.05 mg/kg, which is increased by increments of 5 mg–10 mg/day until the full dosage of 1 mg/kg/day is reached.[297,298] Intravenous administration of the antibiotic should be guided by frequent assessments of renal function. Generally serum creatinine concentrations most reliably indicate amphotericin B toxicity. Impaired renal function is reversible but requires reduction in dose and frequency of the antibiotic.

Coccidioidal meningitis is rarely completely eradicated. Intensive follow-up is necessary, and repeated courses of intraspinal amphotericin B are required to suppress the infection.

HISTOPLASMOSIS

Histoplasmosis, caused by *Histoplasma capsulatum*, is endemic to the northeastern, central, and south central United States.[297] Central nervous system involvement is seen only after disseminated involvement; it occurs in about one-quarter of such cases, and in 7.6% of all *Histoplasma* infections.[302]

Infants and children under three years may have systemic signs, including fever, anemia, hepatosplenomegaly, and less often weight loss, adenopathy, or cough. Neurologic symptoms are usually absent. In older children there may be tetany, or pyramidal tract signs.[302] The CSF is abnormal in all age groups.

Brain changes include the formation of granulomata within the parenchyma or in the perivenous regions, a meningitis, most often involving the basilar regions, and the formation of isolated abscesses.

Skin or complement fixation tests are generally used for the diagnosis of *Histoplasma* infections. They are, however, often negative in patients with central nervous system disease, and a bone marrow biopsy is probably the best diagnostic procedure currently available.[302]

Treatment with amphotericin B is similar to that for coccidioidosis.

CRYPTOCOCCOSIS

Cryptococcosis is one of the most common fungal infections of the nervous system. It is caused by *Cryptococcus neoformans*, an organism which is widely distributed, and often isolated from soil, particularly in the vicinity of pigeon nests.[294]

The pathologic changes in the brain vary. In some areas there may only be minimal inflammation, while in others there may be pseudo-tubercles composed of giant cells, epithelioid cells, and lymphocytes.

The infection is rare in children; adults are more commonly involved because of greater exposure and because of the predilection of cryptococcal infection for individuals debilitated with leukemia and lymphoma, or as a result of therapy with steroids or immune suppressants.

Symptoms usually reflect meningeal involvement, although occasionally neurologic signs or alterations in mental status may predominate.

The diagnosis is difficult. Patients with active cryptococcal disease have a negative cryptococcal antigen skin test in about half of the instances. Complement fixation tests, latex agglutination, fluorescent antibody, and hemagglutination tests have also been employed.[303]

The cerebrospinal fluid in patients with cryptococcal meningitis resembles that of tuberculous meningitis, with a moderate lymphocytic pleocytosis, increased protein, and decreased sugar. The diagnosis depends on culture of organisms from the fluid, or demonstration in CSF of the cryptococcal polysaccharide by latex agglutination tests. There is a high incidence of culture-negative meningitis even in experienced laboratories, although the chance of obtaining a positive culture is higher if the fluid is dripped directly into the culture medium.[304] India ink

TABLE 6-15.
CHARACTERISTICS OF RARER FUNGAL INFECTIONS
OF THE NERVOUS SYSTEM

Organism (Disease)	Major CNS Symptoms	Therapy	Reference
Actinomyces bovis (actinomycosis)	Chronic low grade meningitis, abscesses	Penicillin, tetracycline, surgical drainage	307
Aspergillus niger (aspergillosis)	Multiple brain abscesses, vascular thromboses	Amphotericin B	294, 308
Blastomyces dermatitidis (blastomycosis)	Meningitis	Amphotericin B, 2-hydroxystilbamidine	309
Cephalosporium granulomatis	Meningitis	Amphotericin B	310
Phycomycetes rhizopus (mucormycosis)	Thromboses of cerebral and meningeal arteries	Amphotericin B	311, 312
Nocardia asteroides (nocardiosis)	Meningitis, multiple focal abscesses	Sulfadiazine, tetracycline, erythromycin	313, 314

preparations are positive in 71% of cases.[305] The latex agglutination test may be positive, even when organisms cannot be demonstrated by the other methods.[306]

Untreated cryptococcal meningitis is fatal within a few months. Intravenous or intrathecal amphotericin B has been the antibiotic of choice with a cure rate of the order of 50%.[301] Refractory infections or patients unable to tolerate amphotericin B may respond to 5-fluorocytosine.

The highlights of some of the rarer fungal infections of the nervous system are summarized in Table 6–15.

RICKETTSIAL INFECTIONS

A number of rickettsial organisms invade the nervous system and produce neurologic symptoms. Based on serologic and clinical characteristics, six major rickettsial entities have been recognized:

1. Typhus fever. The epidemic louse-borne form is caused by R. prowazekii, while the endemic murine type is due to R. mooseri.

2. Rocky Mountain spotted fever. In the western hemisphere this illness is caused by R. rickettsii.

3. Scrub typhus due to R. tsutsugamushi and found in Australasia (Japan, India, and Australia).

4. Q fever due to Coxiella burneti.

5. Rickettsialpox, caused by R. akari, with the agent being transmitted to man by the mouse mite.

6. Trench fever transmitted to man by the louse and caused by R. quintana.

ROCKY MOUNTAIN SPOTTED FEVER

In the United States, the commonest rickettsial disease is Rocky Mountain spotted fever. In the western hemisphere this condition has been reported from almost all parts of the United States, notably the Appalachian and the western Rocky Mountain areas. The main vectors for man are the Rocky Mountain wood tick, Dermacentor andersoni, the dog tick, Dermacentor variabilis, which is more prevalent in the Eastern United States; and the Lone Star tick, Amblyomma americanum, prevalent in the Gulf States.[315]

The organisms invade the human following a bite by the vector with fecal contamination. They first enter the nuclei of the capillary endothelial cells where they multiply and destroy the cells. The lesions extend along the blood vessels to the arterioles where smooth muscle cells of the media are invaded and destroyed. Vascular lesions result in scattered thrombosis and extravasation of blood to produce microinfarcts. Within the nervous system the alterations are the most striking of any of the rickettsial diseases. Here there are areas of petechial hemorrhages, perivascular infiltration, glial nodules, and minute sites of focal necrosis. Patches of demyelination are seen throughout the brain.

Clinical Manifestations

Neurologic symptoms are prominent in Rocky Mountain spotted fever. A meningoencephalitis evolves after an incubation period of four to eight days. The acute phase is ushered in with headache, myalgia, fever, and shaking chills. Meningeal signs may be prominent.[316] Mental confusion, hallucination, or delirium may appear, which may progress to coma. Muscular twitchings, fibrillary tremors, fasciculations, and convulsions are common. A variety of neurologic signs including diffuse hyperreflexia, choreoathetosis, sixth nerve palsies, alteration in pupillary size and reflexes, and nystagmus may develop; deafness often occurs during the acute illness.[317] A variety of ophthalmologic signs have been noted including retinal edema, papilledema, and choroiditis. Choked discs may develop in the presence of normal intracranial pressure as a consequence of vasculitis.[318] Intracranial hemorrhage may result from thrombocytopenia and hypofibrinogenemia secondary to intravascular coagulation.[316]

After several days of fever the rash usually begins over the extremities. It spreads centripetally and in two to three days changes from a macular to a maculopapular petechial eruption. Hemorrhagic areas may coalesce to form ecchymotic lesions. At this point myocardial involvement may lead to cardiac failure with hypotension, tachycardia, and shock.[317] Renal and hepatic involvements result in oliguria and hypoproteinemia with generalized edema.

Residual neurologic deficits may not be immediately apparent.[319] At reevaluation after one to eight years, 16% of survivors showed definite neurologic abnormalities, although one-half of this group had no objective changes during the acute phase of the illness. A variety of neurologic residua were observed: mental retardation, behavior disturbances, impairment of coordination, and hypotonia. In one-third of subjects the electroencephalogram was persistently abnormal.[319]

Diagnosis

The diagnosis of Rocky Mountain spotted fever rests in part on a history of exposure and the development of the characteristic rash. The cerebrospinal fluid is normal in 56% of cases. In the remainder white cells may range from 11 to 300/mm^3; only a quarter of these have over 50% polymorphonuclear cells. Modest protein elevations occur in about one-third; the sugar remains normal. Laboratory diagnosis may be made by complement fixation, rickettsial agglutination (Weil-Felix) reaction, or by fluorescent antibody studies.[320,321]

Treatment

Chloramphenicol or tetracycline are the antibiotics of choice. They are continued until at least one week after the patient has become afebrile.

Intravenous tetracycline should be avoided since it may cause hepatic necrosis.[320] Para-aminosalicylic acid is less effective, and sulfonamides appear to aggravate symptoms.

For a discussion of the neurologic complications of typhus and the other rickettsial infections, the reader is referred to papers by Noad and Haymaker[322] on the complications of scrub typhus (tsutsugamushi fever), and by Herman on typhus fever.[323]

SARCOIDOSIS

Nervous system sarcoidosis is unusual in children. The etiology of the disease is still problematic, but for convenience it is classified with infectious diseases. Although it occurs throughout the world, the disease is particularly common in the southeastern portions of the United States where it predominates among blacks. The most affected children are aged 9–15 years.

Pathologically, the disease is characterized by the presence of widely disseminated epithelioid cells, tubercles with little or no necrosis, and giant cells. Tissues most frequently involved are the lymph nodes, lungs, skin, eyes, and bones. While in adults any part of the nervous system may be affected, in particular the cranial nerves, meninges, and musculature,[324,325,356] in children neurologic symptoms are most commonly associated with uveoparotid fever. This syndrome, first described by Heerfordt,[327] is characterized by ocular disturbances, usually uveitis, less commonly, optic neuritis, swelling of the parotid gland, and facial nerve palsy. The latter usually follows a subacute course, appearing after the parotid swelling, and subsiding with it. It occurs in 4% of children with sarcoidosis.[328] Meningeal signs, peripheral neuritis, papilledema, and diabetes insipidus are other rare findings associated with CNS sarcoidosis.[328] The disease has a slowly progressive course, with a tendency to partial or complete spontaneous remissions.

Since facial weakness is rare in mumps, the association of parotid swelling and facial palsy should suggest sarcoidosis. In the rare condition termed Melkersson's syndrome recurrent facial nerve palsy is accompanied by edema of the face or lips.[329] While the Kveim test has been widely used as a diagnostic procedure in sarcoidosis, its unreliability both in terms of false positive and false negative results has prompted biopsy of the peripheral lymph nodes as a diagnostic measure.[330] Hyperglobulinemia, eosinophilia, and hypercalcemia are common associated laboratory findings. The cerebrospinal fluid protein may show an elevation. Rarely, there are signs of meningitis with increased pressure, pleocytosis, and a decreased sugar content.

Treatment with corticosteroids tends to improve ocular and facial nerve involvement.[330]

OTHER NEUROLOGIC DISORDERS WITH PRESUMED INFECTIOUS ETIOLOGY

ENCEPHALOPATHY AND FATTY DEGENERATION OF THE VISCERA (Reye's Syndrome)

This disorder, first described by Reye et al. in 1963, is characterized by fever, profoundly impaired consciousness, convulsions, hypoglycemia, and disordered hepatic function.[331,332]

Etiology and Pathology

The etiology of this condition is obscure. It has accompanied varicella,[331,333] and infectious mononucleosis; in other cases reovirus,[334] influenza B,[335] parainfluenza,[335a]

and ECHO 11 viruses have been isolated.[336] In northern Thailand the condition has been associated with a toxin from *Aspergillus flavus*.[337]

In fatal cases the brain shows severe edema and brain stem herniation. The histopathologic changes are nonspecific. The cortical neurons either are markedly swollen or shrunken and deeply staining. Astrocytes and oligodendroglia are swollen, without microglial proliferation. Some cells are laden with sudanophilic granules.

The liver is enlarged and yellow with fatty infiltration being observed in every cell. Rarely, fatty infiltration of the liver may be minimal.[337a] This extensive fatty change is unassociated with necrosis. On electron microscopy the most striking abnormalities are seen in mitochondria, which are swollen and pleomorphic.[338] Similar changes are seen in the kidney, occasionally in the myocardium and in pancreatic acinar cells. Renal fatty degeneration is most obvious in the proximal convoluted tubules and loops of Henle; glomeruli, vessels, and interstitial tissues are normal, as are the other organs.

Clinical Manifestations

Prodromal symptoms may be mild, or may consist of nonspecific complaints such as malaise, cough, rhinorrhea, or sore throat. Usually after one to three days but sometimes as late as two to three weeks, the child rapidly deteriorates with vomiting and the onset of stupor or coma, sometimes followed by convulsions. Wild delirium and unusual restlessness has been noted in about one-half of patients as the level of consciousness declines. Varieties of seizures occur in about 85% of cases.

With development of coma, the child develops changes in muscle tone, decorticate and decerebrate status, or opisthotonos. The pupils become dilated, unresponsive to light or unequal. Central neurogenic hyperventilation or shallow breathing may occur. Symptoms often correlate with metabolic disturbances, or brain stem herniation. The liver is frequently enlarged.

In the majority of children the blood sugar values may fall to below 50 mg%. Blood urea nitrogen and ammonia levels are often elevated, and liver function tests, particularly serum glutamic-oxalacetic and glutamic-pyruvic transaminases, are elevated. Insulin levels are reduced, and the glucagon response is diminished.[337b,337c]

The clinical course of Reye's syndrome is rapid, and in one series 61% of deaths occurred within 24 hours of the onset of CNS manifestations. Nonfatal cases recover completely within two to three days. The mortality is often as high as 85%; hyperkalemia, hyperpnea, and hematemesis have grave prognostic import.[333]

Diagnosis

The sudden onset of a profound disturbance of consciousness associated with hepatic dysfunction and hypoglycemia suggests the diagnosis of Reye's syndrome. A variety of toxic substances, notably ethanol, may produce a similar picture.

Acute idiopathic encephalopathy[339] differs from Reye's syndrome by the absence of visceral involvement. This entity, also of unknown etiology, is characterized by fever, convulsions, stupor or coma, a decorticate or decerebrate state, and respiratory embarrassment due to central derangement of respiratory mechanisms or asphyxia. The CSF is under increased pressure but otherwise is normal. On pathologic examination brain edema is noted; aside from anoxic changes, no other cellular alteration has been observed.

Treatment

Therapy has been directed to restoring blood sugar levels, controlling cerebral edema with mannitol and dexamethasone, and correction of electrolyte and acid-base imbalances.[331,337] Hydrocortisone and glucose infusions may be helpful, but neither seizures nor the state of consciousness are improved by restoring the blood glucose levels to normal.[331] Exchange transfusion has been suggested as a means of reducing elevated blood ammonia.

BEHCET'S SYNDROME

This rare chronic and relapsing condition is characterized by keratitis, uveitis, recurrent ulcerations of the mouth and genitalia, and a variety of skin lesions. In approximately 25% of patients the nervous system is involved.

A recurrent meningoencephalitis is the most common, while other cases present with an episodic progressive brain stem syndrome, or recurrent encephalitis.[340,341,342,343]

MOLLARET'S MENINGITIS

A recurrent benign, lymphocytic meningitis, presumed to be infectious, was first described by Mollaret.[344] Symptoms recur at intervals of weeks or months over the course of several years.[345,346]

UVEOMENINGOENCEPHALITIC SYNDROME
(Vogt-Koyanagi-Harada)

The uveomeningoencephalitic syndrome is an uncommon condition characterized by the association of uveitis, a meningoencephalitis of variable severity, occasional loss of skin and hair pigmentation, and auditory disturbances.[347]

BENIGN PAROXYSMAL VERTIGO

This condition is characterized by recurrent attacks of vertigo associated with vomiting, pallor, nystagmus, and profuse sweating. Although unaccompanied by loss of consciousness, the child may fall in the course of an attack. Episodes may last a few minutes to several hours, or recur for many weeks or even months, gradually decreasing in severity. The condition is frequently seen in epidemics, and there may be more than one case in a family. The preservation of consciousness during an attack, and abnormalities in labyrinthine function distinguish benign paroxysmal vertigo from temporal lobe epilepsy with a vertiginous component, and from vestibulogenic epilepsy in which an attack is triggered by labyrinthine stimulation.[348,349]

MELKERSSON'S SYNDROME

This condition is characterized by recurrent facial palsy, often associated with swelling of the lips, tongue, cheeks, or eyelids. With each attack facial nerve function becomes progressively more impaired, and paralysis may ultimately be nearly complete.[329]

EPIDEMIC ENCEPHALITIS

This condition, first described by von Economo in 1917,[350] attained epidemic proportions throughout Europe and the United States over the subsequent few years. Since then it has become progressively less common.

The disease presented as an acute encephalitis, often marked by somnolence and oculomotor palsies. The encephalitis cleared completely or left a variety of residua, including mental disturbances and disorders of eye movements. After a quiescent interval of months or years, many of the survivors developed a chronic, progressive extrapyramidal disorder, marked by Parkinsonism, oculogyric crises, tremors, and dystonia.[351]

A common residual finding in children was a postencephalitic behavior syndrome marked by hyperkinesia, shortened attention span, and impaired fine motor function.[352] This picture resembles so-called minimal cerebral dysfunction. As a consequence many children with the latter condition used to be regarded as postencephalitic without any history of encephalitis (see Chapter 13).

REFERENCES

1. Rich, A. R. and McCordock, H. A.: The pathogenesis of tuberculous meningitis, Bull. Hopkins Hosp. 52:5, 1933.
2. Harter, D. H. and Petersdorf, R. G.: A consideration of the pathogenesis of bacterial meningitis. Review of experimental and clinical studies, Yale J. Biol. Med. 32:280, 1960.
3. Ommaya, A. K., et al.: Non-traumatic cerebrospinal fluid rhinorrhea, J. Neurol. Neurosurg. Psychiat. 31:214, 1968.
4. Adams, R. D., Kubik, C. S., and Bonner, F. J.: The clinical and pathological aspects of influenzal meningitis, Arch. Ped. 65:354, 408, 1948.
4a. Burn, C. G. and Finley, K. H.: The role of hypersensitivity in the production of experimental meningitis, J. Exp. Med. 56:203, 1932.
4b. Thomas, V. H. and Hopkins, I. J.: Arteriographic demonstration of vascular lesions in the study of neurologic deficit in advanced *Haemophilus influenzae* meningitis, Develop. Med. Child Neurol. 14:783, 1972.
5. Smith, J. F. and Landing, B. H.: Mechanism of brain damage in *Haemophilus influenzae* meningitis, J. Neuropath. Exp. Neurol. 19:248, 1960.
6. Swartz, M. N. and Dodge, P. R.: Bacterial meningitis: A review of selected aspects. I. General clinical features, special problems, and unusual meningeal reactions mimicking bacterial meningitis, New Eng. J. Med. 272:725, 779, 842, 898, 1965.
7. Dodge, P. R. and Swartz, M. N.: Bacterial meningitis: A review of selected aspects. II.

8. Special neurologic problems, postmeningitic complications and clinicopathological correlations, New Eng. J. Med. 272:954, 1003, 1965.
8. O'Connell, J. E. A.: The clinical signs of meningeal irritation, Brain 69:9, 1946.
8a. Ducker, T. B. and Simmons, R. L.: The pathogenesis of meningitis: Systemic effects of meningococcal endotoxin within the cerebrospinal fluid, Arch. Neurol. 18:123, 1968.
9. Samson, J. H., Apthorp, J., and Finley, A.: Febrile seizures and purulent meningitis, JAMA 210:1918, 1969.
10. Mace, J. W., Peters, E. R., and Mathies, A. W., Jr.: Cranial bruits in purulent meningitis in childhood, New Eng. J. Med. 278:1420, 1968.
11. Rabe, E. F., Young, G. F., and Dodge, P. R.: The distribution and fate of subdurally instilled human serum albumin in infants with subdural collections of fluid, Neurology (Minneap.) 14:1020, 1964.
12. Benson, P., Nyhan, W. L., and Shimizu, H.: The prognosis of subdural effusions complicating pyogenic meningitis, J. Pediat. 57:670, 1960.
13. Dodge, P. R. and Porter, P.: Demonstration of intracranial pathology by transillumination, Arch. Neurol. 5:594, 1961.
14. McLaurin, R. L. and McLaurin, K. S.: Calcified subdural hematomas in childhood, J. Neurosurg. 24:648, 1966.
15. Matson, D. D.: *Neurosurgery of Infancy and Childhood*, 2nd ed., Springfield: Charles C Thomas Publisher, 1969.
16. Shulman, K. and Ransohoff, J.: Subdural hematoma in children: The fate of children with retained membranes, J. Neurosurg. 18:175, 1961.
17. Rabe, E. F., Flynn, R. E., and Dodge, P. R.: Subdural collections of fluids in infants and children: A study of 62 patients with special reference to factors influencing prognosis and efficacy of various forms of therapy, Neurology (Minneap.) 18:559, 1968.
18. Boe, J. and Huseklepp, H.: Recurrent attacks of bacterial meningitis: A "new" clinical problem; report of five cases, Amer. J. Med. 29:465, 1960.
19. Fisher, D. A.: Embryonal rest tumor of the central nervous system, Amer. J. Dis. Child. 99:90, 1960.
20. Smith, C. H., et al.: Hazard of severe infections in splenectomized infants and children, Amer. J. Med. 22:390, 1957.
21. Cherry, J. D. and Sheenan, C. P.: Bacteriologic relapse in *Haemophilus influenzae* meningitis: Inadequate ampicillin therapy, New Eng. J. Med. 278:1001, 1968.
22. Lichtheim, L.: Bei Gehirnkrankheiten durch die Punction der Subarachnoidalräume, Deutsch. Med. Wschr. 19:1234, 1893.
23. Prockop, L. D. and Fishman, R. A.: Experimental pneumococcal meningitis, Arch. Neurol. 19:449, 1968.

24. Menkes, J. H.: The causes for low spinal fluid sugar in bacterial meningitis—another look, Pediatrics 44:1, 1969.

25. Beaty, H. N. and Oppenheimer, S.: Cerebrospinal fluid lactic dehydrogenase and its isoenzymes in infections of the central nervous system, New Eng. J. Med. 279:1197, 1968.

26. Belsy, M. A.: CSF glutamic oxaloacetic transaminase in acute bacterial meningitis, Amer. J. Dis. Child. 117:288, 1969.

26a. Katz, R. M. and Liebman, W.: Creatine phosphokinase activity in central nervous system disorders and infections, Amer. J. Dis. Child. 120:543, 1970.

27. Belagtas, R. C., et al.: Secondary and prolonged fevers in bacterial meningitis, J. Pediat. 77:957, 1970.

28. Kresky, B., Buchbinder, S., and Greenberg, I. M.: The incidence of neurologic residua in children after recovery from bacterial meningitis, Arch. Ped. 79:63, 1962.

29. Sproles, E. T., et al.: Meningitis due to hemophilus influenzae: Long-term sequelae, J. Pediat. 75:782, 1969.

30. Herweg, J.C., Middelkamp, J. N., and Hartmann, A. F.: Simultaneous mixed bacterial meningitis in children, J. Pediat. 63:76, 1963.

31. de Lemos, R. A. and Haggarty, R. J.: Corticosteroids as an adjunct to treatment in bacterial meningitis; a controlled clinical trial, Pediatrics 44:30, 1969.

32. Nyhan, W. L. and Richardson, F.: Complications of meningitis, Ann. Rev. Med. 14:243, 1963.

33. Sell, S. H. W., et al.: Psychologic sequelae of bacterial meningitis: Controlled studies, Pediatrics 49:212, 1972.

34. Wehrle, P. F., Leedom, J. M., and Mathies, A. W.: Treatment of meningococcal meningitis, Mod. Treatm. 4:929, 1967.

35. Margaretten, W. and McAdams, A. J.: An appraisal of fulminant meningococcemia with reference to the Shwartzman phenomenon, Amer. J. Med. 25:868, 1958.

36. Lillehei, R. C., et al.: The modern treatment of shock based on physiologic principles, Clin. Pharmacol. Ther. 5:63, 1964.

37. Williams, D. N. and Geddes, A. M.: Meningococcal meningitis complicated by pericarditis, panophthalmitis, and arthritis, Brit. Med. J. 2:93, 1970.

38: Hardman, J. M. and Earle, K. M.: Myocarditis in 200 fatal meningococcal infections, Arch. Path. 87:318, 1969.

39. Veghelyi, P. V.: Artificial hibernation, J. Pediat. 60:122, 1962.

40. Migeon, C. J., et al.: Study of adrenal function in children with meningitis, Pediatrics 40:163, 1967.

41. Stiehm, E. R. and Damrosch, D. S.: Factors in the prognosis of meningococcal infections, J. Pediat. 68:457, 1966.

42. Page, M. I. and King, E. O.: Infection due to *Actinobacillus actinomycetemcomitans* and *Haemophilus aphrophilus*, New Eng. J. Med. 275:181, 1966.

43. O'Toole, R. D., Goode, L., and Howe, C. V.: Neuraminidase activity in bacterial meningitis, J. Clin. Invest. 50:979, 1971.

44. Winkelstein, J. A. and Drachman, R. H.: Deficiency of pneumococcal serum opsonizing activity in sickle-cell disease, New Eng. J. Med. 279:459, 1968.

45. Pearson, H. A., Spencer, R. P., and Cornelius, E. A.: Functional asplenia in sickle cell anemia, New Eng. J. Med. 281:923, 1969.

46. Ziment, I.: Nervous system complications in bacterial endocarditis, Amer. J. Med. 47:593, 1969.

47. Holt, R.: The classification of staphylococci from colonized ventriculo-atrial shunts, J. Clin. Path. 22:475, 1969.

47a. Shurtleff, D. B., et al.: Ventriculoauriculostomy-associated infection, J. Neurosurg. 35:686, 1971.

48. Becker, D. P. and Nulsen, F. E.: Control of hydrocephalus by valve-regulated venous shunt: Avoidance of complications in prolonged shunt maintenance, J. Neurosurg. 28:215, 1968.

49. Overall, J. C.: Neonatal bacterial meningitis, J. Pediat. 76:499, 1970.

50. Groover, R. V., Sutherland, J. M., and Landing, B. H.: Purulent meningitis of newborn infants: Eleven year experience in the antibiotic era, New Eng. J. Med. 264:1115, 1961.

51. Wise, B. L., Mathis, J. L., and Jawetz, E.: Infections of the central nervous system due to *Pseudomonas aeruginosa*, J. Neurosurg. 31:432, 1969.

52. Blacklock, J. W. S. and Griffin, M. A.: Tuberculous meningitis in children, J. Path. Bact. 40:489, 1935.

53. Critchley, M.: Brain tumors in children: Their general symptomatology, Brit. J. Child. Dis. 22:251, 1925.

54. Lincoln, E. M.: Tuberculous meningitis in children. I. Tuberculous meningitis, Amer. Rev. Tuberc. Pul. Dis. 56:75, 1951.

55. Lincoln, E. H. and Sewell, E. M.: *Tuberculosis in Children*, New York: McGraw-Hill Book Co., 1963.

56. Durfee, N. L., et al.: The treatment of tuberculosis in children, Amer. Rev. Resp. Dis. 99:304, 1969.

57. Freiman, I. and Geefhuysen, J.: Evaluation of intrathecal therapy with streptomycin and hydrocortisone in tuberculous meningitis, J. Pediat. 76:895, 1970.

58. O'Toole, R. D., et al.: Dexamethasone in tuberculous meningitis. Relationship of cerebrospinal fluid effects to therapeutic efficacy, Ann. Intern. Med. 70:39, 1969.

58a. Bhagwati, S. N.: Ventriculo-atrial shunt in tuberculous meningitis with hydrocephalus, J. Neurosurg. 35:309, 1971.

59. Bonforte, R. J., et al.: Tuberculous meningitis

due to primary drug-resistant *Mycobacterium tuberculosis hominis*, Pediatrics 42:969, 1968.

60. Lintermans, J. and Seyhnaeve, V.: Tuberculous meningitis during therapy for pulmonary tuberculosis, Pediatrics 45:715, 1970.

61. Todd, R. M. and Neville, J. G.: Sequelae of tuberculous meningitis, Arch. Dis. Child. 39:213, 1964.

62. Haslam, R. H., Winternitz, W. W., and Howieson, J.: Selective hypopituitarism following tuberculous meningitis, Amer. J. Dis. Child. 118:903, 1969.

63. Drury, M. I., O'Lochlainn, S., and Sweeney, E.: Complication of tuberculous meningitis, Brit. Med. J. 1:842, 1968.

64. Lorber, J.: The results of treatment of 549 cases of tuberculous meningitis, Amer. Rev. Tuberc. Pul. Dis. 69:13, 1954.

65. Lavetter, A., et al.: Meningitis due to *Listeria monocytogenes*, New Eng. J. Med. 285:598, 1971.

66. Levy, H. L. and Ingall, D.: Meningitis in neonates due to *Proteus mirabilis*, Amer. J. Dis. Child. 114:320, 1967.

67. Okoh, O.: Ueber Mima polymorpha Meningitis bei einen 5 Monate alten Saugling und ihre Therapie, Mschr. Kinderheilk. 119:471, 1971.

68. Wilner, E. C. and Fenichel, G. M.: Treatment of *Salmonella* meningitis, Clin. Proc. Child. Hosp. (Wash.) 25:362, 1969.

69. Spivack, A. P., et al.: *Klebsiella* meningitis, Amer. J. Med. 22:865, 1957.

69a.Shackelford, P. G., et al.: Therapy of *Haemophilus influenzae* meningitis reconsidered, New Eng. J. Med. 287:634, 1972.

70. Blattner, R. J.: Infection with *Haemophilus aphrophilus*: Brain abscess, J. Pediat. 66:813, 1965.

71. Krayenbühl, H. A.: Abscess of the brain, Clin. Neurosurg. 14:25, 1966.

72. Clark, D. B.: Brain abscess and congenital heart disease, Clin. Neurosurg. 14:274, 1966.

73. Eberhard, S. J.: Diagnosis of brain abscess in infants and children: A retrospective study of twenty-six cases, N. Carolina Med. J. 30:301, 363, 1969.

74. Heinz, E. R. and Cooper, R. D.: Several early angiographic findings in brain abscess including "the ripple sign," Radiology 90:735, 1968.

75. Kanafani, S. B. and Constantino, G. L.: Perfusion I^{131} macroaggregate brain scanning—a clinical evaluation of its diagnostic efficiency, Amer. J. Roentgen. 106:333, 1969.

75a.Tyler, H. R. and Clark, D. B.: Cerebrovascular accidents in patients with congenital heart disease, Arch. Neurol. Psychiat. 77:483, 1957.

76. Maxwell, J. A. and DeLong, W. B.: Use of micropaque barium in the radiographic visualization of brain abscesses. Case Report, J. Neurosurg. 28:280, 1968.

77. Wright, R. L. and Ballantine, H. T., Jr.: Management of brain abscesses in children and adolescents, Amer. J. Dis. Child. 114:113, 1967.

78. Jennett, W. B., et al.: Effect of anaesthesia on intracranial pressure in patients with space-occupying lesions, Lancet 1:61, 1969.

79. Heusner, A. P.: Nontuberculous spinal epidural infections, New Eng. J. Med. 239:845, 1948.

80. Altrocchi, P. H.: Acute spinal epidural abscess vs. acute transverse myelopathy, Arch. Neurol. 9:17, 1963.

81. MacLaurin, R. L.: Spinal suppuration, Clin. Neurosurg. 14:314, 1966.

82. Raimondi, A. J., Matsumoto, S., and Miller, R. A.: Brain abscess in children with congenital heart disease, J. Neurosurg. 23:588, 1965.

83. Hardy, J. B., et al.: Adverse fetal outcome following maternal rubella after the first trimester of pregnancy, JAMA 207:2414, 1969.

84. Töndury, G. and Smith, D. W.: Fetal rubella pathology, J. Pediat. 68:867, 1966.

85. Dudgeon, J. A.: Fetal infections, J. Obstet. Gynaec. Brit. Comm. 75:1229, 1968.

86. Overall, J. C., Jr. and Glasgow, L. A.: Virus infections of the fetus and newborn infant, J. Pediat. 77:315, 1970.

87. Mims, C. A.: Pathogenesis of viral infections of the fetus, Prog. Med. Virol. 10:194, 1968.

88. Alford, C. A., Jr., et al.: Subclinical central nervous system disease of neonates: A prospective study of infants born with increased levels of IgM, J. Pediat. 75:1167, 1969.

89. Dudgeon, J. A., Marshall, W. C., and Soothill, J. F.: Immunological responses to early and later intrauterine virus infections, J. Pediat. 75:1149, 1969.

90. Rawls, W. E. and Melnick, J. L.: Rubella virus carrier cultures derived from congenitally infected infants, J. Exp. Med. 123:795, 1966.

91. Gregg, N.: Congenital cataract following German measles in the mother, Trans. Ophthal. Soc. Aust. 3:35, 1941.

92. Cooper, L. Z., et al.: Rubella: Clinical manifestations and management, Amer. J. Dis. Child. 118:18, 1969.

93. Plotkin, S. A., et al.: Some recently recognized manifestations of the rubella syndrome, J. Pediat. 67:182, 1965.

94. Desmond, M. M., et al.: Congenital rubella encephalitis: Effects on growth and early development, Amer. J. Dis. Child. 118:30, 1969.

95. Desmond, M. M., et al.: Congenital rubella encephalitis, J. Pediat. 71:311, 1967.

96. Tartakow, I. J.: The teratogenicity of maternal rubella, J. Pediat. 66:380, 1965.

97. Ames, M. D., et al.: Central auditory imperception—a significant factor in congenital rubella deafness, JAMA 213:419, 1970.

98. Cooper, L. Z., et al.: Loss of rubella hemagglutination inhibition antibody in congenital rubella, Amer. J. Dis. Child. 122:397, 1971.

99. Phillips, C. A., et al.: Intrauterine rubella infection following immunization with rubella vaccine, JAMA 213:624, 1970.

100. Forrest, J. M. and Menser, M. A.: Congenital rubella in school children and adolescents, Arch. Dis. Child. 45:63, 1970.

101. Hanshaw, J. B.: Congenital cytomegalovirus infection: A fifteen year perspective, J. Infect. Dis. 123:555, 1971.

102. Hanshaw, J. B.: Developmental abnormalities associated with congenital cytomegalovirus infection, Advances Terat. 4:64, 1970.

103. Stern, H., et al.: Microbial causes of mental retardation. The role of prenatal infections with cytomegalovirus, rubella virus, and toxoplasma, Lancet 2:443, 1969.

104. McCracken, G. H., Jr., et al.: Congenital cytomegalic inclusion disease. A longitudinal study of 20 patients, Amer. J. Dis. Child. 117:522, 1969.

105. Medearis, D. N., Jr.: Observations concerning human cytomegalovirus infection and disease, Bull. Hopkins Hosp. 114:181, 1964.

106. Shinefield, H. R. and Eichenwald, H. F.: In Eichenwald, H. F. (ed.): *Prevention of Mental Retardation Through Control of Infectious Diseases*, Pub. #1692, Gov't Printing Office, 1968.

107. Feigin, R. D., et al.: Floxuridine treatment of congenital cytomegalic inclusion disease, Pediatrics 48:318, 1971.

107a.McKendry, J. B. J. and Bailey, J. D.: Congenital varicella associated with multiple defects, Canad. Med. Ass. J. 108:66, 1973.

108. Robertson, J. S.: Toxoplasmosis, Develop. Med. Child Neurol. 4:507, 1962.

109. Wolf, A., Cowen, D., and Paige, B.: Human toxoplasmosis: Occurrence in infants as an encephalomyelitis verification by transmission to animals, Science 89:226, 1939.

110. Couvreur, J. and Desmonts, G.: Congenital and maternal toxoplasmosis. A review of 300 congenital cases, Develop. Med. Child Neurol. 4:519, 1962.

111. Hafström, T.: Toxoplasmic encephalopathy, Acta Psychiat. Neurol. Scand. 34:311, 1959.

112. Fondu, P. and DeMeuter, F.: Facial palsy, a manifestation of acquired toxoplasmosis, Helv. Paediat. Acta 24:208, 1969.

113. Khanna, K. K., et al.: Acute acquired toxoplasmosis encephalitis in an infant, Canad. Med. Ass. J. 100:343, 1969.

114. Koeze, T. H. and Klingon, G. H.: Acquired toxoplasmosis, Arch. Neurol. 11:191, 1964.

115. Hall, E. G., et al.: Congenital toxoplasmosis in the newborn, Arch. Dis. Child. 28:117, 1953.

115a.Altschuler, G.: Toxoplasmosis as a cause of hydranencephaly, Amer. J. Dis. Child. 125:251, 1973.

116. Eichenwald, H. F.: *Human Toxoplasmosis: Proceedings of the Conference on Clinical Aspects and Diagnostic Problems of Toxoplasmosis in Pediatrics*, Baltimore: Williams & Wilkins Co., 1956.

117. Feldman, H. A.: Congenital toxoplasmosis. Study of one hundred three cases, Amer. J. Dis. Child. 86:487, 1953.

118. Thalhammer, Von O.: Oligosymptomatische toxoplasmose, Helv. Paediat. Acta 9:50, 1954.

119. Feldman, H. A.: Toxoplasmosis, New Eng. J. Med. 279:1370, 1968.

120. Mussbichler, H.: Radiologic study of intracranial calcifications in congenital toxoplasmosis, Acta Radiol. [Diagn.] (Stockholm) 7:369, 1968.

120a.Nahmias, A. J., Tompkins, W. J. F., and Korones, A. J.: Infection of the newborn with herpesvirus hominis, Advances Pediat. 17:185, 1970.

121. Tuffli, G. A. and Nahmias, A. J.: Neonatal herpetic infection, Amer. J. Dis. Child. 118:909, 1969.

121a.Most, H.: Treatment of common parasitic infections of man encountered in the United States, New Eng. J. Med. 287:495, 698, 1972.

122. Dalessio, D. J. and Wolff, H. G.: *Trichinella spiralis* infection of the central nervous system, Arch. Neurol. 4:407, 1961.

123. Gould, S. E.: *Trichinosis*, Springfield: Charles C Thomas Publisher, 1945.

124. Ozere, R. L., et al.: Human trichinosis: Studies on eleven cases affecting two families in Nova Scotia, Canad. Med. Ass. J. 87:1353, 1962.

125. Kramer, M. D. and Aita, J. F.: Trichinosis with central nervous system involvement, Neurology (Minneap.) 22:485, 1972.

126. Reddy, D. and Murty, V. R.: Cerebral cysticercosis. (A detailed clinico-pathological study from four autopsied cases), J. Trop. Med. Hyg. 71:158, 1968.

127. Orman, D. N. and LeRoux, P. A. T.: Cerebral hydatid disease: A radiological review, S. Afr. Med. J. 42:1048, 1968.

128. Chalgren, W. S. and Baker, A. B: The nervous system in tropical disease, Medicine (Baltimore) 26:395, 1947.

129. Thomas, J. D.: Clinical and histopathological correlation of cerebral malaria, Trop. Geogr. Med. 23:232, 1971.

130. Van Bogaert, L. and Janssen, P.: Contribution a l'etude de la neurologie et neuropathologie de la trypanosominiase humaine, Ann. Soc. Belg. Med. Trop. 37:379, 1957.

131. Jorg, M. E. and Orlando, A. S.: Encefalopatia en la tripanosomiasis cruzi cronica: Estudio de dos casos, Prensa Med. Argent. 54:1965, 1967.

132. Duma, R. J., et al.: Primary amoebic meningoencephalitis caused by *Naegleria*; Two new cases, response to amphotericin B and a review, Ann. Intern. Med. (Chicago) 74:923, 1971.

133. Duma, R. J., et al.: Primary amebic meningoencephalitis, New Eng. J. Med. 281:1315, 1969.

134. Orbison, J. A., et al.: Amebic brain abscess: Review of the literature and report of 5 additional cases, Medicine (Baltimore) 30:247, 1951.

135. Chitanondh, H. and Rosen, L.: Fatal eosinophilic encephalomyelitis caused by the nematode *Gnathostoma spinigerum*, Amer. J. Trop. Med. 16:638, 1967.

136. Schochet, S. S.: Human *Toxocara canis* encephalopathy in a case of visceral larva migrans, Neurology (Minneap.) 17:227, 1967.

137. Bird, A. C., Smith, J. L., and Curtin, V. T.: Nematode optic neuritis, Amer. J. Ophthal. 69:72, 1970.

138. Carroll, D. G.: Cerebral involvement in schistosomiasis japonica, Bull. Hopkins Hosp. 78:219, 1946.

139. Zilberg, B.: Bilharzial paraplegia in a child— a case report, S. Afr. Med. J. 41:783, 1967.

140. Oh, S. J.: Bithional treatment in cerebral paragonimiasis, Amer. J. Trop. Med. 16:585, 1967.

141. Oh, S. J.: Roentgen findings in cerebral paragonimiasis, Radiology 90:292, 1968.

142. Shim, J. Y. and Park, C. S.: Cerebral paragonimiasis, Proc. Aust. Ass. Neurol. 5:361, 1968.

142a. Higashi, K., et al.: Cerebral paragonimiasis, J. Neurosurg. 34:515, 1971.

143. Arana-Iniguez, R. and Lopez-Fernandez, J. R.: Parasitosis of the nervous system, with special reference to echinococcosis, Clin. Neurosurg. 14:123, 1966.

144. Melnick, J. L., Wenner, H. A., and Rosen, L.: "Enteroviruses," in Lennette, E. H. and Schmidt, N. J. (eds.): *Diagnostic Procedures for Viral and Rickettsial Infections*, 4th ed., New York: American Public Health Association, 1969.

145. Bodian, D. and Horstmann, D. M.: "Polioviruses," in Horsfall, F. L. and Tamm, I. (eds.): *Viral and Rickettsial Infections of Man*, Philadelphia: J. B. Lippincott Co., 1965.

146. Trueta, J.: Physiologic mechanisms involved in the localization of paralysis, Ann. NY Acad. Sci. USA 61:883, 1955.

147. Heine, J.: *Beobachtungen über Lähmungszustände der untern Extremitäten und deren Behandlung*, Stuttgart: Kohler, 1840.

148. Feigin, R. D., Guggenheim, M. A., and Johnsen, S. D.: Vaccine-related paralytic poliomyelitis in an immunodeficient child, J. Pediat. 79:642, 1971.

149. Baker, A. B., Cornwell, S., and Tichy, F.: Poliomyelitis IX. The cerebral hemispheres, Arch. Neurol. Psychiat. 71:435, 1954.

150. Baker, A. B. and Cornwell, S.: Poliomyelitis X. The cerebellum, Arch. Neurol. Psychiat. 71:455, 1954.

151. Horstmann, D. M. and Paul, J. R.: The incubation period in human poliomyelitis and its implications, JAMA 135:11, 1947.

152. Horstmann, D. M.: Poliomyelitis: Severity and type of disease in different age groups, Ann. NY Acad. Sci. USA 61:956, 1955.

153. Wernstedt, W.: Epidemiologische Studien über die zweite grosse Poliomyelitisepidemie in Schweden 1911–1913, Ergebn. Inn. Med. Kinderheilk. 26:248, 1924.

154. Lawson, R. B. and Garvey, F. K.: Paralysis of the bladder in poliomyelitis, JAMA 135:93, 1947.

155. Minnesota Poliomyelitis Research Commission: The bulbar form of poliomyelitis, JAMA 134:757, 1947, and 135:425, 1947.

156. Baker, A. B., Matzke, H. A., and Brown, J. R.: Poliomyelitis III. Bulbar poliomyelitis: A study of medullary function, Arch. Neurol. Psychiat. 63:257, 1950.

157. Baker, A. B.: Poliomyelitis: A study of pulmonary edema, Neurology (Minneap.) 7:743, 1957.

158. Baker, A. B., Cornwell, S., and Brown, I. A.: Poliomyelitis VI. The hypothalamus, Arch. Neurol. Psychiat. 68:16, 1952.

159. Merritt, H. H. and Fremont-Smith, F.: *The Cerebrospinal Fluid*, Philadelphia: W. B. Saunders Co., 1937.

160. Bodian, D. and Howe, H. A.: Experimental non-paralytic poliomyelitis: Frequency and range of pathological involvement, Bull. Hopkins Hosp. 76:1, 1945.

161. Bukh, N.: Muscle recovery in poliomyelitis, Acta Orthop. Scand. 39:579, 1968.

162. Russell, W. R.: *Poliomyelitis*, 2nd ed., London: Edward Arnold, Ltd., 1956.

163. Moossy, J. and Geer, J. C.: Encephalomyelitis, myocarditis and adrenal cortical necrosis in coxsackie B₃ virus infection, Arch. Path. 70:614, 1960.

164. Kibrick, S. and Benirschke, K.: Severe generalized disease (encephalohepato-myocarditis) occurring in the newborn period and due to infection with coxsackie virus, Group B: Evidence of intrauterine infection with this agent, Pediatrics 22:857, 1958.

165. Walker, S. H. and Togo, Y.: Encephalitis due to group B, type 5 coxsackie virus, Amer. J. Dis. Child. 105:209, 1963.

166. Walters, J. H.: Post-encephalitic Parkinson syndrome after meningoencephalitis due to coxsackie virus Group B, Type 2, New Eng. J. Med. 263:744, 1960.

167. Ravetto, F., Ghidella, G., and Colonna, F.: Acute benign ataxia referable to coxsackie A: 5 cases observed during the summer of 1967, Minerva Pediat. 20:2227, 1968.

168. Marzetti, M. and Balducci, L.: Unilateral paralysis of the third pair of cranial nerves associated with A 9 coxsackie virus infection, Minerva Pediat. 20:943, 1968.

169. Tosphy, D. E., et al.: An epidemic of aseptic meningitis due to ECHO virus Type 30. Epidemiologic features and clinical and laboratory findings, Amer. J. Public Health 60:1147, 1970.

170. Karzon, D. T., et al.: An epidemic of aseptic meningitis syndrome due to ECHO virus Type 6. II. A clinical study of ECHO 6 infection, Pediatrics 29:418, 1962.

171. Forbes, S. J., Brumlik, J., and Harding, H. B.: Acute ascending polyradiculomyelitis associated with ECHO 9 virus, Dis. Nerv. Syst. 28:537, 1970.

172. Simila, S., et al.: Encephalomeningitis in children associated with an adenovirus type 7 epidemic, Acta Paediat. Scand. 59:310, 1970.

173. Burnstine, R. C. and Paine, R. S.: Residual encephalopathy following roseola infantum, Amer. J. Dis. Child. 98:144, 1959.

174. Casals, J. and Clarke, D. H.: "Arboviruses: Group A," in Horsfall, F. L. and Tamm, I. (eds.): *Viral and Rickettsial Infections of Man*, Philadelphia: J. B. Lippincott Co., 1965.

175. Clarke, D. H. and Casals, J.: "Arboviruses: Group B" in Horsfall, F. L. and Tamm, I. (eds.): *Viral and Rickettsial Infections of Man*, Philadelphia: J. B. Lippincott Co., 1965.

176. Monath, T. P. C., et al.: Studies on California encephalitis in Minnesota, Amer. J. Epidem. 92:40, 1970.

177. Thompson, W. H., Kalfayan, B., and Anslow, R. O.: Isolation of California encephalitis group virus from a fatal human illness, Amer. J. Epidem. 81:245, 1965.

178. Young, D. J.: California encephalitis virus: Report of three cases and review of the literature, Ann. Intern. Med. 65:419, 1966.

179. Chun, R. W. M., et al.: California arbovirus encephalitis in children, Neurology (Minneap.) 18:369, 1968.

180. Cramblett, H. G., Stegmiller, H., and Spencer, C.: California encephalitis virus infections in children, JAMA 198:108, 1966.

181. Johnson, K. P., Lepow, M. L., and Johnson, R. T.: California encephalitis. I. Clinical and epidemiological studies, Neurology (Minneap.) 18:250, 1968.

181a. Matthews, C. G., et al.: Psychological sequelae in children with California arbovirus encephalitis, Neurology (Minneap.) 18:1023, 1968.

182. Finley, K. H., et al.: Western encephalitis and cerebral ontogenesis, Arch. Neurol. 16:140, 1967.

183. Earnest, M. P., et al.: Neurologic, intellectual and psychologic sequelae following western encephalitis, Neurology (Minneap.) 21:969, 1971.

184. Robertson, E. G. and McLorinan, H.: Murray Valley encephalitis: Clinical aspects, Med. J. Aust. 1:103, 1952.

185. McCordock, H. A., Collier, W., and Gray, S. H.: The pathologic changes of the St. Louis type of acute encephalitis, JAMA 103:822, 1934.

186. Zentay, P. J. and Basman, J.: Epidemic encephalitis type B in children, J. Pediat. 14:323, 1939.

187. Barrett, F. F., Yow, M. D., and Phillips, C. A.: St. Louis encephalitis in children during the 1964 epidemic, JAMA 193:381, 1965.

188. Ayar, G. J., et al.: Follow-up studies of St. Louis encephalitis in Florida, Amer. J. Public Health 56:1074, 1966.

189. Lawton, A. H., et al.: Follow-up studies of St. Louis encephalitis in Florida: Reevaluation of the emotional and health status of the survivors five years after acute illness, Southern Med. J. 63:66, 1970.

190. Smadel, J. E., Bailey, P., and Baker, A. B.: Sequelae of the arthropod-borne encephalitides, Neurology (Minneap.) 8:873, 1958.

191. Noran, H. H. and Baker, A. B.: Western equine encephalitis: The pathogenesis of the pathological lesions, J. Neuropath. Exp. Neurol. 4:269, 1945.

192. Reeves, W. C. and Hammon, W. M.: *Epidemiology of the Arthropod-borne Viral Encephalitides in Kern County, California 1943–1952*, Berkeley: University of California Press, 1962.

193. Kokernot, R. H., Shinefield, H. R., and Longshore, W. A., Jr.: The 1952 outbreak of encephalitis in California: Differential diagnosis, Calif. Med. 79:73, 1953.

194. Feemster, R. T.: Outbreak of encephalitis in man due to Eastern virus of equine encephalomyelitis, Amer. J. Public Health 28:1403, 1938.

195. Farber, S., et al.: Encephalitis in infants and children caused by the virus of the Eastern variety of equine encephalitis, JAMA 114:1725, 1940.

196. U. S. Dept. H. E. W.: Center for Disease Control Bulletin 20: 310, 1971.

197. Richter, R. W. and Shimojyo, S.: Neurologic sequelae of Japanese B encephalitis, Neurology (Minneap.) 11:553, 1961.

198. Hloucal, L.: Tick-borne encephalitis as observed in Czechoslovakia, J. Trop. Med. Hyg. 63:293, 1960.

199. Clarke, D. H.: Further studies on antigenic relationships among the viruses of the group B tick-borne complex, Bull. WHO 31:45, 1964.

200. Silver, H. K., Meiklejohn, G., and Kempe, C. H.: Colorado tick fever, Amer. J. Dis. Child. 101:30, 1961.

201. Casals, J. and Clarke, D. H.: "Arboviruses Other Than Groups A and B," in Horsfall, F. L. and Tamm, I. (eds.): *Viral and Rickettsial Infections of Man*, Philadelphia: J. B. Lippincott Co., 1965.

202. Plummer, G., et al.: Type 1 and type 2 herpes simplex viruses: Serological and biological differences, J. Virology 5:51, 1970.

203. Dowdle, W. R., et al.: Association of antigenic type of herpes-virus hominis with site of viral recovery, J. Immun. 99:974, 1967.

204. Johnson, R. T. and Mims, C. A.: Pathogenesis of viral infections of the nervous system, New Eng. J. Med. 278:23, 85, 1968.

205. Leider, W., et al.: Herpes-simplex-virus encephalitis: Its possible association with reactivated latent infection, New Eng. J. Med. 273: 341, 1965.

206. Crompton, M. R. and Teare, R. D.: Encephalitis after reduction of steroid maintenance therapy, Lancet 2:1318, 1965.

207. Drachman, D. A. and Adams, R. D.: Herpes simplex and acute inclusion-body encephalitis, Arch. Neurol. 7:45, 1962.

208. Olson, L. C., et al.: Herpesvirus infections of the human central nervous system, New Eng. J. Med. 277:1272, 1967.

208a. Illis, L. S. and Gostling, J. V. T.: *Herpes Simplex Encephalitis*, Bristol: Scientechnica, 1972.

209. Miller, J. K., Hesser, F., and Tompkins, V. N.: Herpes simplex encephalitis: Report of 20 cases, Ann. Intern. Med. 64:92, 1966.

210. Upton, A. and Gumpert, J.: Electroencephalography in diagnosis of herpes-simplex encephalitis, Lancet 1:650, 1970.

211. Johnson, R. T., Olson, L. C., and Buescher, E. L.: Herpes simplex virus infections of the nervous system, Arch. Neurol. 18:260, 1968.

212. Nolan, D. C., Carruthers, M. M., and Lerner, A. M.: Herpes-virus hominis encephalitis in Michigan: Report of 13 cases, including 6 treated with idoxuridine, New Eng. J. Med. 282:10, 1970.

213. Meyer, J. S., et al : *Herpesvirus hominis* encephalitis, Arch. Neurol. 23:438, 1970.

214. Rappel, M.: Treatment of herpesvirus encephalitis, Lancet 1:971, 1971.

215. Marshall, W. J. S.: Herpes simplex encephalitis treated with idoxuridine and external decompression, Lancet 2:579, 1967.

216. Upton, A. R. M., Barwick, D. D., and Foster, J. B.: Dexamethasone treatment in herpes-simplex encephalitis, Lancet 1:290, 1971.

217. Downie, A. W.: Chickenpox and zoster, Brit. Med. Bull. 15:197, 1959.

218. Hope-Simpson, R. E.: The nature of herpes zoster. A long term study and a new hypothesis, Proc. Roy. Soc. Med. 58:9, 1965.

219. Denny-Brown, D., Adams, R. D., and Fitzgerald, P. J.: Pathologic features of herpes zoster. A note on "geniculate herpes," Arch. Neurol. Psychiat. 51:216, 1944.

220. Rose, F. C., Brett, E. M., and Burston, J.: Zoster encephalomyelitis, Arch. Neurol. 11:155, 1964.

221. Keidan, S. E. and Mainwaring, D.: Association of herpes zoster with leukemia and lymphoma in children, Clin. Pediat. (Philadelphia) 4:13, 1965.

222. Merselis, J. G., Jr., Kaye, D., and Hooke, E. W.: Disseminated herpes zoster: A report of 17 cases. Arch. Intern. Med. (Chicago) 113:679, 1964.

223. Pasteur, L.: Methode pour prevenir la rage apres morsure, C. R. Acad. Sci. (Paris) 101:765, 1885.

224. Blattner, R. J.: Bats and rabies, J. Pediat. 46:612, 1955.

225. Constantine, D. G.: Rabies transmission by nonbite route, Public Health Rep. 77:287, 1962.

226. Johnson, H. N.: "Rabies Virus," in Horsfall, F. L. and Tamm, I. (eds.): *Viral and Rickettsial Infections of Man*, Philadelphia: J. B. Lippincott Co., 1965.

227. McKendrick, A. G.: A ninth analytical review of reports from Pasteur Institutes on the results of anti-rabies treatment, Bull. Health Organ. League of Nations, 9:31, 1940.

228. Schindler, R.: Studies on the pathogenesis of rabies, Bull. WHO 25:119, 1961.

229. González-Angulo A., et al.: The ultrastructure of Negri-bodies in Purkinje neurons in human rabies, Neurology (Minneap.) 20:323, 1970.

230. Blatt, M. L., Hoffman, S. J., and Schneider, M.: Rabies: Report of twelve cases, with a discussion of prophylaxis, JAMA 111:688, 1938.

231. Cheetham, H. D., et al.: Rabies with myocarditis. 2 cases in England, Lancet 1:921, 1970.

231a. Hattwick, M. A. W., et al.: Recovery from rabies, Ann. Intern. Med. 76:931, 1972.

232. Cereghino, J. J., et al.: Rabies: A rare disease but a serious pediatric problem, Pediatrics 45:839, 1970.

232a. Ellenbogen, C. and Slugg, P.: Rabies neutralizing antibody: Inadequate response to equine antiserum and duck-embryo vaccine, J. Infect. Dis. 127:433, 1973.

232b. Rubin, P. H., et al.: Human rabies immune globulin, JAMA 224:871, 1973.

233. Kaplan, M. M., et al.: Studies on the local treatment of wounds for the prevention of rabies, Bull. WHO 26:765, 1962.

234. Kreis, B.: "Lymphocytic choriomeningitis," in Debre, R. and Celers, J. (eds.): *Clinical Virology*, Philadelphia: W. B. Saunders Co., 1970.

235. Howard, M. E.: Infection with the virus of choriomeningitis in man, Yale J. Biol. Med. 13:161, 1940.

236. Baker, A. B.: Chronic lymphocytic choriomeningitis, J. Neuropath. Exp. Neurol. 6:253, 1947.

237. Baum, S. G., et al.: Epidemic non-meningitic lymphocytic-choriomeningitis-virus infection, New Eng. J. Med. 274:934, 1966.

238. Lewis, J. M. and Utz, J. P.: Orchitis, parotitis and meningoencephalitis due to lymphocytic choriomeningitis virus, New Eng. J. Med. 265:776, 1961.

239. Green, W. R., Sweet, L. K., and Prichard, R. W.: Acute lymphocytic choriomeningitis: A study of 21 cases, J. Pediat. 35:688, 1949.

240. Adair, C. V., Gauld, R. L., and Smadel, J. E.: Aseptic meningitis, a disease of diverse etiology: Clinical and etiologic studies on 854 cases, Ann. Intern. Med. 39:675, 1953.

241. Gautier-Smith, P. C.: Neurological complications of glandular fever (infectious mononucleosis), Brain 88:323, 1965.

242. Silverstein, A., Steinberg, G., and Nathanson, M.: Nervous system involvement in infectious mononucleosis, Arch. Neurol. 26:353, 1972.

243. Henle, G., Henle, W., and Diehl, V.: Relation of Burkitt's tumor-associated herpes-type virus to infectious mononucleosis, Proc. Nat. Acad. Sci. USA 59:94, 1968.

244. Silver, H K., et al.: Involvement of the central nervous system in infectious mononucleosis in childhood, Amer. J. Dis. Child. 91:490, 1956.

245. Shechter, F. R., Lipsius, E. I., and Rasansky, H. N.: Retrobulbar neuritis. A complication of infectious mononucleosis, Amer. J. Dis. Child. 89:58, 1955.

246. Erwin, W., Weber, R. W., and Manning, R. T.: Complications of infectious mononucleosis, Amer. J. Med. Sci. 238:699, 1959.

247. Nellhaus, G.: Isolated oculomotor nerve palsy in infectious mononucleosis, Neurology (Minneap.) 16 (pt. 2):221, 1966.

248. Pejme, J.: Infectious mononucleosis, Acta Med. Scand. Suppl. 413:51, 1964.

249. Davidsohn, I., Stern, K., and Kashiwagi, C.: The differential test for infectious mononucleosis, Amer. J. Clin. Path. 21:1101, 1951.

250. Karpinski, F. E.: Neurologic manifestations of infectious mononucleosis in childhood, Pediatrics 10:265, 1952.

251. Debre, R., et al.: La maladie des griffes de chat, Sem. Hop. (Paris) 26:1895, 1950.

252. Turner, W., et al.: Hemagglutinating virus isolated from cat scratch disease, J. Bact. 80:430, 1950.

253. Kalter, S. S., Kim, C. S., and Heberling, R. L.: Herpes-like virus particles associated with cat

254. Warwick, W. J.: The cat-scratch syndrome, many diseases or one disease? Progr. Med. Virol. 9:256, 1967.

255. Lyon, L. W.: Neurological manifestations of cat-scratch disease, Arch. Neurol. 25:23, 1971.

256. Steiner, M. W., Vuckovitch, D., and Hadawi, S. A.: Cat-scratch disease with encephalopathy, J. Pediat. 62:514, 1963.

257. Sigurdsson, B.: Rida, a chronic encephalitis of sheep. With general remarks on infections which develop slowly and some of their special characteristics, Brit. Vet. J. 110:341, 1954.

258. Johnson, R. T. and Johnson, K. P.: "Slow and Chronic Virus Infections of the Nervous System," in Plum, F. (ed.): *Recent Advances in Neurology*, Philadelphia: F. A. Davis Company, 1969.

259. Berndt, R. M.: Reaction to contact in the eastern highlands of New Guinea, Oceania 24:206, 1954.

260. Gajdusek, D. C. and Zigas, V.: Kuru, Amer. J. Med. 26:442, 1959.

261. Gajdusek, D. C. and Gibbs, C. J.: Transmission of kuru from man to Rhesus monkey (*Macaca mulatta*) $8\frac{1}{2}$ years after inoculation, Nature 240:351, 1972.

262. Dawson, J. R., Jr.: Cellular inclusions in cerebral lesions of epidemic encephalitis, Arch. Neurol. Psychiat. 31:685, 1934.

263. Bouteille, M., et al.: Sur un cas d'encephalite subaigue a inclusions. Etude anatomo-clinique et ultrastructurale, Rev. Neurol. (Paris) 113:454, 1965.

264. Baublis, J. V. and Payne, F. E.: Measles antigen and syncytium formation in brain cell cultures from subacute sclerosing panencephalitis (SSPE), Proc. Soc. Exp. Biol. Med. 129:593, 1968.

265. Connolly, J. H., et al.: Measles-virus antibody and antigen in subacute sclerosing panencephalitis, Lancet 1:542, 1967.

266. Chen, T. T., et al.: Subacute sclerosing panencephalitis: Propagation of measles virus from brain biopsy in tissue culture, Science 163:1193, 1969.

267. Horta-Barbosa, L., Fuccillo, D. A., and Sever, J. L.: Chronic viral infections of the central nervous system, JAMA 218:1185, 1971.

268. Herndon, R. M. and Rubinstein, L. J.: Light and electron microscopy observation on the development of viral particles in the inclusions of Dawson's encephalitis (subacute sclerosing panencephalitis), Neurology 18 (pt. 2):8, 1968.

269. Koprowski, H., Barbanti-Brodano, G., and Katz, M.: Interaction between papova-like virus and paramyxovirus in human brain cells: A hypothesis, Nature 225:1045, 1970.

270. Brody, J. A. and Detels, R.: Subacute sclerosing panencephalitis: A zoonosis following aberrant measles, Lancet 2:500, 1970.

271. Brody, J. A., Detels, R., and McNew, J.: Evidence that subacute sclerosing panencephalitis is caused by aberrant measles infection followed by a zoonosis, Neurology (Minneap.) 21:439, 1971.

272. Robb, R. M. and Watters, G. V.: Ophthalmic manifestations of sub-acute sclerosing panencephalitis, Arch. Ophthal. 83:426, 1970.

273. Freeman, J. M.: The clinical spectrum and early diagnosis of Dawson's encephalitis, J. Pediat. 75:590, 1969.

274. Cutler, R. W. P., Merler, E., and Hammerstad, J. P.: Production of antibody by the central nervous system in subacute sclerosing panencephalitis, Neurology 18 (pt. 2):129, 1968.

275. Tourtellotte, W. W., et al.: Subacute sclerosing panencephalitis: Brain immunoglobulin-G measles antibody and albumin, Neurology 18 (pt. 2):117, 1968.

276. Lombroso, C. T.: Remarks on the EEG and movement disorder in SSPE, Neurology 18 (pt. 2):69, 1968.

277. Haslam, R. H. A., McQuillen, M. P., and Clark, D. B.: Amantadine therapy in subacute sclerosing panencephalitis, Neurology 19:1080, 1969.

277a. Gajl-Pecksalska, K. J., et al.: B lymphocytes in lepromatous leprosy, New Eng. J. Med. 288:186, 1973.

278. Crawford, C. T.: Neurological lesions in leprosy, Leprosy Rev. 39:9, 1968.

279. Monrad-Krohn, G. H.: *The Neurological Aspect of Leprosy*, Chicago: Chicago Medical Book Co., 1923.

280. Magoro, A., et al.: The condition of the peripheral nerve in leprosy under various forms of treatment, Int. J. Leprosy 38:149, 1970.

281. Dash, M. S.: A study of the mechanisms of cutaneous sensory loss in leprosy, Brain 91:379, 1968.

282. Job, C. K., et al.: Leprous myositis—a histopathological and electron microscopic study, Leprosy Rev. 40:9, 1969.

283. Waters, M. F. R., Rees, R. J. W., and Sutherland, I.: Chemotherapeutic trials in leprosy, Int. J. Leprosy 35:311, 1967.

284. Brown, R. E.: Prevention of leprosy: New ideas out of Africa, Clin. Pediat. (Philadelphia) 6:446, 1967.
285. Hubbert, W. T. and Humphrey, G. L.: Epidemiology of leptospirosis in California: Causes of aseptic meningitis, Calif. Med. 108:113, 1968.
286. Alston, J. M. and Broom, J. C.: *Leptospirosis in Man and Animals*, Edinburgh: E. & S. Livingstone, Ltd., 1958.
287. Ujházyová-Králiková, D. and Veljačiková, Z.: Neurologic aspects of leptospirosis, Bratisl. Lek. Listy 52:573, 1968.
288. Merritt, H. H., Adams, R. D., and Solomon, H. C.: *Neurosyphilis*, New York: Oxford University Press, 1946.
289. Hallgren, B. and Hallstrom, E.: Congenital syphilis: A follow-up study with reference to mental abnormalities, Acta Psychiat. Neurol. Scand. Suppl. 93, 1954.
290. Hunter, E. F., Deacon, W. E., and Meyer, P. E.: An improved FTA test for syphilis, the absorption procedure (FTA-ABS), Public Health Rep. 79:410, 1964.
291. Deacon, W. E., Lucas, J. B., and Price, E. V.: Fluorescent treponemal antibody-absorption (FTA-ABS) test for syphilis, JAMA 198:624, 1966.
292. Alford, C. A., Jr., et al.: Gamma-M-fluorescent treponemal antibody in the diagnosis of congenital syphilis, New Eng. J. Med. 280:1086, 1969.
293. Brown, S. J.: "Syphilis," in Gellis, S. S. and Kagan, B. M. (eds.): *Current Pediatric Therapy*, Philadelphia: W. B. Saunders Co., 1971.
294. Fetter, B. F., Klintworth, G. K., and Hendry, W. S.: *Mycoses of the Central Nervous System*, Baltimore: Williams & Wilkins Co., 1967.
295. Kozinn, P. J., et al.: Candida meningitis successfully treated with amphotericin B, New Eng. J. Med. 268:881, 1963.
296. Roessmann, U. and Friede, R. L.: Candidal infection of the brain, Arch. Path. 84:495, 1967.
297. Conant, N. F.: "Medical Mycology," in Dubos, R. J. and Hirsch, J. G. (eds.): *Bacterial and Mycotic Infections of Man*, Philadelphia: J. B. Lippincott Co., 1965.
298. Caudill, R. G., Smith, C. E., and Reinarz, J. A.: Coccidioidal meningitis. A diagnostic challenge, Amer. J. Med. 49:360, 1970.
299. McCullough, D. C. and Harbert, J. C.: Isotope demonstration of CSF pathways. Guide to antifungal therapy in coccidioidal meningitis, JAMA 209:558, 1969.
300. Reeves, D. L.: Chronic coccidioidal meningitis. Report of two cases, J. Neurosurg. 28:383, 1968.
301. Winn, W. A.: The treatment of coccidioidal meningitis, Calif. Med. 101:78, 1964.
301a. Diamond, R. D. and Bennett, J. E.: A subcutaneous reservoir for intrathecal therapy of fungal meningitis, New Eng. J. Med. 288:186, 1973.
302. Cooper, R. A. and Goldstein, E.: Histoplasmosis of the central nervous system, Amer. J. Med. 35:45, 1963.
303. Gordon, M. A. and Vedder, D. K.: Serologic tests in diagnosis and prognosis of cryptococcosis, JAMA 197:131, 1966.
304. McIntyre, H.: Cryptococcal meningitis. A case successfully treated by cisternal administration of amphotericin B with a review of the recent literature, Bull. Los Angeles Neurol. Soc. 32:213, 1967.
305. Sarosi, G. A., et al.: Amphotericin B in cryptococcal meningitis: Long-term results of treatment, Ann. Intern. Med. 71:1079, 1969.
306. Goodman, J. S., Kaufman, L., and Koenig, M. G.: Diagnosis of cryptococcal meningitis, New Eng. J. Med. 285:434, 1971.
307. Barter, A. P. and Falconer, M. A.: Actinomycosis of the brain, Guy. Hosp. Rep. 104:135, 1955.
308. Iyer, S., Dodge, P. R., and Adams, R. D.: Two cases of Aspergillus infection of the central nervous system, J. Neurol. Neurosurg. Psychiat. 15:152, 1952.
309. Rainey, R. L. and Harris, T. R.: Disseminated blastomycosis with meningeal involvement, Arch. Intern. Med. (Chicago) 117:744, 1966.
310. Papadatos, C., Pavlatou, M., and Alexiou, D.: *Cephalosporium* meningitis, Pediatrics 44:749, 1969.
311. Landau, J. W. and Newcomer, V. D.: Acute cerebral phycomycosis (mucormycosis), J. Pediat. 61:363, 1962.
312. Blodi, F. C., Hannah, F. T., and Wadsworth, J. A.: Lethal orbitocerebral phycomycosis in otherwise healthy children, Amer. J. Ophthal. 67:698, 1969.
313. Carlile, W. K., Holle, K. E., and Logan, G. B.: Fatal acute disseminated nocardiosis in a child, JAMA 184:477, 1963.
314. Ballenger, C. N., Jr. and Goldring, D.: Nocardiosis in childhood, J. Pediat. 50:145, 1957.
315. Woodward, T. E. and Jackson, E. B.: "Spotted Fever Rickettsiae," in Horsfall, F. L. and Tamm, I. (eds.): *Viral and Rickettsial Infections of Man*, Philadelphia: J. B. Lippincott Co., 1965.
316. Bell, W. E. and Lascari, A. D.: Rocky Mountain spotted fever. Neurological symptoms in the acute phase, Neurology (Minneap.) 20:841, 1970.
317. Feigin, R. D., et al.: Rocky Mountain spotted fever. Successful application of new insights into physiologic changes during acute infections to successful management of a severely-ill patient, Clin. Pediat. (Phila.) 8:331, 1969.
318. Raab, E. L., Leopold, I. H., and Hodes, H. L.: Retinopathy in Rocky Mountain spotted fever, Amer. J. Ophthal. 68:42, 1969.
319. Rosenblum, M. J., Masland, R. L., and Harrell, G. T.: Residual effects of rickettsial disease on the central nervous system, Arch. Intern. Med. (Chicago) 90:444, 1952.
320. Haynes, R. E., Sanders, D. Y., and Cramblett, H. G.: Rocky Mountain spotted fever in children, J. Pediat. 76:685, 1970.
321. Hazard, G. W., et al.: Rocky Mountain spotted

fever in the Eastern United States, New Eng. J. Med. 280:57, 1969.

322. Noad, K. B. and Haymaker, W.: Neurological features of tsutsugamushi fever with special reference to deafness, Brain 76:113, 1953.

323. Herman, E.: Neurological syndromes in typhus fever, J. Nerv. Ment. Dis. 109:25, 1949.

324. Jefferson, M.: Sarcoidosis of the nervous system, Brain 80:540, 1957.

325. Symonds, C.: Recurrent multiple cranial nerve palsies, J. Neurol. Neurosurg. Psychiat. 21:95, 1958.

326. Hinterbuchner, C. N. and Hinterbuchner, L. P.: Myopathic syndrome in muscular sarcoidosis, Brain 87:355, 1964.

327. Heerfordt, C. F.: Uber eine, "Febris uveoparotidea sub chronica" an der glandula parotis und der Uvea des Auges lokalisiert und haufig mit Paresen cerebrospinaler Nerven kompliziert, Arch. Ophthal. 70:254, 1909.

328. McGovern, J. P. and Merritt, D H : Sarcoidosis in childhood, Advances Pediat. 8:97, 1956.

329. Stevens, H.: Melkersson's syndrome, Neurology (Minneap.) 15:263, 1965.

330. Jasper, P. L. and Denny, F. W.: Sarcoidosis in children, J. Pediat. 73:499, 1968.

331. Reye, R. D., Morgan, G., and Baral, J.: Encephalopathy and fatty degeneration of the viscera. A disease entity in childhood, Lancet 2:749, 1963.

332. Bradford, W. D. and Parker, J. C.: Reye's syndrome, Clin. Pediat. (Philadelphia) 10:148, 1971.

333. Jenkins, R., Dvorak, A., and Patrick, J.: Encephalopathy and fatty degeneration of the viscera associated with chickenpox, Pediatrics 39:769, 1967.

334. Joske, R. A., et al.: Hepatitis-encephalitis in humans with reovirus infection, Arch. Intern. Med. (Chicago) 113:811, 1964.

335. Norman, M. G., et al.: Encephalopathy and fatty degeneration of viscera in children. II. Report of a case with isolation of influenza B virus, Canad. Med. Ass. J. 99:549, 1968.

335a.Powell, H. C., et al.: Reye's syndrome: Isolation of parainfluenza virus, Arch. Neurol. 29:135, 1973.

336. Golden, G. S. and Duffell, D.: Encephalopathy and fatty change in liver and kidney, Pediatrics 36:67, 1965.

337. Olson, L. C., et al.: Encephalopathy and fatty degeneration of the viscera in northeastern Thailand. Clinical syndrome and epidemiology, Pediatrics 47:707, 1971.

337a.Glasgow, A. M., et al.: Reye's syndrome. II. Occurrence in the absence of severe fatty infiltration of the liver, Amer. J. Dis. Child. 124:834, 1972.

337b.Glasgow, A. M., et al.: Reye's syndrome. I. Blood ammonia and consideration of the nonhistologic diagnosis, Amer. J. Dis. Child. 124:827, 1972.

337c.Glasgow, A. M., et al.: Reye's syndrome. III. The hypoglycemia, Amer. J. Dis. Child. 125:809, 1973.

338. Partin, J. C., Schubert, W. K., and Partin, J. S.: Mitochondrial ultrastructure in Reye's syndrome, New Eng. J. Med. 285:1339, 1971.

339. Lyon, G., Dodge, P. R., and Adams, R. D.: The acute encephalopathies of obscure origin in infants and children, Brain 84:680, 1961.

340. Behcet, H.: Über rezidivierende Aphthose durch ein Virus verursachte Geschwüre am Mund, am Auge und an den Genitalien, Derm. Wschr. 105:1152, 1937.

341. Herrmann, C.: Involvement of the nervous system in relapsing uveitis with recurrent genital and oral ulcers (Behcet's syndrome), Arch. Neurol. Psychiat. 69:399, 1953.

342. Rubinstein, L. J. and Urich, H.: Meningoencephalitis of Behcet's disease: Case report with pathological findings, Brain 86:151, 1963.

343. Wolf, S. M., Schotland, D. L., and Phillips, L. L.: Involvement of nervous system in Behcet's syndrome, Arch. Neurol. 12:315, 1965.

344. Mollaret, P.: La meningite endothelio-leucocytaire multirecurrente benigne. Syndrome nouveau ou maladie nouvelle? Documents humoraux et microbiologiques, Ann. Inst. Pasteur (Paris) 71:1, 1945.

345. Bruyn, G. W., Straathof, L. J. A., and Raymakers, G. M. J.: Mollaret's meningitis, Neurology (Minneap.) 12:745, 1962.

346. Hermans, P. E., Goldstein, N. P., and Wellman, W. E.: Mollaret's meningitis and differential diagnosis of recurrent meningitis. Report of case, with review of literature, Amer. J. Med. 52:128, 1972.

347. Riehl, J. L. and Andrews, J. M.: The uveomeningoencephalitic syndrome, Neurology (Minneap.) 16:603, 1966.

348. Basser, L. S.: Benign paroxysmal vertigo of childhood. (A variety of vestibular neuronitis), Brain, 87:141, 1964.

349. Koenigsberger, M. R., et al.: Benign paroxysmal vertigo of childhood, Neurology (Minneap.) 20:1108, 1970.

350. von Economo, C.: *Encephalitis Lethargica: Its Sequelae and Treatment*. London: Oxford University Press, 1931.

351. Association for Research in Nervous and Mental Disease: *Acute Epidemic Encephalitis*, New York: Paul B. Hoeber, 1921.

352. Hohman, L. B.: Post encephalitic behavior disorders in children, Bull. Hopkins Hosp. 33:372, 1922.

Autoimmune and Postinfectious Diseases

INTRODUCTION

In this section we intend to consider three groups of neurologic diseases. One consists of the neurologic manifestations of systemic autoimmune processes, particularly the collagen vascular diseases, the other two are those chronic disorders of the central or peripheral nervous system characterized by demyelination for which no genetic transmission has been demonstrated. Multiple sclerosis, the postinfectious acute disseminated encephalomyelitides, and postinfectious polyneuritis are the most common entities within the latter two groups. Despite recent progress in the knowledge of autoimmune disorders, the autoimmune etiology of these diseases is based on a superficial clinical and neuropathologic resemblance to experimental allergic encephalomyelitis (EAE) and remains speculative.

Rivers and Schwentker were the first to observe that the repeated injection of cerebral tissue into monkeys produced demyelination.[1] Similar lesions have also been consistently produced in other mammalian species, their appearance enhanced by the addition of Freund's adjuvant, a commonly used emulsion of water, oil, and killed acid-fast organisms added to the antigenic material. Its mode of action is unknown but believed to be due to a slow release of antigen, and the induction of an inflammatory reaction which attracts mononuclear cells. In the original studies of Wolf et al.,[2] 90% of monkeys developed the experimental disease within two to eight weeks after the first of an average of three weekly subcutaneous inoculations. The characteristic clinical features included paresis of the extremities, ataxia, nystagmus, and also blindness. Usually the disease was fatal, but some animals had mild symptoms which often subsided, while others developed a neurologic episode spontaneously and, in the experience of Ferraro and Cazullo, a chronic disease with recurrent relapses.[3]

Multiple focal perivascular areas of demyelination are found throughout the neuraxis. Microscopically these lesions show an extensive infiltration by round cells, mainly lymphocytes and microglial cells, small perivascular hemorrhages, and myelin degeneration with preservation of the axon cylinders. In older lesions, the patches of demyelination are well-defined and marked by varying degrees of gliosis. It is still unclear how perivascular demyelination develops in EAE: Waksman and Adams[4] have postulated that it is directly produced by infiltrating cells. This is borne out of the lack of correlation between the development of brain lesions and the presence of circulating antibody, or the delayed skin reaction to the antigen.[5] Furthermore, passive transfer of EAE can be accomplished by lymphocytes but not by serum. However, serum from animals in whom EAE has been induced has a profound effect on nervous tissue in culture, inhibiting electrical potentials and synthesis of sulfatides.[6] The development of EAE can be suppressed by the administration of corticosteroids, nitrogen mustard, or 6-mercaptopurine. Susceptibility to the induction of the condition depends on a number of factors. Immature animals are relatively more resistant to developing EAE than adult animals, while diets inadequate in vitamin B_{12}, biotin, or folic acid decrease susceptibility. Most important, both highly susceptible and highly resistant genetic lines have been segregated in a number of mammalian species.

The nature of the brain antigen responsible for EAE has been elucidated. Several groups of workers have isolated a relatively pure basic protein with encephalitogenic activity from the central nervous system of a number of mammals, which on the basis of immunofluorescence techniques is believed to be a component of normal myelin sheaths.[7] It contributes about 25% of total myelin proteins of adult white matter and in vivo is probably bound to acidic lipids or proteins.[8] The complete amino acid sequence of the human encephalitic protein has been determined. Encephalitogenic activity is due to a sequence of nine amino acid residues with a tryptophan moiety being essential for development of EAE.[9,10]

Whether there is an antigen responsible for multiple sclerosis, or for the postinfectious encephalomyelitides, which is similar to the basic myelin protein responsible for EAE, or whether the antigen is derived from a virus or viruses, remains to be answered. The basic mechanisms involved in the production of EAE serve, however, for the time being as a model for the pathogenesis of the other disorders in this section.

NEUROLOGIC MANIFESTATIONS OF COLLAGEN VASCULAR DISEASES

The collagen vascular diseases are a group of conditions characterized by diffuse changes in the collagen of the connective tissue. Various clinical syndromes have been described, which include lupus erythematosus, periarteritis nodosa, dermatomyositis, polymyositis, rheumatoid arthritis, rheumatic fever, and scleroderma. Whether these entities are intimately related with respect to etiology is still a matter of conjecture. In any case lesions of the central nervous system, peripheral nerves, and musculature are an important feature of all.

LUPUS ERYTHEMATOSUS

Neurologic complications occur in over 80% of children affected by disseminated lupus erythematosus.[11] These may be focal, diffuse, or both, and are due to multiple ischemic lesions throughout the nervous system, notably in the perisulcal cortical gray matter; these result from a marked intimal proliferation of the smaller cerebral and meningeal arteries.[12]

Despite the multiplicity of abnormal serologic reactions against many different tissue components, especially nuclear proteins, the pathogenesis of lupus remains uncertain, as does the manner in which autoantibodies produce tissue damage.[13]

Clinical Manifestations

The condition occurs predominantly in girls, with onset in the second decade. Central nervous system manifestations may occur at any time in the course of the illness. In order of frequency, three syndromes may be distinguished:

1. An organic brain syndrome resulting from cerebral vascular lesions. This may manifest itself by convulsions, cranial nerve palsies, and hemiplegia. Less commonly there is polyneuritis.

2. A toxic encephalopathy resulting in an organic psychosis may be due to cerebral lesions, electrolyte disturbances resulting from impaired renal tubular function, or, rarely, to steroid therapy. Usually, a psychotic reaction is seen during acute exacerbations of the disease, and improves with improvement of systemic manifestations.[14]

3. A syndrome indistinguishable from systemic lupus is induced by giving anticonvulsants, particularly hydantoins (Dilantin, Ce-

TABLE 7-1.
NEUROLOGIC SYMPTOMS AND SIGNS IN
15 CHILDREN WITH SYSTEMIC
LUPUS ERYTHEMATOSUS*

Symptoms or Signs	Number of Patients
Convulsive seizures (grand mal, akinetic, focal motor)	8
Progressive dementia	3
Recurrent psychotic episodes	3
Papilledema	2
Meningeal irritation	2
Progressive quadriparesis	1
Polyneuritis, progressive	1
Subarachnoid hemorrhage	1
Transverse myelitis	1
Cerebellar ataxia	1

* After Gold and Yahr.[11]

lontin) and trimethadione (Tridione).[15] Symptoms usually subside when the offending medication is discontinued but continued exposure to the drug once symptoms have developed may induce irreversible lupus.

The most common neurologic symptoms and signs of childhood lupus are listed in Table 7-1. In 35% neurologic involvement, usually seizures, was the presenting sign of lupus.

The natural history of childhood lupus is variable. Spontaneous exacerbations and remissions are common, but the ultimate prognosis is poor. In Jacobs' series the average survival time of steroid-treated children was over four years from the onset of symptoms. All the patients whose disease had resolved were those having an anticonvulsant-induced form of lupus.[15]

The diagnosis of lupus erythematosus in the presence of exclusively neurologic symptoms is difficult and rests on either the intermittency of symptoms, or on evidence of systemic involvement including renal abnormalities, notably hematuria and albuminuria. The most specific laboratory test is one that detects antibodies to DNA which, according to Schur,[16] are found in over 61% of patients. The latex nucleoprotein test is positive in only 30% of patients. In some 75% of those afflicted one can find phagocytic polymorphonuclear leukocytes

containing altered nuclear material (LE cells) in bone marrow, or in the buffy coat of peripheral blood. The LE cell preparation may not be positive in a patient who is in clinical remission. The immunofluorescent antinuclear antibody test (ANA) is positive in over 99% of patients but may also be positive in a number of other connective tissue disorders.

Therapy

As is the case for systemic manifestations, adrenal cortical steroids and immunosuppressants may control neurologic symptoms without being biologically curative. Although both seizures and abnormal mental reactions may be induced by hormone therapy, they are more commonly part of the disease process itself, and discontinuation of therapy is usually not indicated.

PERIARTERITIS NODOSA

This is an acute or subacute inflammatory condition of medium and small-sized arteries. There is a fibrinoid or hyaline necrosis of the media, destruction of the internal elastic lamina, and infiltration of all layers by polymorphonuclear leukocytes. Nutrient vessels to voluntary muscles and peripheral nerves are commonly involved, cerebral arteries rarely so; but when they are, infarctions due to ischemia result.[17]

Clinical Manifestations

The disease is uncommon in childhood; the initial clinical picture is either that of a vascular lesion producing hemiplegia, or aphasia or multiple mononeuropathies (mononeuritis multiplex). The latter term refers to involvement of several or many individual nerves at the same or at different times in the course of the disease.[18] The peripheral nerves most frequently affected are the branches of the lateral popliteal nerve.[19] Remissions and relapses of neuropathy are common. Coalescence of the multiple nerve lesions, usually seen at a late stage of the illness, results in a symmetric polyneuritis. Practically every cranial nerve has been reported involved.

The diagnosis of periarteritis nodosa should be considered in patients whose obscure febrile illness is linked with disease of the central or peripheral nervous system. Confirmation may be obtained by biopsy of muscle and its supplying nerve. Since the distribution of the characteristic necrotizing arteritis is irregular, a negative biopsy by no means excludes the diagnosis. A diagnostic procedure that frequently proves conclusive is a biopsy of the peroneus brevis muscle and the musculocutaneous nerve in the lower one-third of the lateral side of the calf.

Therapy

Evaluation of therapy is complicated by the natural fluctuations of the disease. While adrenal cortical steroids are sometimes of temporary benefit, they can aggravate the mononeuritis multiplex, especially when it is accompanied by arthritic symptoms. Sudden reduction or changes in the dosage of steroids also appear to be harmful.

RHEUMATOID ARTHRITIS

A symmetric, ascending, combined sensory and motor polyneuropathy has been seen in some children with rheumatoid arthritis or scleroderma.[20] This condition is probably due to an arteritis of the vasa nervorum and generally carries a poor prognosis. The CSF may often have an increased protein content and, less commonly, a mild pleocytosis. Steroid therapy is of little help and in fact some authorities have ascribed the polyneuritis to a sensitization of the small arteries to cortisone.[21]

RHEUMATIC FEVER (SYDENHAM'S CHOREA)

The principal neurologic manifestation of rheumatic fever is Sydenham's chorea (chorea minor*). This condition was first defined by Sydenham in 1684.[22] It is an acute disease of childhood characterized by gradual or sudden appearance of emotional lability, muscular hypotonia, and choreiform movements of the muscles of the extremities, face, and trunk.

Etiology and Pathology

The relationship of Sydenham's chorea to rheumatic fever was first suggested by Stoll

* For many years the term chorea magna was used to designate chorea of hysterical nature.

in 1780,[23] and gained general acceptance by the medical profession in the nineteenth century. Most cases of chorea are preceded by a streptococcal infection or rheumatic fever. However, the interval between the bacterial infection and the onset of neurologic symptoms is usually so long that, in one study, serologic evidence for the streptococcal infection was absent in 27% of the children who had chorea as the only clinical manifestation of rheumatic disease.[24] In about one-third of choreic patients, rheumatic heart disease or other major manifestations or rheumatic fever develop after the onset of chorea.[25]

Other factors aside from an infection with beta-hemolytic streptococci play a role in the development of chorea. Although a group A streptococcal respiratory infection invariably precedes an attack of rheumatic fever, attacks of rheumatic fever rarely follow streptococcal sore throats, and practically never follow streptococcal infections in other tissues. Host factors determine susceptibility to rheumatic fever, and must also be important in the development of Sydenham's chorea.

A family history of rheumatic fever can be elicited in 26% of choreic patients, while Sydenham's chorea is found in 3.5% of parents and in 2.1% of siblings of choreic patients.[25] Emotional trauma may also be important in the development of chorea, for the onset of neurologic symptoms is often closely correlated with experiences which represent obvious psychic trauma.[26,27]

How these three factors—antecedent streptococcal infection, genetic predisposition, and emotional trauma—interact to induce the movement disorder is completely unknown.

Neuropathologic studies have been singularly uninformative. The few persons that have died during the illness, often due to other rheumatic manifestations, have shown an arteritis, with a mild perivascular cellular infiltration, and a diffuse loss of nerve cells not only from the basal ganglia, but also the cortex and cerebellum. No typical Aschoff bodies have been found in the brain.

These findings do not explain the pathophysiology of chorea. Hodes et al. have found that the H reflex, which cannot be elicited from the hypothenar muscles of normal children after the age of six months, reappears during active Sydenham's chorea.[28] This monosynaptic reflex is normally inhibited by supraspinal mechanisms which are believed to be inactive in Sydenham's chorea. The production of choreiform movements by oral administration of toxic amounts of L-dihydroxyphenylalanine (dopa) raises the possibility that a defect of catecholamine metabolism is implicated in this condition.

Clinical Manifestations

Sydenham's chorea generally has its onset between 3 and 13 years of age and is somewhat more common in girls. There is a saying, cited by Wilson,[29] that the child with Sydenham's chorea is punished three times before the diagnosis is made: once for general fidgetiness, once for breaking crockery, and once for making faces at his grandmother. This illustrates the three major clinical features: spontaneous movements, incoordination of voluntary movements, and muscular weakness.

The involuntary movements mainly affect the face, hands, and arms. At first inconspicuous, and usually best observed under stress, they are abrupt and short but gradually become more frequent and extensive, ultimately being almost continuous, disappearing only during sleep and sedation. Chorea interrupts the voluntary movements and is particularly prominent during skilled motor acts and speech. Muscular weakness may be profound and is sometimes the most prominent aspect of the disorder.

The child with pronounced Sydenham's chorea is not difficult to recognize. He is restless and emotional. Involuntary movements are continuous, quick, and random. They mainly involve the face and the distal portion of the extremities. Speech is jerky, indistinct, and at times completely absent. Willed acts are also performed abruptly; as quickly as the tongue is protruded, it returns into the mouth (chameleon tongue). Muscular hypotonia and weakness result in the characteristic "pronator sign." The patient holds his arms above the head. One notes the outward turning of the palms. Hypotonia can also be demonstrated when the arms are extended in front of the body. The wrist is flexed, and the metacarpophalangeal joints are overextended[29] ("choreic hand," Fig. 7-1). The child is unable to maintain muscular contraction, and the grip waxes and wanes abruptly. The deep tendon reflexes are usually normal, but the patellar reflex is often "hung up." With the legs hanging down the contraction of the quadriceps elicited by the tap is maintained, holding the leg briefly outstretched before it falls back down.

Variants of chorea are occasionally encountered and provide a diagnostic problem. The most common is hemichorea, in which the movements are confined to or are more marked on one side of the body; this was seen in 18% of patients reviewed by Aron et al.[25] In paralytic chorea the hypotonia and muscular weakness are sufficiently pronounced to obscure the presence of choreiform movements.

The duration of chorea ranges from one month to two years. About one-third of patients have a single attack, the remainder up to five or even more recurrences. If the patient has been symptom-free for $1\frac{1}{2}$ to 2 years, there is little likelihood of relapse.

Complications of Sydenham's chorea are rare. There is little evidence for "choreic epilepsy." Rather, it is likely that seizures complicating Sydenham's chorea are a result of concurrent endocarditis and embolization of the central nervous system. Occlusion of the central retinal artery and pseudotumor cerebri are unusual associated conditions.[30]

Complete recovery without neurologic residua is the rule in Sydenham's chorea. Some of the signs, such as the unusual abruptness of voluntary movements, may persist long after the chorea has disappeared.

Diagnosis

Sydenham's chorea is to be distinguished from tics, chorea resulting from perinatal damage to the extrapyramidal system, and from Huntington's chorea.

Unlike true chorea, tics are abrupt, repetitive, and patterned, involving the same muscle groups over and over again. They do not interfere with coordination, and are unassociated with muscular hypotonia. The

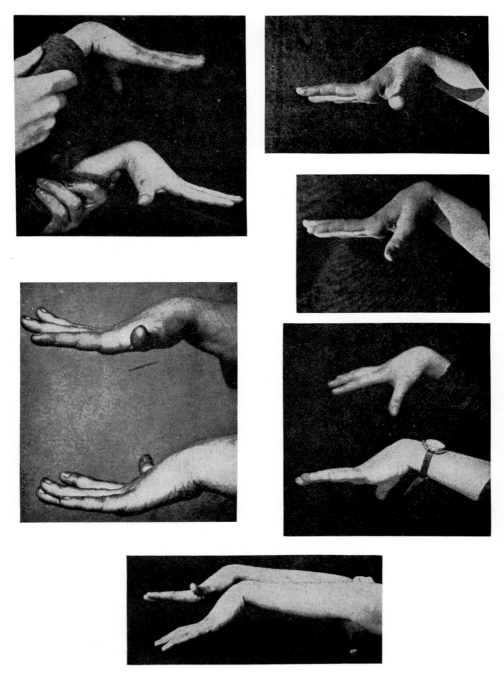

Fig. 7–1. Choreic hand in various characteristic positions. (From Wilson, S. A. K. and Bruce, A. N.: 2nd. ed., *Neurology*, Butterworth, London.)

serologic features of a rheumatic infection are absent.

Choreic movements resulting from perinatal brain damage become apparent between the first and the third year of life (see Chapter 5)—therefore, at an earlier age than Sydenham's chorea. The movements are usually slower and tend to be more evident in the larger proximal musculature. In common with the involuntary movements of Sydenham's chorea, they are exaggerated by fatigue and emotion. In the vast majority of cases, marked choreiform movements are accompanied by other involuntary movements, principally athetosis. The differential diagnosis between children with mild choreiform movements due to Sydenham's chorea and those whose involuntary movements are based on "minimal cerebral dysfunction" (see Chapter 13) is difficult and can often only be determined by continued follow-up of the patient.

Huntington's chorea is rarely seen in children (see Chapter 2). The involuntary movements predominantly involve the proximal musculature and, while abrupt, are more extensive than those of Sydenham's chorea. In particular, the twisting movements of shoulders and trunk are characteristic of Huntington's chorea. Mental deterioration or seizures, commonly found in Huntington's chorea and not observed in Sydenham's chorea, and a history of autosomal dominant transmission are further diagnostic aids.

The ingestion of phenothiazines such as prochlorperazine (Compazine) or of haloperidol (Haldol) may occasionally produce choreiform movements (see Chapter 9). Paroxysmal choreo-athetosis can be distinguished by the sudden onset of choreiform movements in a child who has few if any involuntary movements between attacks (see Chapter 11). Familial benign choreo-athetosis is a rare condition with its onset during the first two decades of life; it is characterized by choreiform movements of hands, shoulders, arms, and legs, and a combined resting and intention tremor.[31] The disorder is transmitted in an autosomal dominant manner and may be related to familial essential tremor. We have also seen a patient with hyperalaninemia (see Chapter 1), who had exacerbations of choreiform movements of the distal portions of his extremities associated with infections.

Treatment

Since Sydenham's recommendation of bleeding and purges, a large number of therapeutic regimens have been suggested for the treatment of chorea. The variability in the duration of untreated chorea makes evaluation difficult, and the effectiveness of salicylates, cortisone, or ACTH in shortening the length of the illness has not been proved.

Currently the optimal form of treatment is bed rest in a darkened, quiet room with sedation, using phenobarbital, chlorpromazine,[25,32] or haloperidol.[32a] Shenker et al. suggest that the last be started at an oral dosage of 0.5 to 1 mg twice daily.[32a] In their experience, improvement occurred within two to three days, and abnormal movements stopped completely within a few weeks. The drug is gradually withdrawn after some two to six months. Should there be a recurrence of symptoms, the medication is restarted.

The subsequent occurrence of rheumatic complications in many patients with Sydenham's chorea dictates the use of antimicrobial agents. Even when streptococci cannot be isolated from throat cultures, a course of penicillin is indicated as soon as the diagnosis of Sydenham's chorea is made. This is achieved by a single intramuscular dose of 1.2 million units of benzathine penicillin (Bicillin), or with an oral penicillin given at a dosage of 200 mg–250 mg four times daily for 10 days.

Prophylaxis against subsequent streptococcal infections can be achieved by the oral administration of 200 mg–250 mg penicillin once or twice a day, or 1.0 gm sulfadiazine per day. The antibiotic is given for several years or at least until the patient has completed high school.

AUTOIMMUNE DISORDERS OF THE CENTRAL NERVOUS SYSTEM

MULTIPLE SCLEROSIS

While multiple sclerosis is one of the most important neurologic problems in the adult population, its rarity among infants and children precludes an extensive discussion of the etiologic factors and symptomatology. The reader is referred to reviews by McAlpine et al.[33,34] The fact that we group this condition with diseases suspected to be of an autoimmune nature should not be construed to imply that its etiology is known.

Multiple sclerosis, also termed disseminated sclerosis, can be defined in clinical terms as a chronic remitting disease characterized by the appearance of neurologic symptoms referable to lesions disseminated in time and in space throughout the neuraxis.

Pathologic Anatomy

The characteristic pathologic features of multiple sclerosis are 1) destruction of the myelin sheath; 2) relative preservation of the axon cylinders and neurons; and 3) a generally perivascular distribution of lesions.[35] While few abnormalities are seen on the external surface of the brain, sections show rounded or irregular areas of grayish gelatinous appearance scattered throughout the neuraxis. While almost any region may be involved, favorite areas include the optic nerves, the centrum ovale, the periaqueductal area of the brain stem, and the spinal cord. Histologically the demyelinated areas, or plaques, are demonstrated most convincingly in sections stained for myelin (Fig. 7–2). The affected areas of absent myelin are sharply punched out. Newly formed plaques can be

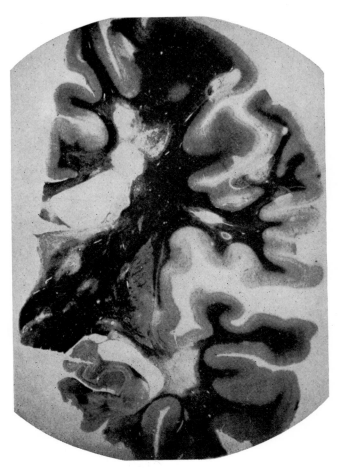

Fig. 7–2. Multiple sclerosis. Disseminated area of demyelination in white and gray matter of cerebral hemispheres. Myelin stain. (From Merritt, H. H.: *Textbook of Neurology*, 4th ed., 1970, courtesy of Lea & Febiger, Philadelphia.)

recognized by their increased cellularity, and by the presence of neutral lipids, representing myelin breakdown products, principally cholesterol esters and triglycerides. Their location in the plaque supports the concept that demyelination develops centrifugally within each plaque. In older lesions, no myelin breakdown products are seen but rather nervous tissue is replaced by a dense glial network.

There is surprisingly little Wallerian degeneration, and only the more extensive plaques show significant axonal destruction.[36] Neurons within plaques are usually normal, or demonstrate changes attributable to intercurrent illness or the malnutrition of chronic disease.

Chemical analyses of the demyelinated areas show several alterations. There is a decreased amount of myelin and a striking alteration in the protein composition of myelin. Normally, there are three types of myelin proteins: acidic proteins, consisting of at least five components; the proteolipid protein; and the basic (encephalitogenic) protein. In multiple sclerosis only traces of the basic protein have been observed.[37,37a] It is not known whether this protein is originally defective and whether its loss is generalized throughout the brain. The alterations in myelin lipids are those characteristic for myelin loss.[38] The concentrations of myelin lipids, notably cholesterol, cerebrosides, and glycerophosphatides, are decreased. White matter cholesterol esters are increased, a possible indication of an increased turnover of the fatty acid components of myelin.

Etiology

Multiple sclerosis is generally considered to be the outcome of either an allergic reaction to an unknown antigen, or of a chronic infestation by a slow acting virus.[39,40] Epidemiologic data gathered by Poskanzer[41] suggests that the disease may be an occasional manifestation of a widespread subclinical infection with a long incubation period, possibly about 21 years. Several groups of workers have found increased antibody to measles in the serum and spinal fluid of patients with multiple sclerosis.[42,43] Its pathogenic significance is still unclear, for the antibody

levels do not vary with progression of the disease or subsequent relapses. The striking increase in measles titer in patients with subacute sclerosing panencephalitis (Dawson-van Bogaert), and the isolation of measles virus from the brain of affected individuals (see Chaper 6) stimulates interest in these immunologic findings. It is, however, likely that a factor or factors other than mere exposure to measles determine the ultimate evolution of multiple sclerosis. In particular, several workers gathered evidence that suggests an underlying disorder in the metabolism or transport of polyunsaturated fatty acids.[44]

Clinical Manifestations

Since the clinical demonstration of scattered lesions within the central nervous system, and remissions and exacerbations of neurologic manifestations are necessary criteria for the diagnosis of multiple sclerosis, the disease is usually only found to have made its first appearance during childhood when its course is viewed retrospectively.

Accepting these limitations, the clinical picture of multiple sclerosis as it occurs in children differs little from that seen in adults.[45,46] Although a few children have had their initial neurologic symptoms prior to 10 years of age, the disease usually first appears after menarche, during adolescence, or during the third decade. The symptoms

TABLE 7-2.
SYMPTOMS DURING THE INITIAL EPISODE OF MULTIPLE SCLEROSIS IN 56 CHILDREN*

Symptoms	Number of Patients
Ataxia or muscle weakness	31
Disturbances of vision (blurring, diplopia, blindness)	19
Numbness or paresthesia	13
Dizziness, headache, vomiting	10
Vertigo	6
Urinary incontinence	2
Facial weakness	1
Hearing loss	1
Focal Jacksonian seizures	1

* Compiled from Low and Carter,[45] Gall et al.,[46] and Isler.[47]

occurring during the initial attack of multiple sclerosis when it appears in childhood are listed in Table 7–2.

Disturbed gait, due to either ataxia or spasticity, and impaired vision are by far the most common presenting complaints. The progression of the illness is completely unpredictable. Some children may only have a single attack during childhood, with subsequent episodes after many symptom-free years, while others have recurrent neurologic episodes before adolescence. In general, prognosis of multiple sclerosis with onset during childhood is not necessarily bad, and relatively severe attacks can be followed by prolonged remission with full restoration of function.[47]

As in adults, neurologic signs may refer to any part of the neuraxis, and to list the possible forms of multiple sclerosis would be tantamount to recounting almost every conceivable neurologic syndrome.

Diagnosis

The diagnosis of multiple sclerosis rests on the demonstration of neurologic symptoms, originating from more than one anatomic area of the brain and tending to remit and recur. Systemic signs are not part of the clinical picture, and seizures and intellectual deterioration are rare during the initial phase of the illness.

The spinal fluid is abnormal at one time or another in more than two-thirds of patients. In Freedman and Merritt's study[48] including patients of all ages, a mild pleocytosis (6–40 cells per cu mm) was seen in 28% of patients; the total protein content was elevated in 24%, and an abnormal colloidal gold curve, either first, or mid-zone, was present in 47%. The most consistent abnormality was a relative or absolute increase in the CSF gamma globulins, present in about two-thirds of cases. None of these abnormalities are pathognomonic of multiple sclerosis, and can only support the diagnosis which is made primarily on the clinical features of the illness.

Multiple sclerosis should be differentiated from other relatively rare neurologic conditions of childhood which spontaneously remit and recur. Recurrent hemiplegia may be seen in cerebral vascular disease, commonly due to disseminated lupus, less often due to homocystinuria. The latter condition can be diagnosed by a positive urinary nitroprusside-cyanide test (see Chapter 1). Neurologic complications of Behcet's disease usually take the form of recurrent meningoencephalitis with iritis, uveitis, oral and genital ulcers, arthritis, and erythema nodosum. The systemic manifestations of Behcet's disease distinguish it from multiple sclerosis. Optic neuritis is often the first manifestation of multiple sclerosis. The optic nerve may be involved proximal to the optic disc, in which case the fundus is normal (retrobulbar neuritis) or, as in papillitis, it may affect the papilla directly, producing an optic disk at times indistinguishable from that seen in early papilledema. While in papilledema the visual field defect is minimal, usually an enlargement of the blind spot, in optic neuritis the field defect is extensive, usually a central scotoma. Optic neuritis may complicate a variety of acute infectious diseases, or be an isolated episode apparently unrelated to multiple sclerosis. About one-third or more of children who suffer an attack of unexplained optic neuritis develop multiple sclerosis within a 10–15 year follow-up period.[49,50]

Treatment

Although many modes of treatment have been proposed for multiple sclerosis, the variable and unpredictable clinical course makes their evaluation a difficult task. It is not unusual for many patients to show some clinical improvement upon the introduction of a new agent, whatever its nature. Rose et al.[51] report that with placebo treatment 62% of subjects gave an overall clinical impression of improvement within four weeks of the start of "therapy," while only 17% were considered worse. Corticosteroids have been suggested for patients whose initial attack is one of retrobulbar neuritis. It is generally agreed that they do not affect the ultimate course of the illness but may shorten the initial period of visual impairment. Swank has suggested that a low-fat diet instituted in the early years of the disease may reduce the frequency and severity of exacerbations and prolong the useful life span of patients.[52]

DIFFUSE CEREBRAL SCLEROSIS
(Schilder's Disease)

This condition was first described by Schilder in 1912,[53] who termed it diffuse periaxial encephalitis. In the intervening years the term Schilder's disease has become considerably confused and has also been applied to a variety of familial demyelinating conditions, particularly those in which sudanophilic lipids accumulate in the demyelinated areas. This includes the familial sudanophilic leukodystrophies first described by Pelizaeus and Merzbacher,[53a] Einarsson and Neel,[54] and the sex-linked recessive form of sudanophilic leukodystrophy associated with adrenal atrophy. These conditions are described in Chapter 2. Poser and van Bogaert,[55] in analyzing the cases compiled by Bouman in his extensive monograph on the disease,[56] found that more than half were leukodystrophies, perinatal encephalopathies, or subacute sclerosing encephalopathy.

We intend to limit the term diffuse sclerosis or Schilder's disease to an acute demyelinating condition, occurring sporadically, related to multiple sclerosis by the morphologic appearance of the demyelinated areas, but differentiated from it by its unremittingly progressive course. Thus defined, the condition is not a common one. Cotrufo et al.[57] have even suggested that all cases of Schilder's disease are either associated with adrenal atrophy, or can be considered as multiple sclerosis.

Pathology

In the sectioned brain the most striking alteration is the gross demyelination of the central white matter. The lesions are most common in the occipital lobe but may involve any part of the cerebral hemispheres, the brain stem, and the cerebellum (Fig. 7–3). Poser and van Bogaert[55] have differentiated two types of alterations; those in which the demyelinated areas are symmetric and involve much of the centrum ovale, and those in which there are both extensive areas of demyelination and small isolated plaques as in multiple sclerosis. They have termed the latter "transitional sclerosis," and emphasize that this condition has an age distribution curve paralleling that of multiple sclerosis, while diffuse sclerosis with widespread symmetric demyelination is mainly seen during the first decade. Even in the most severely affected brain a small band of subcortical white matter is usually spared. Cavitation and ventricular dilatation are not unusual.

Microscopically, the myelin stains confirm the widespread demyelination seen on gross examination. In the demyelinated areas there is dense fibrous gliosis, and enlarged perivascular spaces containing macrophages loaded with neutral, sudanophilic-staining lipids. There is a considerable degree of axonal loss or damage—more than in multiple sclerosis (Fig. 7–4).

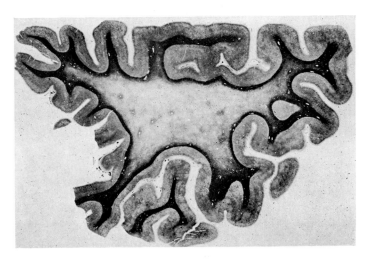

Fig. 7–3. Diffuse sclerosis. Myelin preparation of frontal lobe to demonstrate demyelination. The arcuate fibers are characteristically spared. (Courtesy of Dr. D. B. Clark, University of Kentucky, Lexington.)

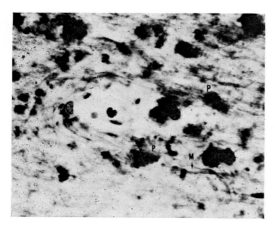

Fig. 7–4. Sudanophilic diffuse sclerosis. Masses of neutral lipids contained within microglial phagocytes (P). The irregularly swollen outline of a degenerated myelin sheath may also be seen (M). (Courtesy of Dr. D. B. Clark, University of Kentucky, Lexington.)

As would be expected from the amount of myelin loss observed on morphologic examination, the chemical analyses of white matter reveal a reduction in the various myelin constituents. Phospholipids, cholesterol, cerebrosides, and sulfatides are all markedly diminished, while as much as 20% of the white matter sterols are in an esterified form.[58]

While the morphologic appearance of the nervous system is not too unlike that seen in experimental allergic encephalopathy, there is insufficient evidence for the etiology of the condition.

Poser and van Bogaert believe that diffuse sclerosis is related to multiple sclerosis, and that the extensive symmetric lesions are a characteristic of the maturational stage of the child, rather than the nature of the inciting factor.[55]

Clinical Manifestations

By definition, diffuse sclerosis is sporadic, with its usual onset between 5 and 12 years of age. Most commonly, a previously healthy child begins to develop intellectual impairment and disturbances of gait. The early appearance of seizures of various types is quite common, and attacks of screaming and crying have also been described. Visual complaints, including cortical blindness due to demyelination of the occipital lobes, were once considered important early features of diffuse sclerosis. In children they are rare during the initial stages of the illness. Occasionally hemiplegia may represent the first indication that the demyelinating process has affected the central white matter. Ataxia and a variety of focal signs, including deafness, retrobulbar neuritis, and sixth nerve palsies are not uncommon during the later stages.[59] Disturbance in swallowing is usually a pseudobulbar palsy due to bilateral involvement of the cerebral hemispheres and occurs in about one-third of cases. Extrapyramidal movements may also be observed. In most cases all neurologic signs progress fairly rapidly, and the disease runs its course to complete deterioration within one to two years. Rarely the condition advances by a series of exacerbations, and we have encountered a patient who showed significant and prolonged improvement after an acute yet classic episode.

In about 10% of children the demyelination process is sufficiently rapid and associated with cerebral edema to produce increased intracranial pressure, including headache, vomiting, and papilledema.

The cerebrospinal fluid may be under increased pressure, even in the absence of clinical evidence for cerebral edema; the protein content is usually elevated and there is a definite lymphocytic pleocytosis.

Diagnosis

When diffuse sclerosis presents with an acute onset of increased intracranial pressure, a space-occupying lesion must be excluded by contrast studies. Once this is done, the diagnosis of diffuse sclerosis can be made with considerable certainty, for no other demyelinating condition progresses with sufficient rapidity to produce massive cerebral edema.

In other cases the diagnosis of diffuse sclerosis can usually not be arrived at without direct examination of the brain. Histologic, histochemical, and biochemical analysis of a biopsy specimen will confirm the presence of a demyelinating process.

Diffuse sclerosis with Addison's disease can be diagnosed by the presence of a family history suggestive of sex-linked recessive transmission, melanoderma, and evidence of adrenal insufficiency. Most often the latter takes the form of diminished urinary output of 17-ketosteroids and 17-hydroxycorticosteroids; excretion of the latter is not enhanced by administration of ACTH.

Treatment

Although long acting ACTH and adrenal cortical steroids have been advocated for treatment of diffuse sclerosis, there is no evidence that this form of therapy is effective and treatment is still symptomatic, being mainly directed toward reduction of cerebral edema in cases with increased intracranial pressure.

BALO'S DISEASE (Encephalitis Periaxialis Concentrica)

This condition is probably identical to diffuse sclerosis, the only distinguishing feature being the bizarre concentric zones of demyelination in central white matter.[60,61] In the few reported cases the clinical picture has been indistinguishable from that of diffuse sclerosis.

NEUROMYELITIS OPTICA (Devic's Disease)

This is a rare entity characterized clinically by optic neuritis and acute transverse myelitis appearing simultaneously or in succession. Pathologically the demyelinating process is particularly marked in white matter of the spinal cord and the optic nerves.[62,63] Whether neuromyelitis optica is distinct from diffuse sclerosis or multiple sclerosis is uncertain.

TRANSVERSE MYELITIS (Progressive Necrotic Myelopathy)

This is a syndrome characterized by the sudden onset of rapidly progressive weakness of the lower extremities, accompanied by loss of sensation and sphincter control, and often preceded by a respiratory infection.

Pathology and Etiology

On pathologic examination the spinal cord is generally softened with the most striking changes occurring in the thoraco-lumbar region. The lesion may be focally transverse or may extend over several cord segments.

In the affected area the spinal cord is often completely necrotic with loss of all nervous elements, which are replaced by a cellular infiltrate or by cavitation.

The etiology of the condition is quite obscure, but both infectious and vascular processes appear to be implicated. Transverse myelitis may occur in association with or after a large variety of infectious illnesses, including measles, mumps, or varicella, following smallpox or rabies vaccination, and in conjunction with systemic lupus erythematosus.[64] In a small number of patients transverse myelitis represents the first bout of multiple sclerosis. In addition, the acute onset of symptoms and the distribution of the lesion suggest that the vascular supply to the spinal cord is compromised, possibly due to occlusion of the anterior spinal artery.[65,66,67]

Clinical Manifestations

About two-thirds of children have a history of a recent or a concurrent acute infection. The presence or absence of an infectious history does not alter the clinical course of the disease.

The earliest symptoms are pain in the back, extremities, or abdomen, or sensory loss.[68] This is followed by a rapidly progressive paraparesis, which preferentially involves the legs, but occasionally may ascend to affect legs and arms sequentially. Fever is present in about half of the children, neck stiffness in about one-third. At first the weakness is flaccid, but gradually evidence of pyramidal tract involvement may be elicited with increased deep tendon reflexes, ankle clonus, and extensor plantar responses usually becoming obvious by the end of the second week of illness.[66] Loss of sphincter tone is almost always present; sensory impairment can be documented in all instances. In most children who can be examined adequately, pain and temperature sensation are primarily affected, while posterior column function (vibration and proprioception) is generally spared. A sensory level can be documented in almost all. It is usually located between T_5 and T_{10}. In about 20% it is in the cervical region, and in 10% in the lumbar region.[68]

Weakness and sensory symptoms evolve

rapidly; in more than 50% of patients the maximum deficit occurs within three days of the onset of symptoms.

Radiographic studies including myelography are unremarkable. In about half of the children there is a cerebrospinal fluid pleocytosis and an elevated protein content of the fluid.[66,68]

Diagnosis

Acute transverse myelitis must be distinguished from acute infectious polyneuritis, and from spinal cord symptoms due to a space-occupying lesion. The diagnosis of acute polyneuritis is not too easy, particularly in the small child whose sensory examination is not reliable. In acute polyneuritis loss of pain sensation is as a rule not as complete as it is in transverse myelitis, and proprioception is the sensory modality most involved. Loss of sphincter function and the appearance of clear-cut pyramidal tract signs argue strongly for transverse myelitis. Neither electric studies nor examination of the CSF will be of much assistance in the differential diagnosis.

Spinal cord neoplasms, epidural abscesses, or vascular malformations of the cord can usually be excluded by myelography, which should be performed in all instances.

Treatment and Prognosis

The prognosis of acute myelitis in children is usually good. About 60% of patients have good return of function, and only some 15% fail to have any significant improvement. There is no evidence that steroids or any other form of therapy has any significant effect on the outcome of the illness.

ACUTE DISSEMINATED ENCEPHALOMYELITIS (Parainfectious or Postvaccinal Encephalomyelitis)

Since the eighteenth century acute encephalitis has been known to occur in the course of various exanthemata, notably measles, chickenpox, and mumps. The mechanism for nervous system involvement is still unknown, but as the clinical and pathologic picture resembles that of experimental allergic encephalomyelitis, these diseases have been grouped together in this section.

Since most cases of uncomplicated exanthe-

matous diseases are not reported, the incidence of parainfectious encephalomyelitis is difficult to estimate. An approximate figure of 1 case of encephalitis per 1000 cases of measles is generally accepted,[69] although there is some evidence that the incidence is higher in some epidemics than in others.

Neurologic complications attending mumps are common but usually mild. On the basis of the clinical picture and abnormalities of the CSF encountered in consecutive patients with mumps, cerebral involvement was documented in about one-third of cases.[70] A similar figure has been derived from the frequency of electroencephalographic abnormalities appearing during the acute and postacute period of the illness.[71]

Frank encephalitis occurs less commonly in other exanthemata, although abnormal electroencephalograms were recorded in 22% of children with chickenpox and in 12% of patients with rubella.[71] It should be stressed, however, that it is still a matter of considerable debate whether transient electroencephalographic changes indicate cerebral involvement.

Pathology

In fatal cases distinctive microscopic abnormalities are detected in all areas of the nervous system, predominantly in white matter. During the early stages of the illness, there is a marked perivascular lymphocytic infiltration, and innumerable foci of perivenous demyelination varying in size up to 1 mm in diameter are seen principally around small and medium-sized veins. Within involved tissue, myelin has generally disappeared leaving behind more or less intact axis cylinders. Microglial cells and macrophages containing neutral lipids abound within the demyelinated areas. The oligodendroglia are usually pyknotic and degenerated, but by contrast with the picture in neurotropic virus infections, neurons remain intact.[35,72]

The mechanism by which the postinfectious encephalitides evolve has not yet been clearly established. Several theories have been advanced:

1. The diseases are due to direct viral invasion of the nervous system. Although

the pathologic changes in postinfectious encephalitis differ from those seen in acute viral encephalitis, Shaffer et al.[73] have reported the recovery of measles virus from the brain of a fatal case of encephalitis, and Adams[74] has observed cytoplasmic and nuclear inclusion bodies characteristic for viral invasion in the majority of cases of measles encephalitis.

2. Activation of a virus latent within the nervous system has also been postulated, but without much evidence to support it.

In view of the similarity between the pathologic picture of postinfectious encephalitis and experimental allergic encephalomyelitis, the concept has evolved that these diseases represent a hypersensitive reaction of the host's nervous system to multiplying virus or to the products of damage induced by virus on the brain. It has been postulated that the virus might share antigenic determinants with some component of brain tissue, or that antibodies are produced against the products of cellular damage induced by the virus as it invades the host's nervous system. A compromise between the postulates of direct viral invasion and an allergic reaction suggests that the virus enters the brain and remains latent within cells until an antigen-antibody reaction destroys both virus and host cells.[75]

Clinical Manifestations

Measles. The most common form of postinfectious encephalomyelitis is that associated with measles. The picture is of varying severity. In the mildest cases, the child, usually between the fourth and the sixth day following onset of the rash,[76,77] becomes irritable, listless, or drowsy and his temperature rises abruptly. Aside from mild meningeal signs no neurologic abnormalities are apparent, although a lumbar puncture, should it be performed, is usually abnormal. In these instances, recovery is rapid and without sequelae.

The spinal fluid in patients with measles encephalitis is almost invariably abnormal. There is a lymphocytic pleocytosis, usually between 10 and 250 cells, and an elevated protein. Colloidal gold curves are usually normal. The sugar content is normal or, rarely, slightly elevated.

In most of the reported series there has been a mortality of about 10 percent. However, at least one-third of children are left with major neurologic residua. These include recurrent seizures, mental retardation, and the syndrome of postencephalitic hyperkinesis and perceptual disorder.[78] Many others, who appear to have made a complete clinical recovery, will show this syndrome once they have reached school age. This results in the relatively common observation that survivors of measles encephalitis will show a progressive deterioration of their IQ scores. In general the older the child, and the shorter the clinical course, the less likely one is to observe this complication. Postencephalitic Parkinsonism has not been observed, although Ford mentions the presence of choreiform movements during recovery in one of his patients.[79]

Aside from symptomatic treatment directed toward the control of convulsions and cerebral edema, the use of gamma globulins and corticosteroids has been advocated. Neither therapy appears to have demonstrable benefits, or to prevent the development of sequelae.[80] Neurologic complications are rare after vaccination with live measles virus; their estimated incidence (1.5 per 1 million vaccine doses) is far lower than the risk of naturally occurring encephalitis following the unattenuated disease.[81,82] Post-measles vaccination encephalitis may present with all the afore-mentioned clinical features, as well as being responsible for the evolution of subacute sclerosing panencephalitis.

Chickenpox. The neurologic complications of varicella occur with approximately the same frequency as those following measles. The interval between the onset of the rash and the encephalitis varies between three and seven days, although rarely encephalitis may accompany or precede the eruption. It is likely, however, that under the latter circumstances encephalitis is the consequence of viremia, and that the pathogenesis differs from a postexanthematous encephalitis.

In general, postvaricella encephalitis follows the clinical pattern already described for measles encephalitis, and there are no pathognomonic features. However, as is evident from Table 7–3, chickenpox encepha-

TABLE 7-3.
COMMON SYMPTOMS AND SIGNS IN PATIENTS WITH MEASLES,
RUBELLA AND VARICELLA ENCEPHALITIS*

| | Percentage of Patients | | |
	Measles	Rubella	Varicella
Convulsions	48	57	17
Ataxia	10	13	34
Coma	45	52	19
Nystagmus	10	10	21
Hemiplegia	12	7	3
Cranial nerve signs	14	15	15
Involuntary movements	12	16	10
Myelitis	4	4	3
Retrobulbar neuritis	2	3	2
Papilledema	2	5	2
Polyneuritis	2	4	7

* After Miller et al.[69]

litis tends to be a milder illness than measles encephalitis. Seizures and coma, which have an ominous prognosis, occur less frequently, and hemiplegia is seen in only about 3% of patients. Ataxia and hypotonia are the most common clinical findings in the series of Boughton[83] and Miller et al.[69] The mortality of postvaricella encephalitis is said to be around 10%; sequelae are somewhat less common than after measles, although careful psychologic follow-up studies have not been performed.

Rubella. Neurologic complications of rubella are definitely less common than those following measles and chickenpox; the most reliable study quotes an incidence of 1 in 5000.[85] The disease tends to be shorter but more severe than the two major postinfectious encephalitides. Coma and seizures are more frequent—57% and 52% respectively (Table 7-3)—and carry a poor prognosis. The mortality is about 20% and most patients die during the first three days of their illness. Recovery is usually complete and in the experience of Margolis et al. as many as 75% of patients had recovered full neurologic function within two weeks of the onset of encephalitis.[86] But no prolonged follow-up studies are available, and the outlook for normal intellect may be less good than is suggested by these figures.

Mumps. While measles, chickenpox, and

rubella encephalitis have a similar clinical picture, mumps encephalitis is quite distinct. Although in this condition the bulk of evidence points to a direct invasion of the nervous system by the mumps virus, it will be covered at this point for the sake of convenience.

Essentially, involvement of the nervous system may take two forms: a leptomeningitis or a meningoencephalitis. The incidence of neurologic involvement in mumps is difficult to estimate, but a cerebrospinal fluid pleocytosis has been observed in 56% of patients with parotitis.[87] In as many as 47% of cases central nervous system symptoms may occur without parotitis but, more commonly, they have their onset from 8 days prior to as late as 20 days following the appearance of parotitis. On the average, leptomeningitis develops about two days after parotitis, and meningoencephalitis develops about nine days after parotitis.[88]

Symptoms

Signs of meningeal irritation, headache, nausea, and vomiting are associated with the benign leptomeningeal form of the disease. Recovery is usually complete.

Signs and symptoms of mumps meningoencephalitis, in order of observed frequency, include fever, vomiting, nuchal rigidity, lethargy, headache, convulsions, and delirium. Vertigo, ataxia, facial nerve palsy, and optic atrophy have also been reported.[89,90]

Mumps infection may result in muscle weakness, most marked in the neck flexors, which becomes evident at the end of the acute phase and can persist for as long as two to five months.

Persistent headache is the commonest sequela of central nervous system involvement. Minor behavioral changes generally clear within a few weeks after the illness. A variety of permanent neurologic residua are encountered after the meningoencephalitic form of mumps. These include optic atrophy, facial palsy, impairment of extraocular muscles, neurogenic deafness, seizures, and behavioral disorders.[91]

The cerebrospinal fluid usually shows a lymphocytic pleocytosis and an elevated protein, which may be accompanied by a reduction in the glucose content.[90,92] The serum amylase is elevated in patients with parotitis or other exocrine gland involvement.

Diagnosis may be established by isolation of the virus from the CSF, demonstration of elevation in complement fixation titer to "S" antigen, rise in complement fixation titer to "V" antigen, or rise in neutralization titer.

Encephalomyelitis Following Other Infections. Very rarely encephalitis may follow viral infections other than the exanthematous diseases already cited. The most common of the other postinfectious encephalomyelitides are those attending infectious mononucleosis,[93] influenza,[94] and smallpox.[95] In all of these, neurologic symptoms may also occur during the acute phase of the illness, probably through direct viral invasion of the nervous system.[75]

Postvaccinal Encephalomyelitis. Neurologic complications may occur after either primary or repeat vaccinations. Their average incidence is 2.9 per 1,000,000 vaccinations, with the highest frequency in the younger vaccinated subjects.[96] They are of two types: postvaccinal encephalomyelitis is pathologically essentially identical to the post-exanthematous encephalitides, and is highlighted by perivascular demyelination. It is an acute illness beginning during the second week

following the successful vaccination of a nonimmune subject.[72,97]

Clinically, it is an acute condition affecting children over three years of age, and involving the cerebrum, brain stem, and spinal cord. It is characterized by the sudden onset of fever and disturbed consciousness, often progressing to coma. Meningism and involuntary movements may also be observed. The cerebrospinal fluid usually shows a lymphocytic pleocytosis and an increased protein content. Except for residual spinal cord signs, recovery is usual and complete within two to three weeks.

The other postvaccinal complication has been termed postvaccinal encephalopathy. It commonly affects infants under two years and will follow a variable incubation period of 1–24 days. The condition is usually heralded by a prolonged generalized convulsion. The spinal fluid is normal, and aside from marked cerebral edema, no striking pathologic alterations are encountered. The outlook for recovery is poor and about one-third of infants succumb during the acute phase of the illness.

Treatment with ACTH or steroids has been advocated for both types of encephalitis. While the effectiveness of treatment is unpredictable, recovery may sometimes set in shortly after it is begun. The use of such agents as dexamethasone, mannitol, or urea to counteract cerebral edema is indicated in the postvaccinal encephalopathy of infants.

Post-Rabies Vaccination Encephalopathy. Since rabies immunization by the use of a duck embryo vaccine, a preparation low in its content of nervous tissue antigen, has become common practice, the incidence of postvaccinal complications has dropped markedly. The current estimated rate is about 1 per 50,000, contrasted with 1 per 300 to 1 per 7000 at a time when the neural vaccines were being used.[98,99]

Neurologic symptoms appear 8–21 days after the first injection of the vaccine. Their onset is marked by chills, fever, headache, vomiting, and changes in mental status. The most common neurologic picture is one of encephalitis, although less frequently patients develop hemiparesis, transverse myelitis, usually involving the thoracic or lumbar segments of the spinal cord, or neuritis of the peripheral or cranial nerves, particularly the facial nerve.[100]

The cerebrospinal fluid usually shows a lymphocytic pleocytosis and increased protein. Although relapses may occasionally be encountered, recovery usually occurs within one to two weeks, and in Applebaum's series was complete in 64% of patients.[101] But other authors report a mortality between 25 and 40%, and major sequelae in about one-third of cases. Permanent residua are usually most marked in patients with transverse myelitis.[100]

Encephalopathy Following Pertussis Vaccination. Although the earliest reports of neurologic complications of pertussis vaccine appeared in 1933, Byers and Moll were the first to document the severe encephalopathy that follows prophylactic vaccination in infants.[102] At first it was not clearly distinguished from the relatively harmless febrile convulsion precipitated by the pyrogenic reaction to the vaccine. The incidence of both febrile convulsions and encephalopathy is about 1 in 6000,[103] and is independent of the type of vaccine used, its dosage, or the interval between injections.

Neurologic symptoms may occur within minutes of the immunization or after a symptom-free interval of as long as three days. Major clinical manifestations include alterations of consciousness and generalized convulsions of varied duration. Hemiplegia was encountered by Byers in about one-quarter of his patients. The cerebrospinal fluid usually shows a mild lymphocytic pleocytosis and a protein elevation. Histologic examination of the brain in fatal cases shows a variable picture. In some cases there is diffuse neuronal destruction, with marked infiltration by macrophages; in others, acute encephalitis with perivascular infiltration, edema, and demyelination.

The prognosis for survival is good, but most children are left with major neurologic residua, retardation, or recurrent seizures. These complications were found in 14 out of 15 cases in the series of Byers and Moll,[102] and in 9 out of 14 cases in Ström's survey,[103] when children with febrile convulsions are excluded.

The relatively high incidence of neurologic complications of pertussis vaccination has been contrasted with the incidence of neurologic complication of pertussis itself. The most severe cases of pertussis encephalopathy occur in small infants, the very population group in whom prophylactic immunization would not be expected to be complete. The advisability of pertussis vaccination, therefore, depends on the risk of exposure to the organism and on the severity of the illness in a given age and population group. While the risk of pertussis immunization is said to be higher in children with convulsive disorders, Melin found that seizures were temporarily or permanently worsened during clinical pertussis.[104] Based on his experience with immunization of 47 children with history of seizures, he believes that even in this selected population group the risk of contracting pertussis and developing complications is higher than that entailed in the immunization procedure.

AUTOIMMUNE DISORDERS OF THE PERIPHERAL NERVOUS SYSTEM

ACUTE INFECTIOUS POLYNEURITIS

Although evidence for the autoimmune nature of this disorder is still incomplete, acute infectious polyneuritis, also termed Landry-Guillain-Barré syndrome, or post-infectious polyneuritis, has been included in this section because of the analogy between its pathologic picture and that of experimental allergic neuritis induced by the injection of peripheral nervous tissue into experimental animals.[105]

Clinically there is progressive weakness, usually appearing a few days after a non-specific infection, and accompanied by mild sensory disturbances and albuminocytologic dissociation (high protein but normal cell count) of the spinal fluid.

The first cases were recorded in 1859 by Landry[106] who noted that the disorder can produce both motor and sensory symptoms, especially the former, that it involves the distal parts of the limbs, and that in some instances it may become generalized by a sequential ascent of the neuraxis. Guillain, Barré, and Strohl[107] stressed the presence of albuminocytologic dissociation. Although for many years the syndromes described by Landry, and later by Guillain, Barré, and Strohl were thought to be distinct, cases fitting both original descriptions are now considered to fall into a single clinical category but are due to many etiologic factors.

Pathology

There is a mononuclear, predominantly lymphocytic inflammatory infiltration of all levels of the peripheral nervous system, from the anterior and posterior roots to the terminal twigs,[108,109,110] and at times also of the sympathetic chain and ganglia and the cranial nerves. Cells are usually clustered around the endoneurial and epineurial vessels, particularly the small veins. There is segmental demyelination in the areas infiltrated by inflammatory cells, while interruption of the axonal cylinders with subsequent Wallerian degeneration is less extensive, usually only where there is an intense inflammation. The number of Schwann cell nuclei is increased, possibly representing a reparative response. Within the central nervous system there are alterations secondary to axonal degeneration. Most commonly there is chromatolysis involving the anterior horn cells, and the cells in the motor nuclei of the cranial nerves. Cases of long-standing show some degeneration of the posterior columns.[110]

Although a number of earlier workers have indicated edema of the peripheral nerves to be the major early alteration,[108] lymphocytic infiltration represents the primary abnormality. Lymphocytes from patients with acute infectious polyneuritis appear to be sensitized to proteins of central and of peripheral neural origin.[111,111a] Sensitized cells may act in conjunction with circulating myelinotoxic factors found in serum. Serum from the large majority of patients produces a primary demyelination of dorsal root ganglion cultures. Immunofluorescent studies show binding of immunoglobulin to the myelin sheaths in affected cultures.[112]

The morphologic alterations resemble those induced by immunization of experimental animals with peripheral nerve in Freund's adjuvant,[105] and indicate a relationship of this disorder to the autoimmune diseases.[110] In experimental allergic neuritis the earliest event is the appearance of lymphocytes within venules of peripheral nerves. Lymphocytes then migrate through the endothelial lining to a perivascular location. In this location they enlarge, their ribosomes increase in number, and RNA production becomes accelerated. The now sensitized lymphocytes contact myelin, and after a lag of at least several hours produce a segmental demyelination, in an as yet unknown manner.[113]

In experimental allergic neuritis, immunization initiates the disease. In acute infectious polyneuritis the precipitating cause is not always obvious. Most commonly, in 80% of Haymaker and Kernohan's fatal cases,[108] an influenzalike illness induced by a variety of pathogenic agents precedes the neurologic symptoms.[114] Influenza A and B, ECHO, and coxsackie viruses have all been implicated in the initial episode. Polyneuritis clinically indistinguishable from acute infectious polyneuritis may also follow any of the exanthematous diseases,[95] vaccination, and immunization against tetanus or rabies.[101]

Currently the most attractive hypothesis is that an antecedent infection indirectly precipitates infectious polyneuritis. The agent may damage the Schwann cell with release of Schwann cell antigen to which the host responds with an immune reaction that attacks the Schwann cell. Alternatively, the infectious agent contains an antigen also found on the Schwann cell, and the immune response is directed against both.

Clinical Manifestations

Acute infectious polyneuritis may occur at any age during childhood but especially between four and nine years.[115] A prodromal respiratory illness or gastroenteritis occurs in about two-thirds of the patients, usually within two weeks before the onset of weakness[115,116] (Table 7–4).

The appearance of neurologic symptoms is usually fairly sudden. In about one-half of patients paralysis is accompanied by pain or paresthesia, while in the majority of the remainder sensory symptoms are not obvious.

The paralysis usually begins in the lower

TABLE 7-4.
CLINICAL CHARACTERISTICS OF 56 CHILDREN WITH ACUTE INFECTIOUS POLYNEURITIS*

	Percent
Antecedent infection	70
Distal weakness predominantly	44
Proximal weakness predominantly	14
Cranial nerve weakness	43
Facial nerve	32
Spinal accessory nerve	21
Papilledema	5
Paresthesia and pain	43
Loss of vibratory and/or position sense	34
Meningeal irritation	17
CSF protein over 45 mg %	88
Mortality	4
Full recovery or mild impairment	77
Relapses	7
Asymmetry of involvement	9

* From Low et al.[115] and Peterman et al.[116]

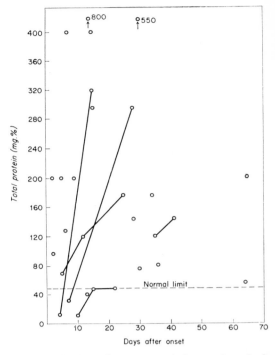

Fig. 7–5. Protein content of the cerebrospinal fluid at various intervals after onset of symptoms. Determinations performed on the same patient are connected by a line. (Courtesy, A. F. Peterman, Reno, Nevada, the editors of Lancet Publications, Inc. and the editors of *Neurology*. From *Neurology* 9:533, 1959.)

extremities, then ascends. Characteristically it is symmetric, although minor differences between the sides are not rare. In about half of the patients the weakness is mostly distal, while in about 15% the proximal musculature is more extensively involved (Table 7-4). Cranial nerve palsies may appear at any time during the illness. The facial nerve is most commonly involved. Papilledema is relatively rare. Its appearance is best correlated with increased cerebrospinal fluid pressure;[117] whether increased pressure is due to interference with the reabsorption of cerebrospinal fluid, or due to an increase in the volume of fluid resulting from the osmotic effect of the high protein content of cerebrospinal fluid, or is caused by cerebral edema remains to be established.

Paralysis of the respiratory muscles is a common complication in severely involved patients, but even in the absence of respiratory symptoms, vital capacity may be impaired with consequent CO_2 retention. Involvement of the sympathetic nervous system may produce a variety of circulatory abnormalities, including cardiac arrhythmias, hypertension, and postural hypotension.[118]

Position sense is the sensory function most frequently impaired, followed by vibration, pain, and touch in descending order of frequency. The deep tendon reflexes are generally absent, although increased reflexes and extensor plantar responses are occasionally recorded during the initial days of the illness.

Characteristic is an elevation in the cerebrospinal fluid protein. This exceeds 45 mg % in 88% of children (Table 7–4), and rises to its maximum by four to five weeks, thereafter gradually returning to normal (Fig. 7–5). The CSF cell count is usually normal, although a significant pleocytosis (100 or more cells) occurs in about 5% of patients.

The electromyogram when tested reveals a picture compatible with involvement of the lower motor neurons or peripheral nerves. The conduction velocity in the motor fibers may be normal or only slightly reduced during the first few weeks of the illness, but during the recovery period it is definitely reduced in the majority of patients.[116]

The neurologic picture described above evolves rapidly and paralysis may be maximal within a few hours of the initial symptoms. More commonly, however, the paralysis becomes more extensive over the course of one to two weeks, often, as in the classical Landry type of paralysis, progressively affecting the trunk, the upper extremities and the cranial nerves. After reaching a plateau, clinical improvement is usually first noted by the second to the fourth week of the illness, and the majority of children experience complete recovery. This is usually achieved within two months, although it may take as long as 18 months.

Diagnosis

The diagnosis of acute infectious polyneuritis rests on a history of a preceding febrile illness, the gradual development of

symmetric muscular weakness, often worse over the distal portion of the lower extremities, and the spinal fluid abnormalities. In the additional presence of sensory changes there usually is little doubt of the diagnosis. When these are absent, however, a number of other entities must be considered. In poliomyelitis the onset of paralysis is accompanied by fever and evidence of a systemic illness. The paralysis is rarely symmetric, and a CSF pleocytosis is common during the initial stages of the illness (see Chapter 6).

Polymyositis may be confused with polyneuritis. The distribution of muscular weakness tends to be proximal, and the CSF protein remains normal. The differential diagnosis of acute transverse myelitis and infectious polyneuritis has already been noted. Other, less common conditions that induce progressive muscular weakness of rapid onset are described in Chapter 12.

Prognosis

In general, the outlook for life and recovery is better in children than in adults. The greatest danger during the acute phase of the illness is respiratory paralysis. Early tracheotomy and the availability of mechanical respirators should eliminate fatalities.

Some children experience one or more relapses over the course of two months to several years.[119] These may be either spontaneous or related to withdrawal of ACTH or steroid therapy.

Other cases possess the clinical features of infectious polyneuritis but have a chronic fluctuating course without complete recovery between exacerbations.[120] In the few children thus affected the motor component of the picture is usually predominant,[121] and weakness is greatest in the distal muscles. On biopsy, peripheral nerves from these patients show a segmental demyelination and increased numbers of Schwann cells, their processes arranged in whorls around the demyelinated axons. The latter structures are termed "onion bulbs." They are characteristic of most chronic recurrent neuropathies, and their presence correlates with the duration of symptoms.[122] A differential diagnosis of chronic polyneuritis of childhood is presented in Table 7–5 together

TABLE 7-5.
DIFFERENTIAL DIAGNOSIS OF CHRONIC POLYNEURITIS OF CHILDHOOD*

Condition	Diagnostic Features
Lead poisoning	Blood lead levels; basophilic stippling of erythrocytes
Arsenic poisoning	Elevated arsenic in hair, nails
Thiamine deficiency	Transketolase deficiency
Periarteritis nodosa	Muscle biopsy
Peroneal muscular atrophy (Charcot-Marie-Tooth)	Familial history
Interstitial hypertrophic polyneuritis (Dejerine-Sottas)	Palpable enlarged nerves; familial history
Refsum's disease (ataxia polyneuritiformis)	Elevated blood phytanic acid
Metachromatic leukodystrophy	Intellectual deterioration; absent urinary and tissue aryl sulfatase
Chronic polyneuritis of unknown cause	Exclusion of above

* After Byers and Taft.[121]

with some salient diagnostic features of each of the major entities. Most children with chronic polyneuritis remain undiagnosed.

Treatment

Treatment of acute infectious polyneuritis is mainly symptomatic. The potential paralysis of the respiratory muscles should be considered in each patient, and facilities for tracheostomy and mechanical respiration should be readily available. As a rule, it is preferable to institute these measures whenever the first indications of impaired vital capacity become apparent, rather than wait until embarrassment of respiration is obvious and the patient has marked difficulty with his air exchange. Most authors have been favorably impressed by the effectiveness of corticotropin or glucocorticoids in the treatment of acute polyneuritis. Reported cases appear to improve or to be arrested after initiation of therapy, but no adequately controlled study is available to prove this impression.[123] The response of patients with the chronic and intermittent forms of polyneuritis appears to be more clear-cut, however.[124] During convalescence, graduated physical therapy including active and passive exercises are indicated.

BELL'S PALSY

An acute paralysis of the face, often following a mild infection, was first described by Bell in 1821.

Cases of this partial paralysis must be familiar to every medical observer. It is very frequent for young people to have what is vulgarly called a blight; by which is meant a slight palsy of the muscles on one side of the face, and which the physician knows is not formidable. Inflammations of glands seated behind the angle of the jaw will sometimes produce this. . . . The patient has a command over the muscles of the face, he can close the lips, and the features are duly balanced; but the slightest smile is immediately attended with distortion, and in laughing and crying the paralysis becomes quite distinct.[125]

Pathology and Etiology

The essential anatomic changes of the seventh nerve in Bell's palsy are still under considerable dispute, and their etiology unknown. Most authors agree that during the acute phase of the illness there is considerable edema of the nerve, and venous congestion in the facial canal. There are a few microscopic hemorrhages but little inflammatory reaction. A genetic predisposition appears to be important[126]; while in 73% of patients there is an antecedent upper respiratory infection or exposure to cold draughts, the latter frequently mentioned as a cause during the nineteenth century.[127]

Clinical Manifestations

In many cases pain localized to the ear or to the surrounding area is the initial symptom. This is followed by a rapid evolution of the paralysis, which reaches its full extent within a few hours. Characteristically, it involves the musculature of the forehead, cheek and the perioral region. In about half of the patients taste sensation is lost. Lacrimation is retained in the great majority of children.[128] The pain usually disappears quickly. In most children recovery begins within a few weeks and reaches its maximum in one to nine weeks.[128]

Recovery can be expected to be complete when the palsy is partial, as is the case in some 80% of children,[129] or when the electric studies show an incomplete denervation of the facial nerve. When denervation is complete, the onset of recovery is delayed for about six weeks, and reaches its maximal extent in six months.[130] In such instances there is usually an incomplete return of muscle function. In 7% of instances the facial paralysis is recurrent.[131] In some of these it is part of the Melkersson syndrome (see Chapter 6).

Diagnosis

The diagnosis of Bell's palsy rests on the exclusion of other causes for isolated facial paralysis. These are listed in Table 6–7.

Facial nerve palsy due to otitis media, with or without mastoiditis, is still relatively common.[130]

A number of intracranial neoplasms, particularly those involving the brain stem, may result in the sudden onset of facial weakness. In some instances transient improvement can

TABLE 7-6.
CAUSES OF ISOLATED FACIAL PARALYSIS
1943-1950*

Cause	Number of Cases	
	Paine	Manning and Adour
Congenital		
Congenital anomaly	15	2
Birth trauma	18	5
Postnatal		
Idiopathic (Bell's)	19	37
With upper respiratory infection	9	
Without upper respiratory infection	10	
Otitis media	16	6
Surgical trauma	2	
Other trauma	3	2
Intracranial tumor	2	
Extracranial tumor	1	
Hypertension	2	
Poliomyelitis	2	
Histiocytosis X		2
Varicella		1
Herpes zoster (Ramsay Hunt)		1
Mumps		1
Postimmunization (DPT and polio)		1

* After Paine[128] and Manning and Adour.[130]

be observed before the appearance of other neurologic signs. Isolated facial nerve palsy can be seen with a variety of viral encephalitides, notably mumps, varicella, and the enteroviruses (see Chapter 6). In children, facial palsy is rarely due to herpes zoster of the geniculate ganglion (Ramsay Hunt syndrome).[130]

Treatment and Prognosis

A number of therapeutic approaches have been suggested. Administration of steroids to reduce the edema within the facial canal has been used for several years. In view of the high recovery rate of untreated children, its evaluation is difficult. In many instances, however, one has the clinical impression that recovery begins soon after the onset of treatment. Steroids are probably reserved for those patients in whom electric studies indicate complete denervation.

Decompression of the facial nerve from the stylomastoid foramen through its pyramidal portion has been advised for patients who show complete denervation. In children there is, however, no evidence that this procedure is effective.[130] In children whose facial function recovers only partially, contractures can be expected. Misdirection of growth results in facial mass action in which attempted activity of one muscle group produces movements in several different muscle groups (synkinesis). It may also result in tics or in the syndrome of "crocodile tears." In the latter the presence of food in the mouth or the smell of food is followed by lacrimation rather than salivation.[132]

Varieties of plastic surgical procedures have been described, but these should be deferred until facial growth has been completed.

POSTINFECTIOUS ABDUCENS PALSY

A painless palsy of the abducens nerve which clears without residua may develop in children of any age 7–21 days after a nonspecific febrile illness or upper respiratory infection. The paralysis is often complete but unassociated with any other cranial nerve palsy or neurologic signs. Improvement becomes evident in three to six weeks, and the palsy clears completely within two to three months. Except for the cerebrospinal fluid which may occasionally show a mild lymphocytosis, all laboratory and radiologic studies are normal.[133]

The diagnosis of this condition is arrived at by exclusion of abducens palsy secondary to increased intracranial pressure, tumors of the brain stem, brain stem encephalitis,[134] and Gradenigo's syndrome.[135] The last is caused by an osteomyelitis of the apex of the petrous bone and is characterized by an abducens palsy following otitis media, and accompanied by pain in the distribution of the homolateral trigeminal nerve.

ACUTE CEREBELLAR ATAXIA

Acute cerebellar ataxia is a relatively common condition first described by Batten in 1907[136] and characterized by the sudden onset of ataxia, often after a nonspecific infectious illness.

Pathologic Anatomy and Etiology

As acute cerebellar ataxia is not a fatal condition, its pathology is unknown. The cause of the condition is probably heterogeneous, with a number of infectious agents being directly or indirectly responsible. Cases caused by polio virus type 1, and others due to influenza A and B have been reported. In other patients ECHO type 9[137] and coxsackie type B have been isolated from cerebrospinal fluid. Ataxia with an acute onset and an identical clinical picture is also seen following a variety of exanthematous diseases, most commonly varicella.[83] Acute and transient cerebellar ataxia may also be the presenting symptom of childhood multiple sclerosis (Table 7–2). The association of acute cerebellar ataxia with occult neuroblastoma has been observed in a number of medical centers, including our own.[138,139] We may therefore conclude that in some instances acute cerebellar ataxia is due to direct viral invasion of the cerebellum, while in others it is the result of an autoimmune response to a variety of agents.

Clinical Manifestations

The condition is seen in children of all ages, although in the experience of Weiss and Carter[140] it occurred most commonly between one and two years of age. By definition, the onset of ataxia is always acute, although about half of the children suffer from a nonspecific infectious illness within three weeks prior to the onset of neurologic symptoms.[140] The clinical picture is marked by severe truncal ataxia resulting in rapid deterioration of gait. Tremor of the extremities, head, and trunk, and hypotonia are seen less invariably. Nystagmus is encountered in 45% of patients,[141] while a number of others may have sudden random motion during voluntary eye movements. Speech is often affected. Other neurologic signs are usually absent, although headache, dizziness, photophobia, and myoclonic movements of the head and arms have occasionally been reported. Constitutional symptoms, including fever, are absent and nuchal rigidity is rare.

The cerebrospinal fluid is usually normal, although a mild pleocytosis was found in 25% of cases.[140,141] The spinal fluid protein may be normal on initial taps but elevated late in the course of the illness.[140]

In the majority of cases, the disease is self-limiting. In about two-thirds of children the ataxia clears completely, with an average duration of cerebellar signs of about two months. Some mildly affected children may recover completely within one week. Persistence of major neurologic deficits is noted in about one-third of children. These include ataxia of trunk and extremities, speech impairment, mental retardation, and behavioral abnormalities.

We have encountered at least two children whose cerebellar ataxia recurred over the course of several years, with exacerbations often preceded by a mild respiratory illness. These bouts could be distinguished from the aggravation of ataxia expected in any incoordinated patient suffering from an acute febrile episode. Both patients were left with mental retardation.

Diagnosis

The diagnosis of acute cerebellar ataxia is made by excluding other conditions producing sudden onset of ataxia. The most important of these are the posterior fossa tumors, acute labyrinthitis, and drug intoxications. Although the onset of ataxia in a posterior fossa tumor is rarely sudden, contrast studies to exclude a mass lesion are almost always indicated in a patient with acute cerebellar ataxia. The presence of papilledema and a history of headache or vomiting point to a posterior fossa tumor.

Ataxia may develop in the course of acute viral diseases of the central nervous system, notably varicella, mumps, and poliomyelitis. The distinction between these cases and the usual patient with acute cerebellar ataxia is difficult and may well be semantic; that is to say, if a causative agent can be proven, one would then term the condition cerebellar encephalitis, but otherwise acute cerebellar ataxia of unknown etiology.

Acute labyrinthitis (vestibular neuronitis or epidemic vertigo) is not easily distinguished from ataxia, particularly in an uncooperative youngster. It is usually associated with nausea, intense vertigo, and abnormal tests of labyrinthine function,[142] particularly an absence of caloric responses.[143]

Acute ataxia may also be seen following the ingestion of a variety of toxins, particularly alcohol, thallium, and organic mercurials (see Chapter 9).

A syndrome of myoclonic encephalopathy has been noted to occur in infants.[144] It is characterized by chaotic irregularity of eye movements and shocklike myoclonic contractions persisting when the affected part is at rest and producing total disorganization of willed movements. The condition is of acute onset and also self-limiting but after many months or years. It is dramatically relieved by ACTH. An indistinguishable clinical appearance, without relief by ACTH, at times represents the remote effect of neuroblastoma.

Acute ataxia, often precipitated by a respiratory infection, accompanies a number of metabolic disorders, including Hartnup's disease, and the intermittent form of maple syrup disease (see Chapter 1). Recurrent attacks of ataxia unaccompanied by aminoacidemia or known specific biochemical abnormalities may be transmitted as a dominant trait.[145]

Ataxia may also develop as a consequence of heat stroke,[146] the result of hyperthermia-induced cerebellar degeneration.

Some children with frequent minor motor seizures may suddenly develop ataxia, probably the result of frequent transitory impairment of consciousness. The presence of striking electroencephalographic signs of a seizure disorder should readily distinguish this entity.

Ataxia associated with the various cerebellar degenerations develops gradually and should cause little confusion. Apparent ataxia may be the consequence of generalized weakness, as seen for instance in acute infectious polyneuritis. In acute cerebellar ataxia hypotonia is associated with normal or increased deep tendon reflexes, while in polyneuritis the reflexes are reduced or absent.

Treatment

Acute cerebellar ataxia is a self-limiting disease, and no specific treatment, including adrenal cortical steroids, appears to be effective. Because of the association of acute cerebellar ataxia and neuroblastoma, children should be surveyed for an inapparent tumor by means of radiographs of skeleton, chest, and spine, an intravenous urograph, a bone marrow aspirate, and a determination of the urinary excretion of catecholamines.[138]

SPASMUS NUTANS

This unusual but benign condition commences in late infancy, often in late winter or early spring, and is marked by anomalous head positions, head nodding, and nystagmus, which is often asymmetric. It is self-limiting, clearing after a period of four months to several years, and unassociated with any permanent residuals. Its cause is unknown, but it may be the sequel to an unknown viral illness.[147]

REFERENCES

1. Rivers, T. M. and Schwentker, F. F.: Encephalomyelitis accompanied by myelin destruction experimentally produced in monkeys, J. Exp. Med. 61:689, 1935.

2. Wolf, A., Kabat, E. A., and Bezer, A. E.: The pathology of acute disseminated encephalomyelitis produced experimentally in the Rhesus monkey and its resemblance to human demyelinating disease, J. Neuropath. Exp. Neurol. 6:333, 1947.

3. Ferraro, A. and Cazullo, C. L.: Chronic experimental allergic encephalomyelitis in monkeys, J. Neuropath. Exp. Neurol. 7:235, 1948.

4. Waksman, B. H. and Adams, P. D.: A histologic study of the early lesion in experimental allergic encephalomyelitis in the guinea pig and rabbit, Amer. J. Path. 41:135, 1962.

5. Alvord, E. C., Jr.: The relationship of hypersensitivity to infection, inflammation and immunity, J. Neuropath. Exp. Neurol. 25:1, 1966.

6. Fry, J. M., Lehrer, G. M., and Bornstein, M. B.: Sulfatide synthesis: Inhibition by experimental allergic encephalomyelitis serum, Science 175:192, 1972.

7. Kies, M. W., Thompson, E. B., and Alvord, E. C., Jr.: The relationship of myelin proteins to experimental allergic encephalomyelitis, Ann. NY Acad. Sci. 122:318, 1965.

8. Eng, L. F., et al.: The maturation of human white matter myelin. Fractionation of the myelin membrane proteins, Biochemistry 7:4455, 1968.

9. Eylar, E. H., et al.: Basic A_1 protein of the myelin membrane, J. Biol. Chem. 246:5770, 1971.

10. Shooter, E. M. and Einstein, E. R.: Proteins of the nervous system, Ann. Rev. Biochem. 40:635, 1971.

11. Gold, A. P. and Yahr, M. D.: Childhood lupus erythematosus, Trans. Amer. Neurol. Ass. 85:96, 1960.

12. Malamud, N. and Saver, G.: Neuropathologic findings in disseminated lupus erythematosus, Arch. Neurol. Psychiat. 71:723, 1954.

13. Glynn, L. E. and Holborow, E. J.: *Autoimmunity and Disease*, Philadelphia: F. A. Davis Co., 1965.

14. O'Connor, J. F. and Musher, D. M.: Central nervous system involvement in systemic lupus erythematosus, Arch. Neurol. 14:157, 1966.

15. Jacobs, J. C.: Systemic lupus erythematosus in childhood, Pediatrics 32:257, 1963.

16. Schur, P. H.: Diagnostic tests for systemic lupus erythematosus, JAMA 214:2201, 1970.

17. Malamud, N.: A case of periarteritis nodosa with decerebrate rigidity and extensive encephalomalacia in a five-year-old child, J. Neuropath. Exp. Neurol. 4:88, 1945.

18. Ford, R. G. and Siekert, R. G.: Central nervous system manifestations of periarteritis nodosa, Neurology (Minneap.) 15:114, 1965.

19. Bleehen, S. S., Lovelace, R. E., and Cotton, R. E.: Mononeuritis multiplex in polyarteritis nodosa, Quart. J. Med. 32:193, 1963.

20. Sundelin, F.: Investigations of the cerebrospinal fluid in cases of rheumatoid arthritis, Amer. J. Med. 2:579, 1947.

21. Pallis, C. A. and Scott, J. T.: Peripheral neuropathy in rheumatoid arthritis, Brit. Med. J. 1:1141, 1965.

22. Sydenham, T.: *The Entire Works of Dr. Thomas Sydenham, Newly Made English from the Originals*, by John Swan, London, printed for E. Cave, 1742.

23. Stoll, M.: Rationis medendi, in Nosocomio practico Vindobonensis, pars tertia, Vol. 7:6, Viennae, sumptibus A. Bernardi, 1780.

24. Taranta, A. and Stollerman, G. H.: Relationship of Sydenham's chorea to infection with group A streptococci, Amer. J. Med. 20:170, 1956.

25. Aron, A. M., Freeman, J. M., and Carter, S.: The natural history of Sydenham's chorea, Amer. J. Med. 38:83, 1965.

26. Chapman, A. H., Pilkey, L., and Gibbons, M. J.: A psychosomatic study of eight children with Sydenham's chorea, Pediatrics 21:582, 1958.

27. Freeman, J. M., et al.: The emotional correlates of Sydenham's chorea, Pediatrics 35:42, 1965.

28. Hodes, R., Gribetz, I., and Hodes, H. L.: Abnormal occurrence of ulnar nerve hypothenar muscle H reflex in Sydenham's chorea, Pediatrics 30:49, 1962.

29. Wilson, S. A. K.: *Neurology*, 2nd ed., Baltimore: Williams & Wilkins Co., 1955.

30. Chun, R. W. M., Smith, N. J., and Forster, F. M.: Papilledema in Sydenham's chorea, Amer. J. Dis. Child. 101:641, 1961.

31. Pincus, J. H. and Chutorian, A.: Familial benign chorea with intention tremor: A clinical entity, J. Pediat. 70:724, 1967.

32. Tierney, R. C. and Kaplan, S.: Treatment of Sydenham's chorea, Amer. J. Dis. Child. 109:408, 1965.

32a. Shenker, D. M., Grossman, H. J., and Klawans, H. L.: Treatment of Sydenham's chorea with haloperidol, Develop. Med. Child Neurol. 15:19, 1973.

33. McAlpine, D., Compston, N. D., and Lumsden, C. E.: *Multiple Sclerosis*, Edinburgh: E. and S. Livingstone, Ltd., 1955.

34. McAlpine, D., Lumsden, C. E., and Acheson, E. D.: *Multiple Sclerosis, A Reappraisal*, Edinburgh: E. and S. Livingstone, Ltd., 1968.

35. Adams, R. D. and Kubik, C. S.: The morbid anatomy of the demyelinative diseases, Amer. J. Med. 12:510, 1952.

36. Greenfield, J. G. and King, L. S.: Observations on the histopathology of the cerebral lesions in disseminated sclerosis, Brain 59:445, 1936.

37. Riekkinen, P. J., et al.: Protein composition of multiple sclerosis myelin, Arch. Neurol. 24:545, 1971.

37a. Einstein, E. R., et al.: Proteolytic activity and basic protein loss in and around multiple sclerosis plaques: Combined biochemical and histochemical observations, J. Neurochem. 19:653, 1972.

38. Alling, C., Vanier, M. T., and Svennerholm, L.: Lipid alterations in apparently normal white matter in multiple sclerosis, Brain Research 35:325, 1971.
39. Alter, M. and Speer, J.: Clinical evaluation of possible etiologic factors in multiple sclerosis, Neurology (Minneap.) 18:109, 1968.
40. Millar, J. H. D.: *Multiple Sclerosis: A Disease Acquired in Childhood*, Springfield: Charles C Thomas Publisher, 1971.
41. Poskanzer, D. C.: Epidemiological Evidence for a Viral Etiology of Multiple Sclerosis, in NINDB Monograph #2, "Slow, Latent and Temperate Virus Infections," Washington: U.S. Dept. of HEW, 1965.
42. Adams, J. M.: Measles antibody in patients with multiple sclerosis, Neurology (Minneap.) 17:707, 1967.
43. Brown, P., et al.: Measles antibodies in cerebrospinal fluid of patients with multiple sclerosis. Proc. Soc. Exp. Biol. Med. 137:956, 1971.
44. Belin, J., et al.: Linoleate metabolism in multiple sclerosis, J. Neurol. Neurosurg. Psychiat. 34:25, 1971.
45. Low, N. L. and Carter, S.: Multiple sclerosis in children, Pediatrics 18:24, 1956.
46. Gall, J. C., et al.: Multiple sclerosis in children, Pediatrics, 21:703, 1958.
47. Isler, W.: Multiple Sklerose im Kindesalter Helv. Paediat. Acta 16:412, 1961.
48. Freedman, D. A. and Merritt, H. H.: The cerebrospinal fluid in multiple sclerosis, A. Res. Nerv. Ment. Dis. Proc. 28:428, 1950.
49. Kennedy, C. and Carter, S.: Relation of optic neuritis to multiple sclerosis in children, Pediatrics 28:377, 1961.
50. Kennedy, C. and Carroll, F. D.: Optic neuritis in children, Arch. Ophthal. 63:747, 1960.
51. Rose, A. S., et al.: Cooperative study in the evaluation of therapy in multiple sclerosis; ACTH vs. placebo in acute exacerbations, Neurology (Minneap.) 18 (pt. 2):1, 1968.
52. Swank, R. L.: Multiple sclerosis: Twenty years on low-fat diet, Arch. Neurol. 23:460, 1970.
53. Schilder, P.: Zur Kenntniss der sogenannten diffusen Sklerose, Z. Ges. Neurol. Psychiat. 10:1, 1912.
53a.Merzbacher, L.: Eine eigenartige familiar-hereditare Erkrankungsform, Z. Ges. Neurol. Psychiat. 3:1, 1910.
54. Einarson, L. and Neel, A.: Contribution to the study of diffuse sclerosis with a comprehensive review of the problem in general and a report of two cases, Acta Jutlandica 14:1, 1942.
55. Poser, C. M. and van Bogaert, L.: Natural history and evolution of the concept of Schilder's diffuse sclerosis, Acta Psychiat. Neurol. Scand. 31:285, 1956.
56. Bouman, L.: *Diffuse Sclerosis*, Bristol: John Wright and Co., Ltd., 1934.
57. Cotrufo, R., et al.: Qu'est-ce que la maladie de Schilder? Riv. Pat. Nerv. Ment. 89:133, 1968.
58. Suzuki, Y., et al.: Ultrastructural and biochemical studies of Schilder's disease, J. Neuropath. Exp. Neurol. 29:405, 1970.
59. Vanden Herrewegen, M. and Chamoles, N.: Nouvelles recherches sur la sclérose diffuse du type Schilder (1912) chez l'enfant, Acta Neurol. Belg. 68:837, 1968.
60. Balo, J.: Encephalitis periaxialis concentrica, Arch. Neurol. Psychiat. 19:242, 1928
61. Patrassi, G.: Diffuse Gehirnentmarkungen und sogenannte Encephalitis periaxialis diffusa, Virchow. Arch. Path. Anat. 98:281, 1931.
62. Ansari, N.: Neuromyelitis optica or Devic's disease (case reports with review of literature), Medicus (Karachi) 35:232, 1968.
63. Walsh, F. B.: Neuromyelitis optica. An anatomical-pathological study of one case; clinical studies of three additional cases, Bull. Hopkins Hosp. 56:183, 1935.
64. Penn, A. S. and Rowan, A. J.: Myelopathy in systemic lupus erythematosus, Arch. Neurol. 18:337, 1968.
65. Lindquist, B.: Syndrome of the anterior spinal artery, Acta Paediat. 46:380, 1957.
66. Paine, R. S. and Byers, R. K.: Transverse myelopathy in childhood, AMA J. Dis. Child. 85:151, 1953.
67. Hoffman, H. L.: Acute necrotic myelopathy, Brain 78:377, 1955.
68. Altrocchi, P. H.: Acute transverse myelopathy, Arch. Neurol. 9:111, 1963.
69. Miller, H. G., Stanton, J. B., and Gibbons, J. L.: Para-infectious encephalomyelitis and related syndromes, Quart. J. Med. 25:427, 1956.
70. Holden, E. M., Eagles, A. Y., and Stevens, J. E., Jr.: Mumps involvement of the central nervous system, JAMA 131:382, 1946.
71. Gibbs, F. A., et al.: Electroencephalographic abnormality in "uncomplicated" childhood diseases, JAMA 171:1050, 1959.
72. DeVries, E.: *Postvaccinal Perivenous Encephalitis*, Amsterdam: Elsevier, 1960.
73. Shaffer, M. F., Rake, G., and Hodes, H. L.: Isolation of virus from a patient with fatal encephalitis complicating measles, Amer. J. Dis. Child. 64:815, 1942.
74. Adams, J. M.: Clinical pathology of measles encephalitis and sequelae, Neurology (Minneap.) 18 (pt. 2):52, 1968.
75. Croft, P. B.: Para-infectious and postvaccinal encephalomyelitis, Postgrad. Med. J. 45:392, 1969.
76. Boughton, C. R.: Morbilli in Sydney. II. Neurological sequelae of measles, Med. J. Aust. 2:908, 1964.
77. Tyler, H. R.: Neurological complications of rubeola (measles), Medicine (Balt.) 36:147, 1957.
78. Meyer, E. and Byers, R. K.: Measles encephalitis: A follow-up study of 16 patients, AMA J. Dis. Child. 84:543, 1952.
79. Ford, F. R.: The nervous complications of measles, Bull. Hopkins Hosp. 43:140, 1928.

80. Karelitz, S. and Eisenberg, M.: Measles encephalitis. Evaluation and treatment with adrenocorticotropin and adrenal corticosteroids, Pediatrics 27:811, 1961.

81. Schneck, S. A.: Vaccination with measles and central nervous system disease, Neurology (Minneap.) 18 (pt. 2):79, 1968.

82. Nader, P. R. and Warren, R. J.: Reported neurologic disorders following live measles vaccine, Pediatrics 41:997, 1968.

83. Boughton, C. R.: Neurological complications of varicella, Med. J. Aust. 2:444, 1966.

85. Sherman, F. E., Michaels, R. H., and Kenny, F. M.: Acute encephalopathy (encephalitis) complicating rubella, JAMA 192:675, 1965.

86. Margolis, F. J., Wilson, J. L., and Top, F. H.: Post-rubella encephalomyelitis, J. Pediat. 23:158, 1943.

87. Russell, R. R. and Donald, J. C.: The neurological complications of mumps, Brit. Med. J. 2:27, 1958.

88. Levitt, L. P., et al.: Central nervous system mumps. A review of 64 cases, Neurology (Minneap.) 20:829, 1970.

89. Azimo, P. H., Cramblett, H. G., and Haynes, R. E.: Mumps meningoencephalitis in children, JAMA 207:509, 1969.

90. Wilfert, C. M.: Mumps meningoencephalitis with low cerebrospinal fluid glucose, prolonged pleocytosis and elevation of protein, New Eng. J. Med. 280:855, 1969.

91. Oldfelt, V.: Sequelae of mumps meningoencephalitis, Acta Med. Scand. 134:405, 1949.

92. Murray, H., Fuld, C. M. B., and McLeod, W.: Mumps meningoencephalitis, Brit. Med. J. 1:1850, 1960.

93. Gautier-Smith, P. C.: Neurological complications of glandular fever (infectious mononucleosis), Brain 88:323, 1965.

94. Hoult, J. G. and Hewett, T. H.: Influenzal encephalopathy and post-influenzal encephalitis, Brit. Med. J. 1:1847, 1960.

95. Marsden, J. P. and Hurst, E. W.: Acute perivascular myelinoclisis in smallpox, Brain 55:181, 1932.

96. Public Health Service Recommendation on Smallpox Vaccination: Vaccination against smallpox in the United States. A reevaluation of the risks and benefits, Center for Disease Control, Morbidity and Mortality, 20:339, 1971.

97. Spillane, J. D. and Wells, C. E. C.: The neurology of Jennerian vaccination, Brain 87:1, 1964.

98. Scott, T. F.: Postinfectious and vaccinal encephalitis, Med. Clin. N. Amer. 51:701, 1967.

99. Cereghino, J. J., et al.: Rabies: Rare disease but serious pediatric problem, Pediatrics 45:839, 1970.

100. Prussin, G. and Katabi, G.: Dorsolumbar myelitis following antirabies vaccination with duck embryo vaccine, Ann. Intern. Med. 60:114, 1964.

101. Applebaum, E., Greenberg, M., and Nelson, J.: Neurological complications following antirabies vaccination, JAMA 151:188, 1953.

102. Byers, R. K. and Moll, F. C.: Encephalopathies following prophylactic pertussis vaccine, Pediatrics 1:437, 1948.

103. Ström, J.: Is universal vaccination against pertussis always justified? Brit. Med. J. 2:1184, 1960.

104. Melin, K. A.: Pertussis immunization in children with convulsive disorders, J. Pediat. 43:652, 1953.

105. Waksman, B. H. and Adams, R. D.: Allergic neuritis: An experimental disease of rabbits induced by the injection of peripheral nervous tissue and adjuvants, J. Exp. Med. 102:213, 1955.

106. Landry, O.: Note sur la paralysie ascendante aiguë, Gaz. Hebd. Med. 6:473, 1859.

107. Guillain, G., Barré, J. A., and Strohl, A.: Sur un syndrome de radiculo-nevrite avec hyperalbuminose du liquide cephalo-rachidien sans reaction cellulaire, Bull. Mem. Soc. Med. Hop. Paris 40:1462, 1916.

108. Haymaker, W. and Kernohan, J. W.: The Landry-Guillain-Barré syndrome, Medicine (Balt.) 28:59, 1949.

109. Wisniewski, H., et al.: Landry-Guillain-Barré syndrome, Arch. Neurol. 21:269, 1969.

110. Asbury, A. K., Arnason, B. G., and Adams, R. D.: The inflammatory lesion in idiopathic polyneuritis, Medicine (Balt.) 48:173, 1969.

111. Caspary E. A., et al.: Lymphocyte sensitization to nervous tissues and muscle in patients with Guillain-Barré syndrome, J. Neurol. Neurosurg. Psychiat. 34:179, 1971.

111a. Birnbaum, G.: Guillain-Barré syndrome: Increased lymphoproliferative potential, Arch. Neurol. 28:215, 1973.

112. Cook, S. D., et al.: Circulating demyelinating factors in acute idiopathic polyneuropathy, Arch. Neurol. 24:136, 1971.

113. Aström, K. E., Webster, H. deF., and Arnason, B. G.: The initial lesion in experimental allergic neuritis. A phase and electron microscopic study, J. Exp. Med. 128:469, 1968.

114. Melnick, S. C. and Flewett, T. H.: Role of infection in the Guillain-Barré syndrome, J. Neurol. Neurosurg. Psychiat. 27:395, 1964.

115. Low, N. L., Schneider, J., and Carter, S.: Polyneuritis in children, Pediatrics 22:972, 1958.

116. Peterman, A. F., et al.: Infectious neuronitis (Guillain-Barré syndrome) in children, Neurology (Minneap.) 9:533, 1959.

117. Morley, J.B. and Reynolds, E. H.: Papilledema and Landry-Guillain-Barré syndrome. Case reports and review, Brain 89:205, 1966.

118. Birchfield, R. I. and Shaw, C. M.: Postural hypotension in the Guillain-Barré syndrome, Arch. Neurol. 10:149, 1964.

119. Thomas, P. K., et al.: Recurrent and chronic relapsing Guillain-Barré polyneuritis, Brain 92:589, 1969.

120. Tasker, W. and Chutorian, A. M.: Chronic polyneuritis of childhood, J. Pediat. 74:699, 1969.

121. Byers, R. K. and Taft, L. T.: Chronic multiple neuropathy in childhood, Pediatrics 20:517, 1957.
122. Pleasure, D. E. and Towfighi, J.: Onion bulb neuropathies, Arch. Neurol. 26:289,1972.
123. Heller, G. L. and DeJong, R. N.: Treatment of the Guillain-Barré syndrome, Arch. Neurol. 8:179, 1963.
124. Austin, J. H.: Recurrent polyneuropathies and their corticosteroid treatment: With 5-year observations of a placebo controlled case treated with corticotrophin, cortisone, and prednisone, Brain 81:157, 1958.
125. Bell, C.: On the nerves; giving an account of some experiments on their structure and functions, which lead to a new arrangement of the system, Trans. Roy. Soc. Lond. 111:398, 1821.
126. Alter, M.: Familial aggregation of Bell's palsy, Arch. Neurol. 8:557, 1963.
127. Zülch, K. J.: " 'Idiopathic' Facial Paresis," in Vinken, P. J. and Bruyn, G. W. (eds.): Handbook of Clinical Neurology, Vol. 8, Pt. 2, New York: Amer. Elsevier Pub. Co., 1968.
128. Paine, R. S.: Facial paralysis in children, Pediatrics 19:303, 1957.
129. Salam, E. A. and Elyahky, W. S.: Evaluation of prognosis and treatment of Bell's palsy in children, Acta Paediat. Scand. 57:468, 1968.
130. Manning, J. J. and Adour, K. K.: Facial paralysis in children, Pediatrics 49:102, 1972.
131. Park, H. W. and Watkins, A. L.: Facial paralysis; analysis o 500 cases, Arch. Phys. Med. 30:749, 1949.
132. Ford, F. R.: Paroxysmal lacrimation during eating as a sequel of facial palsy (syndrome of crocodile tears); report of 4 cases with possible interpretation and comparison with auriculotemporal syndrome, Arch. Neurol. Psychiat. 29:1279, 1933.
133. Knox, D. L., Clark, D. B., and Schuster, F. F.: Benign VI palsies in children, Pediatrics 40:560, 1967.
134. Schain, R. J. and Wilson, G.: Brainstem encephalitis with radiographic evidence of medullary enlargement, Neurology (Minneap.) 21:537, 1971.
135. Gradenigo, G.: A special syndrome of endocranial otitic complications (paralysis of the motor oculi externus of otitic origin), Ann. Otol. 13:637, 1904.
136. Batten, F. E.: Case of acute ataxia, Trans. Clin. Soc. London 40:276, 1907.
137. McAllister, R. M., Hummeler, K., and Correll, L. L.: Acute cerebellar ataxia: Report of case with isolation of type 9 ECHO virus from cerebrospinal fluid, New Eng. J. Med. 261:1159, 1959.
138. Bray, P. F., et al.: Coincidence of neuroblastoma and acute cerebellar encephalopathy, J. Pediat. 75:983, 1969.
139. Korobkin, M., Palubinskas, A. J., and Clark, R. E.: Occult neuroblastoma and acute cerebellar ataxia in childhood, Radiology 102:151, 1972.
140. Weiss, S. and Carter, S.: Course and prognosis of acute cerebellar ataxia in children, Neurology (Minneap.) 9:711, 1959.
141. Cotton, D. G.: Acute cerebellar ataxia, Arch. Dis. Child. 32:181, 1957.
142. Basser, L. S.: Benign paroxysmal vertigo of childhood, Brain 87:141, 1964.
143. Pedersen, E.: Epidemic vertigo: Clinical picture, epidemiology and relation to encephalitis, Brain 82:566, 1959.
144. Kinsbourne, M.: Myoclonic encephalopathy of infants, J. Neurol. Neurosurg. Psychiat. 25:271, 1962.
145. Hill, W. and Sherman, H.: Acute intermittent familial cerebellar ataxia, Arch. Neurol. 18:350, 1968.
146. Freedman, D. and Schenthal, J.: A parenchymatous cerebellar syndrome following protracted high body temperature, Neurology (Minneap.) 3:513, 1953.
147. Norton, W. D. and Cogan, D. G.: Spasmus nutans: Clinical study of 20 cases followed two years or more since onset, AMA Arch. Ophthal. 52:442, 1954.

(Certain reference numbers have been intentionally omitted in the process of updating this chapter.)

CHAPTER 8

John H. Menkes and Ulrich Batzdorf

CRANIOCEREBRAL TRAUMA

In the western world, accidents constitute the major single cause of death between the ages of 1 and 14 years (Table 8–1). In Newcastle-upon-Tyne, England, the number of children admitted to hospitals with head injuries has increased sixfold over the past 20 years, and in 1971 constituted 13.9% of all admissions to pediatric wards.[1a] Most fatal injuries, particularly motor vehicle accidents, involve central nervous system trauma. As a consequence, craniocerebral injuries present a common and serious clinical problem.

TABLE 8-1.
MORTALITY RATES IN CHILDREN

Cause of Death	Age	
	1–4 Years	5–14 Years
All causes	92.9*	42.2
Accidents	31.8	18.7
Motor vehicle accidents	10.5	8.9
Influenza and pneumonia	11.4	2.1
Congenital malformations	10.2	2.8
Malignant neoplasm	8.6	6.5

* Figures are rate per 100,000 for the year 1965. Obtained from the Department of Health, Education, and Welfare, Social and Rehabilitation Service, Children's Bureau.

We here confine ourselves to postnatal injuries, delegating discussion of perinatal injuries to the nervous system to Chapter 5. We are concerned with the diagnosis and nonsurgical management of head injuries, considering first their pathophysiology and pathology, proceeding according to the severity of the craniocerebral trauma, and finally discussing the complications and sequelae of head injuries.

Dynamics and Pathophysiology of Craniocerebral Trauma[1,2,3]

Physical forces act on the head through acceleration, deceleration, or deformation. The brain is injured through compression, tearing, or shearing—alone, in combination, or in succession. Due to its elasticity and ability to undergo a greater degree of deformation, the skull of an infant absorbs the energy of the physical impact and protects the brain better than the skull of older people.

When the stationary head receives a blow it is accelerated and the skull becomes deformed. Deformation, which is both general and localized at the site of impact, may produce a skull fracture. It is greatest on impact of large masses traveling at relatively slow speeds. About 70% of skull fractures are single linear breaks. As a rule, the faster the blow, the more likely is a depressed skull fracture, while low velocity impacts tend to produce linear fractures. However, even fatal intracranial injuries may occur without any skull fracture.

The physical forces already cited distort the brain and cause it to move differentially with respect to the skull, an important antecedent of brain injury. Distortion of the brain stem is particularly important in deceleration injuries, such as occur in falls. Another mechanism is the alteration in intracranial pressure resulting from head trauma. At the site of injury there is a momentary increase in pressure, while negative pressures can be recorded contralaterally.[3] The latter, if sufficiently intense, produce vaporization and cavitation of the brain.[4] Differential movements of the brain, and pressure changes are responsible for the contrecoup injury that frequently occurs when the resting head is suddenly accelerated.[5] Thus, typically, following a blow to the occiput, the major injury is to the frontal and temporal poles. Conversely, when the brain is injured by sudden deceleration, as in falls, cerebral damage is generally greatest near the point of impact. But this generalization does not hold in infants, in whom contrecoup injuries are relatively rare.[5]

CONCUSSION

The physical processes within the skull due to trauma effect numerous changes within the brain. The most common is concussion. According to one widely accepted definition, this is a transient state of neuronal dysfunction, induced by trauma and of instantaneous onset. It is followed by amnesia for the moment of the accident and for a variable period prior to the accident (retrograde amnesia). The pathogenesis of concussion is still under debate. Strich[6] and Symonds[7] have proposed that the shearing forces to which the brain is subjected in an injury induce stretching, compression, and tearing of nerve fibers. Indeed, careful microscopic examination discloses these alterations,[6] together with permanent structural damage and loss of neurons even in cases of cerebral concussion.[3] As the reticular activating system of the central brain stem, particularly the

rostral mesencephalon and diencephalon, is concerned with consciousness, the most significant changes must occur in this area.[8] The exact mechanism through which neuronal dysfunction is induced is also unclear. It is likely, however, that the anatomic alterations of nerve fibers induce a release of acetylcholine and potassium, which may block synaptic transmission in some essential brain stem neurons. Under experimental conditions, head trauma also induces a reduction of oxygen consumption and increased lactate production, suggesting interruptions of the Krebs cycle[9] within the traumatized area.

CONTUSION AND LACERATION

Head injuries, more severe than those resulting in concussion, induce gross and microscopic hemorrhages of the brain substance. Characteristically, contusions represent petechial hemorrhages along the superficial aspects of the brain, occurring at the site of impact (coup injuries), or at contrecoup areas (Fig. 8–1). Points of predilection for contusions are the orbital surfaces of the frontal lobes and the infero-lateral aspect of the temporal lobes.[3] When the impact is on the forehead or vertex, the initial displacement of the brain may cause it to shift downward to-

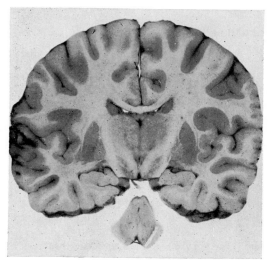

Fig. 8–1. Contusion and cerebral edema in five-year-old following automobile accident. The brain is pale with swelling and flattening of gyri. Hemorrhages and necrosis of left temporal lobe. (Courtesy of Dr. Richard Lindenberg, Baltimore.)

ward and into the tentorial opening. This may result in contusions of the hippocampal gyrus, particularly the uncus, the basal ganglia, and the upper part of the brain stem.[10] Brain damage in the contused area varies in severity depending on the extent of vascular injury. As a rule, contusions are less common in infants and small children than in adults subjected to comparable trauma.[5]

Cerebral lacerations are usually associated with penetrating or depressed skull fractures, although in small children they may also occur without fracture. They frequently involve the frontal and temporal poles, and are associated with tears of the dura, and tears or other injuries of the major vessels, and secondarily, thromboses, hemorrhages, or focal cerebral ischemia.

SECONDARY EFFECTS OF BRAIN TRAUMA

The anatomic alterations secondary to trauma develop as a result of cerebral edema and circulatory disorders. Cerebral edema principally involves the subcortical white matter and the centrum ovale. It may result from a temporary impairment of the water and electrolyte permeability and transport mechanism, located in the injured perivascular astrocytes. Edema in turn induces vascular stasis, anoxia, and further vasodilatation.[11] In infants and small children, massive cerebral edema in the absence of hemorrhages or other evidence of vascular injury, is not unusual. When the additive effects of injury and edema are of sufficient magnitude, a self-perpetuating sequence of events may develop if the progression of edema is not checked. Increased tissue pressure will result in collapse of venules, which in turn induces vascular stasis and tissue anoxia. A loss of selective permeability of of tissue membranes results, with increased loss of fluid from the vascular compartment into the parenchyma, thereby increasing cerebral swelling. Recovery has not been seen when intracranial pressure exceeds arterial pressure, a condition sometimes documented arteriographically (Fig. 8–2). Herniation of the uncus over the tentorial edge compresses the midbrain and often occludes the posterior cerebral arteries. Petechial hemorrhages are

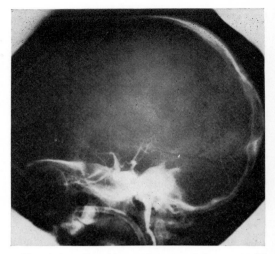

Fig. 8–2. Carotid arteriogram of four-year-old with increased intracranial pressure due to severe cerebral edema following a head injury. Note that carotid flow stops abruptly just above the clinoids. Judging from the arteriogram, the intracranial pressure is sufficiently high to prevent normal cerebral circulation, a circumstance which is almost uniformly fatal.

often found in the midbrain and pons, and infarctions in areas of the basal ganglia supplied by the anterior choroidal artery. A temporary drop in blood pressure, commonly seen with a severe injury, potentiates the vicious circle.

CLOSED HEAD INJURY

Over 90% of major pediatric head injuries are of the nonpenetrating, closed variety, the clinical picture of which is highlighted by alterations in consciousness.[1] As is the case for all head injuries, boys are involved three times more commonly than girls. When the injury is mild, initial unconsciousness is brief and is followed by confusion, somnolence, and listlessness. Vomiting, pallor, and irritability are common, and particularly in infants can occur in the apparent absence of an initial loss of consciousness. By definition, neurologic signs, with the exception of transient nystagmus[12] or extensor plantar responses, are not observed in simple concussion. A lumbar puncture is of little diagnostic value in such cases. Bloody cerebrospinal fluid may be seen with a cerebral contusion or laceration and even with some concussions.

CSF pressure may be increased in cerebral edema associated with contusion or laceration, or as a result of a hematoma which could be epidural, subdural, or intracerebral in location. Thus a lumbar puncture would not clarify the differential diagnosis.

One-third of children with mild head injuries have associated linear fractures of the skull.[1] As a rule their presence does not alter the clinical course or prolong the period of morbidity.[1,13]

Electroencephalographic tracings taken after injury may reveal striking abnormalities, including generalized and focal slowing, prolonged reaction to hyperventilation, and even hypsarhythmia. These changes are generally transient, and correlate neither with the clinical state of the patient nor with subsequent appearance of post-traumatic epilepsy.[14]

In major closed head injuries, consciousness is interrupted more profoundly and for longer periods, and focal neurologic signs point to localized brain contusion. The clinical picture of children with major closed head injuries is outlined in Table 8–2.[15] As a rule the greatest neurologic deficit is found at the time of injury. When new neurologic signs appear subsequently, these indicate progressive cerebral edema or, if localized, secondary intracranial hemorrhage, vasospasm, or thrombosis. The duration of coma depends on the site and severity of injury. The clinical picture may follow one of four courses. The child may die without recovering consciousness. Thus, in one study, there was a 17% mortality for children under 10 years of age, whose coma was of more than 12 hours duration.[16] In another, but smaller, group of patients, coma may persist. Should the child be alive 48 hours after injury, prognosis for survival is relatively good. In half of the surviving children consciousness is regained within one day. Recovery is often complete, although transient sequelae are not unusual. These include a cerebrospinal fluid leak which may be complicated by secondary meningitis, post-traumatic epilepsy, and the development of a carotid artery-cavernous sinus fistula. These complications will be discussed elsewhere in this chapter. Communicating hydrocephalus due to subarachnoid bleeding is more common following postnatal trauma and is referred to in Chapters 4 and 5.

In many instances of severe closed head injury, diagnosis of the injury is performed in parallel with emergency treatment. The former requires careful but not elaborate neurologic examination with particular emphasis on state of consciousness, pupillary size, equality and response to light, extent and symmetry of spontaneous movements, and reflex responses, as well as recording of blood pressure, pulse, and respirations. Of these, the most important are serial determinations of the patient's level of consciousness. The patient's responsiveness is determined in a systematic manner: Does the child verbalize spontaneously or respond only to verbal commands? Does it respond to painful stimuli only, and, if so, in appropriate or decerebrate fashion, or is all response whatsoever lacking? If the older child is able to speak, is it oriented to person, time, and place? The extent of retrograde am-

TABLE 8–2.
CLINICAL FINDINGS IN 4465 CHILDREN WITH HEAD INJURIES*

Finding	Percent	
Initial level of consciousness		
Normal	56.0	
Drowsy, confused	30.2	
Major impairment	13.8	
Vomiting	30.3	
Skull fractures	26.6	
Linear fractures		72.8
Depressed fractures		27.2
Compound fractures		19.7
Seizures	7.4	
Paralyses	3.8	
Retinal hemorrhages	2.3	
Pupillary abnormalities	3.6	
Papilledema	1.5	
Extradural hematoma	0.9	
Subdural hematoma	5.2	
Mortality	5.4	
Major neurologic residua	5.9	

* After Hendrick, et al.[15] This series includes 243 infants with major birth injuries. This group had 50% mortality and a higher incidence of paralyses, retinal hemorrhages, and major residua.

nesia and post-traumatic amnesia is recorded. The latter is a useful prognostic indicator.[17]

Radiographic examination of the skull usually contributes little to the initial management of the major closed head injury and, except in open depressed fractures, can safely be delayed for a few hours until the child's condition has stabilized. Likewise, a diagnostic lumbar puncture is usually not indicated. The use of cerebral angiography in the diagnosis of an intracerebral clot and localized cerebral edema, and for the exclusion of a subdural or epidermal hematoma in patients with focal neurologic signs or steady deterioration of clinical status is well-established.[18]

Treatment

We here confine ourselves to the nonoperative aspects of treatment of closed head injuries. Details of surgical management can be found in textbooks of operative neurosurgery. Following an immediate evaluation of the child's general condition, an adequate airway should be established and maintained. This may require mechanical suction, endotracheal intubation, or artificial respiration. Tracheotomy is performed when indicated to bypass mechanical obstruction of the airway resulting from facial or mandibular injuries. Shock in closed head injuries is usually due to blood loss elsewhere in the body or rarely indicates damage to the medullary cardiovascular centers. In infants, however, subgaleal or subperiosteal hemorrhages may be sufficiently extensive to induce shock. Following completion of the initial emergency measures, the child's neurologic status should be reevaluated. The importance of repeated observations of vital signs and notations of the major parameters of the neurologic status cannot be overemphasized. Slowing of the pulse rate and widening of pulse pressure often accompany increasing intracranial pressure (Cushing effect, see Chapter 10). Irregularities of the respiratory pattern are also common after severe head injuries.[19]

Fluid therapy for the unconscious patient with head trauma generally differs in only a few respects from that required for other intensive care patients. However, an initial period of sodium retention lasting two to four days is a common response to brain injury.[20] Since there may be concomitant water retention as a consequence of an inappropriate excess of antidiuretic hormone, sodium retention may not be reflected by serum electrolyte levels and a mild hyponatremia is common.

These alterations of electrolyte and fluid homeostasis mean that during the early post-traumatic period there is danger of overloading the patient with fluids, which may impair his level of consciousness by increasing cerebral edema. In general, intravenous fluids for the first two to four days should be about 75% of the average calculated daily fluid requirements, even if urine volume remains low.[1] Despite sodium retention in the early post-traumatic period, salt should be administered to avoid hypotonicity of extracellular fluids and increased cerebral edema. The addition of 30 mEq of sodium chloride per liter of calculated fluid meets the usual electrolyte requirements. Potassium generally offers no problem, and extra potassium is not required during the early post-traumatic period.[21]

Less commonly, hypernatremia and dehydration follow closed head injury. This is occasionally seen in a subfrontal injury which has caused hypothalamic damage and diabetes insipidus, or is the result of a failure in the thirst response or inadequate hydration of an unconscious patient.

Cerebral edema can be counteracted by the use of hypertonic solutions.[22] Of these, mannitol and urea are the most commonly employed. Because of its slow transfer across the blood-brain barrier, a high blood urea concentration is unaccompanied by high brain levels, and in this fashion a transient osmotic gradient is established.[23,24] Maximum dehydration occurs within 20–30 minutes after administration of 1.0 gm–1.5 gm urea per kg body weight. Its effect lasts about six hours and is followed by some rebound, that is, an increase of intracranial pressure above the minimum achieved with treatment. Mannitol, given in amounts of 1.5 gm–2.0 gm per kg body weight in the form of a 20% solution, has a slower effect than urea, but maintains the lowered intracranial pressure at its minimum level for two to four hours. These rapidly acting osmotic agents are primarily used to gain time, while patient and operating room are readied for surgery, or diagnostic studies are being performed.

Dexamethasone (Decadron), an anti-inflammatory glucocorticoid, may reduce cerebral edema and it is often desirable to use steroids and osmotic agents simultaneously.[25] A recommended schedule for children is an initial intravenous dose of 0.1 mg/kg body weight, followed by 0.05 mg/kg every six hours for a total daily dose of 0.25 mg/kg body weight. The usefulness of corticosteroids in trauma is controversial, but if they are to be administered, this should be done as soon as possible following injury.

Hypothermia is a useful adjunct for major closed head injuries. It may prevent cerebral damage by reducing the metabolic demands of the brain, and by decreasing the cerebrospinal fluid pressure. Generally, a body temperature of 90°–92°F (32°–33°C) is maintained for at least three days, the period of maximum cerebral edema. In small children, hypothermia is easily induced by the use of ice packs and is maintained with a cooling mattress. Shivering is rarely a problem in the unconscious patient subjected to hypothermia. If present, it can be controlled by chlorpromazine (Thorazine).

Anticonvulsants in the treatment of post-traumatic seizures are discussed in Chapter 11. Intravenous diphenylhydantoin (Dilantin) may control seizures without inducing drowsiness. Intramuscular Dilantin, which may crystallize within muscles, is less reliable. Post-traumatic seizures are rarely intractable, but initial anticonvulsant therapy should be followed by maintenance doses for several years.

Morphine, which aggravates cerebral edema, depresses the level of consciousness and obscures pupillary changes, should be avoided, and other sedatives used sparingly. Paraldehyde is probably the best drug for the overactive, semiconscious child. For pain due to other associated injuries, icebags or small amounts of codeine may be required.

More detailed treatment schedules for the child with a major closed head injury are given by Matson.[22,26]

The treatment of minor closed head injuries requires considerable clinical judgment. Unnecessary hospitalization should be avoided, but the possibility of post-traumatic complications requiring emergency surgery must be kept in mind. In general, children who have suffered only a momentary loss of consciousness are better managed at home. Parents are instructed to note the child's state of alertness and ability to move his extremities at regular intervals, and asked to contact the physician in case of increasing drowsiness or limb weakness. The presence of a linear skull fracture usually does not influence the decision of whether to hospitalize a child. However, if the fracture line crosses the groove of the middle meningeal artery, the lambdoid suture, or the path of the sagittal sinus, the physician may be sufficiently concerned about the possibility of an extradural hemorrhage to prefer to hospitalize such a child for the initial 24 hours.

Prognosis

The outlook for full intellectual function in children suffering minor head injuries—that is, without neurologic manifestations—is excellent.

The prognosis for major head injuries is less certain. Following such trauma, children almost invariably complain of marked tiredness. Their speech may be slurred but speech expression and comprehension are retained. Symonds and Russell found the duration of post-traumatic amnesia a useful prognostic indicator.[17] In patients who were unconscious for 24 hours or longer, Hjern and Nylander[27] found no clear correlation between the duration of unconsciousness and the severity of residual symptoms. However, only some 15% of their cases were free of both neurologic and behavioral abnormalities on follow-up examination. Generally, children with only behavioral abnormalities during the early post-traumatic period tend to achieve complete resolution of symptoms; neurologic abnormalities can continue to improve for as long as three years.[27,28] Decerebrate rigidity, while associated with an early mortality of 25%–50%, by itself does not preclude functional survival of the patient as about one-half of survivors have fair recovery.[28,29]

A high percentage of survivors from major head injuries are mentally retarded. This is not necessarily a consequence of the recent insult to brain function but also reflects the relatively high proportion of mentally subnormal or disturbed children involved in accidents.[30]

SKULL FRACTURES

Because of its flexibility, the immature skull can sustain a greater degree of deformation than that of the adult before incurring a fracture. The great majority of skull fractures are linear. They are generally asymptomatic, and in the older child are readily diagnosed by roentgenography. In infants, the fracture lines are irregular, and it may be difficult to differentiate a fracture from an ununited spheno-occipital suture, metopic or mendosal sutures, or Wormian bones[31] (Fig. 8–3). In early childhood, diastatic fractures are relatively common. These involve a traumatic separation of the cranial bones, usually the lambdoidal suture.

Closed linear fractures generally heal within three to four months and, except for breaks crossing the path of major vessels or entering the paranasal sinuses, do not require special therapy or observations.[13]

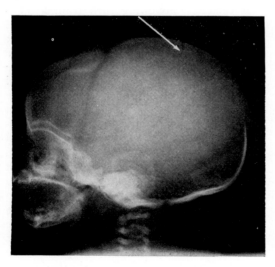

Fig. 8–3. Depressed frontal fracture and linear parietal fracture (arrow) on plain skull films of a newborn infant who had undergone a difficult forceps delivery; associated left-sided epidural hematoma was demonstrated at angiography.

An infrequent complication of a closed head injury associated with a linear fracture is a leptomeningeal cyst.[32] This condition is usually seen when the underlying head injury occurs prior to two or three years of age. This cyst is most commonly located in the parietal area and is associated with an unrecognized dural laceration. It represents a fluid-filled space between the pia mater and the arachnoid, the latter herniating through the dural tear into the fracture separation. The fluid-filled pockets are not completely isolated from the subarachnoid space, so that fluid gradually accumulates, forming a cyst which, however, cannot drain spontaneously into the subarachnoid space and hence enlarges. Through it the pulsations of the brain are transmitted to the inner table of the skull and induce erosion of the overlying bone. The patient with a leptomeningeal cyst may present several months to years after the initial skull trauma with a scalp mass or, less often, a seizure disorder.[33] If the cyst is large, it may not only be palpable but it also may transilluminate. Roentgenographic findings are diagnostic. There is an irregular bony defect, usually with scalloped margins, and some sclerosis of the adjacent bone. Leptomeningeal cysts should be differentiated from encephalocele, which is congenital, usually located in the occipital midline, and associated with a regular bony defect. Treatment consists of excision of the cyst and repair of the dural defect.

Basal skull fractures are relatively uncommon in children. Their presence may be suspected when the child has signs of bleeding from the nasopharynx, or the middle ear, or postauricular ecchymoses (Battle's sign).[33a] It should, however, be pointed out that epistaxis is frequent in head injuries in children, in association with the high incidence of nasal fractures.

Fractures of the base of the anterior fossa may be accompanied by hemorrhage into the orbit with exophthalmos and subconjunctival hemorrhage, while fractures of the mastoid portion of the temporal bone result in postauricular ecchymoses.

Cerebrospinal fluid rhinorrhea may accompany a fracture of the floor of the anterior fossa which has involved the cribriform plate.

It represents a rare complication of head trauma in children, but the higher risk of intracranial infections, 24% as reported by Lewin,[34] makes its recognition and treatment imperative. Cerebrospinal fluid rhinorrhea usually appears within the first two days after injury. If the fluid is clear the presence of glucose will distinguish it from ordinary nasal discharge. In many cases drainage ceases spontaneously within a week or 10 days. If this does not occur, surgical repair of the dural tear responsible is indicated.[34]

A cerebrospinal fluid leak predisposes to meningitis, most often due to pneumococcus, and antibiotic therapy should be directed against this organism.

Injuries to the cranial nerves, particularly the olfactory, acoustic, and facial nerves, may accompany basal fractures. Complete loss of the sense of smell is usually permanent, while 90% of facial nerve injuries recover spontaneously.[35] Deafness may be a temporary or permanent sequel to temporal bone fractures, while labyrinthine disorders are usually transitory. Cerebrospinal fluid otorrhea is seen in about 0.5% of pediatric head injuries but in about 95% of cases stops spontaneously within a week to 10 days. Unlike CSF rhinorrhea, recurrences of discharge are rare.[35] Rarely transient total blindness may follow an apparently mild blunt head injury. The cause for this symptom is uncertain.[36]

The diagnosis of basal fractures often depends on the clinical picture, as in many instances the fracture may not be visible by radiographic examination. In most instances it is academic to demonstrate the extent of the suspected fracture, and special views should not be undertaken if obtaining them delays treating the child. Basal fractures associated with hemotympanum or Battle's sign should be treated with 7–10 days of prophylactic antibiotics, preferably directed against pneumococci and staphylococci. In the case of a cerebrospinal fluid leak, antibiotics are continued well after its cessation. When meningitis is suspected, a diagnostic lumbar puncture should be performed.

Air in the cranial cavity (pneumocele) rarely complicates head injury.[37] It is most common following fracture of the frontal sinuses. It is usually an incidental finding on radiography but as there is a distinct likelihood of meningitis, prophylactic antibiotics are required until the air is resolved spontaneously. Tension pneumocephalus is a rare complication which presents a neurosurgical emergency due to a rapid increase in intracranial pressure.

SCALP LACERATIONS

Scalp lacerations may be the source of considerable blood loss. If any question exists regarding the presence of a scalp injury the child's hair should be clipped. The area around a wound is widely shaved and the wound inspected for evidence of an underlying fracture. Closure should be undertaken after careful debridement with strict adherence to aseptic technique. Tetanus protection should be administered.

Depressed fractures are a common consequence of perinatal injury, often the result of difficult forceps delivery ("Ping-Pong ball fracture," see Chapter 5) but depressed fractures may also occur with any localized skull trauma in later childhood, when they are often associated with a compound fracture and localized cerebral injury. The extent of the bony injury is best diagnosed by roentgenography. If the depression is greater than about 3 mm, the fracture does not reduce itself spontaneously and surgical treatment is recommended as soon as the child's general condition permits it.

Compound fractures of the skull are seen in about 20% of children with major head trauma.[15] In this type of injury medical treatment is limited to an initial cleansing of the scalp, institution of antibiotics, and tetanus prophylaxis. Anticonvulsant therapy, usually diphenylhydantoin (Dilantin), is used routinely when the bony fragments have penetrated beyond the dura.

Complications of Head Injuries

EXTRADURAL HEMATOMA

An extradural or epidural hematoma is a localized accumulation of blood between the skull and the dura. It occurs in about 1% of children hospitalized for head trauma.[15] According to Matson[38] nearly one-half of

TABLE 8-4.
CLINICAL FEATURES OF 116 CASES OF
INFANTILE SUBDURAL HEMATOMA*

Symptom or Finding	Percent of Infants
Tense anterior fontanelle	73
Vomiting	70
Seizures	60
Retinal or subhyaloid hemorrhages	54
Abnormal skull circumference	40
Impaired consciousness	22
Papilledema	12
Skull fracture	13
Other fractures	17

* After Till.[50]

trauma was elicited in 25% of patients. In another 28% there was a history of suspected birth trauma.[49a] In other infants the environmental history or other evidence of recent unreported physical trauma suggests parental abuse.[50] Other known predisposing factors include blood dyscrasias and prematurity.[51]

While there is no characteristic clinical picture, certain features should suggest the presence of this lesion. Convulsions are the most common presenting feature. These occur in about half of the patients and may be either focal or, more commonly, generalized. Vomiting, fever, and hyperirritability or lethargy are other common clinical features (Table 8-4). Most often the history is that of an infant who fails to gain weight, refuses feedings, has frequent episodes of vomiting, some of which might be projectile, becomes irritable, develops progressive enlargement of his head, and ultimately suffers a seizure. Often symptoms are present for several months before a diagnosis is made.

On examination the infant is often febrile, the result of dehydration or blood within the cranial cavity. The head is enlarged and there is a prominent parietal or biparietal bulge. The fontanelle is full, and a "setting sun" sign of the eyes may be noted. The funduscopic examination may reveal retinal hemorrhages, subhyaloid hemorrhages, or, less commonly, papilledema.[52,53] The first

has been found in some 50%–80% of infants.[50,54] Focal neurologic signs, including hemiparesis or facial palsy, are present in some 15%–25% of patients.

Laboratory studies are usually of little help in confirming the presence of a subdural hematoma. About half of the children have anemia. Skull fractures are relatively uncommon, being present in some 10%–15%.

In some other infants, plain skull films may indicate increased intracranial pressure as judged from separation of the sutures. Lumbar puncture is of little diagnostic help. Where the cerebrospinal fluid is abnormal, it may be grossly bloody or xanthochromic and under increased pressure. Red blood cells may be present and the protein elevated. A pleocytosis is also not unusual if the hematoma has been of long-standing. The electroencephalogram is of little assistance in either the diagnosis or the localization of the subdural hematoma and frequently fails to show any focal abnormality. Cerebral angiography will reveal a displacement of the terminal branches of the anterior or middle cerebral arteries from the surface of the skull, leaving an avascular area, the extent of which gives a good indication of the size of the hematoma (Fig. 8–6).

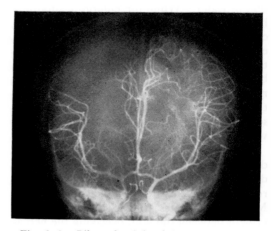

Fig. 8–6. Bilateral subdural hematoma. Angiography demonstrates delayed right-sided filling, and a clear, avascular space between the cerebral surface and the skull, characteristic for a chronic subdural hematoma. There is a slight shift of the vessels to the left suggesting a large hematoma on the right. (Courtesy of Dr. Gabriel Wilson, Department of Radiology, UCLA, Los Angeles.)

Diagnosis

Subdural hematoma should be suspected in an irritable infant who has failed to gain weight and has developed an enlarged head. Characteristically, the head assumes a biparietal bulge, which contrasts with the frontal bulge of early hydrocephalus. Confirmation of the diagnosis rests upon bilateral subdural taps. This procedure should be performed in any infant suspected of harboring a subdural hematoma. Details of the procedure are given by Matson.[55] In essence, aspiration punctures are done through the coronal suture lateral to the margin of the anterior fontanelle at least 3–4 cm from the midline, so as to avoid puncture of the sagittal sinus. Normally, only a few drops of clear fluid can be obtained. In the presence of a subdural hematoma, grossly bloody or xanthochromic fluid is found on subdural puncture. Large amounts of clear fluid with a protein content approaching that of the cerebrospinal fluid suggest the presence of cerebral atrophy, or a porencephalic cyst communicating with the ventricular system. Under these circumstances subsequent pneumoencephalography will delineate any gross cerebral abnormality.

If a concomitant diagnostic lumbar puncture is also deemed advisable in order to exclude the presence of infection or associated subarachnoid bleeding, it should be performed first, so as to avoid its contamination by blood from the subdural space. The extent of the subdural collection is best verified by cerebral angiography (Fig. 8–6). Transillumination of the skull has been suggested as a simple method for the diagnosis of some subdural hematomas of infancy.[56]

Subdural hematomas of infancy are usually not detected by brain scanning, although this procedure is applicable to the chronic hematoma of older children and adolescents.

Treatment

A number of different regimens have been proposed for the treatment of a subdural hematoma in infants who lack a preceding history of meningitis. Based on the classic work of Sherwood[57] and Ingraham and Heyl,[58] Matson has outlined a course of therapy.[55] During the initial phase of treatment the subdural fluid is removed at regular intervals by means of subdural taps. If the subdural effusion does not dry up, these are done daily on alternate sides for about two weeks. This period also allows infants who have sustained a head injury to stabilize with respect to their general condition. Because of the presence of anemia, and the subsequent recurrent loss of fluid having a high protein content, patients may require transfusions or other supportive therapy during this period. During the second stage of therapy exploratory burr holes are performed bilaterally on every infant who at that time still has excessive amounts of blood or xanthochromic subdural fluid. By this means the presence of a subdural membrane can be verified. A subsequent craniotomy serves to evacuate the clot and, if possible, to excise completely both the inner and the outer membranes of the subdural hematoma. Matson has postulated that the membranes are associated with persistent reaccumulation of subdural fluid and are ultimately transformed into inelastic connective tissue which may interfere with the development of the cerebral cortex.[55]

Others, including ourselves, believe that with persistent subdural taps the collection will frequently dry up completely, eliminating the need for surgery. Only when it becomes clear that the subdural fluid continues to re-form between taps do we decide on surgery. Arteriography, a subdural air study, or both, are used to delineate the extent of the subdural space preoperatively. The removal of subdural membranes is always necessary, but even after this major surgical procedure, subdural fluid may re-form. A subduralpleural shunt as originally suggested by Ransohoff[59] serves to reduce the volume of dead space and allows it to be obliterated by the growing brain. Complete disappearance of the subdural membranes, or reduction in vascularity, occurs with time, as long as there is adequate drainage of the subdural space.[60] This can be confirmed by cerebral angiography. The optimal treatment of infantile subdural hematomas, i.e., repeated aspiration, membrane stripping, or shunting, is still a subject of controversy.[60a]

The treatment of a chronic subdural hematoma occurring in older children and adolescents consists of its drainage through burr holes. Since even in this age group the blood clot is frequently bilateral, both sides should always be explored unless arteriography has clearly demonstrated a unilateral lesion.

Prognosis

The prognosis of an infant with a subdural hematoma correlates best with its presumptive cause. Postinfectious subdural effusions, discussed in Chapter 6, have a far better outlook than post-traumatic hematomas. In the experience of Rabe et al.,[61] 80% of infants with postinfectious subdural effusion recovered completely, while only some 40% recovered when the hematoma was secondary to trauma or was of unknown etiology. Rabe et al.[61] furthermore found that there is no difference in the prognosis of infants treated with multiple subdural taps, with taps and exploratory burr holes, or with repeated taps followed by exploratory burr holes and partial excision of the subdural membranes. McLaurin and McLaurin[62] believe that the ultimate outcome depends on the extent of damage sustained by the underlying brain. If this is extensive, expansion will not occur, and the hematoma may calcify or ossify. Removal of a calcified subdural hematoma is of no advantage.

CEPHALHEMATOMA

Cephalhematoma is a traumatic hemorrhage between the scalp and the skull. The hemorrhage is located between the periosteum of the skull (pericranium) and the calvarium, as is usual following a traumatic delivery (see Chapter 5). Less commonly, the hematoma is primarily located between the galea of the scalp and the periosteum. The former lesion is associated with a linear skull fracture in about 25% of infants.[63] Frequently the subperiosteal hematoma is sharply delineated by the suture line, distinguishing it from the subgaleal hematoma which is more diffuse. The fluid collection is usually completely reabsorbed by 3–4 weeks, and aspiration is generally contraindicated because of the danger of infecting the hematoma cavity. Occasionally a subperiosteal hematoma will calcify, but this too should cause little concern, since the calcium deposits are generally

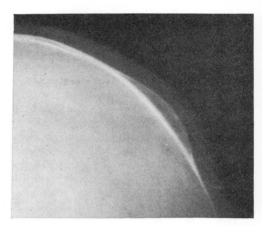

Fig. 8–7. Calcified cephalhematoma. (Courtesy of Dr. Gabriel Wilson, Department of Radiology, UCLA, Los Angeles.)

reabsorbed prior to the end of the first year, leaving no residual asymmetry (Fig. 8–7).

POST-TRAUMATIC EPILEPSY

Seizures associated with trauma have been classified according to the time of onset into the immediate, early, and late types.[64] A few patients suffer a seizure within a second or two following their head trauma. Such immediate seizures are most probably the result of direct mechanical stimulation of cerebral tissue having a low seizure threshold.

In patients who have incurred major cerebral trauma, seizures may appear during the first 24–48 hours after their injury (early post-traumatic seizures). These are due to cerebral edema, or the result of intracranial hemorrhage, contusion, laceration, or necrosis. The convulsions are usually generalized, but unilateral seizures and focal twitching are also seen. In the experience of Hendrick et al.[15] 7.4% of children with head trauma requiring hospitalization had seizures during the early post-traumatic period. The incidence was highest in infants less than one year of age, with patients subjected to perinatal injury being particularly susceptible (Chapter 5). In children suffering from early post-traumatic seizures there is a high incidence of associated skull fractures (24% in the experience of Hendrick et al.).[15] Closed depressed fractures and compound depressed fractures are particularly common, and together account for about half the fractures seen in this group. However in contrast to the experience with adults, seizures are far more likely to occur in children who have sustained relatively minor head trauma.

Late post-traumatic seizures tend to develop within the first two years following the injury; in about half of the instances these appear during the first 12 months.[65] Anatomic and electric studies indicate that the seizures originate from a cerebromeningeal scar with the epileptic focus localized to grossly normal tissue.[66] The overall incidence of late post-traumatic epilepsy is difficult to estimate, as the figure is lowered by the inclusion of mild head injuries in any prospective series.

Two factors determine the likelihood of late post-traumatic epilepsy: the severity of the head injury and its location. In children who did not lose consciousness following head trauma the incidence of post-traumatic epilepsy was only 2%,[65] while it rose to 5%–10% when consciousness was lost for one hour or longer, and was 30% in those children who sustained brain laceration. Generally speaking, if the dura is penetrated in the course of the injury, the incidence of post-traumatic epilepsy rises at least twofold. The site of the injury also influences the incidence of late post-traumatic seizures. Injuries to the parietal lobe and to the anterior medial portion of the temporal lobe are most likely to be followed by this complication.

The clinical appearance of seizures may take several forms. They may be generalized, or generalized but be preceded by an aura which consists of motor phenomena such as clonic movements of an extremity or by somatosensory phenomena. The seizures can also be focal, but petit mal attacks do not occur as a result of trauma. The electroencephalogram has been found to be uniformly unsuccessful in predicting post-traumatic epilepsy.[67]

The diagnosis of post-traumatic epilepsy depends on the antecedent history of head trauma and the absence of any pretraumatic seizure history. The possibility of a subdural hematoma should always be excluded by the use of subdural taps or in older children particularly, by angiography.

Treatment of post-traumatic epilepsy is similar to that employed for focal or generalized seizures of unknown etiology, and is outlined in Chapter 11. In general diphenylhydantoin (Dilantin) is the anticonvulsant of choice at a dose comparable to that used in idiopathic epilepsy. Its prophylactic use has been recommended for patients with penetrating head injury. Generally, the prognosis of post-traumatic seizures is good, and there is a natural tendency for them to regress.[64] Patients with early appearance of convulsions tend to have a better outlook. In about 20%–50% of all patients, seizures gradually become less frequent after the third year and finally cease completely.[65,66] In all instances medical therapy should be given a fair trial, and surgery for excision of the cerebral scar should be reserved for those patients whose seizures persist for three or more years.

MAJOR VASCULAR INJURIES

Injury to the major vessels of the head or neck is relatively uncommon in children suffering from head trauma. Traumatic aneurysms of the internal carotid artery and carotid-cavernous fistulas have occasionally been reported in children.[68] The latter are usually due to a fracture of the sphenoid bone, which lacerates the internal carotid artery as it passes through the cavernous sinus. Symptoms include unilateral pulsating exophthalmos, an intracranial bruit, and paralysis of the cranial nerves, most commonly the sixth.

Traumatic thrombosis of the internal carotid artery has been reported in children as a result of relatively minor injuries to the head or neck, or following puncture of the soft palate by a lollipop stick.[69,70,71] In these cases, early thrombectomy is indicated if the site of obstruction is deemed accessible.[72]

POST-TRAUMATIC MENTAL DISTURBANCES

In the course of recovery from a major head injury almost every child shows some disturbance in behavior or intellect.[72a] This includes post-traumatic amnesia—an inability to recall events following the injury. In most cases, the length of post-traumatic amnesia is proportional to the severity of brain damage.[73,74] One of the common features of concussion injuries is a failure to recall events just prior to the injury (retrograde amnesia). Here too, there is a relationship between the length of impaired memory and the severity of the brain injury. Generally, post-traumatic amnesia is longer than retrograde amnesia. When there is unusually extensive retrograde amnesia, trauma to the limbic system, particularly the hippocampal formation and the mamillary bodies, should be suspected.

As a rule, the rate of recovery is faster in children than in adults. However, in the experience of Harris, major post-traumatic psychologic difficulties persisted in half of the 13% of children who manifested prolonged retrograde amnesia.[75] A true postconcussion syndrome is rare in children and is mainly limited to adolescents. The appearance of major psychiatric disorders, including increased aggressiveness, sleep disturbances, nightmares, and enuresis[76] following head injury is probably unrelated to the injury itself, but reflects the child's family and social environment. It is undoubtedly significant that 30% of children showing these post-traumatic behavior disturbances have had a history of previous accidents requiring medical treatment, and about one-quarter were either mentally retarded or had required psychiatric therapy prior to their head injury. In the experience of Hjern and Nylander[77] the overwhelming majority of children with persistent psychiatric symptoms had similar problems prior to their accident, which only served to aggravate symptoms. Conversely, none of the children who have been free of psychiatric symptoms prior to their accident displayed permanent post-traumatic mental disturbances.

From these data it follows that the psychiatric symptoms of head injury may frequently be avoided by giving parents, particularly mothers, reassurance or extensive supportive therapy at an early stage, preferably as soon as the child is admitted to the hospital.[77]

SPINAL CORD INJURIES

Because of its protected location, a considerable amount of direct trauma is required to injure the spinal cord. In children, therefore, injuries to the spinal cord are most frequently the result of indirect trauma. This is seen in accidents marked by sudden hyperflexion or hyperextension of the neck, or vertical compression of the spine by falls on the head or buttocks, as may occur by diving into shallow water, a fall from a horse, or various other athletic injuries.[78]

Common sites for childhood spinal cord injuries are the twelfth thoracic and first lumbar segments, C_5 and C_6, and the first and second cervical vertebrae. Fractures of the twelfth thoracic and first lumbar vertebrae are relatively common and may produce a conus medullaris and cauda equina syndrome.

Fracture dislocations of the vertebral column are the most frequent immediate cause of spinal cord injuries. Because of the marked mobility of the neck, the lower cervical region is particularly prone to this type of injury. Direct violence along the axis of the vertebral column may produce fractures of the vertebral bodies, and the spinal cord may be injured by fragments of bone entering the vertebral canal. Major spinal cord injuries without radiologic evidence of either fracture or dislocation of vertebrae are not unusual in children.

Pathology

In many patients in whom an accident produced early paraplegia, the spinal cord does not show any gross pathologic abnormality. Such a picture has been termed spinal concussion and is characterized by transient loss of spinal cord function. In other instances the spinal cord, when examined shortly after the injury, is swollen over several segments, and on microscopic examination there are numerous punctate hemorrhages. More extensive confluent hemorrhage is not uncommon, particularly after injuries to the lower cervical region. The major hemorrhages are generally central and extend in the form of a column cephalad and caudad from the site of injury. Extensive damage to the cord can be due to direct compression from without by bone, from within by hematoma, or to interference with its vascular supply. The anterior spinal artery appears particularly vulnerable, with the vascular shed in the upper thoracic cord, and the ventral radicular artery (Adamkiewicz), which usually feeds the cord at approximately T_{10}, representing favorite sites for interruption of the blood supply.[79,80]

When there is prolonged survival after major spinal cord injury, the damaged area is found to be softened, gray and white matter are poorly delineated, the myelin sheaths have been destroyed, and there is extensive loss of all cellular elements. Replacement by cavities or fibrous gliosis occurs ultimately.

Clinical Manifestations

The clinical picture depends on the severity of the injury and its location. Concussion may result from falls on the back and is characterized by temporary and completely reversible loss of function below the injured segment. With more extensive injuries recovery is only partial and permanent residua can be expected.

When transection of the cord is complete, the clinical picture is highlighted by spinal shock affecting the distal segments. This condition represents a transient decrease of synaptic excitability of neurons distal to the injury. It is due to a loss of supraspinal impulses, which normally produce a background of partial depolarization of the spinal neurons. Immediately after the injury there is complete loss of motor and sensory function in the segments caudal to the injury. There is complete areflexia of variable duration usually for at least two to six weeks.[81,82] Should reflex activity not return, the likelihood is that the distal spinal cord has been destroyed, the result of vascular insufficiency. During the first stage of spinal shock, the stage of flaccidity,[82] there is complete bladder paralysis and urinary retention Gradually a muscular response of the lower extremities can be elicited in response to stimulation of the skin or the deeper structures. The earliest movements occur in the legs and are flexor. The deep tendon reflexes reappear and soon become hyperactive. Abdominal reflexes may also return. A typical extensor plantar response can be induced and is often accompanied by flexor withdrawal movements of the foot, ankle, and subsequently the knee

and hip as well. Contraction of the extensor muscles of the crossed limb is a frequent accompaniment to the above mass flexion reflex.[82,83] During this stage the bladder empties automatically, although never completely.

In the majority of patients, extensor reflexes involving the quadriceps and other extensor muscles ultimately appear and become the dominant reflex activity. Stimuli eliciting this reflex are more complicated than those inducing the flexion response and include extension of the thigh, such as is seen when the patient shifts from a sitting to a supine position, or squeezing of the thighs.

Depending on the severity of the spinal cord injury, the final picture may be one of purely reflex activity of the isolated cord. With less extensive injuries there may be return of muscular function or subjective sensation over the course of the next few months up to one year.

The clinical picture of the most common spinal cord injuries is summarized in Table 8–5.

An unusual clinical picture, which occurs exclusively in children, is a transient apparent subluxation of the atlantoaxial joint, which often follows an upper respiratory infection.[84] Children present with a head tilt to the affected side. The neck is tender laterally and posteriorly over C_1 and C_2. It is said that the bulge of the anterior dislocation can be felt through the posterior pharyngeal wall. The condition is only rarely associated with root or cord signs, and resolves spontaneously with traction.

Dislocation of the atlantoaxial joint is seen with particular frequency in mongolism as a consequence of an increased atlantoaxial interval.[84a]

Diagnosis

The history of trauma is usually readily elicitable, and the most common diagnostic problem is to establish the site and extent of the injury. In small children sensory evaluation is usually best performed by demonstrating impairment of autonomic response. Shortly after the injury the dermatomes below the lesion are dry, and often have a defective vasomotor response. Evaluation of

TABLE 8-5.
NEUROLOGIC PICTURES OF SPINAL CORD INJURIES

	Clinical Picture
A. Transverse injuries	
$T_{12} - L_1$	Flaccid paralysis of lower extremities
	Loss of sphincter control
	Loss of sensation below inguinal ligament
$C_5 - C_6$	Flaccid quadriparesis
	Diaphragmatic movements spared
	Sensory level at second rib, with preservation of upper lateral aspect of arm
	Bilateral Horner's syndrome
	Loss of sphincter control
$C_1 - C_2$	Respiratory paralysis complete
	Rapid death
Conus medullaris	
Cauda equina	Urinary retention
	Disturbance of rectal sphincter
	Loss of sensation over lumbosacral dermatomes
	Flaccid paralysis of lower extremities
B. Brown-Sequard syndrome	
	Unilateral muscular paresis
	Contralateral disturbances of superficial sensitivity, especially pain and temperature
	Incomplete forms far more common than classic syndrome
C. Central cord lesion	
	Disproportionately more motor impairment of upper extremities (due to involvement of the more medial segments of the lateral corticospinal tracts)
	Bladder dysfunction (usually urinary retention)
	Varying degrees of sensory loss, usually pain and temperature below level of lesion
	Relatively good prognosis
	Motor power returns first to lower extremities

reflexes and motor function should provide no particular difficulty, since reflex withdrawal will not be seen during the acute phase of spinal shock.

Radiographs of the spine are important for localization of the lesion, but films may be normal and dislocations of the cervical spine may be difficult to interpret (Fig. 8-8). The patient with a suspected cervical spine injury must be moved to the x-ray unit with utmost care. After evaluation of the plain films of the spine, it is usually necessary to establish the presence or absence of a subarachnoid block, which may be due to bone fragments, disc material, hematoma, or swelling of neural tissues. While important to perform, manometric studies must follow initial stabilization of the spine, particularly in cases of cervical injuries. A lumbar puncture is per-

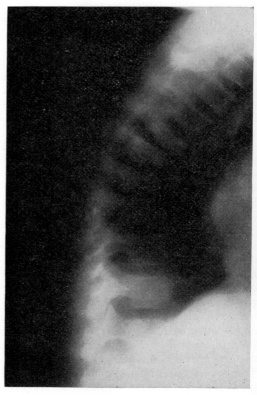

Fig. 8-8. Compression fracture of thoracic spine (T 6, 7 and 8) with anterior displacement of T 6 on T 7. Patient was a nine-year-old girl who fell from a tree and had an immediate total motor and sensory paralysis below the level of the injury.

formed. The column of fluid in the manometer should rise promptly by at least 200 mm H_2O with bilateral jugular compression and should fall promptly on release of pressure. In some instances it may be advantageous to instill a small quantity of iophendylate (Pantopaque) into the subarachnoid space upon completion of the manometric study and perform a limited myelogram.

The severity of the injury frequently cannot be determined immediately. If paralysis is incomplete, the injury is not as severe as when functional loss is complete. In the latter situation, an early return of reflex activity, particularly of extensor movements, is encouraging. In general, sensory changes give a clearer indication of the level of the lesions than do motor changes. In cervical cord injuries, bilateral miosis is a bad prognostic sign, as it indicates extensive cord damage.[85] Incomplete lesions of the central cord type, as described by Schneider et al.,[86] enjoy a better outlook.

Treatment of the child with a spinal cord injury is essentially surgical but not always operative. Since there is a likelihood of aggravating spinal cord injury by excessive movement, special care is required in the handling of the patient and only the absolutely essential diagnostic studies should be carried out. In injuries of the cervical spine, the head should be maintained in neutral position. Skeletal traction, usually by means of tongs inserted into the skull, will be required for hyperflexion injuries of the cervical spine, while mild traction by means of a canvas sling is used in hyperextension injuries. Injuries of the lumbar spine and thoracolumbar junction are best stabilized in slight hyperextension.

All open wounds of the spine, all injuries in which bony fragments appear to be within the spinal canal by x ray and all patients with a total manometric or myelographic block should undergo surgery including debridement, removal of bone fragments, laminectomy, and dural repair if necessary. Any patient whose neurologic deficit increases following initial assessment, either by cephalad extension or by becoming more complete, should have the benefit of an exploratory laminectomy. Dislocations of the spine which cannot be reduced adequately by traction and immobilization, and injuries of the spine, known by past experience to be unstable, require surgical intervention, although this often need not be done immediately. Reduction of dislocations and internal stabilization are then carried out as indicated.

The chronic care of the paraplegic child is beyond the scope of this book. It is reviewed by Harris[80] and Walsh.[87]

The following require attention:

1. Care of the skin overlying the paralyzed part and prevention of decubitus lesions.

2. Care of the bladder. During the acute phase urinary retention is treated by intermittent catheterization or insertion of an indwelling catheter, preferably one with a separate irrigating arm (three-way Foley).

3. Fecal retention requires regular enemas. Automatic sphincter function may develop. Ileus, when present, can be relieved with neostigmine, or by an indwelling rectal tube.

Prognosis

The ultimate outlook for spinal cord function after injury depends on the completeness of the transection. The immediate loss of function is due to both anatomic alteration and impaired physiologic function of the cord. In general, most of the improvement occurs during the first six months after the injury, and little or none after one year.

HERNIATED INTERVERTEBRAL DISC

Although common in the adult, this is rare in children, with most cases occurring during adolescence, usually after trauma.

Injuries at L_4-L_5 and at L_5-S_1 occur with about equal frequency. Many of the children have an underlying malformation of the vertebral column, most often spondylolisthesis or spina bifida. Herniation of intervertebral discs has also been noted in achondroplasia. Since extradural neoplasms may present with a similar picture, myelography is indicated with all of suspected disc lesions.[88]

INJURIES OF THE PERIPHERAL NERVES

Peripheral nerve injuries are relatively uncommon in childhood. The most common postnatal injuries are of the brachial plexus and are due to severe trauma to the shoulder or sudden traction to the arm. Other injuries include division of the ulnar and median nerves at the wrist, the result of pushing the hand through a pane of glass, division of the radial nerve in the upper arm associated with fracture of the humerus, division of the ulnar nerve with fracture or dislocation of the medial epicondyle, injury of one or both branches of the sciatic nerve as a consequence of injections into the buttocks, and division of the common peroneal nerve in fractures at the neck of the fibula.

Pathology

The pathologic changes in an injured peripheral nerve depend on whether or not the axon remains intact. When the axon is destroyed at the site of injury, Wallerian degeneration is induced in the peripheral segment of the nerve. The pathologic, neurophysiologic, and biochemical alterations accompanying Wallerian degeneration are beyond the scope of this book.[89,90,91,92]

Stretch injuries of the peripheral nerves result from damage to the perineurium and to the blood vessels (vasa nervorum), while the ischemic peripheral nerve injuries are also produced by impairment of the blood supply to the nerves via these vessels. Regeneration of the injured nerve starts from the proximal end of the axon and begins after a short interval following injury, proceeding in children at about 2.5–3.0 mm per day. The speed and extent of recovery depends on whether the sheaths of the nerve remain intact. These provide a continuous channel for the young neurites sprouting from the proximal axonal end. When the gap between nerve ends is wide, and particularly when the ends are separated by fibrous tissue, a neuroma may form proximally, and spontaneous anastomosis may be delayed or impossible.

Clinical Manifestations

The salient clinical features of the most frequent peripheral nerve lesions of childhood are presented in Table 8–6.

Generally speaking, symptoms consist of weakness and sensory disturbances in the area supplied by the individual nerve. Muscular weakness and wasting are characteristic for peripheral nerve injuries. Contractures develop through overaction of unopposed muscle groups. Causalgia is rare in childhood. As first defined by Mitchell,[93] it consists of the presence of spontaneous burning pain over the denervated area. It is most common when the nerve division is incomplete.

When a nerve regenerates, manual pressure on the nerve at the level to which axons have regrown may induce a tingling pain referred distally to an area which is still anesthetic (Tinel's sign). Pain and paresthesia may be generalized or may be referred to one locality along the course of the nerve. These symptoms are aggravated by touch or by muscular contractions.

Deep tendon reflexes are diminished or abolished in the affected area. A number of vasomotor symptoms including mottling and thinning of the skin, edema, cyanosis, and impaired sweating, are also observed.

Diagnosis

Examination of the child with a peripheral nerve injury is directed toward the cause and the anatomic site of the injury. Several manuals detail the neurologic examination of such a patient.[94] Generally, evaluation of motor function and sensory deficits is more important in the diagnosis of peripheral nerve injuries than is the status of reflexes, as the latter are not dependent on the integrity of one single nerve.

Tinel's sign, which originally was believed to be evidence of regeneration, does not have much prognostic significance during the first month of injury, unless the most distal point at which it can be elicited moves down over the course of the nerve trunk on progressive examinations.

Electric studies may be used to delineate the extent of the nerve injury. Electromyography will indicate fibrillation potentials of denervated muscles. Nerve conduction times are either impossible to elicit or reduced. The ability of the nerve below the lesion to respond to direct electric stimulation despite motor paralysis indicates absence of Wallerian degeneration and is a favorable

TABLE 8-6.
CLINICAL FEATURES OF COMMON PERIPHERAL NERVE INJURIES

Nerve Injury	Predisposing Factors	Clinical Features
Brachial plexus upper root (Erb-Duchenne)	Sudden traction to arm	Arm internally rotated at shoulder, pronated at forearm Paralysis of spinati, deltoid, biceps, brachialis, brachioradialis, extensor carpi radialis Sensory disturbance minimal or absent Biceps and supinator jerks lost, triceps preserved
Lower root (Klumpke)	Violent upward pull of shoulder	Arm flexed at elbow, forearm supinated, fingers extended, edema and cyanosis of hand Paralysis of small muscles of hand, finger flexors Sensory loss of ulnar aspect of fingers, hand, and forearm Horner's syndrome if root evulsed
Long thoracic nerve	Carrying heavy weights on shoulder Postimmunization	Paralysis of serratus magnus, with or without trapezius No sensory symptoms
Circumflex nerve	Fracture of humerus "crutch palsy"	Paralysis of deltoid Sensory loss of upper and outer part of arm
Radial nerve	Fracture of humerus "Saturday night palsy"	Paralysis of triceps uncommon, only if nerve damaged in axilla Paralysis of brachioradialis, extensors of wrist and fingers Sensory loss inconstant
Median nerve	Cuts at wrist	Atrophy of thenar eminence Paralysis of pronation beyond mid-position Paralysis of flexor of index finger, impaired flexion, and opposition of thumb Sensory loss of radial aspect of palm
Ulnar nerve	Fractures at lower end of humerus Pressure palsy at elbow	Flattened hypothenar eminence, "claw hand" Paralysis of ulnar flexors at wrist and fingers, interossei, adductor of thumb Sensory loss of ulnar side of arm, hand
Sciatic nerve (common peroneal and posterior tibial nerves[97])	Intramuscular injuries (common peroneal component injured more frequently)	Foot drop, paralysis of peronei, anterior tibials, extensors of toe Sensory loss of anterior aspect of lower leg and foot Absent ankle jerk
Femoral nerve[98]	Hemorrhagic diseases (hemophilia)	Paralysis and atrophy of quadriceps Defective sensation anterior and anterior medial aspect of thigh
Common peroneal nerve	Fractures at neck of fibula Incorrectly fitted leg cast	Stepping gait Loss of dorsiflexion (anterior tibial) eversion at ankle (peronei), extensors of toe Sensory deficit dorsum of foot and outer side of leg Achilles tendon reflex lost or reduced

prognostic sign. In the course of regeneration, the conduction times, which initially were impossible to determine are slow at first, and subsequently regain as much as 40%– 60% of the original velocity.[95]

Treatment

Surgical treatment is not required during the early phase of peripheral nerve injuries, and nothing is gained by immediate exploration of the site of injury. If the nerve presents readily in the wound, a single stainless steel marking suture may facilitate subsequent repair. Secondary disability such as contractures or injury of the paralyzed muscles by excess stretching should be prevented by splinting the affected limb. Electrostimulation of the paralyzed muscles is of no advantage. A severed nerve should be explored and reapproximated three weeks after injury, provided the wound is healed. At this time the extent of nerve injury can be defined more clearly and suture is technically more satisfactory. A nerve which is known to have been traumatized but not severed should be explored if recovery of motor and sensory function does not take place or is less than anticipated. External and internal neurolysis of such a nerve trunk may be followed by further recovery of function. A neuroma in continuity may require resection and reanastomosis if nerve function is absent or poor. For causalgia, sympathectomy at the appropriate cervical or lumbar level is the procedure of choice.

Prognosis

The prognosis depends on the extent and nature of the nerve injury. Pressure palsies almost invariably recover. If electric studies indicate Wallerian degeneration of the distal segment, recovery will be delayed until the regenerating fibers have reached the muscles which they innervate. If no recovery can be documented after three months by either clinical or electric examinations, the ultimate prognosis is poor, and only few patients benefit from surgical exploration. Different nerves have different capacities for regeneration. As a rule, radial nerve injuries fare best, and sciatic, worst. Spontaneous recovery from sciatic nerve injuries may be extremely slow but may continue for as long as one to two years.

INJURIES BY PHYSICAL AGENTS

INJURIES OF THE NERVOUS SYSTEM BY X-RAY IRRADIATION

Radiation damage to the central nervous system may occur prior to birth and may result in a variety of gross and microscopic malformations of the brain. These are discussed in Chapter 4.

In older children therapeutic irradiation for intracranial tumors may damage the brain. Even standard doses induce temporary or permanent epilation, while excessive irradiation may necrose the scalp, the skull, and underlying brain. While these complications are preventable by the use of multiple ports of entry, occasionally neurologic symptoms are encountered after a latent interval ranging from several weeks to years.[99] The pathologic picture is one of diffuse collagenous thickening of the smaller blood vessels, with fibrinous necrosis and thrombosis. Cortical neurons disappear, and fibrillary gliosis extends from the cortical surface into the deeper layers of the gray matter.

The clinical picture is variable. Symptoms may appear suddenly, progress to a point and become arrested, or they may come on gradually and progress inexorably to death.[100] The amount of radiation required to produce brain necrosis ranges between 2000 and 2400 r administered as a single dose. Tolerance to radiation is greater when the exposure takes place over a prolonged period of time.

SUNSTROKE (Heatstroke)

This condition results from prolonged exposure to direct sunlight and heat, with subsequent failure of the heat regulating mechanism. It is to be distinguished from symptoms due to sodium loss as a consequence of excessive sweating, of which hyperpyrexia is not a feature.

The clinical and pathologic picture of sunstroke results from a combination of hyperpyrexia and shock. Sunlight contributes to the heat load but probably does not affect the brain directly. In fatal cases, examination of the brain reveals degeneration of cerebellar neurons, particularly the Purkinje cells, with lesser degrees of neuronal loss in other areas of the neuraxis.[101]

Clinically, there is sudden onset of coma, cyanosis, impaired sweating, generalized or focal seizures, and hyperpyrexia. Upon recovery, cerebellar symptoms may be evident. These usually improve considerably with time.

Treatment of the acute condition involves removing the child from the sun, reducing body temperature, and providing intravenous fluids.

ELECTRIC INJURIES OF THE NERVOUS SYSTEM

Electric injuries to children may be due to household current, or lightning. The latter is responsible for about one-quarter of all fatal electric accidents. Generally, the patient either dies at once or recovers without neurologic aftereffects. In a few patients one may observe a variety of neurologic symptoms, mostly transitory.[102] These include hemiparesis, paraplegia, and various other focal neurologic signs.[103]

NEUROLOGIC COMPLICATIONS OF BURNS

About 14% of children develop encephalitic symptoms soon after they sustain severe burns. These include changes in level of consciousness, seizures, aphasia, extrapyramidal disorders, and impaired intellectual function.[104] Pathologic examination reveals cerebral edema, and nerve cell loss in the dentate nucleus, the olivary nucleus, and damage to the Purkinje cells.[105]

Hypoxia, hypovolemia, hyponatremia, sepsis, and cerebrovascular accidents contribute to the evolution of the neurologic picture. In the majority of children, there is full neurologic recovery.[106]

REFERENCES

1. Mealey, J.: *Pediatric Head Injuries*, Springfield: Charles C Thomas Publisher, 1968.
1a. Craft, A. W., Shaw, D. A., and Cartlidge, N. E. F.: Head injuries in children, Brit. Med. J. 4:200, 1972.
2. Courville, C. B.: *Forensic Neuropathology*, Mundelein, Illinois: Callaghan and Co., 1964:
3. Gurdjian, E. S., et al.: Mechanism of head injury, Clin. Neurosurg. 12:112, 1964.
4. Gross, A. G.: A new theory on the dynamics of brain concussion and brain injury, J. Neurosurg. 15:548, 1958.
5. Courville, C. B.: Contrecoup injuries of the brain in infancy, Arch. Surg. (Chicago) 90:157, 1965.
6. Strich, S. J.: Shearing of nerve fibers as a cause of brain damage due to head injury: A pathological study of twenty cases, Lancet 11:443, 1961.
7. Symonds, C.: Concussion and its sequelae, Lancet 1:1, 1962.
8. Ward, A. A., Jr.: The physiology of concussion, Clin. Neurosurg. 12:95, 1964.
9. Meyer, J. S., et al.: Cerebral hemodynamics and metabolism following experimental head injury, J. Neurosurg. 32:304, 1970.
10. Lindenberg, R.: Significance of the tentorium in head injuries from blunt forces, Clin. Neurosurg. 12:129, 1964.
11. Langfitt, T. W., Tannanbaum, H. M., and Kassell, N. F.: The etiology of acute swelling following experimental head injury, J. Neurosurg. 24:47, 1966.
12. Davey, L. M.: Labyrinthine trauma in head injury, Conn. Med. 29:250, 1965.
13. Burkinshaw, J.: Head injuries in children: Observations on their incidence and causes with an enquiry into the value of routine skull X-rays, Arch. Dis. Child. 35:205, 1960.
14. Kellaway, P.: Head injury in children, Electroenceph. Clin. Neurophysiol. 7:497, 1955.
15. Hendrick, E. B., Harwood-Hash, D.C.F. and Hudson, A. R.: Head injuries in children: A survey of 4465 consecutive cases at the Hospital for Sick Children, Toronto, Canada, Clin. Neurosurg. 11:46, 1963.
16. Carlsson, C. A., von Essen, C., and Löfgren, J.: Factors affecting the clinical course of patients with severe head injuries, J. Neurosurg. 29:242, 1968.
17. Symonds, C. P. and Russell, W. R.: Accidental head injuries, Lancet 1:7, 1943.
18. Schechter, M. M.: Angiography in head trauma, Clin. Neurosurg. 12:193, 1964.
19. Plum, F. B. and Posner, J. B.: *The Diagnosis of Stupor and Coma*, Philadelphia: F. A. Davis Company, 1966.
20. McLaurin, R. L.: Metabolic changes accompanying head injury, Clin. Neurosurg. 12:143, 1964.
21. Stern, W. E.: Problems in fluid replacement and cerebral edema in the management of surgical lesions of the central nervous system, Amer. J. Surg. 100:303, 1960.
22. Matson, D. D.: Treatment of cerebral swelling, New Eng. J. Med. 272:626, 1965.
23. Stern, W. E.: The contribution of the laboratory to an understanding of the cerebral edemas: A review of recent progress, Neurology (Minneap.) 15:902, 1965.

24. Stern, W. E., Abbott, M. L., and Cheseboro, B. W.: A study of the role of osmotic gradients in experimental cerebral edemas, J. Neurosurg. 24:57, 1966.

25. Kurze, T. and Pitts, F. W.: Management of closed head injuries, Surg. Clin. N. Amer. 48:1271, 1968.

26. Matson, D. D.: "Head Injury—General Considerations," in: *Neurosurgery of Infancy and Childhood*, Springfield: Charles C Thomas Publisher, 1969, p. 271.

27. Hjern, B. and Nylander, I.: Late prognosis of severe head injuries in childhood, Arch. Dis. Child. 37:113, 1962.

28. Richardson, F.: Some effects of severe head injury: A follow-up study of children and adolescents after protracted coma, Develop. Med. Child Neurol. 5:471, 1963.

29. Scarcella, G. and Fields, W. S.: Recovery from coma and decerebrate rigidity of young patients following head injury, Acta Neurochir. (Wien) 10:134, 1962.

30. Berfenstam, R.: Accidents in childhood, Med. Press 239:451, 1958.

31. Taveras, J. M. and Wood, E. H.: *Diagnostic Neuroradiology*, Baltimore: Williams & Wilkins Co., 1964.

32. Taveras, J. M. and Ransohoff, J.: Leptomeningeal cysts of the brain following trauma with erosion of the skull, J. Neurosurg. 10:233, 1953.

33. Matson, D. D.: "Leptomeningeal Cysts," in: *Neurosurgery of Infancy and Childhood*, Springfield: Charles C Thomas Publisher, 1969, p. 304.

33a. Battle, W. H.: Hunterian Lectures, Royal College of Surgeons of England (1890).

34. Lewin, W.: Cerebrospinal fluid rhinorrhea in nonmissile head injuries, Clin. Neurosurg. 12:237, 1966.

35. Hughes, B. J.: "The Results of Injury to Special Parts of the Brain and Skull," in Rowbotham, G. F. (ed.): *Acute Injuries of the Head, Their Diagnosis, Treatment, Complications and Sequels*, Baltimore: Williams & Wilkins Co., 1964. p. 406.

36. Griffith, J. F. and Dodge, P. R.: Transient blindness following head injury in children, New Eng. J. Med. 278:648, 1968.

37. Dandy, W. E.: Pneumocephalus (intracranial pneumatocele or aerocele), Arch. Surg. (Chicago) 12:949, 1926.

38. Matson, D. D.: "Extradural Hematoma" in: *Neurosurgery of Infancy and Childhood*, Springfield: Charles C Thomas Publisher, 1969, p. 316.

39. McKissock, W., et al.: Extradural hematoma: Observations on 125 cases, Lancet 2:167, 1960.

40. Lemmen, L. J. and Schneider, R. C.: Extradural hematomas of the posterior fossa, J. Neurosurg. 9:245, 1952.

41. Cronqvist, S. and Kohler, R.: Angiography in epidural hematomas, Acta Radiol. [Diagn.] (Stockholm) 1:42, 1963.

42. Helfer, R. E. and Kemp, C. H.: *The Battered Child*, Chicago: The University of Chicago Press, 1968.

43. Silber, D. L. and Bell, W. E.: The neurologist and the physically abused child, Neurology (Minneap.) 21:991, 1971.

44. Banker, B. Q., Barrows, L. J., and Hunter, F. T.: The nature and clinical significance of pigments in the cerebrospinal fluid, Brain 78:59, 1955.

45. Rabe, E. F., Young, G. F., and Dodge, P. R.: The distribution and fate of subdurally instilled human serum albumin in infants with subdural collections of fluid, Neurology (Minneap.) 14:1020, 1964.

46. Shulman, K. and Ransohoff, J.: Subdural hematoma in children: The fate of children with retained membranes, J. Neurosurg. 18:175, 1961.

47. Herzberger, E., Rotem, Y., and Braham, J.: Remarks on thirty-three cases of subdural effusion in infancy, Arch. Dis. Child. 31:44, 1956.

48. McLaurin, R. L. and Tutor, F. T.: Acute subdural hematoma: Review of ninety cases, J. Neurosurg. 18:61, 1961.

49. Rahme, E. S. and Green, D.: Chronic subdural hematoma in adolescence and early adulthood, JAMA 176:424, 1961.

49a. Ingraham, F. D. and Matson, D. D.: Subdural hematoma in infancy, Advances Pediat. 4:231, 1949, and J. Pediat. 24:1, 1944.

50. Till, K.: Subdural haematoma and effusion in infancy, Brit. Med. J. 3:400, 1968.

51. Moyes, P. D.: Subdural effusions in infants, Canad. Med. Ass. J. 100:231, 1969.

52. Hollenhorst, R. W., et al.: Subdural hematoma, subdural hygroma and subarachnoid hemorrhage among infants and children, Neurology (Minneap.) 7:813, 1957.

53. Govan, C. D., Jr. and Walsh, F. B.: Symptomatology of subdural hematoma in infants and in adults, Arch. Ophthal. 37:701, 1947.

54. Russell, P. A.: Subdural haematoma in infancy, Brit. Med. J. 2:446, 1965.

55. Matson, D. D.: "Subdural Hematoma" in: *Neurosurgery of Infancy and Childhood*, Springfield: Charles C Thomas Publisher, 1969.

56. Dodge, P. R. and Porter, P.: Demonstration of intracranial pathology by transillumination, Arch. Neurol. 5:594, 1961.

57. Sherwood, D.: Chronic subdural hematoma in infants, Amer. J. Dis. Child. 39:980, 1930.

58. Ingraham, F. D. and Heyl, H. L.: Subdural hematoma in infancy and childhood, JAMA 112:198, 1939.

59. Ransohoff, J.: Chronic subdural hematoma treated by subdural-pleural shunt, Pediatrics 20:561, 1957.

60. Collins, W. T. and Pucci, G. L.: Peritoneal drainage of subdural hematomas in infants, J. Pediat. 58:482, 1961.

60a. Yashon, D., et al.: Traumatic subdural hematoma of infancy, Arch. Neurol. 18:370, 1968.

61. Rabe, E. F., Flynn, R. E., and Dodge, P. R.: Subdural collection of fluid in infants and children, Neurology (Minneap.) 18:559, 1968.

62. McLaurin, R. L. and McLaurin, K. S.: Calcified subdural hematomas in childhood, J. Neurosurg. 24:648, 1966.

63. Kendall, N. and Woloshin, H.: Cephalhematoma associated with fracture of the skull, J. Pediat. 41:125, 1952.

64. Walker, A. E.: "Post-traumatic Epilepsy," in: Rowbotham, G. F. (ed.): *Acute Injuries of the Head, Their Diagnosis, Treatment, Complications and Sequels*, Baltimore: Williams & Wilkins Co., 1964.

65. Jennett, W. B.: *Epilepsy after Blunt Head Injuries*, Springfield: Charles C Thomas Publisher, 1962.

66. Walker, A. E.: Posttraumatic epilepsy: An inquiry into the evolution and dissolution of convulsions following head injury, Clin. Neurosurg. 6:69, 1959.

67. Walton, J. W., Barwick, D. D., and Longley, B. P.: "The Electro-encephalogram in Brain Injury," in Rowbotham, G. F. (ed.): *Acute Injuries of the Head, Their Diagnosis, Treatment, Complications and Sequels*, Baltimore: Williams & Wilkins Co., 1964.

68. Dandy, W. E. and Follis, R. H., Jr.: On the pathology of carotid-cavernous aneurysms (pulsating exophthalmos), Amer. J. Ophthal. 24:365, 1941.

69. Frantzen, E., Jacobsen, H. H., and Therkelsen, J.: Cerebral artery occlusions in children due to trauma to the head and neck: A report of six cases verified by cerebral angiography, Neurology (Minneap.) 11:695, 1961.

70. Braudo, M.: Thrombosis of internal carotid artery in childhood after injuries in the region of soft palate, Brit. Med. J. 1:665, 1956.

71. Pitner, S. E.: Carotid thrombosis due to intraoral trauma: An unusual complication of a common childhood accident, New Eng. J. Med. 274:764, 1966.

72. Bruetman, M. E., et al.: Cerebral hemorrhage in carotid artery surgery, Arch. Neurol. 9:458, 1963.

72a. Black, P., et al.: "The Post-Traumatic Syndrome in Children," in: Walker, A. E., Caveness, W. F., and Critchley, M. (eds.): *The Late Effect of Head Injury*, Springfield: Charles C Thomas Publisher, 1969, p. 142.

73. Russell, W. R.: "The Traumatic Amnesias," in: Vinken, P. J. and Bruyn, G. W. (eds.): *Handbook of Clinical Neurology*, Vol. 3, Amsterdam: North-Holland Publishing Co., 1969.

74. Symonds, C.: Disorders of memory, Brain 89:625, 1966.

75. Harris, P.: Head injuries in childhood, Arch. Dis. Child. 32:488, 1957.

76. Dillon, H. and Leopold, R. L.: Children and the post-concussion syndrome, JAMA 175:86, 1961.

77. Hjern, B. and Nylander, I.: Acute head injuries in children: Traumatology, therapy and prognosis, Acta Paediat. Suppl. 152, 1964.

78. Schafer, E. R. and Weber, H. J.: "Verletzungen des Ruckenmarks," in Bushe, K. A. and Glees, P. (eds.): *Chirurgie des Gehirns und Ruckenmarks im Kindes und Jugendalter*, Stuttgart: Hippokrates Verlag, 1968.

79. Bischof, W. and Nittner, K.: Zur Klinik und Pathogenese der vaskular bedingten Myelomalazien, Neurochirurgie 8:215, 1965.

80. Harris, P.: Symposium on spinal injuries, J. Roy. Coll. Surg. Edinb. 9:77, 1963.

81. Sherrington, C. S.: Experiments in examination of the peripheral distribution of the fibers of the posterior roots of some spinal nerves: Part IV. Spinal reflex action, Trans. Roy. Soc. Lond. 190B:128, 1898.

82. Riddock, G.: The reflex functions of the completely divided spinal cord in man, compared with those associated with less severe lesions, Brain 40:264, 1917.

83. Kuhn, R. A.: Functional capacity of the isolated human spinal cord, Brain 73:1, 1950.

84. Sullivan, A. W.: Subluxation of atlanto-axial joint, J. Pediat. 35:451, 1949.

84a. Tishler, J. and Martel, W.: Dislocation of atlas in mongolism, Radiology 84:904, 1965.

85. Jefferson, G.: Concerning injuries of the spinal cord, Brit. Med. J. 2:1125, 1936.

86. Schneider, R. C., Cherry, G., and Pantek, H.: The syndrome of acute central cervical spinal cord injury with special reference to the mechanism involved in hyperextension injuries of the cervical spine, J. Neurosurg. 11:546, 1954.

87. Walsh, J. J.: *Understanding Paraplegia*, London: Tavistock Publications, 1964.

88. Epstein, J. A. and Lavine, L. S.: Herniated lumbar intervertebral disks in teenage children, J. Neurosurg. 21:1070, 1964.

89. Lee, J. C.: Electron microscopy of Wallerian degeneration, J. Comp. Neurol. 120:65, 1963.

90. Sunderland, S.: *Nerves and Nerve Injuries*, Edinburgh: E. and S. Livingstone, Ltd., 1968.

91. Bubis, J. J. and Wolman, M. L.: Hydrolytic enzymes in Wallerian degeneration, Israel J. Med. Sci. 1:410, 1965.

92. Berry, J. F., Cevallos, W. H., and Wade, R. R.: Lipid class and fatty acid composition of intact peripheral nerve and during Wallerian degeneration, J. Amer. Oil Chem. Soc. 42:492, 1965.

93. Mitchell, S. W.: *Injuries of Nerves and Their Consequences*, Philadelphia: J. B. Lippincott Co., 1872.

94. Nerve Injury Committee: "Peripheral Nerve Injuries," Her Majesty's Stationery Office, London, 1954.

95. Hodes, R., Larrabee, M. G., and German, W.: The human electromyogram in response to nerve stimulation and the conduction velocity of motor axons: Studies on normal and on injured peripheral nerves, Arch. Neurol. Psychiat. 60:340, 1948.

96. Bateman, J. E.: *Trauma to Nerves in Limbs*, Philadelphia: W. B. Saunders Co., 1962.

97. Gilles, F. H. and French, J.: Post-injection sciatic nerve palsies in infants and children, J. Pediat. 58:195, 1961.

98. DeBolt, W. L. and Jordan, J. C.: Femoral neuropathy from heparin hematoma: Report of two cases, Bull. Los Angeles Neurol. Soc. 31:45, 1966.

99. Pennybacker, J. and Russell, D. S.: Necrosis of the brain due to radiation therapy, J. Neurol. Neurosurg. Psychiat. 11:183, 1948.

100. Rider, W. D.: Radiation damage to the brain: A new syndrome, J. Canad. Ass. Radiol. 14:67, 1963.

101. Malamud, N., Haymaker, W., and Custer, R. P.: Heat stroke: A clinicopathologic study of 125 fatal cases, Milit. Surg. 99:397, 1946.

102. Critchley, M.: The effects of lightning with special reference to the nervous system, Bristol Med. Chir. J. 49:285, 1932.

103. Silversides, J.: The neurological sequelae of electrical injury, Canad. Med. Ass. J. 91:195, 1964.

104. Warlow, C. P. and Hinton, P.: Early neurologic disturbances following relatively minor burns in children, Lancet 2:978, 1969.

105. Harbauer, H.: Neuro- und psychopathologische Spatbefunde nach Verbrennungskrankheit beim Kind, Deutsch. Med. Wschr. 88: 1281, 1963.

106. Antoon, A. Y., Volpe, J. J., and Crawford, J. D.: Burn encephalopathy in children, Pediatrics 50:609, 1972.

Toxic Disorders and Neurologic Manifestations of Diseases Arising Outside the Nervous System

CHAPTER 9

TOXIC DISORDERS

Almost all poisons induce neurologic symptoms if ingested in sufficiently large amounts. In this section we will only consider toxins which have the central nervous system as a primary site of action. They will be discussed in ascending order of their chemical complexity. Poisons which are less commonly encountered by the practitioner will not be considered, and the reader is referred to the following references for a discussion of their neurologic complications and treatment:

Alcohol—(Dickerman et al.,[1] Cummins,[2] MacLaren et al.[3])
Aminophylline—(White and Daeschner[4])
Antihistamines—(Judge and Dumars[5])
Atropine—(Priest[6])
Boric acid—(Valdes-Dapena and Arey[7])
Carbon monoxide—(Garland and Pearce[8])
Dexamphetamine—(Espelin and Done[9])
Ferrous sulfate—(Whitten et al.,[10] James[11])
Imipramine—(Monnet et al.[12])
Organic phosphate esters—(Kopel et al.,[13] Hayes[13a])

Piperazine—(Parsons[14])
Tetracycline—(Wilson and Dally[15])

Metallic Toxins

LEAD POISONING

Although some of the toxic actions of lead have been known since antiquity, we owe our understanding of the clinical picture of lead poisoning to the classic studies of Tanquerel des Planches,[16] Blackfan,[17] and Holt.[18] Despite considerable advances in preventing exposure to lead, neurologic symptoms induced by acute or chronic ingestion of the metal are still far from rare and take two main forms: lead encephalopathy and polyneuritis. The first occurs in younger and the second occurs in older children.

Pharmacology

Most cases of lead poisoning are in pica-prone toddlers of low socioeconomic status living in homes built prior to the 1940s, a time when lead was commonly used for

339

interior paint. Lead is ingested by chewing wood coated with old paint, or eating crumbling plaster or flaked-off paint. Less than 10% of ingested lead is absorbed by the gastrointestinal tract. Constipation encourages absorption; diarrhea has the reverse effect. Following absorption, lead first becomes distributed in liver, kidney, and on the surface of erythrocytes.[19,20] Ultimately the metal is deposited in the epiphyseal portion of growing bone as an insoluble and nontoxic lead triphosphate.[19] A high phosphate and high vitamin D intake favors skeletal storage of lead, while parathormone, low phosphate intake and acidosis promote its release into the blood stream. Almost all the lead is excreted into urine; fecal lead represents the unabsorbed fraction. The rate of excretion is so slow that only a slight increase in the average daily intake above the maximum permissible level for adults of 0.3 mg/day can ultimately induce poisoning.

The levels of lead in blood and urine are an index of the degree of exposure to the toxin. In whole blood the "normal" range is said to be between 0.015 mg% and 0.040 mg%.[20a,22] Concentrations of 0.050 mg% or higher indicate potentially toxic exposure even in asymptomatic children,[20a,21] whereas levels of 0.2 mg% or higher are invariably accompanied by clinical symptoms. Normally, lead levels in the cerebrospinal fluid are below 0.01 mg%.

Almost all organs are affected by the poisoning, with damage as a result of heavy metal inhibition of numerous sulfhydryl enzymes. One of the cardinal manifestations of lead intoxication is anemia, induced by a disturbance in heme synthesis, and shortening of the red cell life span. Lead impairs heme synthesis at least at three points.[23] These include the condensation of glycine with succinyl CoA to form δ-aminolevulinic acid, a reaction catalyzed by δ-aminolevulinic acid synthetase; the condensation of δ-aminolevulinic acid to form porphobilinogen, and the formation of heme from iron and protoporphyrin IX. Globin synthesis is also disordered, and an excess of its β-chains exists in the free form.[23a] How these blocks induce an increase in coproporphyrin III output is still unclear, although porphyrinuria was already demonstrated in plumbism by Garrod in 1892.[24]

Pathology[25]

Within the central nervous system, the characteristic changes of lead poisoning take about one week or longer to develop. In subacute or chronic intoxications a striking and generalized cerebral edema is the most prominent pathologic feature. On microscopic examination neuronal degeneration and proliferation of the vascular endothelium with obliteration of the smaller caliber vessels is found throughout the cerebral parenchyma. The peripheral nerves undergo a segmental parenchymatous degeneration of the myelin sheath and axis cylinders. Occasionally the anterior horn cells are also degenerated.

Pathologic changes within other organs, notably the liver and kidney, have been described by Blackman.[26]

Clinical Manifestations[27]

The incidence of lead poisoning is at its highest between 12 and 35 months of age.[22] Pica is common, and its history can be elicited in at least one-half of cases.[28] In more than 90% of children the overt clinical picture is that of lead encephalopathy.[28] Symptoms develop insidiously, becoming first apparent in late summer in about 80% of instances.[29] This is perhaps a consequence of increased lead absorption in the presence of vitamin D and actinic rays at that time. Even before the child comes to his physician's attention there is usually a prodromal period of several weeks or months during which he is pale, irritable, listless and has lost his appetite. Epigastric pain, vomiting, and constipation are common. These nonspecific symptoms are often interrupted by the sudden onset of a series of generalized convulsions or depression of consciousness (Table 9–1).[30,31]

Seizures are common and resistant to anticonvulsant therapy. They may be followed by hemiplegia or other neurologic sequelae.

On physical examination the child with lead encephalopathy has all the signs of increased intracranial pressure. These include papilledema, a bulging fontanelle, and separation of the sutures, indicated by a tympanitic note or a cracked-pot sound on percussion of

TABLE 9-1.
SIGNS AND SYMPTOMS OF LEAD POISONING
IN CHILDREN (CHICAGO)*

Prodromal Symptoms No. of Cases		Overt Symptoms No. of Cases	
Irritability	20	Convulsions	11
Pallor	16	Lethargy	7
Vomiting	16	Sixth nerve	
Constipation	11	palsy	7
Weight loss	7	Ataxia	2

Two-Year Follow-up

13/46	Fatal
3/14	Retarded motor development
7/14	Retarded language development

* From Mellins and Jenkins[30] and Jenkins and Mellins.[31]

the skull (Macewen's sign). Less frequently patients develop cerebellar ataxia and palsies of the sixth and seventh cranial nerve. Nuchal rigidity is fairly common and may be related to tonsillar herniation. In some parts of the world there is a high incidence of optic neuritis with profound visual loss, acute communicating hydrocephalus, and tremors.[32]

In children, peripheral neuritis is a far less common form of lead poisoning. Turner has observed that in contrast to adults, children develop foot drop early, and that the legs are usually more involved than the arms.[27] A lead line is rarely seen in children. When it appears it takes the form of a bluish-black line at the margin of the gums or at the anus, the result of the deposition of lead sulfide.

Anemia usually accompanies the neurologic symptoms. Red cells in peripheral blood and bone marrow may show basophilic stippling, and the presence of a large percentage of such cells is almost invariable in chronic poisoning due to inorganic lead, although not in poisoning with organic (tetraethyl) lead. This finding, however, is not specific for lead intoxication.

Many patients have deranged renal tubular function. This may result in glycosuria and a generalized aminoaciduria, and less commonly in hypophosphatemia and x-ray evidence of renal rickets.[33]

In lead encephalopathy the cerebrospinal fluid is under increased pressure. Pleocytosis

is common, and the great majority of patients have a cell count of 10–60. The protein content is usually increased.

Radiologic findings are characteristic.[34] Most prominent is the presence of a dense, radiopaque band at the metaphyses of numerous long bones. Less commonly there are radiopaque particles within the gastrointestinal tract, evidence of recent plaster ingestion.

Diagnosis

Seizures and increased intracranial pressure should suggest the diagnosis of lead poisoning. Posterior fossa tumors rarely produce seizures, while tumors of the cerebral hemispheres are rare in infants of toddler age. Lead lines on radiographic examination, and basophilic stippling in a blood smear, offer a presumptive diagnosis even in the absence of a history of pica.

A number of screening procedures have been proposed to detect unsuspected cases of lead poisoning. Measurement of whole blood lead is the most reliable indicator of exposure to the metal, but the determination requires venous blood and lead-free equipment, and is too complex and expensive for use in routine screening. Serum levels and urinary excretion of δ-aminolevulinic acid are elevated in lead poisoning,[35] but this procedure is also inadequate for rapid screening. A very sensitive index of subclinical lead poisoning is the assay for δ-aminolevulinic acid dehydratase in erythrocytes. As a rule, there is an inverse correlation between enzyme activity and blood lead concentrations.[36] Current assays are, however, too sensitive for prospective screening of large populations.[37] Chisholm has proposed the microphotofluorometric assay for capillary blood protoporphyrins[38] as the most sensitive and yet practical indicator of lead toxicity. The determination can be done reproducibly on finger-stick samples, and is therefore applicable to screening of large populations.[39] The urinary output of coproporphyrins can be estimated semi-quantitatively, using a relatively easy method described by Benson and Chisholm.[39a] This test, however, is not specific. Aside from lead poisoning, a striking increase in coproporphyrin excretion is also seen in hepato-

Clinical Manifestations

Clinical symptoms of barbiturate intoxication are mainly those of CNS depression. In severe intoxication the child is comatose, the deep tendon reflexes may however persist, and the plantar reflex is often positive. Respiration is affected early, and breathing becomes slow and shallow. A fall in blood pressure is due to direct action of the drug on the myocardium, and depression of the medullary centers. A central antidiuretic action depresses urine formation. Hypoxia and pulmonary complications are common with severe barbiturate poisoning. Neuropathologic findings in fatal cases closely resemble those of fatal anoxia.

Treatment

If the drug is ingested shortly before the child is seen, gastric lavage is used. When respirations are depressed, an airway is instituted and artificial respiration is used whenever necessary to maintain normal blood CO_2 and pH levels. Care is also taken to prevent circulatory collapse, the chief cause of death in barbiturate intoxication, by the use of plasma expanders, or whole blood. Vasopressors are of relatively little value except in the initial management of severe hypotension.[54] Renal failure and hypothermia are other potentially serious complications of barbiturate intoxication.[55]

In severe intoxication, hemodialysis or peritoneal dialysis are the most effective means of removing the drug from the blood stream. Over the past years the use of analeptics such as picrotoxin has been abandoned as they were found to induce cardiac arrhythmias and convulsions.

PHENOTHIAZINES

The principal neurotoxic action of phenothiazines takes the form of extrapyramidal movements. These may appear at both toxic and therapeutic doses. Although all phenothiazines may produce these symptoms, in children they are seen most commonly with prochlorperazine (Compazine), haloperidol (Haldol), and chlorpromazine (Thorazine).[56,57]

Several types of movement disorders may be encountered. The most common are sudden episodes of opisthotonus accompanied by marked deviation of the eyes, and torticollis, but without loss of consciousness. Dystonic movements of the tongue, face and neck muscles, drooling, trismus, ataxia, tremor, episodic rigidity, and oculogyric crises are also seen. Seizures are rare and may be mimicked by violent dystonic movements. Drowsiness is common in patients ingesting toxic doses of phenothiazines but rare when symptoms are due to an idiosyncrasy for the drug. Persistence of the dyskinesias following withdrawal of the drug is relatively common in young adults but rare in children.[58]

Diagnosis of phenothiazine intoxication rests on the history of drug ingestion. The most common picture—namely, episodes of opisthotonus, trismus, and dystonic posturing—is distinctive. Paroxysmal choreo-athetosis may present a similar picture, but its onset is gradual and there is a prolonged history of recurrent attacks. The presence of a positive urine ferric chloride test (light pink to lilac color) is common in chronic intoxication but rare after acute drug ingestion.

Diphenylhydramine (Benadryl) 2 mg/kg, given intravenously, over the course of five minutes is an effective antidote and often produces a dramatic response.

Poisoning with psychedelic drugs is uncommon in small children. As a rule, this form of intoxication is not life-threatening. Observation of the intoxicated youngster is usually sufficient, although a variety of barbiturates or phenothiazines may be used for sedation.

HEXACHLOROPHENE TOXICITY

At present, the question whether hexachlorophene is toxic to the nervous system has not been completely resolved. This chlorinated phenolic compound, until recently a widely used antiseptic, has been found to induce seizures when ingested or absorbed through burned or extensively excoriated skin. However, small amounts are also absorbed through the intact skin.

Rats fed large amounts of hexachlorophene (25 mg/kg/day) showed a highly vacuolated white matter throughout the brain and spinal cord.[58a] On electron microscopy the vacuolation was seen to represent splitting of the interperiod lines of the myelin sheath, which appeared to be filled with fluid. Similar spongiform changes in the myelinated tracts of the brain stem have been seen in brains of premature infants who have repeatedly been exposed to 3% hexachlorophene. All infants showing these abnormalities weighed less than 1400 gm, had a gestational age from 26 to 32 weeks, and had rashes, abrasions, or wounds.[58b] In at least one other nursery, which has used 3% hexachlorophene extensively, these cystic changes in white matter have not been observed,[58c] and Gilles has presented evidence suggesting that the pathologic alterations in white matter represent fixation artefacts caused by the presence of hexachlorophene within the brain.[58d]

NEONATAL DRUG ADDICTION

The increasing prevalence of drug abuse among women of childbearing age has led to the relatively common problem of the neonate born to a mother addicted to heroin or other opiates.

The clinical picture in the neonate is the result of withdrawal from opiates. About two-thirds of infants born to heroin-addicted mothers develop symptoms.[59] These generally become apparent during the first 48 hours of life and, in order of frequency, consist of irritability, tremors, vomiting, high-pitched cry, sneezing, hypertonia, and abnormal sleep patterns.[60] Seizures are relatively uncommon.[59] The severity of the clinical course is related to the length of maternal addiction and to the magnitude of the drug dosages taken.

Untreated, the syndrome has a significant mortality. The administration of diazepam (Valium) is of considerable benefit. One to two mg are given intramuscularly, with the exact amount depending on the size of the infant and the severity of symptoms. The dosage is repeated every eight hours. When symptoms are fully controlled, the amount is tapered by decreasing the dosage and increasing the interval between injections.[61] Chlorpromazine, phenobarbital, and paregoric have also been recommended.

KERNICTERUS

The term "kernicterus," originally coined by Schmorl in 1903,[62] has been used both pathologically and clinically. Pathologically it indicates a canary-yellow staining of circumscribed areas of the basal ganglia, brain stem, and cerebellum, while clinically it comprises a syndrome consisting of athetosis, impaired vertical gaze, and auditory loss or imperception.

Pathology and Pathogenesis

On gross inspection, deposition of deep yellow pigment is noted in the meninges, the choroid plexus, and in numerous areas of the brain itself.[63] Although almost any portion may be involved at one time or other, the regions most commonly affected are the basal ganglia, particularly the globus pallidus, the dentate nucleus, the cerebellar vermis, the hippocampus, and the nuclei of the medulla. Except for gliosis, the cochlear nuclei and their pathways are usually unaffected despite the frequent finding of a central hearing loss. On microscopic examination the pigment is seen within neurons, their processes, and the surrounding glial cells. Neurons are in various stages of degeneration, the severity depending on the age of the patient; a marked neuronal loss with demyelination and astrocytic replacement is observed in patients who die after the first month.

Although the exact pathogenesis of kernicterus is far from clear, several factors are involved. The first is an elevated blood level of indirect bilirubin of approximately 20 mg per 100 ml or more. This can be due to Rh incompatibility, prematurity, or any other condition which might induce a marked rise in the infant's indirect serum bilirubin levels.[64] The etiology of neonatal hyperbilirubinemia has been reviewed by Brown.[65]

Other factors aside from an elevated serum bilirubin level are essential for the development of neurologic symptoms. Evidence for this has been accumulating: in the premature infant kernicterus can develop at a lower level than it does in the full-term infant; on the other hand, in the latter group the likelihood of kernicterus with bilirubin levels of 30 mg per 100 ml or higher is no greater than one in two. Furthermore, kernicterus is extremely rare in the adult, even with massive elevation of indirect serum bilirubin. Patients who have a congenital deficiency of glucuronyl transferase (Crigler-Najjar syndrome) and whose indirect bilirubin levels consistently range from 10 mg to 44 mg per 100 ml, have been known to be free of neurologic symptoms for many years before developing a rapidly progressive extrapyramidal disorder.[66]

These facts are consistent with the theory that antecedent or concomitant damage to the central nervous system is a prerequisite for the clinical and neuropathologic picture of kernicterus. A number of factors, present singly or in combination, may act as noxious agents. Some of these—Rh hemolytic disease and ABO incompatibility—may damage the vascular endothelium of the brain, while pre- and perinatal anoxia, sepsis, and acidosis may damage the nerve cells directly. Drugs such as vitamin K, and sulfisoxazole (Gantrisin) can contribute to the development of kernicterus by interfering with the binding of bilirubin to albumin, so that more bilirubin becomes ultrafilterable. Vitamin K, in addition, may also increase erythrocyte hemolysis. Since the sites of bilirubin deposition closely resemble the areas of neuronal damage in patients succumbing to anoxic damage, as in neonatal asphyxia, Lucey et al. have suggested that kernicteric staining locates areas of abnormal neuronal metabolism, and that bilirubin converts a transient cellular injury into a permanent one.[67]

Although bilirubin itself has toxic properties and interferes with neuronal oxygen consumption and oxidative phosphorylation, the applicability of these findings to the pathogenesis of kernicterus is questionable, as Vogel, among others, has shown that the injection of bilirubin in experimental animals will produce deposition of bile pigments in the brain but no neuronal damage.[68]

Clinical Manifestations

The jaundiced infant developing kernicterus becomes drowsy by the second to fifth day of life and begins to nurse poorly. He develops fever, his cry is monotonous, and the Moro reflex becomes unobtainable.[69] By two weeks of age there usually is marked

TABLE 9-2.
CLINICAL PICTURE OF PATIENTS WITH KERNICTERUS*

Number of children with severe neonatal jaundice due to Rh factor	248
Athetosis	93%
Gaze palsy	91%
Dental enamel dysplasia	83%
Auditory imperception	43%
Extrapyramidal rigidity	5%

* From Perlstein.[70]

hypertonia, with opisthotonus, extensor spasms, and in about 10% of infants clonic convulsions. Over the ensuing months the infant becomes hypotonic, and by four years of age the syndrome characteristic for kernicterus has evolved. The striking constancy of neurologic symptoms in the older child with kernicterus is evident from Table 9–2.[70]

The great majority of children are mentally retarded. Athetosis is almost invariably present, often with dystonia, rigidity, and tremors. Gaze palsy may involve movements in all directions, but vertical gaze is by far the most commonly involved. Auditory imperception may take the form of a hearing loss, a receptive aphasia, or a combination of the two. In a number of patients the vestibular portion of the eighth nerve is also involved.[71]

Diagnosis

The combination of extrapyramidal signs, ocular disturbances, and impaired hearing, while characteristic for kernicterus due to isoimmunization, may also be seen in children who were only mildly jaundiced but who have a history of prematurity and perinatal anoxia. The diagnosis of kernicterus during the neonatal period rests on changes in body tone, abnormalities in eye movements, loss of the Moro reflex, and an abnormal cry, all in the presence of hyperbilirubinemia.

Treatment and Prognosis

The treatment of kernicterus rests on the prevention of severe hyperbilirubinemia. The role of exchange transfusions, multiple intrauterine transfusions, phenobarbital, the use of artificial blue light in the current treatment of isoimmunization and hyperbilirubinemia is discussed by Crigler and Gold[72] and Schaffer and Avery.[73] There is little doubt that erythroblastotic infants who receive an exchange transfusion when their bilirubin exceeds 20 mg% have only a slight chance of developing kernicterus. In the premature infant, replacement transfusions should probably be done when bilirubin levels exceed 15 mg%.[64,74] There is less need to perform an exchange transfusion on a full-term infant with nonhemolytic hyperbilirubinemia and no evidence of neurologic symptoms.

Bacterial Toxins

The most potent nerve poisons known are produced by two anaerobic, spore-forming bacteria, *Clostridium botulinum* and *Clostridium tetani*.

BOTULISM

Botulism is food poisoning which follows the ingestion of preserves and other canned goods in which *Clostridium botulinum* has grown and produced toxin.

The toxins produced by *Clostridium botulinum* have the lowest lethal dose/kg of any of the known poisons; calculated from data obtained on mice, the lethal dose for an adult is approximately 0.12 mg per ingestion. Chemically, botulism toxin A, the most studied substance, is a simple protein, the toxicity of which is lost on heat denaturation. It acts on the terminal unmyelinated motor nerve fibrils so as to block transmission of the nerve impulse, producing a myastheniclike syndrome.[75] Since a lag period with a high temperature coefficient is observed in isolated nerve-muscle preparations exposed to botulism toxin, the toxin probably acts chemically to inhibit an enzyme essential to the propagation of the nerve impulse.

Symptoms appear between 12 and 48 hours after ingestion of contaminated food. A prodromal period of nonspecific gastrointestinal symptoms is followed by the evolution of the neurologic picture.[76] Initial symptoms include blurring of vision, impaired pupillary reaction to light, diplopia, and progressive weakness of the bulbar musculature. Paralysis of the major skeletal muscles follows, with death in respiratory arrest. In nonfatal cases, convalescence is slow, and complete recovery of a totally paralyzed muscle may take as long as one year. Botulism is distinguished from various viral encephalitides by the early appearance of internal and external ophthalmoplegia, ptosis, and paralysis of the pupillary accommodation reflex. In botulism the electrocardiogram will often indicate a toxic myocarditis, and the diagnosis can be confirmed by demonstrating the presence of toxin in serum prior to treatment.[77]

Treatment relies on a polyvalent serum prior to the development of symptoms. Guanidine (350 mg/kg) appears to be beneficial in botulism due to type A toxin,[78] but not for type B, which may be more rapidly and more tightly bound to tissues.[75] Symptomatic therapy consists of tracheotomy, artificial respiration, and nasogastric feeding. The mortality rate remains about 65%.

TETANUS

Tetanus is the result of an infection of wounded or damaged tissue by the spores of *Clostridium tetani*. Under anaerobic conditions the spores germinate and the vegetative forms multiply to produce two toxins, a hemolysin and a neurotoxin.

Crystalline tetanus toxin is a protein ranking second in potency only to botulism toxin. When treated with formalin, two molecules of protein polymerize to form toxoid, a nontoxic dimer with intact antigenicity which is used for immunizations.

The toxin acts on both the central and peripheral nervous systems. The major symptoms, paroxysmal muscle spasms, are due to fixation of the toxin by gray matter gangliosides[79] and consequent depression of inhibitory synapses along polysynaptic pathways.[80,81] Monosynaptic reflexes remain intact. Sustained muscular rigidity is due to the action of the toxin on the myoneural junction. In addition, elevation of serum creatine phosphokinase and fluorescent binding techniques provide evidence that the toxin produces direct injury to skeletal muscle.

Most commonly, symptoms appear about one week after injury. A number of authors

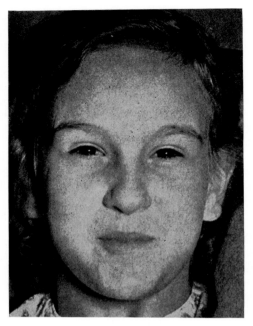

Fig. 9–1. Tetanus. Risus sardonicus. There is increased tone of all facial muscles. (From Ford, F. R.: *Diseases of the Nervous System in Infancy, Childhood and Adolescence*, 5th ed., 1966, Courtesy of Charles C Thomas Publisher, Springfield.)

have noted that the shorter the incubation period, the graver the infection. Trismus, or stiffness of the neck and back are generally the earliest symptoms. A characteristic retraction of the angles of the mouth has been termed risus sardonicus (Fig. 9–1). Rigidity becomes generalized and tetanic spasms develop. These may be induced by various sensory stimuli, passive movements of the limbs, or can occur spontaneously. Sudden respiratory failure, obstruction of the airway, and bronchopneumonia account for most deaths.

In some patients muscular rigidity is initially localized to the area of the wound and only slowly extends to other muscles.

Tetanus due to clostridial otitis media is distinctive in that trismus and risus sardonicus predominate over generalized spasms and rigidity.

Tetanus neonatorum, due to clostridial infection of the umbilical stump, is a major health hazard in some underdeveloped countries.[82,83] Trismus, with consequent in-

ability to nurse, and striking nuchal rigidity are the initial symptoms in some 70% of infants. Generalized tetanic spasms occur less often and indicate a more severe form of the disease.

Stiff-man syndrome, a condition characterized by progressive muscular stiffness and intermittent spasms, may represent a mild form of tetanus.[84]

Despite the widespread use of tetanus toxoid, antitoxin, and antibiotics, mortality in children developing typical symptoms has not improved greatly, and is still about 40%–50%. The mortality in neonatal tetanus is even higher and approaches 100%. Initial treatment includes the use of massive doses of antitoxin, even though once toxin is fixed in the central nervous system antitoxin is relatively ineffective in neutralizing its action. Supportive therapy includes sedation, the use of muscle relaxants, debridement of the site of infection, and maintenance of respiratory exchange. Problems of treatment are discussed by Pinheiro.[82]

Prophylaxis is by use of tetanus toxoid, and administration of antitoxin following any puncture wound.[85,86] Recovery from tetanus is slow. About one-quarter of patients have major sleep disturbances for about one to three years. In about one-half, seizures, often accompanied by myoclonus, may occur one to two months after apparent recovery, and persist for six months to one year, with an average frequency of one major attack every two months.[87]

Animal Venoms

Neurologic symptoms induced through the bite or sting of venomous animals are usually due to impaired neuromuscular transmission and take the form of muscular weakness or painful muscle spasm. They are reviewed in Table 9–3, where pertinent literature references discussing treatment are also cited.

METABOLIC ENCEPHALOPATHIES

Extracerebral diseases may interfere with normal brain function either by impairing the necessary supply of oxygen and glucose, or by disturbing the ionic environment of neurons, glia, and cell processes.

TABLE 9-3.
NEUROLOGIC SYMPTOMS OF ANIMAL VENOMS

Animal	Symptoms	Action of Venom	Reference
Coelenterata jellyfish	Muscular weakness, respiratory paralysis	Unknown	Flecker[88]
Mollusca bivalve (infected by flagellate plankton, paralytic shellfish poisoning)	Ataxia, ascending paralysis, paresthesia	Unknown	Meyer[89]
Reptiles Crotalidae (rattlesnakes, water moccasins, copperheads)	Progressive paralysis	Direct action on central nervous system, inhibits neuromuscular transmission at motor end plate, damage to muscle	Chapman[90]
Elapidae (coral snakes, cobras)	Progressive paralysis		
Arthropods spiders, *Latrodectus* (black widow)	Local pain, abdominal rigidity, muscle spasms, convulsions	Nerve endings	Greer[91]
Centruroides (scorpion)	Muscle spasms, convulsions	Action on motor end plate	Stahnke[92]
Wood tick	Ascending paralysis, or ataxia	Defect in acetylcholine liberation	Lagos and Thies,[93] McCue et al.[94]
Chordata Chondrichthyes (stingray)	Pain, reflex spasms, paresthesia, rarely paralysis	Unknown	Russell[95]
Osteichthyes (stonefish)	Local pain, paralysis, convulsions, slow recovery		
Puffers (ingestion of ovaries, liver)	Ataxia, paresthesias, muscular twitching, paralysis	Neuromuscular block, inhibition of acetylcholine release, paralysis of bulbar centers	Halstead,[96] Scholz[97]

TABLE 9-6.
CONDITIONS PRODUCING HYPOCALCEMIA AND HYPOMAGNESEMIA
AND NEUROLOGIC SYMPTOMS

Conditions	Symptoms	Reference
Premature infants, infants of diabetic mothers infants born after abnormal pregnancies	Onset in first 48 hours of life, generalized neuromuscular hyperexcitability, convulsions, spontaneous attacks of apnea and cyanosis, hollow or squeaky cry, hyperactivity alternating with immobility	Craig and Buchanan[120]
Transient neonatal hypoparathyroidism, decreased urinary excretion of phosphate (neonatal tetany)	Seen mainly in bottle-fed infants; appears 7–14 days of age, convulsions and generalized neuromuscular hyperexcitability	Gardner[127]
Maternal hyperparathyroidism	Major motor convulsions, refractory to anticonvulsants; appears in second week of life	Hartenstein and Gardner[128]
Vitamin D deficiency	Convulsions, laryngospasm, carpopedal spasm, muscular hypotonia, appears 3–12 months of age	Eliot and Park[129]
Hypoparathyroidism	Cataracts, photophobia, increased density of bones, ridging of teeth and nails, tetany and convulsions, increased intracranial pressure, mental deterioration, extrapyramidal disorder, calcification of basal ganglia	Simpson[130]
Pseudohypoparathyroidism	Obesity, dysmorphic appearance, round facies, stubby short hands and fingers, tetany and convulsions (88%), mental retardation (60%), syndrome unaltered by parathormone	Cohen and Donnell[131]
Renal disease	Tetany, muscle cramps, fasciculations associated with moderate to severe acidosis, elevated serum potassium/calcium ratio, often unresponsive to calcium or magnesium administration	Tyler[132]
Hypomagnesemic tetany of infancy	Recurrent convulsions, appears first month of life, impaired magnesium absorption across G.I. tract	Paunier et al.[133]

Two forms of neonatal hypocalcemia are seen most frequently. One occurs during the first two days of life in premature or low birth weight infants, or offspring of a pregnancy complicated by maternal diabetes or toxemia. The exact mechanism of this form of hypocalcemia is obscure.

The second form of neonatal hypocalcemia is the classic "neonatal tetany," the mechanism of which was first elucidated by Bakwin in 1937.[122] It occurs between the fifth and tenth day of life and results in part from intake of cow's milk which induces an increased phosphate load, and probably also from a transient hypoparathyroidism. In this form of hypocalcemia, hyperphosphatemia is usually present.

Less often maternal hyperparathyroidism, congenital absence of the parathyroid glands, or disturbed renal function may induce neonatal hypocalcemia (Table 9–6). Neonatal hypomagnesemia has been recorded in the association with hypocalcemia due to maternal hyperparathyroidism.[123] It may also be the result of a selective malabsorption of magnesium[133] (Table 9–6).

In some nurseries, neonatal tetany is one of the major causes for infantile convulsions.[124] There is nothing in the nature of the attack to distinguish neonatal convulsions due to hypocalcemia from those due to other causes. The classic signs of tetany seen in the older child are usually absent. Carpopedal spasm was rare, and stridor due to laryngospasm and Chvostek's sign were not noted in any of the hypocalcemic infants reported by Keen.[125]

The treatment of seizures due to neonatal tetany is covered in the section on neonatal seizures in Chapter 11. The long-term outlook of children who have suffered from seizures due to neonatal hypocalcemia is better than that of infants with hypoglycemic seizures. In Keen's series, 80% developed normally. Nothing in the neonatal period distinguished the remainder who were retarded or had seizures.[125]

In older infants and in children, neurologic symptoms of hypocalcemia include tetany and seizures. Tetany is characterized by episodes of muscular spasms and paresthesias mainly involving the distal portion of the peripheral nerves. Episodes appear abruptly and are precipitated by hyperventilation or ischemia. There is no alteration of consciousness. Carpopedal spasm and laryngospasm are the two most frequent examples of tonic muscular spasms. Chvostek's sign, a brief contraction of the facial muscles elicited by tapping the face over the seventh nerve, is not diagnostic of tetany, being seen also in normal infants. Seizures may occur in the absence of tetany and are occasionally focal. Headaches and extrapyramidal signs are less common and confined to older patients with hypoparathyroidism.[126] In this condition, x rays may show symmetric bilateral punctate calcifications of the basal ganglia, although only in 50% is there an association between this finding and the occurrence of extrapyramidal signs.[126]

Pseudohypoparathyroidism is characterized by obesity, moon-shaped facies, mental retardation, cataracts, short, stumpy digits, and enamel defects. Calcifications of the basal ganglia are seen in about one-third of instances. The condition tends to be familial and is due to an inability of renal tubules to respond to parathormone.[131]

HYPERCALCEMIA

Aside from hyperparathyroidism, which is rare, hypercalcemia of childhood takes two forms, mild and severe idiopathic hypercalcemia. Patients with mild idiopathic hypercalcemia usually show a sudden failure to thrive between three and seven months of age. The condition is reversible with restriction of calcium and vitamin D intake. In the severe form, patients have an unusual, "elfin-like" facies. There is marked physical and mental retardation. An aortic systolic murmur is heard, most commonly due to supravalvular aortic stenosis. The condition has a prenatal onset, and patients may succumb to azotemia, or may spontaneously become normocalcemic, while the cardiac murmur, characteristic facies, and mental retardation persist.[134] On pathologic examination, the brain is microcephalic, with paucity of gray matter neurons and foci of ectopic gray matter. These abnormalities point to a neurologic disturbance occurring during the late months of pregnancy or early infancy.[135]

While the mild form is probably due to ex-   hemorrhage.   Focal neurologic signs are the

defect in oxygen utilization. In part, this may be due to nonspecific increases in brain permeability and disordered membrane function, which could allow the accumulation of toxic products and alter function of the sodium-potassium ion pump. Disorders in blood and CSF electrolytes may aggravate the clinical picture, as may bouts of acute hypertensive encephalopathy.

Clinical Manifestations

The principal neurologic symptoms of uremia are abnormalities in mental status, asterixis, convulsions, and muscular cramps.[132] Peripheral neuritis occurs fairly commonly in patients in prolonged uremia. It may begin with sensory symptoms in the lower extremities and can progress slowly to total flaccid quadriparesis. Less commonly, patients develop cranial nerve palsies and choreoathetosis. Signs of hypocalcemia are often present. In hypertensive encephalopathy, such as is seen with acute glomerulonephritis, patients develop symptoms and signs of increased intracranial pressure, with headache, vomiting, disturbance of vision, and papilledema. Seizures, transient focal cerebral syndromes, including hemiparesis, and cortical blindness, are also common.

Treatment and Prognosis

Treatment of uremia involves correction of electrolyte disturbance and maintenance of normal plasma composition. This has been greatly assisted by the use of dialysis. In some instances, neurologic symptoms can become aggravated following peritoneal dialysis or hemodialysis. It has been suggested that urea in the brain does not equilibrate freely with urea in blood, so that water enters the brain along an osmotic gradient. Gradual changes in blood electrolytes and earlier dialysis will prevent some neurologic complications. Generally, motor symptoms tend to improve once the blood urea levels are lowered, while sensory symptoms tend to remain fixed. The sensory neuropathy will, however, respond to renal transplant.

Complications of Treatment of Chronic Uremia

As a consequence of the various methods of therapy currently available for what up to recently was considered to be irreversible renal disease, various neurologic complications have been encountered.

As a rule, neurologic complications are seen more frequently following hemodialysis than peritoneal dialysis.[144] Restlessness, headache, nausea, and vomiting are relatively common following more extreme adjustments of urea levels or acidosis. Seizures followed by impaired consciousness were seen in some 8% of patients subjected to dialysis prior to 1965 but are now less common.[144] These symptoms have been attributed to the osmotic gradient established when, as a consequence of the blood-brain barrier, urea is removed more rapidly from the blood than from the brain.

Cerebral hemorrhages are a less common complication of hemodialysis.

With repeated dialyses a variety of syndromes are encountered which have been attributed to a deficiency of vitamins or other nutritional factors. These include a peripheral sensory-motor neuropathy ("burning feet syndrome"), which at times has responded to vitamin supplementation;[144] central pontine myelinolysis;[141] and Wernicke's encephalopathy.[145]

The neurologic complications attending renal homotransplants are mainly due to immune suppressant therapy.

They include fungal infections, notably due to *Aspergillus* or *Candida*,[146] and cytomegalovirus and herpes simplex infections.[147] The clinical picture of these secondary infections is highlighted by disturbances of behavior and seizures. Fungal infections, in particular, are seen in as many as 45% of boys who have been on prolonged immunosuppressive therapy, and their appearance is unrelated to preexisting treatment with antibiotics. In most patients an antemortem diagnosis is impossible, although it is likely that CSF abnormalities should suggest this complication.[146]

About 6% of renal homograft recipients, followed up to eight years, have developed neoplasms. Three-quarters of these have involved the central nervous system, and include reticulum cell sarcomas and lymphomas.[148,149] The relationship between immunosuppressive therapy and carcinogenesis is currently the subject of intense investigation.

NEUROLOGIC COMPLICATIONS OF CARDIAC DISEASE

In addition to the neurologic effects of hypoxia, cerebral complications may be encountered in a significant proportion of children with congenital or acquired heart disease.

CONGENITAL HEART DISEASE

Left-to-Right Shunts

In the absence of congestive heart failure, neurologic complications are relatively uncommon in these conditions. Perhaps the most likely entity to be encountered is cerebral embolization as a consequence of bacterial endocarditis. Currently, most cases of bacterial endocarditis are due to congenital heart disease, but with the widespread prophylactic use of antibiotics for dental surgery, and for the treatment of bacterial infections, and with progressively earlier surgical correction of most cardiac malformations, this entity is only rarely seen.

Relatively current experience indicates that about one-half of children with bacterial endocarditis develop emboli in the course of their illness.[150] Most frequently these emboli are to the lungs or the brain. Evidence for cerebral embolization may be a sudden disturbance of consciousness, hemiparesis, or aphasia. Most patients show hematuria, the result of embolization to the kidneys. Rarely, cerebral embolization may be the first sign of bacterial endocarditis.

The diagnosis of the condition rests upon the demonstration of sepsis by means of repeated blood cultures. Treatment consists of adequate antibacterial therapy against the invading organism, most commonly alpha- or gamma-streptococcus, or staphylococcus.

Coarctation of Aorta

The association of coarctation of the aorta with intracranial arterial aneurysms has been well-documented. While this complication is seen only in a small percentage of children with coarctation, it accounts for about one-quarter of aneurysms in childhood.[151] Like arterial aneurysms in general, these are located around the circle of Willis and its major branches, particularly the anterior communicating artery.

The subject of arterial aneurysms is discussed in Chapter 4.

A rare complication of surgery for repair of the coarctation is spinal cord damage. This may result in residuals ranging from mild weakness to complete paraplegia, with transsection usually at the midthoracic level. As a rule, children in whom the period of aortic occlusion was the longest are more liable to this complication, but other factors including the degree of compromise to the circulation of the spinal cord and variations in the anatomy of the blood supply to the spinal cord, play an important role.[152,153]

Cyanotic Congenital Heart Disease

The three principal neurologic complications of cyanotic congenital heart disease are cyanotic attacks, brain abscesses, and cerebrovascular accidents.

Episodic cyanosis and dyspnea followed by loss of consciousness is seen in 10%–20% of cyanotic children, particularly in those with severe anoxia. Attacks occur most frequently between six months and three years, and are precipitated by feeding, bowel movements, or undue exertion. In about half of the children, severe cyanotic attacks are followed by a generalized convulsion.[154] The electroencephalogram during such an attack shows high voltage slow wave activity but no spike discharges.[155]

Brain abscesses are seen in older children, usually after two years of age. With increased longevity the incidence of this complication has risen considerably. The diagnosis and treatment of brain abscesses in children with cyanotic heart disease is discussed more extensively in Chapter 6.

Cerebrovascular accidents are seen most often in those forms of cyanotic congenital heart disease in which hypoxia is most extreme. Their incidence is highest (11%) in patients with transposition of the great vessels.[154] About three-quarters of the attacks occur during the first 20 months of life.[156] The majority of cerebral infarcts in children with cyanotic heart disease are due to vascular occlusions, most often in the distribution of the middle cerebral artery. Venous thrombi are perhaps somewhat more common than arterial occlusions.[157] Hypoxia, dehydration, fever, cardiac surgery, iron deficiency anemia and, in older children, polycythemia—all seem to play a role in the evolution of cerebrovascular accidents.[156,156a]

The clinical picture of a cerebrovascular accident is one of a sudden onset of hemiplegia or aphasia. Seizures may accompany the acute episode, or in some 10% of children may follow the attack after a latent period of some six months to five years. In the experience of Tyler and Clark, these have been most difficult to control. About 20% of children suffering a cerebrovascular accident are left with mental retardation.[156]

The differential diagnosis of hemiplegia and seizures in a child with cyanotic congenital heart disease is covered in the section on brain abscess (Chapter 6). We should point out that in cyanotic children, funduscopy is of little help in ascertaining the presence of increased intracranial pressure. Retinal changes consisting of markedly dilated and tortuous veins and blurring of the disc margins can be observed in the majority of these children. This retinopathy is related to decreased oxygen tension and secondary polycythemia, rather than to retention of carbon dioxide or increased venous pressure.[158]

A neurologic syndrome associated with cyanotic congenital heart disease is that of congenital facial paralysis, abnormalities of the external ear, with tetralogy of Fallot or a ventricular septal defect.[159]

ACQUIRED HEART DISEASE

The principal neurologic complications of acute rheumatic fever and rheumatic heart disease are Sydenham's chorea (see Chapter 7), and cerebral embolization secondary to bacterial endocarditis or cardiac irregularities.

Neurologic complications due to hypertension, whether due to renal disease or essential hypertension, are covered more fully in a text on adult neurology. The interested reader is referred to the paper of Still and Cottom[160] covering hypertensive encephalopathy in a pediatric population. The association of hypertension with a lower motor neuron facial nerve palsy has been noted by several clinicians.[161] The association of hypertension with pheochromocytoma and neurofibromatosis is also well-recognized (Chapter 10).

Congestive heart failure has been observed in neonates secondary to cerebral arteriovenous malformations.[162] Although this condition is readily delineated by cerebral angiography, the clinical recognition is often difficult. Audible bruits over the cranium can be heard in many of these patients but also in about 15% of normal infants under one year of age.[163] Cutaneous abnormalities around the head and neck, and dilated scalp veins, are perhaps more reliable indications of the diagnosis[162] (see also Chapter 4).

NEUROLOGIC COMPLICATIONS OF CARDIAC SURGERY

The past few years have witnessed an increased aggressiveness in the surgical approach to the management of the child with heart disease. With this, the incidence of neurologic complications attending cardiac surgery has risen considerably.

Currently, cerebral disturbances are seen in more than one-half of patients undergoing open-heart surgery. These are mainly due to two processes: impaired cerebral blood flow and embolization.[164] Several factors are responsible for impaired cerebral blood flow. Hypotensive episodes may occur in relation to the operative procedure. In addition, there is considerable evidence that the use of cardiopulmonary bypass may result in a significant depression of cerebral blood flow and metabolism, which is not immediately reversible postoperatively.[165] The presence of large numbers of microparticles in blood after passage through a pump oxygenator may be responsible for this phenomenon. If so, it can probably be avoided by adequate filtration of the blood. In the experience of most centers, impaired cerebral blood flow results in alterations of consciousness, behavioral changes, and defects of intellectual function, particularly of recent memory, and those modalities pertaining to perception and synthesis of visual patterns.[164] As a rule, these symptoms improve in the course of several days to three weeks and ultimately clear completely. When anoxic brain damage has been extensive, patients do not recover consciousness postoperatively. They often experience focal or generalized seizures. On examination they are in extensor rigidity with papilledema and fixed, dilated pupils. Focal signs may be evident, even though on autopsy there are widespread anoxic changes throughout both hemispheres.

Macroembolization of the CNS is much less common and now is mainly due to fat particles. Fat emboli have been found in about three-quarters of open-heart cases coming to autopsy, and in 37% of bypass cases.[166] Less often, embolization results from detachment of mural thrombi, or calcified material from diseased heart valves.[164,167] Symptoms of cerebral emboli include hemiplegia, visual field defects, and seizures.[164] These deficits are less likely to clear up spontaneously, and permanent residua are not unusual.

Injuries to the brachial plexus may result from traction in the course of surgery. A postoperative polyneuropathy has been encountered. This complication may be related to the duration of hypothermia used in the course of surgery.

NEUROLOGIC COMPLICATIONS OF HEMATOLOGIC DISEASES

ANEMIA

Neurologic symptoms accompanying anemia are due to cerebral hypoxia. They include irritability, listlessness, and impaired intellectual function. Specific neurologic complications seen with some of the anemias are considered below:

Congenital Aplastic Anemia (Fanconi's Anemia)

This syndrome is characterized by the association of pancytopenia and bone marrow hypoplasia with a variety of congenital anomalies. These include skeletal defects, seen in some 68% of children, growth retardation, microcephaly, microphthalmus, ptosis, strabismus, deafness, and malformations of ears, kidneys, and heart.[168] A patchy, brown pigmentation has been observed in about 75% of cases. The condition is said to be transmitted as an autosomal recessive trait with a variable penetrance.[169]

Hereditary Hemoglobinopathies

Sickle cell disease is characterized by the presence of sickle hemoglobin (hemoglobin S) in erythrocytes. It is almost exclusively found in Negroes.

In about one-third of patients, neurologic symptoms become apparent prior to five years of age. These are the consequence of excessive blood destruction and the tendency for intravascular sickling and thromboses. The pathologic findings include perivascular hemorrhages, focal dilatation of arterioles, and multiple microinfarcts of white matter.

Neurologic symptoms are seen in about one-third of patients and may be the presenting signs.[170] Their onset is generally sudden and accompanies sickle cell crises. A variety of factors are known to induce sickling, particularly fever, infections, dehydration, and surgical procedures. Neurologic symptoms include generalized or psychomotor seizures, headaches, meningeal signs, and changes in consciousness. The most obvious neurologic findings are hemiparesis, paresthesias of the extremities, ataxia, homonymous hemianopsia, and a variety of reflex abnormalities. Multiple lesions are common. The cerebrospinal fluid may be grossly bloody. Occlusion of the larger arteries or veins can be demonstrated by cerebral angiography.[171] The electroencephalogram may reveal slow wave foci. The neurologic symptoms may be irreversible. The prognosis for patients with major neurologic lesions is poor and recurrent cerebral infarctions with progressively more extensive deficits can be expected.

Neurologic symptoms can be suspected as being caused by sickle cell disease when the sickling phenomenon is demonstrable in vitro. This test should be performed routinely on all black children with conditions simulating meningitis, encephalitis, or cerebrovascular disease. The neurologic symptoms are usually part of vaso-occlusive crises, and diagnostic angiography is contraindicated in the early stages, since the contrast medium may aggravate any vascular occlusions.

Treatment includes prompt hydration, correction of acidosis—which, when present, may aggravate sickling—administration of oxygen, and multiple transfusions of packed erythrocytes, which are intended to dilute the number of sickle cells in the circulation.[172] Anticoagulants and urea have also been recommended, but their effectiveness is still unproven.

The association of sickle cell disease and pneumococcal meningitis is well-known.[172a] The high incidence of this infection may be related to a decreased phagocytic ability of the reticuloendothelial system.

Similar neurologic symptoms have been encountered in about 25% of patients with sickle cell-hemoglobin C disease.

The incidence of neurologic symptoms in children with sickle cell trait is low (6.4%).[171] Seizures have been observed after otherwise uncomplicated surgical procedures. Transient subarachnoid hemorrhages and visual impairment due to vitreous and retinal hemorrhages have also been reported.[171]

Several forms of congenital hemolytic anemia have been associated with neurologic deficits, most commonly developmental retardation. Deficiency of erythrocyte phosphoglycerate kinase is a sex-linked recessive disorder, causing hemolytic anemia of variable severity and accompanied by slowly progressive extrapyramidal disease characterized by a resting tremor, dystonic posturing of the extremities, and hyperlordosis.[172b]

In thalassemia neurologic symptoms are rare, but some 20% of patients, homozygous for β-thalassemia have myalgia, a myopathy with weakness of the proximal muscles in the lower extremities, hyporeflexia, and a myopathic EMG pattern.[172c]

LEUKEMIA

With the advent of more effective anti-leukemic chemotherapy, the incidence of neurologic complications in children with acute leukemia has increased, and their diagnosis and treatment has become a major medical problem.[173] In the experience of the Children's Cancer Research Foundation, the incidence of central nervous system involvement rose from 10% in the years 1947 to 1953 to 40% in 1960.[173]

Neurologic complications are due to leukemic infiltrations of the meninges, brain, and cranial or peripheral nerves, and as the result of intracranial hemorrhage and infections. Meningeal leukemia is seen in all forms of acute leukemia. The complication may occur at any stage of the disease; one-third to one-half of children being in complete hematologic remission.[174,175] The reason for this phenomenon is not clear, although generally it has been stated that it reflects a failure of antimetabolites to cross the "blood-brain barrier," allowing leukemic cells in the brain and the cerebrospinal fluid to survive and proliferate.

The presenting symptoms and signs of meningeal leukemia are depicted in Table 9–7. They include increased intracranial pressure with vomiting, headache, and papilledema. Nuchal rigidity, while not noted by Hardisty and Norman,[175] has been present in our experience. Cranial nerve palsies are relatively common. They are a result of the leukemic infiltration of the basilar meninges. The most common nerves to be affected are the facial, abducens, and auditory nerves. Increased appetite and sudden weight gain, an indication of hypothalamic infiltration, has also been noted.[175]

X rays of the skull often show splitting of the sutures. The cerebrospinal fluid is diagnostic. In almost every instance there is an increased cell count, with the cells often being recognized on stained smears as blast cells. The sugar content is reduced in about

TABLE 9-7.
PRESENTING SYMPTOMS AND SIGNS IN 50 EPISODES OF MENINGEAL LEUKEMIA OCCURRING IN 29 PATIENTS*

Neurologic Symptom or Sign	Percentage of Episodes
Vomiting	80
Headache	70
Papilledema	70
Increased appetite and weight gain	26
Cranial nerve palsies	16
Seizures	8
Visual disturbance	4
Ataxia	4

* From Hardisty and Norman.[175]

60% of cases, and the protein content is increased in about 50% of children.[174]

Currently, the treatment of choice for meningeal leukemia is the intrathecal administration of methotrexate. In our institution we administer approximately 12 mg/m² diluted to a concentration of 1 mg/ml with sterile water, containing no preservatives. The medication is injected rapidly into the lumbar subarachnoid space, the rapid injection allowing good dispersal of the medication.[175,176] Concurrent intramuscular injection of folinic acid (Leukovorin) (12 mg/m²) is intended to prevent symptoms of vitamin deficiency, which may take the form of confusion, ataxia, and seizures.[176a] Injections are repeated twice weekly until the cell count has dropped to below 10/mm³. Acute symptoms of meningeal leukemia may be relieved by dexamethasone (0.2 mg/kg/day) with the first dose being given intravenously, and subsequent doses orally every six hours for about two days.[177] Radiation therapy may be employed concurrently for infiltrations of the nerve roots.[178] Remissions may last for several months, and subsequent retreatment is often very effective. Recurrences are common, however, particularly in patients with high cerebrospinal fluid cell counts. There is no evidence that the survival time is signficantly reduced by the development of meningeal leukemia.

The most frequent neurologic complication in acute leukemia is massive cerebral hemorrhage caused by thrombocytopenia. The hemorrhage may be intracerebral, intraventricular, or subarachnoid. Subdural hematomas are relatively rare.[179] Intracranial hemorrhage is often a terminal event, triggered by infection, with concurrent hemorrhages outside of the central nervous system usually being evident. This complication occurs in the terminal stages of the disease, and the average duration of life after its onset is but a matter of days.[174]

Infections of the central nervous system may be due to a variety of organisms, with *Staphylococcus aureus*, *Pseudomonas*, *E. coli* and a variety of fungi, notably *Monilia*, being the most common invaders. Herpes zoster encephalitis has been reported in association with leukemia with greater than chance frequency.[174]

Vincristine Neuropathy

The widespread use of vincristine as an effective agent in the treatment of leukemia necessitates a brief description of the neurologic side effects of the drug. In the main, these are a dose-dependent peripheral neuropathy with initial effect of the drug being on the muscle spindle. The Achilles tendon reflexes are depressed or lost in almost all cases. Less often, there is paroxysmal abdominal pain, weakness of the distal musculature of the lower extremities, and paresthesias in a glove and stocking distribution. Cranial nerve involvement, most often ptosis, ophthalmoplegia, and facial palsy, have also been noted but less often, and almost always in association with muscle weakness and atrophy. Their appearance in a leukemic child treated with vincristine should suggest meningeal infiltration, and is an indication for a lumbar puncture.[180] The cerebrospinal fluid is normal in leukemic children without meningeal infiltrates and in vincristine neuropathy.[180,181] Motor nerve conduction times are normal in the early stages of vincristine toxicity. Improvement has been noted within two to six weeks after discontinuation of drug therapy.

LYMPHOSARCOMA AND HODGKIN'S DISEASE

The neurologic complications of lymphomas are generally the result of an infiltration of the central nervous system and meninges. Symptoms and signs of increased intracranial pressure are present. A peripheral neuropathy has also been encountered.[182]

Neurologic complications of Hodgkin's disease are relatively unusual in childhood. They may take the form of infiltrations along the floor of the cranial cavity and the overlying meninges with an extension to the cranial nerves. Intracranial granulomata are rare.[183] Progressive multifocal encephalopathy, an acute disseminated demyelination encountered in Hodgkin's disease and lymphosarcoma, and associated with intranuclear inclusions of viruslike particles, is more common in older subjects[184] but has also been seen in children with acute leukemia dying either in clinical relapse or remission.[184a]

COAGULATION DISORDERS

Intracranial hemorrhage is the leading cause of death in hemophilias (Factor VIII deficiency).[185] About 10% of subjects experience an intracranial hemorrhage, almost always the result of trauma. In about one-half of instances, the site of bleeding is within the subdural or epidural spaces. When neurologic symptoms develop in a hemophiliac child, a diagnostic lumbar puncture will often be required. To avoid epidural or subarachnoid bleeding, this procedure should be deferred until factor VIII replacement therapy has been completed.[186]

Patients with factor IX deficiency show a clinical picture which is essentially identical to hemophilia. Intracranial hemorrhages occur rarely but apparently spontaneously in factor IX (plasma thromboplastin antecedent) deficiency, factor VII deficiency, and in von Willebrand's disease.[187]

THROMBOCYTOPENIC PURPURAS

Idiopathic thrombocytopenic purpura occurs as an acute, self-limiting form or, less often, as a chronic disease with remissions and exacerbations. Intracranial hemorrhages are rare in both forms. In the latter group of patients, learning disorders and behavior problems are common, and significant electroencephalographic abnormalities are seen in about 50% of cases. Minute, multiple capillary bleeding is believed to account for these findings.[188]

Neurologic complications are rare in Schönlein-Henoch purpura, although cases with fatal subarachnoid and intracranial hemorrhages have been encountered.[189]

In thrombotic thrombocytopenic purpura, a rare condition usually confined to adult life, intracapillary and intraarteriolar thrombi are widespread throughout the brain and produce a variety of neurologic symptoms, which have been reviewed by O'Brien and Sibley.[190]

NEUROLOGIC COMPLICATIONS OF ENDOCRINE DISORDERS

THYROID GLAND

Pathology

Brain and thyroid act reciprocally on each other. The anterior hypothalamus controls the thyrotropic function of the pituitary by regulating TSH secretion, which in turn is rendered feedback control by blood thyroxine or T_3 concentrations. Thyroid hormone is believed to stimulate brain protein synthesis, and assist in the differentiation of neural tissue during the later stages of development in utero. Sokoloff and associates have distinguished two in vivo effects of thyroid on protein synthesis.[191] An initial stimulatory effect of thyroid occurs shortly after its administration, and requires the presence of mitochondria. It probably represents stimulation of the translational activity of ribosomes, occurring independently of new RNA synthesis. A second, delayed effect, occurs independently of mitochondria, probably due to increased ribosomal synthesis. In the human fetus, thyroxine is synthesized after 10–14 weeks' gestation. Since thyroxine is unable to cross the placenta to any significant degree, inability of the fetus to initiate or maintain thyroid synthesis may affect brain development.[192] The degree of thyroid deficiency suffered by the athyrotic fetus will therefore influence the extent of intellectual retardation.

Structural abnormalities in the brain of hypothyroid individuals often incorporate characteristics of the immature organ. The size and number of cortical neurons is reduced, axons and dendrites are hypoplastic and myelination is retarded. Both cerebrum and cerebellum partake of the developmental delay.

HYPOTHYROIDISM

Clinical Manifestations

The clinical picture of hypothyroidism depends on the degree of thyroid insufficiency and the time of its onset. With respect to neurologic symptoms, five clinical forms may be distinguished.

In neonatal nongoitrous hypothyroidism the thyroid gland is absent or too small to keep the patient euthyroid. At birth these infants are usually of normal size, although their birth weights are somewhat greater than normal, and they have retarded osseous development. Symptoms arise in the first few months of life. Infants are placid, with diminished spontaneous movements, generalized hypotonia, and a husky, grunting cry. The head appears large with coarse, lusterless hair, and widely open sutures and fontanelle. Motor and intellectual development is delayed. One-third of patients have spasticity, incoordination and cerebellar ataxia.[193] The electroencephalogram also reflects delayed development of the brain.[194] Congenital goitrous cretinism may be familial and due to intrathyroid enzyme defects. The degree of hypothyroidism varies widely, as does the impairment of intelligence. The association of deafness due to a defect in nerve conduction, with goitrous hypothyroidism has been termed Pendred's syndrome. It is transmitted as an autosomal recessive disorder.[195]

When hypothyroidism develops after three years of age, intelligence is not irreversibly damaged. Impaired memory, poor school performance, and generalized slowing of movement and speech are prominent. The muscles are weak and pseudohypertrophic. There is a significant reduction in the speed of muscular contraction and relaxation, which can be demonstrated electromyographically, and may be visible to the examiner.

Mental retardation, deaf-mutism, and spasticity are seen in children with endemic goitrous cretinism. In some areas of the world nerve deafness may be the sole neurologic abnormality.[195]

Kocher in 1892[196] and more recently Debré and Semelaigne[197] have described infants with an unusual combination of diffuse muscular hypertrophy and congenital thyroid deficiency. The muscular hypertrophy is unexplained, for neither fiber enlargement nor an infiltrative process have been found on light or electron microscopy.[198,199]

Diagnosis

The diagnosis of hypothyroidism is often considered in the evaluation of a child with developmental retardation. The infantile facies, protuberant abdomen, and dry hair and skin evoke the suspicion of the condition.[200] This is confirmed by finding retarded osseous development, delayed growth, and infantile bodily proportions. Even more specific is the determination of serum thyroxine by means of column fractionation, or

by measurement of the serum PBI. In a few cases of goitrous hypothyroidism due to thyroiditis, the PBI and bone age may be normal. Failure in the uptake of radio-iodine will indicate the absence of a functioning thyroid gland.

Treatment and Prognosis

The use of desiccated thyroid in the treatment of hypothyroidism has gone virtually unchallenged. While somatic growth is usually correctable, the prognosis as far as mental function is concerned is less good.

In the study by Smith et al.[201] only 15% of children with severe symptoms of hypothyroidism present during infancy achieved an IQ of 90 or better, and 41% were grossly retarded (IQ of less than 50). While the ultimate results are better in those infants whose therapy is begun prior to six months of age or even earlier,[202] there is considerable evidence that there is often some degree of intra-uterine thyroid deficiency and that this contributes significantly to the poor prognosis of severe cretinism.

HYPERTHYROIDISM

Clinical Manifestations

The association of hyperthyroidism with neuromuscular disease is much more frequent in adults than children. The condition is more common in girls, a recently quoted sex ratio being 6:1. Neuromuscular disorders seen in the course of hyperthyroidism include exophthalmic ophthalmoplegia, thyrotoxic myopathy, myasthenia gravis, and periodic paralysis.[203] Cerebral symptoms begin insidiously and at first are nonspecific. The child is irritable, nervous, unable to concentrate, has a short attention span, and does poorly in school. Exophthalmos is the most characteristic sign. It may be unilateral early in the disease and, when severe, is accompanied by papilledema and central scotomata. Tremor and increased deep tendon reflexes are seen in the more toxic children. Cranial nerve palsies, and muscular disorders are rare in childhood. Thyrotoxicosis is occasionally associated with myasthenia gravis or with familial periodic paralysis (see Chapter 12).

Diagnosis

In thyrotoxic children, the thyroid gland is nearly always enlarged. Useful laboratory measurements are serum PBI, or when there has been exposure to inorganic iodides, butanol-extractable iodine (BEI), and estimation of thyroxine iodide by column chromatography. Also useful is the measurement of radioactive iodine uptake by the thyroid gland.

Thyroiditis, which may simulate the behavior pattern of thyrotoxicosis, is suggested by the presence of a symptomatic goiter in a euthyroid child. The clinical picture of thyroiditis is variable and may run the gamut of symptoms suggesting hyperthyroidism to those of hypothyroidism.

Treatment

The optimal treatment of thyrotoxicosis is still controversial. Once thyroid function returns to normal neuromuscular symptoms remit.

PARATHYROID GLAND

The neurologic symptoms of hypo- and hyperparathyroidism are the direct or indirect result of disordered calcium metabolism and are therefore discussed under the disturbances of electrolyte metabolism.

ADRENAL GLAND

Neurologic symptoms accompanying disorders of the adrenal gland are generally the result of disturbed serum electrolytes and osmolarity. They are referred to in another portion of this chapter. The association of Addison's disease with sudanophilic leukodystrophy has been reported in several families (see Chapter 2). The association of papilledema with Addison's disease has been recorded.[204]

PITUITARY GLAND

Neurologic symptoms associated with disorders of pituitary function usually result from direct involvement of the perisellar and hypothalamic regions by a mass originating from the pituitary gland or neighboring structures (see Chapter 10). Less commonly, the neurologic picture evolves in conjunction with a destructive lesion affecting this area, such as occurs with histiocytosis X, sarcoidosis, and other granulomatous diseases, or with direct trauma. A hypertrophic neuropathy is a rare but distinct complication of acromegaly.[205]

A syndrome of cerebral gigantism appears not to be very rare. Patients are mentally retarded, their facies are unusual with frontal bossing, hypertelorism, macrocrania, and prognathism. Birth weights are usually above the ninetieth percentile, and for the first four to five years children experience a growth spurt, which subsequently subsides. Convulsions and sexual precocity are occasionally present. Plasma growth hormone levels are normal, and the cause for this syndrome is unknown.[206]

Some of the conditions in which delayed growth accompanies mental retardation are outlined in Table 9–8. The reader is also referred to a recent review by Smith[221] and a book by Smith.[222]

DIABETES

Of the neurologic complications of diabetes in children, the most common is peripheral neuropathy. This condition is usually asymptomatic, although careful neurologic examination of diabetics may reveal slight distal weakness in the lower extremities, wasting of the interossei muscles, and diminished deep tendon reflexes. Conduction velocity in the peroneal nerve is abnormally slow in 11% of diabetics between the ages of 8 and 15 years. Eeg-Olofsson and Petersen believe that the appearance of the neuropathy correlates with the duration of the diabetes and is more commonly seen in children who have been under poor control.[223]

We have not observed involvement of the cranial nerves or cerebral vascular disease in diabetic children.

The cause of neurologic impairment in diabetic keto-acidosis is not well understood. For some time it has been known that under these circumstances cerebral oxygen uptake is reduced by some 40%,[224] and that cerebral blood flow is decreased, but the role of the various metabolic abnormalities present in diabetic coma in causing these changes has not been completely clarified.

It is unlikely that accumulation of ketone bodies is solely responsible, as the cerebro-

TABLE 9-8.
SYNDROMES OF SHORT STATURE ASSOCIATED
WITH MENTAL RETARDATION

Condition	Symptoms	Reference
Prader-Willi syndrome	Hypotonia, cryptorchidism, hypoplastic scrotum, obesity, high incidence of diabetes mellitus	Zellweger and Schneider[207]
Smith-Lemli-Opitz syndrome	Microcephaly, ptosis, broad upturned nares, hypospadias, cryptorchidism, history of persistent vomiting	Smith et al.[208]
Cornelia de Lange syndrome	Low birth weight, growling cry, anteverted nostrils, carplike mouth, micromelia, or low position of thumbs, hirsutism	Vischer[209]
Bird-headed dwarf	Low birth weight, craniosynostosis, dislocation of joints, numerous bony defects, unusual facies	McKusick et al.[210] Seckel[211]
Kinky-hair disease	Failure to thrive, focal and generalized seizures, stubby white hair, transmitted as sex-linked recessive, probably due to defect of copper absorption	Menkes et al.[212] Danks et al.[212a]
Cockayne's syndrome	Impaired hearing, retinal degeneration, aged appearance, cataracts, intracranial calcifications, peripheral neuropathy	McDonald et al.[213] Moosa and Dubowitz[214]
Leprechaunism	Large nares, low-set ears, sunken eyes, absent subcutaneous adipose tissue, short limbs	Dekaban[215]
Rubenstein's syndrome	Narrow nose, slanting palpebral fissures, maxillary hypoplasia, broad thumbs and toes	Rubenstein and Taybi[216]
Lowe's syndrome	Cataracts, glaucoma, hypotonia, aminoaciduria, organic aciduria, choreo-athetosis, sex-linked recessive transmission	Richards et al.[217]
Sjögren (type II) syndrome	Congenital cataracts, autosomal recessive transmission	Engels[218]
Börjeson syndrome	Seizures, hypogonadism, obesity, swelling of subcutaneous tissue of face, narrow palpebral fissures, large ears	Börjeson et al.[219]
de Sanctis-Cacchione syndrome	Xeroderma pigmentosum, microcephaly, autosomal recessive transmission	Reed et al.[220]

spinal fluid concentrations of beta-hydroxy butyrate and acetoacetate vary widely at the time when obtundation first becomes apparent.[225] Cerebrospinal fluid pH is normal or even elevated in severely acidotic patients. The most consistent alteration is an increase in the osmolality of cerebrospinal fluid. As a rule, the hyperosmolality of cerebrospinal fluid is more striking than that of plasma and returns more slowly to normal with treatment.[225] The production of sorbitol and fructose by brain during hyperglycemia may contribute to cerebrospinal fluid hyperosmolality.[226]

A number of deaths from irreversible cerebral edema have occurred in the course of apparently adequate treatment of diabetic keto-acidosis.[227] A rapid reduction of blood hyperosmolality with treatment, and a slower change in the cerebral hyperosmolality may result in the entrance of water into the brain and consequent cerebral edema. Diagnosis of this complication is difficult, since characteristic clinical or biochemical features are lacking. Rather it is a failure of the patient to recover consciousness despite adequate treatment with insulin and fluids, that points to the presence of cerebral edema. The presence of high blood sugar levels and, according to Young and Bradley,[227] of hyperpyrexia should alert the clinician to the imminence of this complication. A gradual correction of hyperglycemia will in most instances prevent cerebral edema. Dexamethasone has been used in its treatment, but in our experience it is usually given too late to be effective.

Intracellular dehydration associated with hyperosmolality is presumed to be responsible for neurologic symptoms in nonketotic hyperglycemic coma.[228]

The neurologic complications of hypoglycemia are discussed at another point in this chapter.

NUTRITIONAL DISORDERS OF THE NERVOUS SYSTEM

Nutritional disorders are due to a conjunction of environmental and internal metabolic factors. Grossly reduced quantities of food, dietary imbalances, poor protein intake, lack of essential fatty acids and vitamins, climate, intercurrent bacterial or parasitic infections, and emotional deprivation all combine to produce the symptoms of nutritional diseases.

PROTEIN-CALORIE MALNUTRITION

Malnourished children comprise about 75% of the preschool population in the underdeveloped countries. There are two interrelated food deficiency syndromes which in their most severe stages of development are distinct with different etiologies and different metabolic pictures. One, primarily due to caloric insufficiency, has been termed infantile marasmus, and is seen when infants are weaned before the end of their first year, or when the amount of breast milk becomes markedly reduced. It is characterized by emaciation and growth failure.[229]

The other condition, due to a diet containing adequate calories but insufficient protein, goes under the name of kwashiorkor and is most common in children weaned between two and three years of age.[230] In many areas of the world, symptoms of kwashiorkor develop in a child who already is suffering from caloric deficiency, producing the clinical picture of kwashiorkor in a child who is also emaciated and has retarded growth.

In mild to moderate forms of protein-calorie malnutrition, a clinical distinction between the two syndromes is impossible. In certain areas of the world, diets giving rise to kwashiorkor may also be deficient in one or more vitamins, and signs of vitamin deficiency occur inconstantly in the more advanced stages. In west Africa, for instance, riboflavin deficiency is common, while in southeast Asia thiamin deficiency may induce a mixed picture of protein-calorie malnutrition and beri-beri.

Certain changes in protein metabolism, notably a reduced serum albumin concentration, a reduced serum concentration of all essential amino acids except phenylalanine and histidine, and a normal or even higher than normal concentration of nonessential amino acids, are characteristic for kwashiorkor and can be used in making a diagnosis.

Children with kwashiorkor demonstrate edema, dyspigmentation of hair and skin, dermatitis, and hepatomegaly. Apathy is the most constant and earliest neurologic feature and is usual in children whose weight is less than 40% of the expected value.[231]

Psychologic studies on malnourished infants show them to have cognitive inadequacies resulting in delay in learning, particularly of reading and writing.[232,233,234] The medical and social aspects of treatment are reviewed by deSilva.[229]

About one-fifth of children with kwashiorkor become drowsy within three to four days after being started on a normal diet. While the condition is most often self-limited, it is occasionally accompanied by asterixis and can progress to coma with fatal outcome.[235] The nature of this complication is unknown but it may reflect hepatic failure resulting from the use of relatively large amounts of protein. Even more rarely, a transient syndrome marked by coarse tremors, Parkinsonian rigidity, bradykinesia, and myoclonus may appear in children with kwashiorkor six days to several weeks after the starting of the corrective high-protein diet.[236] This condition is distinct from the infantile tremor syndrome.[236a] The latter entity is seen in Indian infants aged 7 months to $2\frac{1}{2}$ years. Many of the children have had a history of slow development. Symptoms commence between May and July, and include a tremor, which may be generalized or confined to one or more extremities. The tremor is rapid, rhythmic and coarse, and disappears during sleep. It may be accompanied by myoclonic jerks, epilepsia partialis continua, or choreiform movements. The cause of infantile tremor syndrome is unknown, but the condition does not accompany dietary correction, and is self-limiting. Although symptoms subside within four to six months, most affected infants remain mentally retarded.

Follow-up studies on children who suffered from protein-calorie malnutrition indicate that the younger the child at the time of his hospitalization for malnutrition, the less likely he is to achieve intellectual parity.[237,238]

The effects of undernutrition on the immature nervous system have been the subject of recent intensive investigation.[239] Neuropathologic studies have almost all been performed on patients dying as a consequence of a combination of infection and caloric and protein deprivation. Their brains are small for the infants' chronologic age, and there is a reduction in the number of neurons, the degree of myelination, and the total cerebral lipid content.[240,241] However, recent studies showing that children whose nutrition is adequate during the first two years of life do not have a greater head circumference at the same height than their malnourished siblings suggest that malnutrition in early life has no apparent selective effect on head growth, and possibly on brain size as well.[242]

Animal experiments indicate that a severe nutritional insult in the early course of brain development may induce a permanent adverse effect on cerebral structure and function. Periods of CNS growth spurt, in man between 15 and 20 weeks' gestation, when neuronal multiplication is maximal, and between 30 weeks' gestation and the end of the first year of extra-uterine life when glial division occurs, are times when the brain is particularly vulnerable to nutritional deficiency.[239,243]

As yet we are unable to correlate these data with clinical experience. The intellectual inadequacy which is a residuum of malnutrition in early life may not only be the result of protein-calorie deficiency but may have developed because the infant's nervous system was inadequate from birth on and interfered with his ability to feed and to interact emotionally with his mother.[238]

VITAMIN DEFICIENCIES

The action of a vitamin in intermediary metabolism can be disturbed by its deficiency, by abnormally high vitamin requirements, and by the inhibitory action of various antivitamin substances. An alteration in the configuration of the apoenzyme protein is probably the cause for vitamin B_6 (pyridoxine) dependency, a condition characterized by seizures and an increase in the minimum pyridoxine requirements.[244] Dietary factors antagonistic to the action of a vitamin include avidin, found in raw egg white, an antagonist to biotin, and the enzyme thiaminase, present in raw fish, which destroys dietary thiamine.

While a deficiency in almost any of the vitamins may directly or indirectly affect the central nervous system, only components of the B complex group are known to be directly involved in brain function.

Deficiency of vitamin A can produce increased intracranial pressure, reversed by dietary treatment. Chronic vitamin A intoxication will also induce increased intracranial pressure which is accompanied by craniotabes, and cortical hyperostosis.[245,246]

Vitamin E (tocopherol) deficiency is encountered in severe cases of cystic fibrosis of the pancreas. Occasionally it induces focal necrosis of striated muscle, degeneration of the dorsal columns of the spinal cord, and dystrophic changes in axons.[247]

Thiamine Deficiency

The discovery of how thiamine participates in cerebral metabolism forms an important part of the early history of neurochemistry and is reviewed by Peters.[248] Thiamine functions in the form of its pyrophosphate, and acts at three points in the intermediary metabolism of carbohydrates. These are the decarboxylation of pyruvate and alpha-ketoglutarate, two integral steps of the Krebs cycle, and the conversion of five-carbon to six-carbon sugars by means of the enzyme transketolase. In thiamine deficiency, oxidation of pyruvate and alpha-ketoglutarate by the brain is reduced. As a consequence, cerebral oxygen and glucose consumption are lowered, and the concentrations of the two keto-acids are increased in various tissues, including blood.[249] When a thiamine-deficient individual is presented with a glucose load, the concentration of serum keto-acids rises to abnormal levels, and remains elevated for several hours. Transketolase has been found to be more susceptible to thiamine deprivation than the keto-acid decarboxylases, and the fall in transketolase activity during induced thiamine deficiency is greater than that of pyruvate decarboxylase.[250] While Dreyfus and Hauser[251] have postulated that failure in transketolase represents the basic biochemical lesion of thiamine deficiency, the rise in transketolase activity with administration of thiamine was insufficient to account for the clinical improvement.[250]

An excellent diagnostic test for thiamine deficiency is the reduction of whole blood transketolase, described by Dreyfus.[252]

Thiamine deficiency is seen mainly in breast-fed infants, whose mothers may have had beriberi during pregnancy or the puerperium. The condition occurs principally in Asia, where the milling of rice grain or the use of soda in the baking of bread excludes the vitamin from the diet. Two symptom complexes are seen: infantile beriberi and Wernicke-Korsakoff's encephalopathy. Infantile beriberi appears suddenly, often following a bout of gastroenteritis, and is marked by weakness due to acute peripheral neuritis, neck stiffness, aphonia, and cardiac symptoms.[253] A neurologic picture resembling that seen in adults with Wernicke-Korsakoff's syndrome is rare in childhood.[254] The experience of Haridas in Malaya[255] and deSilva in Ceylon[229] illustrate differential diagnosis and treatment.

A familial neurologic degenerative disease with pathologic changes reminiscent of Wernicke's disease has been termed pseudo-Wernicke's syndrome, Leigh's syndrome, or infantile subacute necrotizing encephalopathy. It is referred to in Chapter 1.

Pyridoxine Deficiency

Pyridoxine (vitamin B_6) in the form of its aldehyde derivative, pyridoxal-5-phosphate, is a coenzyme for numerous essential metabolic reactions within the nervous system. Decarboxylation of glutamic acid to gamma-aminobutyric acid (GABA), a neurotransmitter, and transamination of glutamic acid to alpha-ketoglutaric acid are both impaired in animals receiving a pyridoxine-deficient diet, and a disturbance in the normal ratio of glutamic acid to gamma-aminobutyric acid has been postulated to be responsible for the seizure disorder seen in pyridoxine deficient infants. Tower has reviewed the relationship of pyridoxine to cerebral amino acid metabolism.[256]

Pyridoxine deficiency causes seizures and hyperirritability. At least two conditions are encountered in which pyridoxine is related to the appearance of seizures. A familial pyridoxine dependency syndrome causes seizures at birth or shortly thereafter.[244,257] These are arrested by the administration of the vitamin. The dose required to control seizures and reverse the electroencephalographic abnormalities (2–15 mg/day) is about 10 times the minimum daily requirements. The cause of this condition is unknown, but a structural variation in one of the apoenzymes requiring pyridoxine as cofactor has been postulated. This alteration would produce a diminished affinity of coenzyme for apoenzyme which can only be overcome by increasing the tissue concentration of the coenzyme.

Pyridoxine deficiency appears between 1 and 12 months of age in a significant number of infants whose intake of the vitamin is below 0.1 mg/day. Aside from seizures, other symptoms of vitamin deficiency, notably anemia, can sometimes be documented.[258] Isolated pyridoxine deficiency is rarely encountered even in the underdeveloped countries. A rash of cases was seen in the United States between 1952 and 1953 and occurred in a small percentage of infants who were fed a pyridoxine-deficient proprietary formula.[259] Treatment with penicillamine, isoniazide, or with other hydrazides capable of reacting with the aldehyde group of pyridoxal may also induce deficiency symptoms.[260]

A disorder of tryptophan metabolism has been encountered in some patients with infantile minor motor seizures. Even though the relationship between the abnormal tryptophan tolerance shown by these patients to a relative pyridoxine deficiency is poorly established, administration of very high doses of pyridoxine (6–14 mg/kg/day) has relieved the seizure disorder in some of these patients.[261]

Pellagra

Although pellagra is considered a multiple deficiency disease, the main clinical manifestations—dermatitis, diarrhea, and diffuse cerebral disease—respond to nicotinic acid therapy. About one-half of man's minimal daily requirements are synthesized from tryptophan, either in tissues, or in the intestinal tract by microorganisms. The condition is endemic to those areas where corn, a poor source of nicotinic acid, forms the staple food, and where meat intake, which provides tryptophan for the biosynthesis of nicotinic acid, is also low.[262]

In the brain, nicotinic acid largely takes the form of phosphopyridine nucleotides, which serve as cofactors for numerous metabolic reactions.

Mildly affected children are irritable or apathetic. With severe involvement, children are delirious, or obtunded, and may show spasticity, coarse tremors of face and hands, polyneuritis, and optic atrophy.[263] Histologic examination of the brain shows degeneration of the Betz cells of the motor cortex and, to a lesser extent, of the cerebellar Purkinje cells. In the spinal cord there is degeneration of the posterior columns, and the pyramidal and spino-cerebellar tracts. Demyelination of the peripheral nerves is common.[264]

The experiences of Spies et al. in Alabama illustrate differential diagnosis and therapy.[263]

Subacute Combined Degeneration

Degeneration of the posterior and lateral columns of the spinal cord due to deficiency of vitamin B_{12} is a rare condition in childhood. When seen, it may accompany congenital pernicious anemia, a genetic disorder characterized by a failure to secrete gastric intrinsic factor, or it may be associated with intestinal disease, regional ileitis, or celiac syndrome. The condition presents with ataxia, spasticity, weakness of the lower extremities, loss of vibratory sensation, and mental retardation.[265,266]

A megaloblastic anemia is always present when subacute combined degeneration appears in childhood. The neurologic abnormalities can be arrested or partly improved with administration of vitamin B_{12}. In the experience of Pearson et al., folic acid therapy often aggravates the neurologic symptoms.[267]

REFERENCES

1. Dickerman, T. D., Bishop, W., and Marks, J. F.: Acute ethanol intoxication in a child, Pediatrics 42:837, 1968.
2. Cummins, L. H.: Hypoglycemia and convulsions in children following alcohol ingestion, J. Pediat. 58:23, 1961.
3. MacLaren, N. K., Valman, H. B., and Levin, B.: Alcohol-induced hypoglycemia in childhood, Brit. Med. J. 1:278, 1970.

4. White, B. H. and Daeschner, C. W.: Amino-phylline poisoning in children, J. Pediat. 49:262, 1956.

5. Judge, D. J. and Dumars, K. W.: Diphenydramine (Benadryl) and tripelennamine (Pyribenzamine) intoxication in children, AMA J. Dis. Child. 85:545, 1953.

6. Priest, J. H.: Atropine response of eyes in mongolism, Amer. J. Dis. Child. 100:869, 1960.

7. Valdes-Dapena, M. A. and Arey, J. B.: Boric acid poisoning: Three fatal cases with pancreatic inclusion and review of literature, J. Pediat. 61:511, 1962.

8. Garland, H. and Pearce, J.: Neurological complications of carbon monoxide poisoning, Quart. J. Med. 36:445, 1967.

9. Espelin, D. and Done, A.: Amphetamine poisoning, New Eng. J. Med. 278:1361, 1968.

10. Whitten, C. F., et al.: Studies in acute iron poisoning. I. Desferrioxamine in the treatment of acute iron poisoning: Clinical observations, experimental studies, and theoretical considerations, Pediatrics 36:322, 1965.

11. James, J. A.: Acute iron poisoning: Assessment of severity and prognosis, J. Pediat. 77:117, 1970.

12. Monnet, P., et al.: L'intoxication par l'imipramine et ses derives en pediatrie, Rev. Lyon. Med. 19:845, 1970.

13. Kopel, F. B., et al.: Acute parathion poisoning: Diagnosis and treatment, J. Pediat. 61:898, 1962.

13a. Hayes, W. J.: Epidemiology and general management of poisoning by pesticides, Pediat. Clin. N. Amer. 17:629, 1970.

14. Parsons, A. C.: Piperazine neurotoxicity: "Worm wobble," Brit. Med. J. 4:792, 1971.

15. Wilson, S. G. F. and Dally, W. J.: Meningeal irritation due to tetracycline administration, Arch. Dis. Child. 41:691, 1966.

16. Dana, S. L.: Lead Diseases, a Treatise from the French of L. Tanquerel des Planches, Lowell, Mass. D. Bixby Co., 1848.

17. Blackfan, K. D.: Lead poisoning in children with especial reference to lead as a cause of convulsions, Amer. J. Med. Sci. 153:877, 1917.

18. Holt, L. E.: Lead poisoning in infancy, Amer. J. Dis. Child. 25:229, 1923.

19. Canterow, A. and Trumper, M.: Lead Poisoning, Baltimore: Williams & Wilkins Co., 1944.

20. Kehoe, R. A.: The metabolism of lead in man in health and disease, J. Roy. Inst. Public Health 24:81, 101, 177, 1961.

20a. U.S. Public Health Service: Medical aspects of childhood lead poisoning, Pediatrics 48:464, 1971.

21. Chisholm, J. J., Jr. and Harrison, H. H.: Exposure of children to lead, Pediatrics 18:943, 1956.

22. Chisholm, J. J.: Poisoning due to heavy metals, Pediat. Clin. N. Amer. 17:591, 1970.

23. Chisholm, J. J.: Disturbances in the biosynthesis of heme in lead intoxication, J. Pediat. 64:174, 1964.

23a. White, J. M. and Harvey, D. R.: Defective synthesis of α and β globin chains in lead poisoning, Nature 236:71, 1972.

24. Garrod, A. E.: The occurrence and detection of haematoporphyrin in the urine, J. Physiol. 13:598, 1892.

25. Cumings, J. N.: Heavy Metals and the Brain, Oxford: Blackwell Scientific Publications, 1959.

26. Blackman, S. S.: Intranuclear inclusion bodies in the kidney and liver caused by lead poisoning, Bull. Hopkins Hosp. 58:383, 1936.

27. Turner, A. J.: Lead poisoning among Queensland children, Australasian Med. Gaz. 16:475, 1897.

28. Freeman, R.: Chronic lead poisoning in children: A review of 90 children diagnosed in Sydney 1948–1967. 2. Clinical features and investigations, Med. J. Aust. 1:648, 1970.

29. Tanis, A. L.: Lead poisoning in children, Amer. J. Dis. Child. 89:325, 1955.

30. Mellins, R. B. and Jenkins, C. D.: Epidemiologic and psychological study of lead poisoning in children, JAMA 158:15, 1955.

31. Jenkins, C. D. and Mellins, R. B.: Lead poisoning in children, Arch. Neurol. Psychiat. 77:70, 1957.

32. Mirando, E. H. and Ranasinghe, L.: Lead encephalopathy in children: Uncommon clinical aspects, Med. J. Aust. 2:966, 1970.

33. Chisholm, J. J., et al.: Aminoaciduria, hypophosphatemia, and rickets in lead poisoning, Amer. J. Dis. Child. 89:159, 1955.

34. Park, E. A., Jackson, D., and Kajdi, L.: Shadows produced by lead in the X-ray pictures of the growing skeleton, Amer. J. Dis. Child. 41:485, 1931.

35. Feldman, F., et al.: Serum delta-aminolevulinic acid in plumbism, J. Pediat. 74:917, 1969.

36. Weissberg, J. B., Lipschutz, F., and Oski, F. A.: δ-aminolaevulinic acid dehydratase activity in circulating blood cells, New Eng. J. Med. 284:565, 1971.

37. Hernberg, S., et al.: Erythrocyte δ-aminolevulinic acid dehydratase in new lead exposure, Arch. Environ. Health (Chicago) 25:109, 1972.

38. Chisholm, J. J.: Screening for lead poisoning in children, Pediatrics 51:280, 1973.

39. Piomelli, S.: The FEP (free erythrocyte porphyrins) test: A screening micromethod for lead poisoning, Pediatrics 51:254, 1973.

39a. Benson, P. F. and Chisholm, J. J., Jr.: A reliable qualitative urine coproporphyrin test for lead intoxication in young children, J. Pediat. 56:759, 1960.

40. Coffin, R., et al.: Treatment of lead encephalopathy in children, J. Pediat. 69:198, 1966.

41. Bessman, S. P., Ried, H., and Rubin, M.: Treatment of lead encephalopathy with calcium disodium versenate. Report of a case, Med. Ann. DC 21:312, 1952.

42. Chisholm, J. J., Jr.: The use of chelating agents in the treatment of acute and chronic lead intoxication in childhood, J. Pediat. 73:1, 1968.

42a. de la Burde, B. and Choate, M. S.: Does asymptomatic lead exposure in children have latent sequelae? J. Pediat. 81:1088, 1972.

42b. Barltrop, D.: Chronic neurological sequelae of lead poisoning, Develop. Med. Child Neurol. 15:365, 1973.

43. Grossman, H.: Thallotoxicosis: Report of a case and a review, Pediatrics 16:868, 1955.

44. Chamberlain, P. H., et al.: Thallium poisoning, Pediatrics 22:1170, 1958.

45. Reed, D., et al.: Thallotoxicosis: Acute manifestations and sequelae, JAMA 183:516, 1963.

46. Bank, W. J., et al.: Thallium poisoning, Arch. Neurol. 26:456, 1972.

47. Russell, D. S.: Changes in the central nervous system following arsphenamine medication, J. Path. Bact. 45:357, 1937.

48. Woody, N. C. and Kometani, J. T.: BAL in the treatment of arsenic ingestion in children, Pediatrics 1:372, 1948.

49. Cheek, D. B.: Pink disease (infantile acrodynia), J. Pediat. 42:239, 1953.

50. McCoy, J. E., Carre, I. J., and Freeman, M.: A controlled trial of edathamil calcium disodium in acrodynia, Pediatrics 25:304, 1960.

50a. Bakir, F., et al.: Methylmercury poisoning in Iraq, Science 181:230, 1973.

51. Kurland, L. T., Faro, S. N., and Siedler, H.: Minimata disease, World Neurol. 1:370, 1960.

52. Snyder, R. D.: Congenital mercury poisoning, New Eng. J. Med. 284:1014, 1971.

53. Mark, L. C.: Metabolism of barbiturates in man, Clin. Pharmacol. Ther. 4:504, 1963.

54. Mann, J. B. and Sandberg, D. H.: Therapy of sedative overdosage, Ped. Clin. N. Amer. 17:617, 1970.

55. Matthew, H. and Lawson, A. A. H.: Acute barbiturate poisoning: Review of two years' experience, Quart. J. Med. 35:539, 1966.

56. Gupta, J. M. and Lovejoy, F. H., Jr.: Acute phenothiazine toxicity in childhood: A five-year survey, Pediatrics 39:771, 1967.

57. Cohlan, S. Q.: Convulsive seizures caused by phenothiazine tranquilizers, GP 21:136, 1960.

58. Schmidt, W. R. and Jarcho, L. W.: Persistent dyskinesias following phenothiazine therapy, Arch. Neurol. 14:369, 1966.

58a. Kimbrough, R. D.: Review of recent evidence of toxic effects of hexachlorophene, Pediatrics 51:pt. II, 391, 1973.

58b. Powell, H., et al.: Hexachlorophene myelinopathy in premature infants, J. Pediat. 82:976, 1973.

58c. Plueckhahn, V. D.: Hexachlorophene and the control of staphylococcal sepsis in a maternity unit in Geelong, Australia, Pediatrics 51:pt. II, 368, 1973.

58d. Gilles, F. H.: Discussion of the use of hexachlorophene in the nursery. Pediatrics 51: pt. II, 408, 1973.

59. Zelson, C., Rubio, E., and Wasserman, E.: Neonatal narcotic addiction: 10-year observation, Pediatrics 48:178, 1971.

60. Schulman, C.: Alterations of the sleep cycle in heroin addicted and suspect newborns, Neuropaediatrie 1:89, 1969.

61. Nathenson, G., Golden, G. S., and Litt, I. F.: Diazepam in the management of the neonatal narcotic withdrawal syndrome, Pediatrics 48:523, 1971.

62. Schmorl, G.: Zur Kenntnis des Ikterus neonatorum insbesondere der dabei auftretenden Gehirnveränderungen, Verh. Deutsch. Ges. Path. 6:109, 1903.

63. Haymaker, W., et al.: "Pathology of Kernicterus and Post Icteric Encephalopathy," in American Academy for Cerebral Palsy: Kernicterus and Its Importance in Cerebral Palsy, Springfield: Charles C Thomas Publisher, 1961, p. 21.

64. Gartner, L. M., et al.: Kernicterus: High incidence in premature infants with low serum bilirubin concentrations, Pediatrics 45:906, 1970.

65. Brown, A. K.: Management of neonatal hyperbilirubinemia, Obstet. Gynec. 7:985, 1964.

66. Blumenschein, S. D., et al.: Familial nonhemolytic jaundice with late onset of neurological damage, Pediatrics 42:786, 1968.

67. Lucey, J. F., et al.: Kernicterus in asphyxiated newborn rhesus monkeys, Exp. Neurol. 9:43, 1964.

68. Vogel, F. S.: Studies on the pathogenesis of kernicterus. With special reference to the nature of kernicteric pigment and its deposition under natural and experimental conditions, J. Exp. Med. 98:509, 1953.

69. Boreau, T., Mensch-Dechene, J., and Roux-Doutheret, F.: Etude clinique de 34 cas d'ictere nucleaire par maladie hemolytique neo-natale et leur evolution, Arch. Franc. Pediat. 21:43, 1964.

70. Perlstein, M. A.: "The Clinical Syndrome of Kernicterus," in American Academy for Cerebral Palsy: Kernicterus and Its Importance in Cerebral Palsy, Springfield: Charles C Thomas Publisher, 1961, p. 268.

71. Johnston, W. H., et al.: Erythroblastosis fetalis and hyperbilirubinemia: Five year follow-up with neurologic, psychologic and audiologic evaluation, Pediatrics 39:88, 1967.

72. Crigler, J. F., Jr. and Gold, N. I.: Effect of sodium phenobarbital on bilirubin metabolism in an infant with congenital, non-hemolytic, unconjugated hyperbilirubinemia, and kernicterus, J. Clin. Invest. 48:42, 1969.

73. Schaffer, A. J. and Avery, M. E.: Diseases of the Newborn, 3rd ed., Philadelphia: W. B. Saunders Co., 1971.

74. Ackerman, B. D., Dyer, G. Y., and Leydorf, M. M.: Hyperbilirubinemia and kernicterus in small premature infants, Pediatrics 45:918, 1970.

75. Cherington, M. and Ginsberg, S.: Type B botulism: Neurophysiologic studies, Neurology (Minneap.) 21:43, 1971.

151. Matson, D. D.: Intracranial arterial aneurysms in childhood, J. Neurosurg. 23:578, 1965.
152. Schuster, S. R. and Gross, R. E.: Surgery for coarctation of the aorta. A review of 500 cases, J. Thorac. Cardiov. Surg. 43:54, 1962.
153. Albert, M. L., Greer, W. E. R., and Kantrowitz, W.: Paraplegia secondary to hypotension and cardiac arrest in a patient who has had previous thoracic surgery, Neurology (Minneap.) 19:915, 1969.
154. Tyler, H. R. and Clark, D. B.: Incidence of neurological complications in congenital heart disease, AMA Arch. Neurol. Psychiat. 77:17, 1957.
155. Kalyanaraman, K., et al.: The electroencephalogram in congenital heart disease, Arch. Neurol. 18:98, 1968.
156. Tyler, H. R. and Clark, D. B.: Cerebrovascular accidents in patients with congenital heart disease, AMA Arch. Neurol. Psychiat. 77:483, 1957.
156a.Martelle, R. R. and Linde, L. M.: Cerebrovascular accidents with tetralogy of Fallot, Amer. J. Dis. Child. 101:206, 1961.
157. Berthrong, M. and Sabiston, D. C., Jr.: Cerebral lesions in congenital heart disease, Bull. Hopkins Hosp. 89:384, 1951.
158. Peterson, R. A. and Rosenthal, A.: Retinopathy and papilledema in cyanotic congenital heart disease, Pediatrics 49:243, 1972.
159. Cayler, G. C.: Cardiofacial syndrome: Congenital heart disease and facial weakness, hitherto unrecognized association, Arch. Dis. Child. 44:69, 1969.
160. Still, J. L. and Cottom, D.: Severe hypertension in childhood, Arch. Dis. Child. 42:34, 1967.
161. Lloyd, A. V. C., Jewitt, D. E., and Still, J. D. L.: Facial paralysis in children with hypertension, Arch. Dis. Child. 41:292, 1966.
162. Holden, A. M., et al.: Congestive heart failure from intracranial arteriovenous fistula in infancy, Pediatrics 49:30, 1972.
163. Moore, R. Y. and Baumann, R. J.: Intracranial bruits in children, Develop. Med. Child Neurol. 11:650, 1969.
164. Gilman, S.: Cerebral disorders after open-heart operations, New Eng. J. Med. 272:489, 1965.
165. Brennan, R. W., Patterson, R. H., and Kessler, J.: Cerebral blood flow and metabolism during cardio-pulmonary bypass: Evidence of microembolic encephalopathy, Neurology (Minneap.) 21:665, 1971.
166. Aguilar, M. J., Gerbode, F., and Hill, J. D.: Neuropathologic complications of cardiac surgery, J. Thorac. Cardiov. Surg. 61:676, 1971.
167. Stephens, J. W.: Neurological sequelae of congenital heart surgery, Arch. Neurol. 7:450, 1962.
168. Minagi, H. and Steinbach, H. L.: Roentgen appearance of anomalies associated with hypoplastic anemias of childhood: Fanconi's anemia and congenital hypoplastic anemia (erythrogenesis imperfecta), Amer. J. Roentgen. 97:100, 1966.

169. McDonald, R. and Goldschmidt, B.: Pancytopenia with congenital defects (Fanconi's anemia), Arch. Dis. Child. 35:367, 1960.
170. Baird, R. L., et al.: Studies in sickle cell anemia. XXI. Clinico-pathological aspects of neurological manifestations, Pediatrics 34:92, 1964.
171. Greer, M. and Schotland, D.: Abnormal hemoglobin as a cause of neurologic disease, Neurology (Minneap.) 12:114, 1962.
172. Pearson, H. A. and Diamond, L. K.: The critically ill child: Sickle cell disease crises and their management, Pediatrics 48:629, 1971.
172a.Logothetis, J., et al.: Thalassemia major (homozygous beta-thalassemia), Neurology (Minneap.) 22:294, 1972.
172b.McCarthy, D. J., et al.: Erythrocyte phosphoglycerate kinase (PGK) deficiency in brothers with associated neurologic disorder, Pediat. Res. 6:425, 1972.
173. Evans, A. E.: Central nervous system involvement in children with acute leukemia, Cancer 17:256, 1964.
174. Pierce, M. I.: Neurologic complications in acute leukemia in children, Pediat. Clin. N. Amer. 9:425, 1962.
175. Hardisty, R. M. and Norman, P. M.: Meningeal leukemia, Arch. Dis. Child. 42:441, 1967.
176. Evans, A. E., D'Angio, G. J., and Mitus, A.: Central nervous system complications of children with acute leukemia, J. Pediat. 64:94, 1964.
176a.Kay, H. E. M., et al.: Severe neurological damage associated with methotrexate therapy, Lancet 2:542, 1971.
177. Mitus, A.: Dexamethasone: Its effectiveness in treatment of acute symptoms of meningeal leukemia, Amer. J. Dis. Child. 117:307, 1969.
178. Sullivan, M. P.: Leukemic infiltration of meninges and spinal nerve roots, Pediatrics 32:63, 1963.
179. Hunt, W. E., Bouroncle, B. A., and Meagher, J. N.: Neurologic complications of leukemias and lymphomas, J. Neurosurg. 16:135, 1959.
180. Sandler, S. G., Tobin, W., and Henderson, E. S.: Vincristine induced neuropathy, Neurology (Minneap.) 19:367, 1969.
181. Evans, A. E.: Cerebrospinal fluid of leukemic children without central nervous system manifestations, Pediatrics 31:1024, 1963.
182. Sparling, H. J., Jr., Adams, R. D., and Parker, F., Jr.: Involvement of the nervous system by malignant lymphoma, Medicine (Balt.) 26:285, 1947.
183. Sohn, D., Valensi, Q., and Miller, S. P.: Neurologic manifestations of Hodgkin's disease, Arch. Neurol. 17:429, 1967.
184. Morecki, R. and Porro, R. S.: Progressive multifocal leukoencephalopathy, Arch. Neurol. 22:253, 1970.
184a.Jamieson, P. A. and Price, R. A.: Nonleukemic disease of the central nervous system in childhood lymphocytic leukemia, Proc. Amer. Ass. Cancer Res. 14:127, 1973.

185. Singer, R. P. and Schneider, R. C.: The successful management of intracerebral and subarachnoid hemorrhage in a hemophilic infant, Neurology (Minneap.) 12:293, 1962.

186. Olsen, E. R.: Intracranial surgery in hemophiliacs, Arch. Neurol. 21:401, 1969.

187. Smith, C. H.: *Blood Diseases of Infancy and Childhood*, St. Louis: C. V. Mosby Co., 1966.

188. Matoth, Y., Zaizov, R., and Frankel, J. J.: Minimal cerebral dysfunction in children with chronic thrombocytopenia, Pediatrics 47:698, 1971.

189. Lewis, I. C. and Philpott, M. G.: Neurological complications in the Schönlein-Henoch syndrome, Arch. Dis. Child. 31:369, 1956.

190. O'Brien, J. L. and Sibley, W. A.: Neurologic manifestations of thrombotic thrombocytopenic purpura, Neurology (Minneap.) 8:55, 1958.

191. Sokoloff, L., et al.: Mechanisms of stimulation of protein synthesis by thyroid hormones in vivo, Proc. Nat. Acad. Sci. USA 60:652, 1968.

192. Fisher, D. A., et al.: Thyroid function in the preterm fetus, Pediatrics 46:208, 1970.

193. Wilkins, L.: The effects of thyroid deficiency upon the development of the brain, Ass. Res. Nerv. Ment. Dis. Proc. 39:150, 1962.

194. Schultz, M. A., et al.: Development of electroencephalographic sleep phenomena in hypothyroid infants, Electroenceph. Clin. Neurophysiol. 25:351, 1968.

195. Batsakis, J. G. and Nishiyama, R. H.: Deafness with sporadic goiter: Pendred's syndrome, Arch. Otolaryng. (Chicago) 76:401, 1962.

196. Kocher, T.: Zur Verhutung des Cretinismus und cretinoider Zustande nach neuen Forschungen, Deutsch. Z. Chir. 34:556, 1892.

197. Debré, R. and Semelaigne, G.: Syndrome of diffuse muscular hypertrophy in infants causing an athletic appearance. Its connection with congenital myxedema, Amer. J. Dis. Child. 50:1351, 1935.

198. Cross, H. E., et al.: Familial agoitrous cretinism accompanied by muscular hypertrophy, Pediatrics, 41:413, 1968.

199. Spiro, A. J., et al.: Cretinism with muscular hypertrophy (Kocher-Debré-Semelaigne syndrome): Histochemical and ultrastructural study of skeletal muscle, Arch. Neurol. 23:340, 1970.

200. Andersen, H. S.: Studies in hypothyroidism in children, Acta Paediat. Suppl. 125, 1961.

201. Smith, D. W., Blizzard, R. M., and Wilkins, L.: The mental prognosis in hypothyroidism of infancy and childhood, Pediatrics 19:1011, 1957.

202. Klein, A., Meltzer, S., and Kenny, F. M.: Improved prognosis in congenital hypothyroidism treated before three months, J. Pediat. 81:912, 1972.

203. Mosier, H. D.: "Hyperthyroidism," in Gardner, L. I. (ed.): *Endocrine and Genetic Diseases of Childhood*, Philadelphia: W. B. Saunders Co., 1969, p. 268.

204. Jefferson, A.: A clinical correlation between encephalopathy and papilloedema in Addison's disease, J. Neurol. Neurosurg. Psychiat. 19:21, 1956.

205. Stewart, B. M.: The hypertrophic neuropathy of acromegaly, Arch. Neurol. 14:107, 1966.

206. Milunsky, A., Cowie, V. A., and Donoghue, E. C.: Cerebral gigantism in childhood, Pediatrics 40:395, 1967.

206a. Ott, J. E. and Robinson, A.: Cerebral gigantism, Amer. J. Dis. Child. 117:357, 1969.

207. Zellweger, H. and Schneider, H. J.: Syndrome of hypotonia, hypomentia-hypogonadism-obesity (HHHO) or Prader-Willi syndrome, Amer. J. Dis. Child. 115:588, 1968.

208. Smith, D. W., Lemli, L., and Opitz, J. M.: A newly recognized syndrome of multiple congenital anomalies, J. Pediat. 64:210, 1964.

209. Vischer, D.: Typus degenerativus Amstelodamensis (Cornelia de Lange syndrome), Helv. Paediat. Acta 20:415, 1965.

210. McKusick, V. A., et al.: Seckel's birdheaded dwarfism, New Eng. J. Med. 277:279, 1967.

211. Seckel, H. P. G.: *Bird-headed Dwarfs*, Springfield: Charles C Thomas Publisher, 1960.

212. Menkes, J. H., et al.: A sex-linked recessive disorder with retardation of growth, peculiar hair, and focal central and cerebellar degeneration, Pediatrics 29:764, 1962.

212a. Danks, D., et al.: Menkes's kinky hair syndrome, Pediatrics 50:188, 1972.

213. McDonald, W. B., Fitch, K. D., and Lewis, I. C.: Cockayne's syndrome: A heredofamilial disorder of growth and development, Pediatrics 25:997, 1960.

214. Moosa, A. and Dubowitz, V.: Peripheral neuropathy in Cockayne's syndrome, Arch. Dis. Child. 45:674, 1970.

215. Dekaban, A.: Metabolic and chromosomal studies in leprechaunism, Arch. Dis. Child. 40:632, 1965.

216. Rubenstein, J. H. and Taybi, H.: Broad thumbs and toes and facial abnormalities: A possible mental retardation syndrome, Amer. J. Dis. Child. 105:588, 1963.

217. Richards, W., et al.: Oculocerebrorenal syndrome of Lowe, Amer. J. Dis. Child. 109:185, 1965.

218. Engels, H. J.: Oligophrenia combined with congenital cataract: Contribution on metabolic anomaly of Sjögren's syndrome, Arch. Psychiat. 208:91, 1966.

219. Börjeson, M., Forssman, H., and Lehmann, O.: An X-linked, recessively inherited syndrome characterized by grave mental deficiency, epilepsy, and endocrine disorder, Acta Med. Scand. 171:13, 1962.

220. Reed, W. R., May, S. B., and Nickel, W. R.: Xeroderma pigmentosum with neurological complications, Arch. Derm. (Chicago) 91:224, 1965.

221. Smith, D. W.: Compendium on shortness of stature, J. Pediat. 70:463, 1967.

222. Smith, D. W.: *Recognizable Patterns of Human Malformation*, Philadelphia: W. B. Saunders Co., 1970.

223. Eeg-Olofsson, O. and Petersen, I.: Childhood diabetic neuropathy, Acta Paediat. Scand. 55:163, 1966.

224. Kety, S. S., et al.: The blood flow and oxygen consumption of the human brain in diabetic acidosis and coma, J. Clin. Invest. 27:500, 1948.

225. Ohman, J. L., et al.: The cerebrospinal fluid in diabetic ketoacidosis, New Eng. J. Med. 284:283, 1971.

226. Clements, R. S., Prockop, L. D., and Winegrad, A. I.: A mechanism to explain acute cerebral edema during the treatment of diabetic acidosis, Diabetes 17:299, 1968.

227. Young, E. and Bradley, R. F.: Cerebral edema with irreversible coma in severe diabetic ketoacidosis, New Eng. J. Med. 276:665, 1967.

228. Danowski, T. S. and Nabarro, J. D. N.: Hyperosmolar and other types of nonketoacidotic coma in diabetes, Diabetes 14:162, 1965.

229. deSilva, C. C.: Common nutritional disorders of childhood in the tropics, Advances Pediat. 13:213, 1964.

230. Trowell, H. C., Davies, J. N. P., and Dean, R. F. A.: *Kwashiorkor*, London: Edward Arnold, Ltd., 1954.

231. Udani, P. M.: Neurological manifestations in kwashiorkor, Indian J. Child Health, 9:103, 1960.

232. Cravioto, J., DeLicardie, E. R., and Birch, H. G.: Nutrition, growth and neurointegrative development. An experimental and ecologic study, Pediatrics 38:319, 1966.

233. Dean, R. F. A.: The psychological changes accompanying kwashiorkor, Courrier 6:3, 1956.

234. Eichenwald, H. F. and Fry, P. C.: Nutrition and learning, Science 163:644, 1969.

235. Balmer, S., Howells, G., and Wharton, B.: The acute encephalopathy of kwashiorkor, Develop. Med. Child Neurol. 10:766, 1968.

236. Kahn, E. and Falcke, H. C.: A syndrome simulating encephalitis affecting children recovering from malnutrition (kwashiorkor), J. Pediat. 49:37, 1956.

236a.Garg, B. K. and Srivastava, J. R.: Infantile tremor syndrome, Indian J. Pediat. 36:213, 1969.

237. Cravioto, J. and Robles, B.: Evolution of adaptive and motor behavior during rehabilitation from kwashiorkor, Amer. J. Orthopsychiat. 35:449, 1965.

238. Birch, H. G., et al.: Relation of kwashiorkor in early childhood and intelligence at school age, Pediat. Res. 5:579, 1971.

239. Elliott, K. and Knight, J. (eds.): *Lipids, Malnutrition and the Developing Brain.* CIBA Foundation Symposium, London: Churchill, 1972.

240. Winick, M.: Malnutrition and brain development, J. Pediat. 74:667, 1969.

241. Fox, J. H., et al.: The effect of malnutrition on human central nervous system myelin, Neurology (Minneap.) 22:1213, 1972.

242. Graham, G. G. and Adrianzen, B. T.: Growth, inheritance and environment, Pediat. Res. 5:691, 1971.

243. Dobbing, J.: Undernutrition and the developing brain, Amer. J. Dis. Child. 120:411, 1970.

244. Scriver, C. R. and Hutchison, J. H.: Vitamin B$_6$ deficiency syndrome in human infancy: Biochemical and clinical observations, Pediatrics 31:240, 1963.

245. Keating, J. P. and Feigin, R. D.: Increased intracranial pressure associated with probable vitamin A deficiency in cystic fibrosis, Pediatrics 46:41, 1970.

246. Persson, B., Tunell, R., and Ekengren, K.: Chronic vitamin A intoxication during first half year of life: Description of five cases, Acta Paediat. Scand. 54: 49, 1965.

247. Sung, J. H.: Neuroaxonal dystrophy in mucoviscidosis, J. Neuropath. Exp. Neurol. 23:567, 1964.

248. Peters, R. A.: "Significance of Thiamine in the Metabolism and Function of the Brain," in Elliott, K. A. C., Page, I. H., and Quastel, J. H. (eds.): *Neurochemistry*, Springfield: Charles C Thomas Publisher, 1962, pp. 267–275.

249. Shimojyo, S., Scheinberg, P., and Reinmuth, O.: Cerebral blood flow and metabolism in the Wernicke-Korsakoff syndrome, J. Clin. Invest. 46:849, 1967.

250. McCandless, D. W. and Schenker, S.: Encephalopathy of thiamine deficiency: Studies of intracerebral mechanisms, J. Clin. Invest. 47:2268, 1968.

251. Dreyfus, P. M. and Hauser, G.: The effect of thiamine deficiency on the pyruvate decarboxylase system of the central nervous system, Biochim. Biophys. Acta 104:78, 1965.

252. Dreyfus, P. M.: The clinical applications of blood transketolase determinations, New Eng. J. Med. 267:596, 1962.

253. Haridas, L.: Infantile beriberi in Singapore, Arch. Dis. Child. 22:23, 1947.

254. de Wardener, H. E. and Lennox, B.: Cerebral beriberi, Lancet 1:11, 1947.

255. Haridas, G. J.: Brit. Med. Ass., Malayan branch 1:26, 1937. Cited by Spillane, J. D.: *Nutritional Disorders of the Nervous System*, Edinburgh: E. and S. Livingstone, Ltd., 1947 pp. 53–54.

256. Tower, D. B.: "Cerebral Amino Acid Metabolism and Vitamin B$_6$," in *Neurochemistry of Epilepsy*, Springfield: Charles C Thomas Publisher, 1960.

257. Scriver, C. R.: Vitamin B$_6$ dependency and infantile convulsions, Pediatrics, 26:62, 1960.

258. Bessey, O. A., Adam, D. J. D., and Hansen, A. E.: Intake of vitamin B$_6$ and infantile convulsions, Pediatrics 20:33, 1957.

259. Molony, C. J. and Parmelee, A. H.: Convulsions in young infants as a result of pyridoxine (vitamin B$_6$) deficiency, JAMA 154:405, 1954.

260. Jaffe, K. A., Altman, K., and Merryman, P.: The antipyridoxine effect of penicillamine in man, J. Clin. Invest. 43:1869, 1964.

261. French, J. H., et al.: Pyridoxine and infantile myoclonic seizures, Neurology (Minneap.) 15:101, 1965.

262. Spillane, J. D.: *Nutritional Disorders of the Nervous System*, Edinburgh: E. and S. Livingstone, Ltd., 1947.

263. Spies, T. D., Walker, A. A., and Wood, A. W.: Pellagra in infancy and childhood, JAMA 113:1481, 1939.

264. Meyer, A.: On parenchymatous systemic degeneration mainly in the central nervous system, Brain 24:47, 1901.

265. Reisner, E., et al.: Juvenile pernicious anemia, Pediatrics 8:88, 1951.

266. McNicholl, B. and Egan, B.: Congenital pernicious anemia: Effects on growth, brain, and absorption of B_{12}, Pediatrics 42:149, 1968.

267. Pearson, H. A., Vinson, R., and Smith, R. T.: Pernicious anemia with neurologic involvement in childhood, J. Pediat. 65:334, 1964.

Tumors of the Nervous System

CHAPTER 10

Incidence

Tumors of the nervous system occur relatively frequently during the early years of life. Their nature and distribution differ in major respects from those of brain tumors in adults.

Brain tumors were found in 2.2% of consecutive autopsies performed at the Great Ormond Street Children's Hospital, the highest incidence being between 5 and 10 years of age.[1] This frequency is about twice that expected in the general population.

Earlier studies on the incidence of intracranial space-occupying lesions indicate that the relative frequencies of their pathologic varieties has changed over the past forty to fifty years. Critchley (1925)[2] found tuberculoma to be the most common intracranial tumor of childhood. The more recent surveys of Bailey et al.[3] and of Cuneo and Rand (Table 10–1)[4] stressed the preponderance of gliomas. Meningiomas and neurinomas were virtually absent, except in association with neurofibromatosis.[4a] Tuberculomas are now rare in the West, but a series of 107 cases was reported from India as recently as 1965.[5]

Subtentorial tumors constitute 60%–70% of all intracranial space-occupying lesions in children. In adults only 25%–30% of tumors originate below the tentorium. However, in the first year of life, supratentorial tumors are, as in adults, in the majority, but in

TABLE 10-1.
FREQUENCY OF BRAIN TUMORS IN CHILDREN
(Percent of Total Patients in Series)

	Bailey, Buchanan, and Bucy (1939)[3]	Cuneo and Rand (1952)[4]
Subtentorial		
Cerebellar astrocytoma	24	21
Medulloblastoma	19	29
Ependymoma	7	4
Brain stem glioma	14	4
Supratentorial		
Cerebral astrocytoma	1	9
Glioblastoma and sarcoma	9	3
Intraventricular		
Ependymoma	0	4
Papilloma of choroid plexus	1	4
Craniopharyngioma	5	11
Optic glioma	10	3
Pinealoma	5	4
Meningioma	3	3
Metastatic tumor	0	3

infancy these are largely based on neoplastic change in malformed brain.

Pathogenesis

The basic mechanisms of neoplasia, at whatever age, are as yet little understood. In children, genetic factors determine the development of some tumors, as in tuberose sclerosis, neurofibromatosis, and retinoblastoma, traits transmitted by dominant inheritance. Craniopharyngiomas and some of the medulloblastomas are of congenital origin, and arise from an area of maldevelopment, the former from persistent remnants of the craniopharyngeal (Rathke's) pouch, the latter usually from primitive cell rests in the posterior medullary velum.

Postnatal factors, such as trauma, have not proven significant in the development of brain tumors in children.

General Symptomatology

Neurologic symptoms produced by brain tumors are general, due to increased intracranial pressure, the direct result of the progressive enlargement of the tumor within the limited volume of the cranial vault, and local, resulting from the effects of the tumor on contiguous areas of the brain.

Increased Intracranial Pressure. An intracranial mass produces cerebral compression by its intrinsic volume, by encroaching on the ventricular system to obstruct the flow of cerebrospinal fluid and produce ventricular dilatation and, when malignant, by producing edema in white matter adjacent to the expanding mass.

As the tumor enlarges there is an initial compression of intracranial contents, primarily of the ventricular spaces. The duration of the initial asymptomatic period depends on the rate of tumor expansion and on whether it is so located as to compromise the circulation of cerebrospinal fluid.

When the intracranial pressure approaches or equals the systemic arterial pressure it evokes an increase in the latter. Cushing noted that systemic hypertension was accompanied by bradycardia, and slow, irregular respirations, the "Cushing triad."[6,7] Compression of the venous channels, primarily those at the base of the brain, will reduce

cerebral blood flow. The resulting cerebral anoxia in turn produces vascular dilatation and a further increase in intracerebral volume and pressure.[7a]

While a number of experiments have borne out Cushing's contention that the pressure threshold for the induction of the vasopressor response is reached when intracranial pressure is at the level of systemic arterial pressure, clinical experience suggests that arterial hypertension first appears at lower pressures, particularly when there is a marked pressure differential above and below the tentorium. In these instances the pressure response may be triggered by local ischemia of the cerebral hemispheres or by distortion of the brain stem and subsequent medullary ischemia. With a further increase in intracranial pressure, the vasopressor mechanism fails, ar-

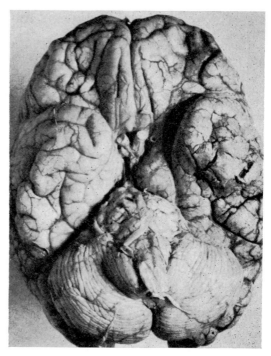

Fig. 10–1. Photograph of brain showing unusually large herniations of left hippocampal gyrus and cerebellar tonsils. The ridge clearly seen on the left uncus is due to pressure by the tentorium. A ridge on the right uncus is also seen but the herniation of this structure is minor. (From Zimmerman, H. M., Netsky, M. G., and Davidoff, L. M.: *Atlas of Tumors of the Nervous System*, 1956, courtesy of Lea & Febiger, Philadelphia.)

pseudotumor cerebri. (Courtesy of Dr. Robert Hepler, Department of Ophthalmology, UCLA, Los Angeles.)

* Adapted from Low et al.[14]

terial pressure falls, and cerebral blood flow   when sutures can be split, an enlarging head.
is substantially reduced.[8],[9]   *Headache.* Headache, a constant feature of

posterior fossa. Psychomotor seizures are the
most common seizure types seen with intracranial masses, and the temporal lobe is the
most common site for tumors producing
seizures early in the course of illness (Table
10–2).[14]

While mental disturbances or psychiatric
disorders are fairly common with brain
tumors in adults and point to lesions of the
frontal or temporal lobes, they are rarely observed in children. Children may occasionally develop drowsiness, changes in personality and irrational behavior. This suggests
hypothalamic or thalamic involvement, while
changes in sleep patterns or in appetite are
relatively common in frontal tumors.

Diagnostic Procedures

Radiologic Studies

PLAIN SKULL FILMS. Even when the patient's symptoms leave little doubt as to the
presence of an intracranial mass, radiologic
procedures are necessary to confirm the
clinical diagnosis, and to define the tumor's
extent and location. About 75% of children
who have had increased intracranial pressure
longer than six weeks show definite radiographic abnormalities. Separation of sutures, erosion or enlargement of the sella
turcica, and osteoporosis, especially thinning
of the sphenoid ridge, are the most common

TABLE 10-3.
**RADIOLOGIC EFFECTS OF INCREASED
INTRACRANIAL PRESSURE***

	Age in Years			
	2–4	5–8	9–12	13–16
Sella eroded, sutures normal	0	1	6	9
Sutures spread, sella normal	13	13	5	1
Sutures spread, sella eroded	10	14	11	2

* After du Boulay.[16]

radiologic changes[15],[16] (Fig. 10–3). Separation of sutures is rare in children over 10
and is practically nonexistent beyond the age
of 20. In estimating the width of the suture
line, Taveras has found the top of the coronal
suture, as seen in the lateral view, most
reliable. A width greater than 2 mm is
considered to be abnormal in a child aged
three years or more. Erosion of the sella is
inconspicuous in the first decade (Table
10–3).[16] In young children, sutures may
spread after a history as brief as 10 days but
this takes longer to develop in older children.
As expected, erosion of the sella is not observed until at least six weeks after the onset

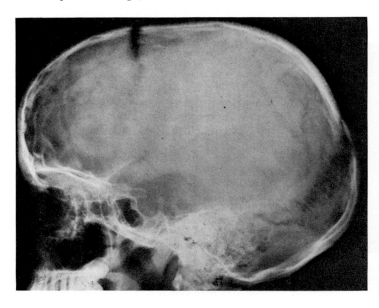

Fig. 10–3. Medulloblastoma.
Marked splitting of coronal and
lambdoidal sutures in this 12-
year-old boy. (Courtesy of Dr.
Gabriel Wilson, Department of
Radiology, UCLA, Los Angeles.)

of symptoms but also tends to occur earlier in infants than in older children. In young children erosion of the sella with suture separation suggests a perisellar destructive process.

Radiographic evidence of calcification may be seen in as high as 15%–20% of intracranial tumors of childhood, mostly in the form of clusters of multiple specks. About 50% of oligodendrogliomas, a rare tumor in childhood, develop radiologic signs of calcification.[16a] Although calcification in astrocytomas and ependymomas is much less common, these tumors are by far the leading causes of gliomatous calcification in the cerebral hemispheres. The most common tumor to produce suprasellar calcification is the craniopharyngioma, and it does so in about 70%–80% of cases, usually along the superior aspect of the mass. In tuberose sclerosis multiple calcifications varying in size from specks up to 1 cm are usually located along the ventricular walls, less often within the cerebrum and the posterior fossa.

BRAIN SCAN. Brain scanning has become an established procedure for the diagnosis of intracranial masses. Currently technetium (Tc^{99}) in the form of the pertechnetate (TcO_4) is the isotope of choice.[17] The accuracy of the scan depends on the site of the mass lesion, its nature, and its size. Tumors of the cerebral hemisphere are successfully localized by their isotope uptake in about 86% of cases.[18] Suprasellar tumors are identified in about 50% of patients, while only about one-third of posterior fossa tumors can be detected.

In general, malignant gliomas are most apt to be visualized by this method, while the frequency of negative scans is highest in astrocytomas of low-grade malignancy.[19] As a rule, tumors smaller than 2–3 cm are not detectable.[19a] Occasionally, the uptake of pertechnetate by the choroid plexus may interfere with the interpretation of the scan. The uptake may be blocked by administering iodide in the form of Lugol's solution 24 hours prior to injection of the isotope, or preferably by the use of potassium perchlorate given one hour prior to the procedure.

Although brain scan primarily detects and localizes tumors, other intracranial lesions may also be demonstrated (Table 10–4).[20]

ECHOENCEPHALOGRAPHY. The use of ultrasound in the diagnosis of intracranial masses was first introduced by Dussik in 1942.[21] The current method is based on the finding that sound waves are reflected from interfaces created within organs by contiguous media with different acoustic properties. Within the brain the most prominent echoes are those produced by interfaces between the cerebrospinal fluid and the brain.

High frequency pulsed sound at 0.5–18 Mc/sec is produced by piezoelectric transducers. With the commonly employed one-dimensional technique (A-scan), the transducer is kept in a fixed position and also serves as receiver of the reflected waves. The echo is displayed as a vertical deflection of the horizontal sweep of the cathode ray beam. This allows a measurement of the distance of the interface source of the echo to the face of the transducer.

In two-dimensional echoencephalography (B-scan) the transducer is moved mechanically in a direction perpendicular to the ultrasound beam, and a two-dimensional picture of the reflecting surfaces is formed on the screen.[22]

The presence of an intracranial mass is detected by a shift in the midline structures, particularly the 3rd ventricle, and in the case of a posterior fossa lesion producing obstruc-

TABLE 10-4.
THE DISTRIBUTION OF POSITIVE PERTECHNETATE SCANS IN NON-NEOPLASTIC LESIONS*

Lesion	Positive Scans
Arteriovenous malformation	14 (14/14)†
Subdural and epidural hematoma	9 (9/9)†
Vascular occlusion	18 (18/22)†
Intracerebral hematoma	8 (8/9)†
Abscess	1
Encephalitis	2
Contusion	1
Craniectomy defect	5
Subarachnoid hemorrhage	2
Meningitis	1
Sturge-Weber disease	1

* From Witcofski et al.[20]
† Proven by angiography, surgery, or autopsy.

tive hydrocephalus, by the increased size of the lateral ventricles.

ELECTROENCEPHALOGRAPHY. A somewhat less valuable adjunct to the localization of an intracranial mass lesion is the electroencephalogram. This procedure is most applicable to supratentorial tumors, particularly those within the frontal and parietal regions, which are relatively uncommon lesions in children.[23] Areas of focal slowing often correspond to the position of the tumor. When the tumor is in the posterior fossa, or the suprasellar region, two favorite sites for tumors occurring in infancy and childhood, normal tracings are common, and when abnormalities occur they are related to an increase in intracranial pressure and to impaired consciousness. A normal EEG in the presence of severe papilledema is suggestive of a posterior fossa tumor. The EEG is perhaps of greatest value in detecting temporal lobe tumors in children with temporal lobe seizures. In such patients the prominence of local slow wave activity, overshadowing spike and sharp wave activity usually associated with seizures, suggests an expanding lesion.

CEREBROSPINAL FLUID. The dangers attending lumbar puncture in the presence of increased intracranial pressure should be weighed against the value of the information gained by examining the cerebrospinal fluid.[23a] Abnormalities of the cerebrospinal fluid encountered in children harboring brain tumors include an increase in pressure and an elevated protein content.

In 70% of children with brain tumors intracranial pressure is increased, although in general, pressure readings are not as high as those seen in purulent meningitis. In 70% the protein is increased. Pleocytosis occurs in only 30%. This contrasts with the 75% incidence of pleocytosis seen in brain abscesses. In general the pleocytosis is not striking and counts greater than 100 are uncommon.[24]

In about one-third of cases, most commonly in tumors within or in close relation to the ventricular system, the cerebrospinal fluid is xanthochromic indicating an exceptionally high protein level.

Cerebrospinal fluid sugar is almost always normal, except that it is reduced in some children with leukemic or lymphosarcomatous infiltration of the meninges, and in meningeal carcinomatosis secondary to an ependymoma, a melanosarcoma, or a malignant tumor of the meninges.[25]

Cytology can be obtained on the cerebrospinal fluid after centrifugation and can assist in determining whether there has been spread to the meninges or to the spinal subarachnoid space, as may occur in a medulloblastoma.

The concentration of cerebrospinal fluid desmosterol is increased in patients with intracranial tumors.[26] Desmosterol, a precursor of cholesterol, is a normal constituent of growing brain but is hardly detectable in the mature organ. Total sterol synthesis is increased in neoplastic nervous tissue, and incorporation of labeled precursors into desmosterol is greatest in the more malignant tumors. A biochemical test for the diagnosis of brain tumors, based on the elevation of CSF desmosterol after five days of oral triparanol administration, has been proposed by Fumagalli and Paoletti.[26] The usefulness of this test in determining whether a tumor has been completely removed by surgery or irradiation is still under study.[27]

ARTERIOGRAPHY. The visualization of cerebral blood vessels by the injection of radiopaque dyes was introduced by Moniz in 1927.[27a] Currently various techniques are used for arteriography in children, most commonly cannulation of the brachial or femoral arteries under direct visualization. The exact amount injected depends on the size of the child, but generally 8–20 cc of 50% Hypaque are injected by reflux, and filling of both the carotid and vertebral-basilar system is obtained. Lateral and anterior-posterior views of the skull are taken simultaneously or with successive injections. Tumors of the cerebral hemispheres are localized by the distortion of the normal vascular patterns of the carotid arterial or venous system, or by the presence of abnormal vasculature.[15]

In posterior fossa lesions, displacement of the vertebral-basilar system is used for diagnosis. In children the incidence of complications, most of which are related to the presence of atheromatous vascular disease, is less than in adults. However, temporary occlusion of the artery as a result of intramural injection of contrast medium is not rare but can be avoided by obtaining scout films. The induction of an arteriovenous fistula resulting in the loss of a forearm has been reported.

PNEUMOENCEPHALOGRAPHY AND VENTRICULOGRAPHY. In 1918 Dandy[28] introduced the technique of visualizing the cerebral ventricles and subarachnoid spaces by the injection of air into the lumbar spinal canal. For the technique of this procedure the reader is referred to the monographs of Taveras and Wood[15] and Robertson.[29]

In general, localization of intracranial neoplasms relies on the presence of abnormalities in ventricular size and location.

In children with increased intracranial pressure, ventriculography appears to be a safer procedure than pneumoencephalography. Within recent years some have expanded the indications for pneumoencephalography in the belief that the dangers of cerebellar herniation, the most feared complication, are relatively slight when small amounts of air are injected fractionally without withdrawing any spinal fluid, and that sudden deterioration of a patient with a posterior fossa tumor may also occur spontaneously.[30] However, in 8% of tumor patients, the presence of a posterior fossa tumor may, by impaction of the cerebellar tonsils in the foramen magnum, block the entry of air into the skull and in this manner prevent filling of the ventricles.

Often introduction of air into the ventricular system produces a cellular reaction the intensity of which depends in part on the amount of air introduced. The count may reach 500 monocytes per mm^3 within 24 hours after the procedure, but the protein and sugar content remain normal or may decrease.[30a] Other complications of pneumoencephalography include hypotensive episodes, particularly after extensive fluid-air exchange, and focal or generalized seizures. Transient increases in neurologic deficits may result from the anesthesia employed in the procedure.

Which contrast study to use in a given patient with an intracranial mass is often difficult to decide. Hemisphere lesions generally require arteriography, while midline lesions, such as craniopharyngiomas, and posterior fossa tumors when uncomplicated by increased intracranial pressure, as is usually the case for pontile gliomas, are best visualized with pneumoencephalography. When there is increased intracranial pressure, a ventriculogram is indicated. Whenever both arteriography and air studies are contemplated, the former should be done first, since the occasional exacerbation of neurologic symptoms following the latter will require prompt surgery. Furthermore, arteriography by itself will show the presence of hydrocephalus, tentorial or tonsillar herniations, and midline shifts.

Differential Diagnosis

Increased intracranial pressure is encountered not only in brain tumors, but also in various other mass lesions within the cranium. The most common of these are brain abscesses (Table 10–5).[31] As described in greater detail in Chapter 6, they may result from the direct spread of bacteria from an

TABLE 10-5.
DIFFERENTIAL DIAGNOSIS OF INTRACRANIAL TUMORS*

Patients Suspected of Tumor	
Condition	Number
Pseudopapilledema	1
Optic neuritis	1
Tuberculous meningitis	1
Postvaccinal encephalitis	1
Sudanophilic diffuse sclerosis (Schilder's)	1
Hysteria	1

Patients with Mistaken Diagnosis of Tumor	
Condition	Number
Brain abscess	5
Lead poisoning	2
Occlusion of foramina of Magendie and Luschka	2
Hemangioma	1
Subdural hematoma	1
Aqueductal atresia	1
Tuberculoma	1
Venous sinus thrombosis	1

* After Bailey et al.[3]

when this is followed by radiotherapy. Medulloblastomas are very radiosensitive, and the whole cerebrospinal axis is irradiated with a minimum total dose of 3500 R–4000 R to the posterior fossa[42] over the course of some six weeks. Prophylactic treatment of the spinal cord should use about 2500 R–3000 R.

With this amount of radiation, bone marrow depression is not unusual, and may require brief interruption of treatment. Epilation will always occur, but the hair will usually regrow within two to six months. With large doses of radiation, headache, vomiting, general lassitude, and impairment of consciousness are common. Occasionally there is a transitory aggravation of neurologic manifestations, appearing within one day to six weeks after the start of radiation.[43] These symptoms have been attributed to an accumulation of fluid in the extracellular spaces[44] and increased intracranial pressure, although there is little clinical or experimental evidence documenting the latter.[45] Side effects are treated symptomatically with dexamethasone, chlorpromazine, or a combination of the two. The usefulness of antitumor agents appears to be quite limited, although vincristine may have a place in the management of recurrent tumors.[46]

With the newer method of irradiation the 5- and 10-year survival rate has been as high as 77% and 50% respectively,[42] with none of the long-term survivors having clinical evidence of recurrence.

While ependymomas can ordinarily not be totally removed since they involve the vital floor of the 4th ventricle, they grow so slowly that with relief of increased intracranial pressure through a shunting procedure and irradiation, long-term survivals are relatively common, as for instance in 5 out of 19 cases of Ingraham and Matson's series.[41]

TUMORS OF THE BRAIN STEM

Tumors of the brain stem produce a clinical picture which is quite variable in its initial presentation but uniform in its progression to a fatal termination. Regardless of their actual histology, these tumors are for practical purposes malignant, since, due to their location, they are inaccessible to surgery and they are only transiently responsive to irradiation.

Pathology

Most commonly this tumor arises from the pons and presents as a symmetric enlargement of the brain stem, bulging into the floor of the 4th ventricle, a pathologic feature termed "pontile hypertrophy." On microscopic examination, the glioma is seen to be composed of elongated bipolar cells, resembling a fibrillary astrocytoma.[32] Characteristically cells grow by insinuating themselves between preexisting structures, separating but not destroying them (Fig. 10–9). Like astrocytomas of the cerebral hemispheres, and in contrast to cerebellar astrocytomas, these tumors tend to anaplasia, and certain areas, primarily those in the depth of the tumor, ultimately resemble glioblastoma multiforme. Metastasis and invasion of the meninges are rare.

Clinical Manifestations

Brain stem tumors are characterized by the combined presence of four major features: cranial nerve palsies, pyramidal tract signs, cerebellar signs, and progression to advanced stages, usually without increase in intracranial pressure.[47]

In contrast to the comparatively uniform evolution of the clinical picture in cerebellar tumors, the initial symptoms of a brain stem neoplasm are quite variable.

Symptoms appear between 2 and 12 years of age, with peak incidence at six years. Vomiting and disturbances of gait are the most common presenting complaints. Less frequent is the gradual or rapid onset of a hemiparesis, or evidence of cranial nerve involvement, especially facial weakness, strabismus, or difficulties in swallowing. The presence of a head tilt and changes in personality are other relatively common early signs (Table 10–8).[47]

Vomiting, unaccompanied by headache, is another common early symptom, due not to increased intracranial pressure but to direct infiltration of the medullary vomiting center. Impairment of gait is in part due to involvement of the cerebellum or its peduncles, and in part the result of hemiparesis. The inci-

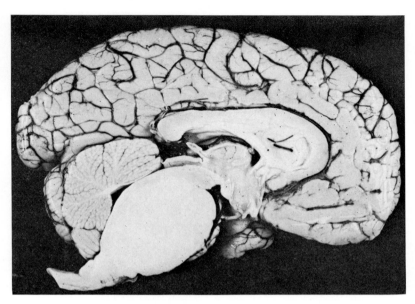

Fig. 10–9. Glioma of the brain stem. Tumor has diffusely infiltrated the brain stem, producing "hypertrophy." Note relative lack of dilatation of lateral ventricles. (Courtesy of Dr. P. Cancilla, Department of Pathology, UCLA, Los Angeles.)

TABLE 10-8.
INCIDENCE OF NEUROLOGIC SYMPTOMS IN 48 CHILDREN WITH BRAIN STEM TUMORS*

Symptom	Number
Gait disturbance	47
Squint	25
Vomiting	22
Headache	21
Dysarthria	19
Facial weakness	15
Personality change	11
Dysphagia	10
Drowsiness	10
Head tilt	5
Hearing loss	4

* From Bray et al.[47]

TABLE 10-9.
INCIDENCE OF NEUROLOGIC SIGNS IN CHILDREN WITH BRAIN STEM TUMORS*

Neurologic Signs	Number
Pyramidal tract signs	41/48
Cranial nerve involvement	
VII	64/78
IX and X	54/78
VI	48/78
V (sensory)	38/78
V (motor)	13/48
XII	13/48
VIII	12/78
Cerebellar signs	62/78
Nystagmus	
Horizontal	26/48
Vertical	14/14
Papilledema	24/78
Gaze paralysis	
Horizontal	22/48
Vertical	5/48
Hemisensory deficit	5/48

* From Bray et al.[47] and Ingraham and Matson.[41]

dence of various neurologic signs found in affected children are listed in Table 10–9. They result from involvement of the major structures within the brain stem: the pyramidal tracts, the nuclei of the various cranial nerves, and the cortico-ponto-cerebellar fibers. Corticospinal tracts are usually involved early. Patients develop a spastic hemiparesis, increased deep tendon reflexes, and an extensor plantar response.

The cranial nerves most commonly affected by the neoplasm are the seventh and the sixth. Since the nucleus of the facial nerve is involved, facial weakness is almost invariably of lower motor neuron type. Dysfunction of the ninth and tenth nerves leads to drooling, difficulty in swallowing, and, not rarely, to insidious loss of weight. Sixth nerve weakness is often associated with horizontal conjugate gaze palsy, and is thus due to involvement of the brain stem and not a false localizing sign associated with increased intracranial pressure.

Functions of some of the other structures within the brain stem, notably the sensory pathways within the medial lemniscus, appear to be more resistant to tumor encroachment, and hemisensory deficits are rare. Occasionally infiltration of the reticular substances will produce alterations in personality, changes in eating and sleeping patterns, drowsiness, and coma without increased intracranial pressure.

The progression of symptoms is relentless. As one after the other of the cranial nerves become involved, patients become unable to swallow or speak, the extremities become completely paralyzed, and finally impairment of consciousness with deepening coma, and respiratory or cardiac irregularities terminate the course. The average survival time is about nine months from the date of the patient's first hospitalization.

Diagnosis

The clinical features of a brain stem neoplasm are usually confirmed by x-ray studies. The cerebrospinal fluid pressure at the time of pneumoencephalography is almost always normal; there is no pleocytosis, and the protein level is rarely increased. On radiography of the skull, evidence for increased intracranial pressure is usually absent, and the tumor does not calcify. Satisfactory pneumoencephalograms with tomography of the posterior fossa will demonstrate a normal or only slightly dilated ventricular system, with the aqueduct of Sylvius and the floor of the 4th ventricle displaced upward and posteriorly (Fig. 10–10).

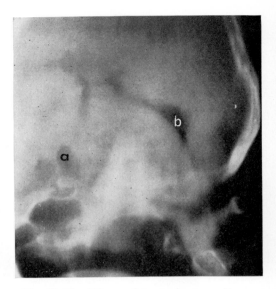

Fig. 10–10. Glioma of the brain stem. Pneumoencephalogram, lateral view. The brain stem is markedly enlarged, as the cisterna pontis (a) is pushed forward, and the floor of the fourth ventricle (b) is pushed up. (Courtesy of Dr. Gabriel Wilson, Department of Radiology, UCLA, Los Angeles.)

Occasionally contrast studies cannot establish the diagnosis beyond reasonable doubt. Under these circumstances it is advisable to proceed to suboccipital craniotomy, visualization, and, if possible, biopsy of the tumor. Very rarely classic symptoms and signs of a brain stem glioma have receded spontaneously with complete recovery, a condition termed brain stem encephalitis.[47a] Cysts located anterior to the brain stem, and conceivably amenable to surgery, may also produce a similar clinical picture.[48]

Treatment

The location of the tumor makes a surgical approach impossible. Radiation therapy has produced transient clinical remissions in about 60% of children. The initial improvement is first noted about three to six weeks after the onset of treatment, most commonly as partial clearing of the cranial nerve signs. Bray and co-workers have found that, on the average, radiotherapy prolongs survival by about six months.[47] Survival time correlates with histologic diagnosis, with the average survival for astrocytomas being $2\frac{1}{2}$ years, but only six months for anaplastic tumors.[48a] The response to a second course of irradiation is usually poor.

MIDLINE TUMORS

A number of pathologically diverse tumors arising from the midline of the supratentorial region will here be grouped together since their initial clinical picture has common features. These include the insidious development of increased intracranial pressure, visual impairment, abnormalities of endocrine or metabolic function, and alterations of consciousness or personality.

Most common are the craniopharyngioma and the glioma of the optic nerve. Other tumors such as pinealomas, and various intraventricular neoplasms such as colloid cysts of the 3rd ventricle, papillomas of the choroid plexus, and ependymomas of the lateral or 3rd ventricle are much rarer (Table 10–1).

CRANIOPHARYNGIOMA

Pathology

The craniopharyngioma is located in the suprasellar region in 43% of patients, and both intra- and suprasellar in 53%. Purely intrasellar craniopharyngiomas are therefore rare in childhood. The tumor is believed to arise from small rests of squamous cells, normally encountered at the junction of the stalk with the pars distalis of the pituitary gland, and considered to represent remnants of the embryonal Rathke's pouch. The tumor would then already be present at birth, but due to its slow growth symptoms may be delayed for years to several decades. As the tumor expands forward it begins to compress the optic chiasm. With downward expansion the pituitary gland is compressed, and with upward expansion the 3rd ventricle becomes distorted (Fig. 10–11). Large tumors are partly or completely cystic and contain a cloudy, brown fluid with a high concentration of cholesterol. Micro-

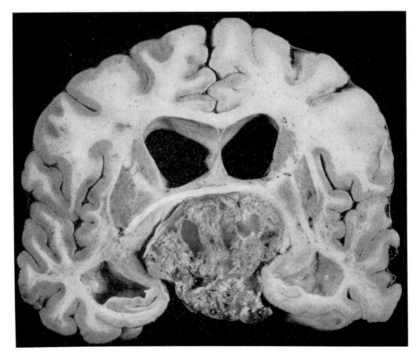

Fig. 10–11. Craniopharyngioma. Large tumor obstructing third ventricle and causing hydrocephalus. (From Merritt, H. H.: *A Textbook of Neurology*, 4th ed., 1970, courtesy of Lea & Febiger, Philadelphia.)

pituitary are extremely rare in childhood, and unless they produce gigantism or acromegaly are usually not diagnosed before the operation or autopsy. Suprasellar meningiomas are equally rare in children. Pinealomas, particularly those with extensions or implantations into the anterior portion of the 3rd ventricle, may be mistaken for suprasellar cysts. These tumors tend to compress the upper part of the mesencephalon and produce paralysis of upward gaze, impaired pupillary light reaction, and precocious puberty. At other times they may present with increased intracranial pressure due to meningeal invasion.

Chordomas, arising from the base of the sphenoid bone, may involve the chiasm.[53] Radiography reveals marked destruction of the pyramids and clivus, thus differentiating this lesion from a craniopharyngioma. When tumors of the anterior 3rd ventricle produce symptoms during infancy, the diencephalic syndrome is produced. Its outstanding features, as described by Russell,[54] are marked emaciation in spite of normal food intake, hypoglycemia, hyperkinetic behavior, vomiting, a characteristic pale, elflike facies and exceptional alertness or euphoria. Visual impairment becomes evident during the latter months of the illness. Contrast studies will be diagnostic and reveal a filling defect in the 3rd ventricle. Tumors producing this syndrome are usually astrocytomas of the 3rd ventricle, or optic gliomas.

Treatment and Prognosis

In favorable cases, complete surgical removal of the craniopharyngioma is possible.[55] Puncture of the cyst and evacuation of its content produce temporary relief. Radiotherapy or the instillation of radioactive gold (Au[198]) may be beneficial in those cases in which subtotal removal is impossible but may also aggravate endocrine disturbances by damaging the surrounding tissue.[56]

Following surgery endocrine disturbances are generally exacerbated. When diabetes insipidus develops transiently, correction by fluid replacement is usually adequate. For prolonged or permanent diabetes insipidus, injection of pitressin is indicated.[57] Other endocrine abnormalities may occur post-

operatively. Their correction and the schedule of preoperative endocrine therapy are reviewed by Kenny and associates.[58]

Craniopharyngiomas grow so slowly that even without operation the average life expectancy is three to four years from the onset of symptoms. Forty percent of operated patients survive eight years or longer.

GLIOMAS OF THE OPTIC NERVE

Pathology

This tumor arises from the optic nerve within or outside the orbit, as a fusiform dilatation of the nerve. Neoplasms arising within the orbit tend to spread through the optic foramina and expand into the cranium in a dumbbell fashion. Tumors arising from the optic chiasm may invade the 3rd ventricle and hypothalamus, or grow inferiorly to compress the pituitary gland.[59] The neoplasm consists of a mixture of astrocytes, like those seen in cerebellar astrocytomas and oligodendroglia.[32] Many optic nerve tumors are associated with neurofibromatosis. Here the neoplasm is usually a glioma, less often a meningioma of the optic sheath.[4a]

Clinical Manifestations

The various signs and symptoms seen in patients with this tumor are depicted in Table 10–11.[60] In about one-half of the patients poor vision is the initial symptom. In infancy, this may become evident as searching nystagmus, or failure to fix on and follow objects. Deterioration of eyesight may progress so insidiously that children may present with an apparent sudden loss of vision. When the tumor grows anteriorly, exophthalmos develops. Since this is easily recognized, patients with this symptom have a relatively shorter illness prior to hospitalization than those whose tumor expands into the 3rd ventricle.

Other ocular symptoms such as strabismus are less frequent presenting symptoms, and are usually secondary to impaired vision. Between 10% and 50% of patients have either the clinical features or a family history of neurofibromatosis. Increased intracranial pressure and such endocrine abnormalities

TABLE 10-11.
SYMPTOMS AND SIGNS IN 56 CHILDREN WITH OPTIC GLIOMA*

	Initial Symptom	Presenting Sign
Diminished visual acuity	28	53
Exophthalmos	25	29
Nystagmus	8	14
Strabismus	6	17
Field cut	1	12
Disc change		
Pallor		36
Pallor and blurring		11
Blurring		8
Increased intracranial pressure	3	15
Enlarged head	1	4
Multiple café-au-lait spots		12
Hemiparesis		4

* From Chutorian et al.[60]

as precocious puberty, diabetes insipidus, and growth retardation are uncommon early symptoms of optic gliomas. They indicate that the tumor has extended into the area surrounding the 3rd ventricle, and are therefore associated with a poor prognosis.

Almost all children have abnormalities of the optic discs. These consist of primary optic atrophy, papilledema, or a mixture of the two. These findings accompany a variety of visual field defects.

Diagnosis

The most constant radiologic abnormality seen in gliomas of the optic nerve is enlargement of one optic foramen. In about 10% of patients both optic foramina are enlarged (Fig. 10–14). In patients with normal foramina, the tumor is either entirely within the orbit, or within the cranium. A characteristic pear or J-shaped deformity of the sella, produced by the erosion of the tuberculum sellae and the anterior clinoid processes, is seen in about 50% of children.[61] This radiographic abnormality is not diagnostic of an optic glioma, since a somewhat similar deformity is seen in children with Down's syndrome, Hurler's disease, and in some 5%

of normal population. Pneumoencephalography will confirm the retrograde spread of the tumor. Calcifications within the tumor are rare and are usually indicative of meningiomas of the optic sheath.

Treatment and Prognosis

When the tumor is confined to the optic nerve, the prognosis is excellent, while the outlook is uncertain when tumors have extended into the 3rd ventricle. Partial resection of the tumor through a transcranial approach has been advocated, but radiotherapy alone often arrests the slow growth of the tumor and can partially restore vision.[62] On follow-up examinations tumor size can be estimated in the older child by repeated visual field charting and measurement of the diameter of the optic foramina. In the very young repeated brain scans or pneumoencephalography may be necessary.

PINEALOMAS

On histologic examination at least four types of neural tumors can be distinguished: 1) pinealomas, which arise from the pineal parenchyma cells; 2) teratomas, the most frequent intracranial site of which is the pineal body or structures immediately surrounding it; 3) epidermoid cysts; and 4) gliomas. Russell and Sachs consider atypical teratomas to be the most common pineal tumor.[63]

Clinical Manifestations

Pinealoma occurs predominantly in males. The tumor induces increased intracranial pressure, which often arises acutely as a result of aqueductal obstruction or meningeal infiltration. Other neurologic signs are those caused by pressure on the corpora quadrigemina, notably limitation of conjugate upward gaze, impaired pupillary light reaction, and central deafness. Cerebellar signs, resulting from transmitted pressure, and finally endocrine dysfunction are also observed. Diabetes insipidus, the most common endocrine abnormality, is seen in 32% of patients (Table 10–12).[64] Precocious puberty is present in about 40% of patients under the age of 15 years, almost all of these being males. Seventy percent of patients with this abnor-

TABLE 10-12.
EYE SIGNS IN PINEAL TUMORS*

Signs	Percent
Dilated pupils	31
Impaired light reaction	50
Diplopia	25
Nystagmus	38
Limitation of upward gaze	31
Papilledema	56
Abducens palsy	25

* From Posner and Horrax.[64]

mality have other signs of hypothalamic disturbance, including obesity, somnolence, polyphagia, and diabetes insipidus.

Diagnosis

Impaired upward gaze and precocious puberty in a male should always suggest a hypothalamic tumor. However, the exact histologic diagnosis of the lesion often cannot be determined on clinical grounds alone. Occasionally radiograms of the skull may help. A calcified pineal is normally rarely seen before the age of 10. Calcium deposits in the pineal area at an earlier age, or extensive calcifications at any age should suggest a pinealoma.

Treatment and Prognosis

The direct surgical approach to these tumors is hazardous, and fatalities in the immediate postoperative period are high. Radiotherapy preceded by a shunting procedure, such as 3rd ventriculostomy, or perforation of the anterior wall of the 3rd ventricle is more promising. Nine out of eleven of Davidoff's patients treated in this manner were alive 9–24 years after diagnosis.[65]

TUMORS OF LATERAL AND THIRD VENTRICLES

Intraventricular tumors are rare in children. The most common histologic types encountered are ependymomas, papillomas of the choroid plexus and lateral ventricles, and colloid cysts arising from the 3rd ventricle.

The clinical picture is usually one of progressive increase in intracranial pressure.

In some instances of 3rd ventricular colloid cysts, particularly those located in the vicinity of the foramen of Monro, symptoms may appear acutely or intermittently with paroxysmal attacks of headache and vomiting, terminated by a brief period of unconsciousness, with complete but transient recovery.[66,67]

TUMORS OF THE CEREBRAL HEMISPHERES

Tumors of the cerebral hemispheres are less frequent in children than in adults. In children it is often difficult to arrive at an early diagnosis, since increased intracranial pressure appears late, focal signs are hard to elicit, and the high incidence of idiopathic epilepsy in childhood makes the appearance of seizures at that time less alarming than subsequently. Tumors of the cerebral hemispheres may therefore grow to enormous size before a diagnosis is made, and surgical treatment often fails.

Pathology

Most tumors in this area are gliomas. Astrocytomas in pure form, or in conjunction with other cell types such as oligodendrogliomas, or the malignant glioblastomas, are histologically the most frequent. In contrast to adults, meningiomas in children are rare, and meningeal tumors are usually highly malignant meningeal sarcomas. A number of patients have clinical or pathologic evidence of tuberose sclerosis. Metastatic tumors are rare in childhood; the only form that seeds into the central nervous system with any frequency is the neuroblastoma.

Clinical Manifestations

The clinical picture depends on the location of the tumor rather than on its histologic characteristics.[14] Signs of increased intracranial pressure, headaches, and vomiting occur in about one-half of patients, and are the initial complaints in about 25% of children. Seizures occur in about 50% of patients, most commonly in temporal lobe tumors. Many patients exhibit a combination of different seizure patterns; nearly one-half of seizure patients experience psychomotor seizures either alone, or in combination with generalized seizures, or generalized

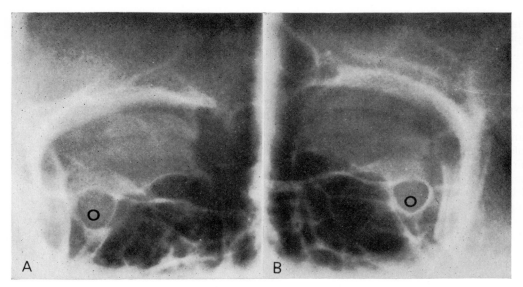

Fig. 10–14. Optic glioma. Views of optic foramina. (A) Right foramen; (B) left foramen. In this 12-year-old boy, both optic foramina (O) are quite large. The right measures almost 9 mm in its greatest diameter, and the left $7\frac{1}{2}$ mm. There is no evidence of erosion. At that age an optic foramen is considered to be enlarged if it measures over $6\frac{1}{2}$ cm in diameter or if it measures 2 mm more than the one on the opposite side. (Courtesy of Dr. Gabriel Wilson, Department of Radiology, UCLA, Los Angeles.)

TABLE 10-13.
CHARACTERISTICS OF SEIZURES IN 49 PATIENTS WITH TUMORS OF THE CEREBRAL HEMISPHERES*

	Percent
Seizure Type	
Generalized	49
Generalized with focal components	25
Psychomotor	39
Focal	39
Petit mal	0
Other seizure forms	6
Duration of Seizures before Diagnosis of Tumor	
Less than 6 months	39
6–12 months	6
1–3 years	18
3–5 years	12
5–10 years	20
Longer than 10 years	2
Location of Tumor Producing Seizures	
Temporal lobe	36
Frontal lobe	7
Parietal lobe	29
Other sites or diffuse	29

* Adapted from Low et al.[14]

seizures with a focal component. Petit-mal attacks are rarely seen (Table 10–13). A prolonged history of seizures may precede demonstration of a tumor[69] (see Chapter 11). Other symptoms are related to the presence of hemiparesis. Hemisensory signs and aphasia are rare. About 15% of patients show ataxia, usually the outcome of involvement of the fronto-ponto-cerebellar pathways but often misinterpreted as a posterior fossa mass.

Diagnosis

Plain skull films often confirm the clinical diagnosis of a cerebral hemisphere tumor. Signs of intracranial pressure, notably separation of the sutures, are seen in about one-half of patients. Calcifications were found in 23% of tumors reported by Low et al.[14] Contrast studies are usually definitive, although in some children, particularly those presenting with seizures, the tumor may be so small that initial contrast studies may be normal, the tumor only becoming evident subsequently. Arteriography is the procedure of choice on suspicion of hemisphere tumors.

Electroencephalography may be helpful in localizing a structural lesion, particularly in the case of tumors of the temporal lobe. The spinal fluid may be under increased pressure, with increased protein content.

Treatment

Astrocytomas of the cerebral hemispheres, even when localized to the periphery of the cerebrum and appearing well-circumscribed, infiltrate adjacent tissues so readily that complete surgical removal is usually impossible. Frontal lobe tumors can be treated by lobectomy and therefore have a better prognosis. Most gliomas are radiosensitive, and in many instances a course of radiotherapy is followed by prolonged symptomatic relief. The outlook for the patient with malignant glioblastoma or sarcoma is even poorer. Neurologic deterioration is rapid and radiotherapy may give either transitory relief or none.

SPINAL CORD TUMORS

In childhood, spinal cord neoplasms are about one-fifth as common as intracranial neoplasms. Their infrequency and the relative subtlety of neurologic signs during the early phases hinder the physician from making the diagnosis at a time when removal without paraplegia or other irreparable damage is still possible.

Pathology

Tumors may arise anywhere along the spinal cord.[70] They may be extradural, extramedullary, or intramedullary. A great variety of tumor types are encountered, with a relative frequency that differs considerably in the various reported series. Benign tumors, such as neurofibromas, dermoid cysts, and teratomas are usually extradural or extramedullary, while ependymomas and astrocytomas arise from within the spinal cord (Fig. 10–15). Intramedullary tumors are occasionally associated with syringomyelia. The interrelationship between the two conditions is still problematic, and the various hypotheses have been discussed by Poser.[71]

Clinical Manifestations

Presenting symptoms depend on whether the tumor originates within or outside the spinal cord (intra- or extramedullary). Intramedullary lesions usually produce symmetric weakness and atrophy of the affected segments, while extramedullary tumors tend to begin with unilateral pain in segmental distribution. In both types of tumors impaired gait and stiffness and pain in the back or the legs are common early complaints, although in extramedullary lesions the weakness tends to be unilateral.[72] The condition progresses to urinary incontinence and sensory deficits.

Two types of neurologic findings may be elicited: those due to segmental spinal cord

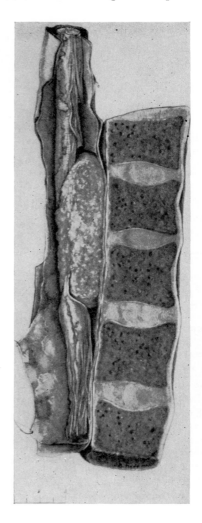

Fig. 10–15. Drawing of subdural spinal meningioma showing compression of the spinal cord. (From Zimmerman, H. M., Netsky, M. G., and Davidoff, L. M.: *Atlas of Tumors of the Nervous System*, 1956, courtesy of Lea & Febiger, Philadelphia.)

involvement, and those resulting from interruption of ascending and descending tracts within the cord. Segmental weakness, atrophy, hyporeflexia, and sensory changes result from involvement of nerve roots. Spasticity, sensory deficits to a definable spinal cord level, and sphincteric involvement are due to interruption of long tracts. Extramedullary tumors may cause a Brown-Sequard syndrome. Classically this syndrome follows hemisection of the spinal cord and includes homolateral weakness, spasticity, and ataxia, and contralateral loss of pain and temperature sensation.

In infants and small children an absolute loss of response to pin prick below a specific spinal level can usually not be established. However diminished or absent sweating below the appropriate level is frequently demonstrable on examination or by the iodine-starch sweat test, particularly in intramedullary lesions.[73] Deep tendon reflexes below the level of the lesion are exceptionally brisk in tumors compressing the spinal cord. Impaired bladder function is a late finding, which dictates emergency surgery. Initial bladder symptoms are increased urgency, followed by incontinence or retention of urine.[74,75]

Papilledema is a rare finding in spinal cord tumors and is usually related to a high cerebrospinal fluid protein. Nystagmus may accompany high cervical cord tumors.

Diagnosis

The diagnosis of a spinal cord tumor in a child rests in part on the clinical examination of the patient. The presence of pain in the back, elicited by tapping vertebral tips with a reflex hammer, or in the extremities, accompanied by either bladder or bowel dysfunction, impaired gait, muscular weakness, or curvature of the spine indicate further diagnostic studies. These should be done swiftly for the expanding tumor may compromise circulation through the anterior spinal artery, and produce sudden and irreversible paraplegia.

Plain radiograms of the spine may often suffice to confirm the diagnosis of a spinal cord tumor. In Austin's experience nearly 40% of tumors were so diagnosed.[70] One

may see gross bone destruction, erosion of spinal pedicles or vertebral bodies, and widening of the interpedicular spaces. The normal interpediculate distance varies considerably with age but norms have been compiled by Schwartz.[76]

If the presence of a cord tumor is suspected, a myelogram should be done at the time of diagnostic lumbar puncture. This is because withdrawal of spinal fluid may be followed by rapid worsening of symptoms, and there is an increased incidence of technically inadequate myelograms within the first few days following a lumbar puncture. In the presence of a block superior to the usual site for a lumbar puncture, drainage of CSF induces the collapse of the subarachnoid sac and obliteration of the subarachnoid space. The presence of a subarachnoid block is indicated by a positive Queckenstedt's test. Since this test is not without risks, and since pressure readings are difficult to obtain in children under the conditions required for it, it has largely been abandoned. Myelography will yield all the information obtained from Queckenstedt's test, and when adequate to visualize the spinal segments suspected of harboring the tumor, it is almost always diagnostic.[77] The spinal fluid protein is usually elevated, with levels proportional to the degree of block in cerebrospinal fluid circulation. When spinal cord symptoms have evolved over a period of hours or one to two days, often following a mild antecedent infection, and plain radiographs of the spine are normal, the most likely diagnosis is transverse myelitis. Under such circumstances myelography may worsen the neurologic manifestations.[78]

Therapy and Prognosis

Extramedullary tumors which can be totally removed have an excellent prognosis. However, even tumors which can be only partly removed are compatible with long periods of partial or complete symptomatic relief, particularly when surgery is followed by radiotherapy.[79] Intramedullary tumors are not suitable for surgical removal. However, here too decompression and x-ray therapy may generally give fairly long symptomatic relief. Patients with malignant tumors such as neuroblastomas and sarcomas do poorly regardless of the relationship of the tumor to the spinal cord.

THE PHAKOMATOSES
(Neurocutaneous Syndromes)

The phakomatoses are a group of hereditary diseases due to an unknown abnormality of germ plasm. They are characterized by a tendency for malformations and tumors to arise in numerous organs, notably in skin and central nervous system.

The following conditions, ranked in order of their frequency, are usually included in this group: neurofibromatosis, tuberose sclerosis, Sturge-Weber disease, von Hippel-Lindau disease, and ataxia-telangiectasia. Each will be considered in turn. Each of these conditions is distinct, and their documented appearance in combination with each other is explicable on a chance basis.

NEUROFIBROMATOSIS
(von Recklinghausen's Disease)

Neurofibromatosis is characterized by multiple tumors within the central and peripheral nervous system, cutaneous pigmentation, and lesions of the vascular system and viscera. Although it was first described in the eighteenth century, von Recklinghausen first combined the various features of the condition and termed it neurofibromatosis in 1882.[80] The disease has a frequency of approximately 1 in 2000, and is transmitted as a dominant trait with frequent incomplete or abortive forms. The classic syndrome occurs slightly more commonly in males than females.[81]

Pathology

The basic disorder is considered to be hyperplasia and neoplasia of neuroectodermal elements associated with hyperplasia of mesodermal tissues. The tumor has a multiple cell origin, as is shown by the presence of both A and B type glucose-6-phosphate dehydrogenase. A hormonal change which induces the oncogenetic mechanism in a number of cells simultaneously has been postulated.[81a] Neurofibromata occur along the major peripheral and cranial nerves.

Among the latter, the acoustic and optic nerves are most commonly involved. Multiple meningiomas, and gliomas of the cerebral and cerebellar hemispheres and spinal cord occur less often.[82] The association of neurofibromatosis with pheochromocytomas has also been established. While generally benign, both central and peripheral tumors may undergo malignant change.

Clinical Manifestations

Almost every organ can be a site for the disease process. When peripheral lesions are many, there tend to be few lesions within the central nervous system, and the reverse is also true.

Among skin lesions the most common are the café-au-lait spots. These are numerous light brown areas, usually located over the trunk, with either geographical or regular punched-out borders. According to Crowe and associates, at least six of such lesions are necessary for a diagnosis of neurofibromatosis.[81] Less frequent are diffuse freckling, freckling under the armpits, and large areas of faintly increased pigmentation (melanoderma). These pigmentary abnormalities, while usually present prior to the onset of neurologic symptoms, are not striking during infancy but intensify with age, particularly after puberty.

Various types of cutaneous tumors may be found. The most characteristic for neurofibromatosis are the pedunculated molluscum fibrosum and the subcutaneous neurofibromata. The latter are located singly or in groups along nerve trunks. As a rule these tumors tend to enlarge slowly throughout life. Plexiform neuromas may occur in all affected tissues and may lead to hypertrophy of one or more extremity, exophthalmos, or defects of the skull and orbit.

Various skeletal abnormalities have been described. Of these scoliosis is the most common, occurring in about 40% of patients. Rarely it is sufficiently severe to produce paraplegia. Bony rarefactions, ascribed to the presence of subperiosteal neurofibromas, may arise within the spine, pelvis, or skull, and may induce pathologic fractures. Bony overgrowth, often with adjacent elephantiasis, is seen in about 10% of patients.

TABLE 10–14.
NEUROLOGIC MANIFESTATIONS IN 92 PATIENTS WITH NEUROFIBROMATOSIS*

Patients without neurologic manifestations	49
Patients with neurologic manifestations	43
Intracranial tumors	15
Optic glioma	5
Bilateral acoustic tumors	1
Multiple tumors	6
Intraspinal tumors	14
Multiple tumors	6
Associated with intracranial tumors	5
Peripheral nerve tumors	10
Seizures	11
Intracranial tumors	5
Mental retardation	9
Radicular pain	4

* After Canale et al.[84]

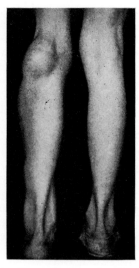

Fig. 10–16. Neurofibromatosis. Posterior view of left leg to show spherical mass in popliteal space and general enlargement of lower part of leg. Note café-au-lait spot about right popliteal area. (From Zimmerman, H. M., Netsky, M. G., and Davidoff, L. M.: *Atlas of Tumors of the Nervous System*, 1956, courtesy of Lea & Febiger, Philadelphia.)

Some patients with neurofibromas develop hypertension, due to the presence of pheochromocytomas, or occasionally to an intense subintimal proliferation within arteries of small and medium caliber.

Neurologic manifestations can be grouped into four major categories. Their incidence is presented in Table 10–14.[83,84,85,86,87,88,89]

1. Mental retardation: About 10% of patients with neurofibromatosis are mentally retarded. This symptom is related to cortical heterotopias and other malformations of cerebral architecture.

2. Intracranial tumors: These may arise at any time of life, the optic nerve being the most common and the earliest site of involvement. Bilateral acoustic neuromas occur less frequently. Their hereditary transmission has been noted in a number of families with neurofibromatosis. Focal or generalized seizures may appear early in childhood. Since nearly one-half of patients with seizures and neurofibromatosis are ultimately found to have intracranial tumors, a child with cutaneous neurofibromatosis and seizures must be suspected to have a tumor.

3. Tumors of the peripheral nerves may arise at any age and may involve any of the major nerves (Fig. 10–16). Even though these tumors are occasionally painful, surgical removal must be carefully weighed against the possibility of producing considerable neurologic deficit. Malignant degeneration of neurofibromas occurs in less than 3% of patients. Tumors may also arise within the autonomic nerve supply of various viscera. According to Kissel and Schmitt, the stomach, tongue, mediastinum, large intestines, and adrenal medulla are the most common sites.[88]

4. Intraspinal tumors: These are generally slower to develop than intracranial tumors; the youngest patient with an intraspinal tumor in Canale's series was 20 years of age,[84] while Nellhaus has seen patients aged 10 and 12 years.[78] About one-half of intraspinal tumors are multiple, and occasionally they are accompanied by malformations such as syringomyelia.

Diagnosis

The diagnosis of neurofibromatosis is not difficult in patients with the characteristic skin lesions, and multiple subcutaneous nodules. Although a solitary café-au-lait

14

spot may occur in normal individuals, the normal incidence of more than four such lesions is low, and in the absence of other symptoms of neurofibromatosis may indicate a forme fruste of the disease.[90] Conversely, some 75% of individuals with proven neurofibromatosis have six or more café-au-lait spots 1 cm or more at the largest diameter.[81]

Treatment and Prognosis

Therapy is symptomatic. Surgical removal of centrally located tumors is often lifesaving. When tumors are confined to peripheral nerves, the long-term prognosis is generally good. The outlook for intracranial tumors depends on their location, and on whether they are single or multiple.

TUBEROSE SCLEROSIS

Although the earliest report of a patient with this condition is said to have been by von Recklinghausen in 1863,[91] its first complete, albeit mainly pathologic, description is attributed to Bourneville in 1880[92] who also first called it tuberose sclerosis. This is a protean disorder, chiefly manifested by mental deficiency, epilepsy, and skin lesions. It occurs with a frequency of 1 in 30,000, and is transmitted as an autosomal dominant, with variable penetrance. A parent who only has adenoma sebaceum has a one in two risk of an affected child. No family of two or more affected siblings has been encountered in whom one parent did not have adenoma sebaceum or some other skin lesion characteristic for tuberose sclerosis.[93] It occurs two or three times more often in males than in females.

Pathology

As with the other phakomatoses, the basic cause for tuberose sclerosis is unknown. Genetic studies have shown this condition to be distinct from neurofibromatosis, but like the latter it also is a disorder of early embryogenesis.

Abnormalities may be found in the brain, eyes, skin, kidneys, bones, heart, and lungs.

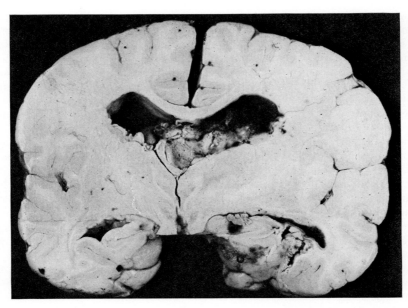

Fig. 10–17. Tuberose sclerosis. There is a large intraventricular tuber, producing increased intracranial pressure, flattening of the gyri, and herniation of the right temporal uncus (U). (Courtesy of Dr. P. Cancilla, Department of Pathology, UCLA, Los Angeles.)

The characteristic gross abnormality is the presence of numerous hard areas of gliotic tissue of varying size, the tubers, after which this condition is named. They may be located in the convolutions of any part of the cerebral hemispheres (Fig. 10–17). Multiple small tumorlike nodules project into the lateral and 3rd ventricles to give a "candle-drippings"-like appearance on pneumoencephalography. The sclerotic areas consist of an overgrowth of astrocytes, and groups of large, bizarre, and frequently vacuolated "monster cells." Blood vessels in the sclerotic regions show hyaline degeneration of their walls. Calcium is deposited within the gliotic areas sufficiently extensively to be visible radiologically.

Myelination is usually diminished in the gliotic areas. Tumors may arise from either cortical or subependymal tubers, and transitions between gliosis and astrocytomas are common. The subependymal tumors are usually located in the walls of the lateral ventricles, or on the surface of the basal ganglia, and while only rarely malignant, may often obstruct the foramen of Monro. Tumors may also arise from various viscera. In the heart the characteristic lesion is the rhabdomyoma. Eighty percent of patients develop multiple renal tumors, usually of mixed embryonal type. Lungs are rarely involved, but when there are lesions in the organ, they are usually of cystic or fibrous nature. Other organs may be the seat of fibrocellular hamartomas.[32]

Clinical Manifestations

Symptoms of tuberose sclerosis vary considerably with respect to age of onset, severity and rate of progression. There are four main types: mental retardation, seizures, cutaneous lesions, and tumors in various organs including the brain. The frequency of the major symptoms is given in Table 10–15.[94]

The degree of mental retardation varies widely. About one-third of patients diagnosed as tuberose sclerosis on the basis of other clinical manifestations maintain a normal intelligence. In others development, notably of speech, is slowed. Fifteen percent of retarded patients studied by Borberg[83] developed normally for the first few years of

TABLE 10-15.
CLINICAL PICTURE IN 71 PATIENTS WITH TUBEROSE SCLEROSIS*

Manifestation	Number of Patients
Patients with Mental Retardation	43
Seizures	43
Major motor seizures	19
Minor seizures	6
Major and minor seizures	7
Seizure onset before one year of age	28
Seizure onset before five years of age	38
Adenoma sebaceum	37
Appearance of skin lesion before two years of age	17
Appearance of skin lesion after nine years of age	2
Retinal tumors	21
Intracranial calcifications	20
Patients with Average Intelligence	26
Seizures	26
Major motor seizures	6
Minor seizures	5
Major and minor seizures	3
Seizure onset before one year of age	4
Seizure onset before five years of age	8
Adenoma sebaceum	22
Appearance of skin lesions before two years of age	9
Appearance of skin lesions after nine years of age	3
Retinal tumors	13
Intracranial calcifications	15

* From Lagos and Gomez.[94]

life, only showing the first signs of intellectual deterioration between 8 and 14 years of age.

Seizures are the most common presenting complaint in all patients with tuberose sclerosis, and occur at one time or other in all those who are retarded. Massive minor motor seizures (infantile spasms) are most common during infancy.[95] Later on generalized convulsions, or focal seizures may occur. Seizures can appear as early as the first week of life. Their severity and response to anticonvulsant medication is unpredictable, but as a rule there is little correlation between the frequency of attacks and the degree of mental retardation.[96]

Adenoma sebaceum (angiofibroma) are the characteristic cutaneous lesion of tuberose sclerosis (Fig. 10–18). They consist of a red, papular rash over the nose, chin, cheeks, and the malar region, appearing between one and five years of age. Depigmented nevi, resembling vitiligo, in the form of oval areas with irregular margins ("ash-leaf") over the trunk and extremities, are equally common, and as a rule appear earlier than the adenoma sebaceum, sometimes at birth.[97,98] Unlike vitiligo, these lesions do not lack melanin completely. In light-skinned children they may only be demonstrable under Wood's light.

Of the other cutaneous abnormalities, flattened fibromata are the most common; they appear in a variety of areas, including the trunk, gingivae, and periungual regions. In some infants fibromata are found along the hairline or eyebrows. Another striking but less common lesion is the shagreen patch. This is an uneven thickening of skin, grayish-green or light brown in color, raised above

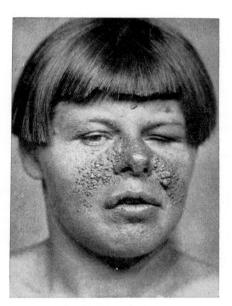

Fig. 10–18. Tuberose sclerosis. Characteristic facial adenoma sebaceum. (From Merritt, H. H.: *A Textbook of Neurology*, 4th ed., 1970, Lea & Febiger, Philadelphia.)

the surrounding surface, usually in the posterior lumbosacral region. Café-au-lait spots are also seen but far less frequently in tuberose sclerosis than in neurofibromatosis.

Intracranial tumors are less frequent in tuberose sclerosis than in neurofibromatosis but occurred in 15% of the series of Kapp and co-workers.[99] Although, strictly speaking, the numerous intraventricular nodules are tumors, they usually do not grow to the extent of producing increased intracranial pressure. Tumors are found in the neighborhood of the foramen of Monro, arising from either the walls of the lateral ventricles, or the anterior portion of the 3rd ventricle.

The usual symptoms indicating the presence of an expanding mass in a patient with tuberose sclerosis are headache, vomiting, and diminished vision. Papilledema is common and occasionally lateralizing signs such as hemiparesis may develop. In as many as 50% of patients tumors are detected in the retina, where they usually arise from the nerve head.[100] Other common retinal anomalies are hyaline or cystic nodules.[101] Other sites for neoplasms include the skin, lung, kidneys, and bone.[102,103] A variety of endocrine abnormalities have also been found. These include abnormal glucose tolerance, hypothyroidism, and a reduced excretion of 17-hydroxycorticosteroid.[104]

Diagnosis

The diagnosis of tuberose sclerosis is based on the characteristic skin lesions, seizures, and intellectual impairment or deterioration. In infants the combination of depigmented skin areas, infantile spasms, and delayed development is diagnostic. On radiography multiple scattered calcium deposits varying in size up to several centimeters, and located close to the wall of the lateral and 3rd ventricles are seen in about 50% of patients (Fig. 10–19). In distinction to the intracranial calcifications due to toxoplasmosis, cytomegalic inclusion disease, and Sturge-Weber disease, they tend to appear in late childhood and according to Taveras, their presence prior to five years of age is distinctly unusual.[105] About 40% of patients in Holt and Dickerson's series had localized areas of increased density in the cranial vault.[106]

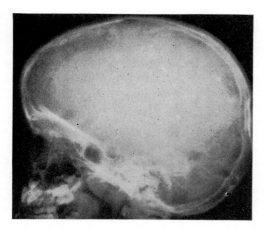

Fig. 10–19. Tuberose sclerosis. Intracranial calcifications. Deposits tend to be rounded and are found along the ventricular walls. (Courtesy of Dr. Gabriel Wilson, Department of Radiology, UCLA, Los Angeles.)

Even more diagnostic are the cystlike foci in the phalanges in about two-thirds of subjects. These are not present at birth but appear around puberty. On air encephalography multiple nodular projections into the lateral ventricles are often noted ("candle-drippings").

The spinal fluid protein may be elevated, particularly in those patients in whom intraventricular nodules have expanded to interfere with cerebrospinal fluid circulation.

Numerous patients with incomplete forms of tuberose sclerosis have been recognized by means of genetic surveys. These include subjects with isolated adenoma sebaceum, adenoma sebaceum with intracranial tumors but no seizures or intellectual deterioration, and visceral tumors without cerebral involvement.[93,94,96]

A syndrome, characterized by the triad of a midline sebaceous nevus, mental retardation, and seizures, should be distinguished from tuberose sclerosis. The skin lesions are present at birth, and there are no intracranial calcifications.[106a]

Treatment and Prognosis

There is no specific treatment. Seizures are managed with the usual anticonvulsant medications. Intraventricular tumors should be considered for surgical resection. In view of the long survival of patients who do not receive radiation therapy for their mass lesions, we cannot draw any conclusions as to its usefulness as an adjunct to surgery.

STURGE-WEBER DISEASE

The classic picture of Sturge-Weber disease, as described by Sturge in 1879[107] and Kalischer in 1897,[108] is characterized by a port wine vascular nevus on the upper part of the face, generalized or contralateral focal seizures, contralateral hemiparesis or homonymous hemianopsia, ipsilateral intracranial calcifications, and a high incidence of mental retardation. The condition is transmitted by a dominant gene with variable penetrance, although a recessive inheritance has been postulated for a number of families.[109]

Pathology

The essential pathologic feature of the condition is a leptomeningeal angiomatosis, with a predilection for the occipital or occipitoparietal regions of one cerebral hemisphere.[110] The affected vessels are mainly venous and lie deep in the subarachnoid space. Cortical calcifications are usually found in the degenerated cortex underneath the vascular malformations, while in the less affected areas they are localized to the cortical tissue surrounding the walls of the smaller blood vessels. Calcification of microglia and neurons is a less common finding. The mechanism for calcium deposition is still not clear, but the phenomenon may be related to an enhanced capillary permeability, resulting from the hypoxia of cortical tissues beneath the angiomatoses. The vascular malformation may relate to a defect in cerebral vascularization early in gestation and prior to the separation of the embryonic vasculature into superficial and deep beds.

Clinical Manifestations

The cutaneous port wine nevus is present at birth, and involves at least one eyelid or the supraorbital region of the face.[111] Commonly the angiomata may also affect the mucous membranes of the pharynx, and other viscera. An angioma of the choroid mem-

brane of the eye is often associated with unilateral congenital glaucoma and buphthal-
mos.   Bilateral facial nevi are not rare.
Ninety percent of affected patients develop
focal or generalized seizures; these are usually
the initial neurologic manifestation and almost always begin in the first year of life.
Seizures may become progressively more refractory to medication and may be followed
by transient or permanent hemiparesis.
Hemiparesis, often with homonymous hemianopsia, will ultimately develop in about 30%
of patients.[112]   About 80% of patients are
mentally retarded.   Glaucoma may be present at birth, or develop over the years in 25%
of patients.   Less commonly, there are symptoms due to hemangiomata involving the viscera.   These include hematuria and gastrointestinal hemorrhages.   Intracranial hemorrhages are rare.

Diagnosis

The coincidence of a facial vascular nevus
and seizures suggests Sturge-Weber disease.
On radiography intracranial calcifications
may be seen.   These are rarely present at
birth but are evident in nearly 90% of patients by the end of the second decade of
life.[113]   Characteristically, calcifications are
arranged in parallel lines (railroad tracks) or
serpentine convolutions which are most
striking in the occipital and parietooccipital
areas (Fig. 10–20).   Rarely, characteristic
intracranial calcifications and seizures may
be unaccompanied by a facial nevus.

On arteriography about one-half of patients show some abnormality, including
visualization of the venous angiomata, thrombotic lesions, and other vascular anomalies.[114]
The extent of the vascular lesion may also be
disclosed by a brain scan.

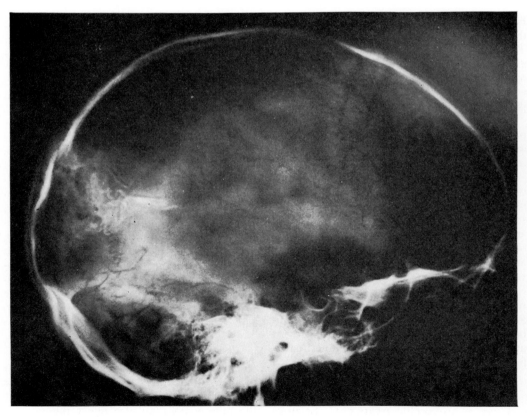

Fig. 10–20.   Sturge-Weber disease.   Intracerebral calcifications most marked in the
occipital and posterior parietal areas.

Treatment and Prognosis

Many patients deteriorate. Seizures are often difficult to control and may require surgical resection of the affected lobe, or even complete hemispherectomy.[115] Postoperative follow-up suggests that surgery improves the control of seizures and behavior, but usually has no effect on the hemiparesis.

VON HIPPEL-LINDAU DISEASE

The association of cerebellar hemangioblastomas with angiomata of the spinal cord, multiple congenital cysts of the pancreas and kidney and renal carcinoma was first recorded by Lindau in 1926,[116] although retinal hemangiomas had already been described by Treacher Collins[117] and more definitely by von Hippel in 1904.[118] The condition is transmitted as a dominant trait with variable penetrance.

Symptoms are delayed until the second decade and may be referred to the eye with sudden intraocular hemorrhage, or to the posterior fossa with increased intracranial pressure or cerebellar signs. Only about 20% of patients with cerebellar hemangioblastomas have the complete symptom complex, while only 25% of patients with retinal angiomata develop neurologic complications.

A high spinal fluid protein is seen in the majority of subjects, while about 50% of patients with cerebellar tumors have polycythemia. A more complete discussion is to be found in the cited literature.[118a,118b]

ATAXIA-TELANGIECTASIA

This recently recognized clinical entity has been considered to be one of the phakomatoses. It is characterized by slowly progressive cerebellar ataxia, choreo-athetosis, and telangiectasis of the skin and conjunctivae. It was first described by Syllaba and Henner in 1926[119] and more definitively, in 1941 by Louis-Bar[120] and in 1958 by Boder and Sedgwick.[120a]

All of the autopsied patients have had cerebellar cortical atrophy involving both Purkinje and internal granular cells. Demyelination of the posterior column and dorsal spinocerebellar tracts has also been noted, but may be due to nutritional deficiencies incurred by subjects during the terminal stages of their illness.[121] Examination of the peripheral nerves may reveal lipid inclusions in Schwann cells, and a slight degree of axonal degeneration.[121a] Vascular malformations have not been consistently

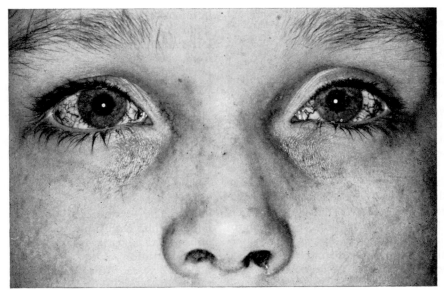

Fig. 10–21. Ataxia telangiectasia. Telangiectases in the bulbar conjunctiva. (From Merritt, H. H.: *A Textbook of Neurology*, 4th ed., 1970, courtesy of Lea & Febiger, Philadelphia.)

22. Hovind, K. H., Galicich, J. H., and Matson, D. D.: Normal and pathological intracranial anatomy revealed by two-dimensional echo-encephalography, Neurology (Minneap.) 17: 253, 1967.

23. Hill, D. and Parr, G.: *Electroencephalography*, New York: The Macmillan Co., 1963, pp. 317–326.

23a. Menkes, J. H.: To tap or not to tap, Pediatrics 50:560, 1972.

24. Merritt, H. H.: The cerebrospinal fluid in cases of tumors of the brain, Arch. Neurol. Psychiat. 34:1175, 1935.

25. Berg, L.: Hypoglycorrhachia of non-infectious origin, Neurology (Minneap.) 3:811, 1953.

26. Fumagalli, R. and Paoletti, D.: Sterol test for human brain tumors: Relationship with different oncotypes, Neurology (Minneap.) 21:1149, 1971.

27. Weiss, J. F., Ransohoff, J., and Kayden, J. H.: Cerebrospinal fluid sterols in patients undergoing treatment for gliomas, Neurology (Minneap.) 22:187, 1972.

27a. Moniz, E.: L'encephalographie arterielle, son importance dans la localisation des tumeurs cerebrales, Rev. Neurol. (Paris) 2:72, 1927.

28. Dandy, W. E.: Ventriculography following the injection of air into the cerebral ventricles, Ann. Surg 68:5, 1918.

29. Robertson, E. G.: *Pneumoencephalography*, Springfield: Charles C Thomas Publisher, 1957.

30. Prince, D. and Wiener, L. M.: Pneumoencephalography in patients with brain tumor, Neurology (Minneap.) 14:677, 1964.

30a. Levine, M. C.: Changes in the CSF during pneumoencephalography, Neuroradiology 5:1, 1973.

31. Loeser, E., Jr. and Scheinberg, L.: Brain abscesses, Neurology (Minneap.) 7:601, 1957.

32. Russell, D. S. and Rubinstein, L. J.: *Pathology of Tumors of the Nervous System*, Baltimore: Williams & Wilkins Co., 1963.

32a. Rubinstein, L. J.: Cytogenesis and differentiation of primitive central neuroepithelial tumors, J. Neuropath. Exp. Neurol. 31:7, 1972.

33. Fokes, E. C. and Earle, K. M.: Ependymomas: Clinical and pathological aspects, J. Neurosurg. 30:585, 1969.

34. Cushing, H.: Experiences with the cerebellar astrocytomas, Surg. Gynec. Obstet. 52:129, 1931.

35. Cushing, H.: Experiences with the cerebellar medulloblastomas, Acta Path. Microbiol. Scand. 7:1, 1930.

36. Fincher, E. F., Jr. and Coon, P. G.: Ependymomas: A clinical and pathologic study of eight cases, Arch. Neurol. Psychiat. 22:19, 1929.

37. Stewart, T. G. and Holmes, G.: Symptomatology of cerebellar tumors: A study of forty cases, Brain 27:522, 1904.

38. Boldrey, E. and Miller, E. R.: Calcified ependymoblastoma of the fourth ventricle in a four year old girl: Roentgen demonstration, Radiology 38:495, 1942.

39. Grant, F. C.: Cerebellar symptoms produced by supratentorial tumors: A further report, Arch Neurol. Psychiat. 20:292, 1928.

40. Oppenheimer, D. R.: A benign tumor of the cerebellum, J. Neurol. Neurosurg. Psych. 18:199, 1955.

41. Ingraham, F. D. and Matson, D. D.: *Neurosurgery in Infancy and Childhood*, Springfield: Charles C Thomas Publisher, 1954.

42. Hope-Stone, H. F.: Results of treatment of medulloblastomas, J. Neurosurg. 32:83, 1970.

43. Boldrey, E. and Sheline, G.: Delayed transitory clinical manifestations after radiation therapy of intracranial tumors, Acta Radiol. [Ther.] (Stockholm) 5:5, 1966.

44. Cervós-Navarro, J.: Time course of brain edema after irradiation, Acta Neurochir. (Wien) 22:43, 1970.

45. Redmond, D. E., Rinderknecht, R. H., and Hudgins, P. T.: The effect of total-brain irradiation on cerebrospinal fluid pressure, Radiology 89:727, 1967.

46. Lampkin, B. C., Mauer, A. M., and McBride, B. H.: Response of medulloblastoma to vincristine sulfate: A case report, Pediatrics 39:761, 1967.

47. Bray, P. F., Carter, S., and Taveras, J. M.: Brainstem tumors in children, Neurology (Minneap.) 8:1, 1958.

47a. Schain, R. T. and Wilson, G.: Brainstem encephalitis with radiographic evidence of medullary enlargement. Neurology (Minneap.) 21:537, 1971.

48. Lassiter, K. R. L., et al.: Surgical treatment of brain stem gliomas, J. Neurosurg. 34:719, 1971.

48a. Panitch, H. S. and Berg, B. O.: Brain stem tumors of childhood and adolescence, Amer. J. Dis. Child. 119:465, 1970.

49. Northfield, D. W. C.: Rathke-pouch tumors, Brain 80:293, 1957.

50. Bingas, B. and Wolter, M.: Das Kraniopharyngiom, Fortschr. Neurol. Psychiat. 36:117, 1968.

51. Bailey, P.: Concerning the cerebellar symptoms produced by suprasellar tumors, Arch. Neurol. Psychiat. 11:137, 1924.

52. Russell, R. W. R. and Pennybacker, J. B.: Craniopharyngioma in the elderly, J. Neurol. Neurosurg. Psychiat. 24:1, 1961.

53. Poppen, J. L. and King, A. B.: Chordoma: Experience with 13 cases, J. Neurosurg. 9:139, 1952.

54. Russell, A.: A diencephalic syndrome of emaciation in infancy and childhood, Arch. Dis. Child. 26:274, 1951.

55. Matson, D. D. and Crigler, J. F., Jr.: Management of craniopharyngioma in childhood, J. Neurosurg. 30:377, 1969.

56. Bond, W. H., Richards, D., and Turner, E.: Experiences with radioactive gold in treatment of craniopharyngioma, J. Neurol. Neurosurg. Psychiat. 28:30, 1965.

57. Wise, B. L.: Management of postoperative diabetes insipidus, J. Neurosurg. 25:416, 1966.

58. Kenny, F. M., et al.: Iatrogenic hypopituitarism in craniopharyngioma. Unexplained catch-up growth in three children, J. Pediat. 72:766, 1968.

59. Martin, P. and Cushing, H.: Primary gliomas of chiasm and optic nerves in their intracranial portion, Arch. Ophthal. 52:209, 1923.

60. Chutorian, A. M., et al.: Optic gliomas in children, Neurology (Minneap.) 14:83, 1964.

61. Holman, C. B.: Roentgenologic manifestations of glioma of the optic nerve and chiasm, Amer. J. Roentgen. 82:462, 1959.

62. Taveras, J. M., Mount, L. A., and Wood, E. H.: The value of radiation therapy in the management of glioma of the optic nerves and chiasm, Radiology 66:518, 1956.

63. Russell, W. O. and Sachs, E.: Pinealoma: A clinicopathologic study of seven cases with a review of the literature, Arch. Path. 35:869, 1943.

64. Posner, M. and Horrax, G.: Eye signs in pineal tumors, J. Neurosurg. 3:15, 1946.

65. Davidoff, L. M.: Some considerations in therapy of pineal tumors, Bull. NY Acad. Med. 43:537, 1967.

66. Teng, P. and Papatheodorou, C.: Tumors of cerebral ventricles in children, J. Nerv. Ment. Dis. 142:87, 1966.

67. Yenermen, M. H., Bowerman, C. I., and Haymaker, W.: Colloid cyst of the third ventricle, Acta Neuroveg. (Wien) 17:211, 1958.

68. Koos, W., Laubichler, W., and Valencak, E.: Les tumeurs du troisieme ventricule chez l'enfant, Neurochirurgie 12:645, 1966.

69. Page, L. K., Lombroso, C. T., and Matson, D. D.: Childhood epilepsy with late detection of cerebral glioma, J. Neurosurg. 31:253, 1969.

70. Austin, G.: "Tumors—Intraspinal," in Jackson, I. J. and Thompson, R. K.: Pediatric Neurosurgery, Springfield: Charles C Thomas Publisher, 1959.

71. Poser, C. M.: Relationship Between Syringomyelia and Neoplasm, Springfield: Charles C Thomas Publisher, 1956.

72. Richardson, F. L.: A report of 16 tumors of the spinal cord; the importance of spinal rigidity as an early sign of disease, J. Pediat. 57:42, 1960.

73. Buchanan, D. N.: Tumors of the spinal cord in infancy, Arch. Neurol. Psychiat. 63:835, 1950.

74. Haft, H., Ransohoff, J., and Carter, S.: Spinal cord tumors in children, Pediatrics 23:1152, 1959.

75. Ross, A. T. and Bailey, O. T.: Tumors arising within the spinal canal in children, Neurology (Minneap.) 3:922, 1953.

76. Schwartz, G.: The width of the spinal canal in the growing vertebra with special reference to the sacrum. Maximum interpediculate distances in adults and children, Amer. J. Roentgen. 76:476, 1956.

77. Rubin, P.: Extradural spinal cord compression by tumor, Radiology 93:1243, 1969.

78. Nellhaus, G.: Personal communication (1971).

79. Wood, E. H., Berne, A. S., and Taveras, J. M.: The value of radiation therapy in the management of intrinsic tumors of the spinal cord, Radiology 63:11, 1954.

80. von Recklinghausen, F. D.: "Ueber die multiplen Fibrome der Haut und ihre Beziehung zu den multiplen Neuromen," Berlin: A. Hirschwald, 1882.

81. Crowe, F., Scholl, W., and Neel, J.: Clinical, Pathological and Genetic Study of Multiple Neurofibromatosis, Springfield: Charles C Thomas Publisher, 1956.

81a. Fialkow, P. J., et al.: Multiple cell origin of hereditary neurofibromatosis, New Eng. J. Med. 284:289, 1971.

82. Pearce, J.: The central nervous system pathology in multiple neurofibromatosis, Neurology (Minneap.) 17:691, 1967.

83. Borberg, A.: Clinical and genetic investigation into tuberous sclerosis and Recklinghausen's neurofibromatosis: Contribution to elucidation of interrelationship and eugenics of the syndromes, Acta Psychiat. Neurol. Scand. Suppl. 71:3, 1951.

84. Canale, D., Bebin, J., and Knighton, R. S.: Neurologic manifestations of von Recklinghausen's disease of the nervous system, Confin. Neurol. 24:359, 1964.

85. Chao, D. H.: Congenital neurocutaneous syndromes in childhood. I. Neurofibromatosis, J. Pediat. 55:189, 1959.

86. Frézal, J. and Rey, J.: "Genetique des Phakomatoses," in Michaux, L. and Feld, M. (eds.): Les Phakomatoses Cerebrales, Paris: Droust, 1963.

87. Habib, R.: "Les Lesions Vasculaires de la Neurofibromatose de Recklinghausen," in Michaux, L. and Feld, M. (eds.): Les Phakomatoses Cerebrales, Paris: Droust, 1963.

88. Kissel, P. and Schmitt, J.: "Les Formes Viscerales des Phakomatose," in Michaux, L. and Feld, M. (eds.): Les Phakomatoses Cerebrales, Paris: Droust, 1963.

89. Rodriguez, H. A. and Berthrong, M.: Multiple primary intracranial tumors in von Recklinghausen's neurofibromatosis, Arch. Neurol. 14:467, 1966.

90. Whitehouse, D.: Diagnostic value of the café-au-lait spot in children, Arch. Dis. Child. 41:316, 1966.

91. von Recklinghausen, F. D.: Ein Herz von einen Neugeborenen, Verh. Berl. Ges. Geburt. 15:73, 1863.

92. Bourneville, D. M.: Contribution a l'etude de l'idiotie. III. Sclerose tubereuse des circonvolutions cerebrales, Arch. Internat. Neurol. (Paris) 1:81, 1880.

93. Bundey, S. and Evans, K.: Tuberous sclerosis: A genetic study, J. Neurol. Neurosurg. Psychiat. 32:591, 1969.

94. Lagos, J. C. and Gomez, M. R.: Tuberose sclerosis: Reappraisal of a clinical entity, Mayo Clin. Proc. 42:26, 1967.

95. Roth, J. C. and Epstein, C. J.: Infantile spasms and hypopigmented macules: Early manifestations of tuberous sclerosis, Arch. Neurol. 25:547, 1971.

96. Critchley, M. and Earl, C. J. C.: Tuberose sclerosis and allied conditions, Brain 55:311, 1932.

97. Gold, A. P. and Freeman, J. M.: Depigmented nevi: The earliest sign of tuberose sclerosis, Pediatrics 35:1003, 1965.

98. Hurwitz, S. and Braverman, I. M.: White spots in tuberose sclerosis, J. Pediat. 77:587, 1970.

99. Kapp, J. P., Paulson, G. W., and Odom, G. L.: Brain tumors with tuberose sclerosis, J. Neurosurg. 26:191, 1967.

100. McLean, J. M.: Glial tumors of the retina in relation to tuberous sclerosis, Amer. J. Ophthal. 41:428, 1956.

101. Grover, W. D. and Harley, R. D.: Early recognition of tuberous sclerosis by funduscopic examination, J. Pediat. 75:991, 1969.

102. Dawson, J.: Pulmonary tuberose sclerosis, Quart. J. Med. 47:113, 1954.

103. Reed, W. B., Nickel, W. R., and Campion, G.: Internal manifestations of tuberous sclerosis, Arch. Derm. (Chicago) 87:715, 1963.

104. Sareen, C. K.: Tuberose sclerosis, Amer. J. Dis. Child. 123:34, 1972.

105. Taveras, J. M.: Personal communications (1967).

106. Holt, J. F. and Dickerson, W. W.: The osseous lesions of tuberous sclerosis, Radiology 58:1, 1952.

106a. Lovejoy, F. H. and Boyle, L. E.: Linear nevus sebaceous syndrome: Report of two cases and a review of the literature, Pediatrics 52:382, 1973.

107. Sturge, W. A.: A case of partial epilepsy apparently due to a lesion of one of the vasomotor centres of the brain, Clin. Soc. Lond. Trans. 12:162, 1879.

108. Kalischer, S.: Demonstration des Gehirns eines Kindes mit Teleangiectasie der linksseitgen Gesichts-Kopfhaut und Hirnoberflache, Berl. Klin. Wchnschr. 48:1059, 1897.

109. Koch, G.: "Considerations Nouvelles sur l' Heredite des Maladies de Sturge-Weber et de von Hippel-Lindau," in Michaux, L. and Feld, M. (eds.): *Les Phakomatoses Cerebrales*, Paris: Droust, 1963.

110. Wohlwill, F. J. and Yakovlev, P. I.: Histopathology of meningo-facial angiomatosis (Sturge-Weber Disease), J. Neuropath. Exp. Neurol. 16:341, 1957.

111. Alexander, G. L. and Norman, R. M.: *The Sturge-Weber Syndrome*, Bristol: John Wright and Co., Ltd., 1960.

112. Chao, D. H. C.: Congenital neurocutaneous syndromes of childhood. III. Sturge-Weber disease, J. Pediat. 55:635, 1959.

113. Nellhaus, G., Haberland, C., and Hill, B. J.: Sturge-Weber disease with bilateral intracranial calcifications at birth and unusual pathological findings, Acta Neurol. Scand. 43:314, 1967.

114. Poser, C. M. and Taveras, J. M.: Cerebral angiography in encephalo-trigeminal angiomatosis, Radiology 68:327, 1957.

115. Falconer, M. A. and Ruschworth, R. G.: Treatment of encephalotrigeminal angiomatosis (Sturge-Weber Disease) by hemispherectomy, Arch. Dis. Child. 35:433, 1960.

116. Lindau, A.: Studien uber Kleinhirncysten: Bau, Pathogenese und Beziehungen zur Angiomatosis retinae, Acta Path. Microbiol. Scand. Suppl. 1:1–128, 1926.

117. Collins, E. T.: Intra-ocular growths. I. Two cases, brother and sister, with peculiar vascular new growth, probably primarily retinal, affecting both eyes, Trans. Ophthal. Soc. UK 14:141, 1894.

118. von Hippel, E.: Ueber eine sehr seltene Erkrankung der Netzhaut, Arch. Ophthal. 59:83, 1904.

118a. Macmichael, I. M.: Von Hippel–Lindau's disease of the optic disc. Trans. Ophthal Soc. UK 90:877, 1970.

118b. Grizzard, H. T., et al.: Angiomatosis retinae, J. Tenn. Med. Ass. 63:34, 1970.

119. Syllaba, L. and Henner, K.: Contribution a l'independance de l'athetose double idiopathique et congenitale, Rev. Neurol. (Paris) 45:541, 1926.

120. Louis-Bar, D.: Sur un syndrome progressif comprenant des telangiectasies capillaires cutanees et conjonctivale symetriques a disposition naevoide et des troubles cerebelleux, Confin. Neurol. 4:32, 1941.

120a. Boder, E. and Sedgwick, R. P.: Ataxia-telangiectasia. A familial syndrome of progressive cerebellar ataxia, oculocutaneous telangiectasia and frequent pulmonary infection, Pediatrics 21, 526, 1958.

121. Solitare, G. B. and Lopez, V. F.: Louis-Bar's syndrome (ataxia-telangiectasia): Neuropathologic observations, Neurology (Minneap.) 17:23, 1967.

121a. Jerusalem, F. and Bischoff, A.: Ataxia teleangiectatica: Elektronenmikroskopische Biopsiebefunde des Nervus suralis von 2 Fallen, Z. Neurol. 202:128, 1972.

122. Reed, W. B., et al.: Cutaneous manifestations of ataxia-telangiectasia, JAMA 195:746, 1966.

122a. Sedgwick, R. P. and Boder, E.: "Ataxia-telangiectasia," in Vinken, P. J., and Bruyn, G. W. (eds.): *Handbook of Clinical Neurology*, Vol. 14, Amsterdam: North-Holland Publishing Co., 1972, pp. 267–339.

123. Peterson, R.D.A., Kelly, W. D., and Good, R. A.: Ataxia-telangiectasia: Its association with a defective thymus, immunologic-deficiency disease and malignancy, Lancet 1:1189, 1964.

124. Strober, W., et al.: Immunoglobulin metabolism in ataxia telangiectasia, J. Clin. Invest. 47:1905, 1968.

125. Schalch, D. S., McFarlin, D. E., and Barlow, M. H.: An unusual form of diabetes mellitus in ataxia telangiectasia, New Eng. J. Med. 282:1396, 1970.

126. Quincke, H.: "Ueber Meningitis serosa Volkmann's Sammlung klinischer Vortrage," N.F. 1893, Nr. 67; cited in Quincke, H.: Ueder

Meningitis Serosa und verwandte Zustande, Deutsch. Z. Nervenheilk. 9:149, 1897.

127. Gills, J. P., Kapp, J. P., and Odom, G. L.: Benign intracranial hypertension: Pseudotumor cerebri from obstruction of dural sinuses, Arch. Ophthal. 78:592, 1967.

128. Greer, M.: Benign intracranial hypertension. IV. Menarche, Neurology (Minneap.) 14:569, 1964.

129. Foley, J.: Benign forms of intracranial hypertension—"toxic" and "otitic" hydrocephalus, Brain 78:1, 1955.

130. Greer, M.: Benign intracranial hypertension. I. Mastoiditis and lateral sinus obstruction, Neurology (Minneap.) 12:472, 1962.

131. Rose, A. and Matson, D. D.: Benign intracranial hypertension in children, Pediatrics 39:227, 1967.

132. Feldman, M. H. and Schlezinger, N. S.: Benign intracranial hypertension associated with hypervitaminosis A, Arch Neurol. 22:1, 1970.

133. Walker, A. E. and Adamkiewicz, J. J.: Pseudotumor cerebri associated with prolonged corticosteroid therapy: Reports of four cases, JAMA 188:779, 1964.

133a. Grant, D. N.: Benign intracranial hypertension, Arch. Dis. Child. 46:651, 1971.

134. Guidetti, B., Giuffre, R., and Gambacorta, D.: Followup study of 100 cases of pseudotumor cerebri, Acta Neurochir. (Wien) 18:259, 1968.

the discharge takes the form of spike and wave complexes, occurring at an average frequency of three per second. This electric picture is associated with petit mal epilepsy. Bilaterally synchronous spike discharges are seen in those forms of grand mal epilepsy not due to a cortical focus.

On electroencephalography the diffuse dysrhythmias are recognized by the presence of multiple, usually disorganized paroxysmal discharges, most commonly slow and sharp waves and multiple spike and wave patterns. The term hypsarhythmia was applied by Gibbs and co-workers[8] to this pattern when present in early childhood. Usually it is associated with minor motor seizures, particularly infantile spasms.

Etiology of Seizures

The processes leading to the appearance of recurrent seizures can be viewed from several aspects: a genetic predisposition, alterations in neuronal metabolism, abnormalities of electrophysiology, and neuropathologic changes. Each of these factors will be considered in turn.

Genetic Factors. Numerous studies indicate a high incidence of seizures among relatives of children with idiopathic epilepsy. Metrakos and Metrakos found an incidence of seizures among parents and siblings of children with petit mal epilepsy of centrencephalic origin of 12%, while 45% of siblings had an abnormal electroencephalogram. This suggests that this electroencephalographic abnormality is an expression of an autosomal dominant gene with nearly complete penetrance during childhood, and low penetrance in infancy and adult life.[9]

Electroencephalographic abnormalities are also transmitted in a dominant manner with age-dependent penetrance in families with temporal lobe spike discharges and psychomotor seizures.[10] In other forms of epilepsy the genetic factors, while demonstrable through controlled twin studies, are not as striking. However, even in petit mal epilepsy, in which the genetic factor is most prominent, the overall risk of developing seizures is only 8% for siblings of affected patients, and only 2% in an as yet unaffected sibling older than six years.[11]

Biochemical Factors. The biochemical abnormality responsible for an uncontrolled electric discharge of neurons is still unknown, but a seizure may result from numerous metabolic alterations and, in turn, produce other biochemical changes.

The common characteristic of seizure-prone gray matter may be an impairment of cellular metabolism which produces a partial depolarization of neurons, and decreases the gap between the resting potential and the level of the membrane potential required to generate an action potential. Tissue from human epileptogenic cortex contains reduced intracellular potassium and increased intracellular sodium during the interictal period,[12] indicating that the seizure-prone neurons may exist in a partially depolarized state. A variety of alterations of cellular metabolism could produce partial neuronal depolarization.[13]

1. Imbalance of excitatory and depressant amino acids, as for instance an increase in the ratio of glutamic acid/gamma-amino butyric acid (GABA). This is found in pyridoxine deficiency in which the conversion of glutamic acid to GABA is impaired.

2. Interference with the conversion of glutamic acid to glutamine with a resulting increase in glutamic acid.

3. Anoxia decreasing ATP production to a level insufficient to maintain the normal resting membrane potential.

4. Hypoglycemia with a reduction in normal Krebs cycle function and a shift to the utilization of GABA as a substrate for energy production.

5. Interference with the binding of acetylcholine, a known excitatory transmitter.

All but two of these mechanisms directly or indirectly involve an alteration in the ratio of the concentrations of glutamic acid to GABA.[14] GABA has been shown to transmit inhibitory postsynaptic activity in crayfish nerve and may be the principal inhibitory transmitter in the mammalian brain as well, acting to stabilize neuronal membrane potentials.[15] The suggestion that GABA concentrations in human epileptogenic cortex are reduced lends support to this hypothesis.[16]

An increased glutamic acid/GABA ratio may also occur in pyridoxine deficiency where it results from impaired activity of glutamic acid decarboxylase. This, in turn, diminishes GABA synthesis and increases the concentration of glutamic acid. Increased utilization of GABA is seen in hypoglycemia when the GABA shunt, which normally provides up to 40% of the total energy consumed by the brain, is required to take up the entire responsibility for energy production.

In some instances an abnormality of acetylcholine metabolism may be responsible for the initiation and propagation of seizures. Normally acetylcholine is present in cortex in a bound state, but in epileptic cortex it is present in an unbound form.[16] The inhibition of acetylcholine esterase by parathione induces an accumulation of acetylcholine and is responsible for the occurrence of seizures in organo-phosphate poisoning.

During a brief seizure the brain undergoes several biochemical alterations. Cerebral oxygen and glucose consumption increases strikingly, but with maintenance of adequate ventilation the increase in cerebral blood flow is sufficient to meet the increased metabolic requirements of the brain.

A generalized convulsion, lasting 30 minutes or more, is usually accompanied by apnea, inducing hypoxia and carbon dioxide retention. As a result of the energy demands of the convulsing muscles, the subject becomes hypoxic and hyperpyrexic.[16a] There is a fall of oxygen tension within the brain, a shift towards anaerobic metabolism, and an accumulation of lactic acid.[17] These chemical alterations, aggravated by hyperpyrexia and arterial hypotension, are probably the most important factors in the production of cellular damage which attends prolonged convulsions.[16b]

Experimental evidence indicates that if adequate ventilation is maintained and the subject's muscles are paralyzed, cerebral venous oxygen tension does not fall and there is no increase in cerebral venous lactic acid.[18]

Electrophysiologic Factors. Physiologically an epileptic seizure has been defined as an alteration of central nervous system function resulting from spontaneous electric discharge in a diseased neuronal population of cortical gray matter or brain stem. As a consequence of a standing partial depolarization, the epileptic neuron has increased electric excitability in response to a variety of physiologic stimuli, including changes in cellular hydration, synchronous cerebral discharges such as occur during sleep, and afferent volleys which produce a series of high voltage spike or sharp wave discharges. These activate surrounding normal cells and distant, synaptically related cells. As a result of continuous bombardment, the latter may be transformed into secondary epileptic foci. In man secondary foci are usually contralateral to the primary focus, or in synaptically related subcortical nuclei.[19] These secondary foci do not have the same functional significance as the primary focus for the production of seizures, for surgical removal of the primary lesion may often be successful in causing the disappearance of secondary spike foci.

Schmidt and Wilder[13] suggest that with the involvement of subcortical neurons by the epileptic discharge, a positive excitatory feedback circuit is established between the cortex and the subcortical neurons inducing discharges at a rate of 10 to 40 cycles per second, and being responsible for the tonic phase of the focal motor seizure. As inhibitory neurons are recruited, a negative inhibitory feedback circuit develops which periodically interrupts the excitatory activity and produces the clonic phase of the seizure. When the negative feedback wins ascendancy the seizure will cease. There is considerable evidence that postictal (Todd's) paralysis, a common sequel to a focal seizure, is due to a persistence of the active inhibitory state rather than to a metabolic exhaustion of epileptic neurons.[20]

Once the neuronal excitation derived from the epileptic focus spreads to involve the brain stem, particularly the midbrain and pontine reticular formation, a generalized seizure develops almost instantly. These areas, known as the centrencephalic system, are responsible for the dissemination of epileptic potentials.[21,22,23] This process has been termed secondary subcortical epilepsy, with the EEG correlate being secondary bilateral synchrony. This type of epileptic discharge is distinct from centrencephalic epilepsy with an EEG correlate of primary bilateral synchrony.

A number of areas including the temporal, frontal, and prefrontal cortex have particularly strong corticofugal projections to the centrencephalic system, and focal lesions within them may induce a generalized seizure discharge.[24,25,26] The importance of focal epileptogenic lesions has become increasingly evident with the use of direct brain recording and the realization of the marked disparities that may exist between scalp EEG and records made directly from brain.[27]

Three factors determine whether a focal seizure will become generalized. The first is the excitability of the epileptic neurons, the second the ease with which an electric discharge can be propagated from the focus to the centrencephalic system, and finally, the threshold of the brain stem centers for disseminating an electric discharge. The last is believed to reflect in part a genetic predisposition and in part the frequency with which it is activated by the primary epileptic focus.

Discharges may originate spontaneously from the centrencephalic system or may be triggered by a cortical focus which is often undetected by electroencephalographic and clinical examination.[28] Clinically such a discharge produces grand mal or petit mal epilepsy. In the latter condition a quick excitation of a neuronal inhibitory system prevents a prolonged clinical seizure and the development of the tonic-clonic components.

These seizures can occur without known cerebral injury or disease but, as indicated previously, have a high rate of genetic transmission.

Neuropathologic Factors. There is no specific pathology for epilepsy. Seizures may occur in patients with almost any pathologic process that can affect the brain. There are also a large number of patients whose brains, after a lifetime of recurrent epileptic attacks, show no gross abnormalities. Because of surgical excisions for psychomotor seizures with temporal lobe foci, the best pathologic data available are for patients with this condition. The data of Falconer and associates on the pathogenesis of temporal lobe epilepsy as ascertained from surgically removed specimen are presented in Table 11–3.[29]

Incisural sclerosis (mesial temporal sclerosis) is an atrophic lesion of the hippocampal gyrus and deep temporal lobe structures believed to result from tentorial herniation of these structures at birth or due to cerebral edema induced by prolonged grand mal convulsions.

Both conditions are believed to induce transient interruption of the blood supply.[30] In other areas of the brain, malformations such as heterotopias of gray matter or "cryptic tubers" may be the cause for focal epilepsy.[31,32] We should emphasize that all pathologic brain tissue, whether it be atrophic, malformed, or neoplastic, is elec-

TABLE 11-3.
POSSIBLE ETIOLOGIC FACTORS IN TEMPORAL LOBE EPILEPSY*

	Mesial Temporal Sclerosis 47 Cases	Small Tumors 21 (24)† Cases	Miscellaneous Lesions 10 (13) Cases	Equivocal Lesions 22 Cases	Totals 100 Cases
Positive family history	6	0	2 (4)	0	8
Difficult or precipitate birth alone	7	4	3	7	21
Infantile convulsions alone	13	1	1	1	16
Both factors together	6	1	0	0	7
Head injury	5	6	3 (5)	5	19
Other factors‡	11	1 (2)	4	4	20
None of above factors	5	10	2	7	—

* After Falconer et al.[29]
† The figures without parentheses refer to pure cases of each subgroup and those with parentheses to cases with a dual pathology including mesial temporal sclerosis.
‡ E.g., meningitis, mastoid disease, febrile illnesses in infancy without convulsions, etc.

trically inert and that epileptogenic neurons, functioning but having an abnormal cellular metabolism, are located around the periphery of the various lesions.

Clinical Manifestations

In order to facilitate presentation of the clinical manifestations of seizures, which are varied even in one given patient, each of the common seizure types will be taken up in turn. We then plan to cover briefly a miscellaneous group of less common seizure forms, with literature references for more extensive reading. Finally, the discussion will turn to febrile convulsions and the problem of seizures during the neonatal period.

Grand Mal (Major Motor). A grand mal seizure occurring by itself or in combination with other seizure forms is the most common epileptic manifestation of childhood (Table 11–2).

The seizure may occur without warning or may be preceded by an aura. Occasionally the child may be irritable or manifest unusual behavior for several hours prior to the seizure. From the standpoint of localizing the epileptic focus, the aura offers the most important clinical clue—more reliable at times than the EEG; the examining physician should always try to elicit its history. The most common epileptic aura is a sensation of dizziness or an unusual feeling of ascending abdominal discomfort. These sensations have been attributed to a discharge in the area of visceral sensory representation but offer less evidence for the site of the epileptic focus than do focal sensory symptoms.[33]

In the classic form of an attack the aura may be followed by rolling up of the eyes and loss of consciousness. There is a generalized tonic contraction of the entire body musculature and the child may utter a piercing, peculiar cry, after which he becomes apneic and cyanotic. With the onset of the clonic phase of the convulsion, the trunk and extremities undergo rhythmic contraction and relaxation. As the attack ends, the rate of clonic movements slows and finally they cease abruptly. The duration of a seizure varies from a few seconds to as long as half an hour or more. A series of attacks at intervals too brief to allow the child to regain con-

sciousness from one attack before the onset of the next is known as status epilepticus. Since status epilepticus is one of the few neurologic conditions requiring emergency treatment, it will again be referred to in the section on therapy.

Following the seizure the child may remain semiconscious and then confused for several hours. When examined soon after an attack, the child is poorly coordinated, with mild impairment of fine movements. There may be truncal ataxia, increased deep tendon reflexes, clonus, and extensor plantar responses. Occasionally the child appears blind and speechless. Postictally he may vomit or complain of severe headache.

There are numerous variations of the major motor attack. Occasionally, particularly when drug therapy has been partly effective, a typical aura occurs but is not followed by a seizure. In other patients either the tonic or the clonic phase is too brief to be noted. Attacks can occur at any time of the day or night, although their frequency is somewhat greater shortly before or after the child falls asleep or awakens. As a rule, patients who for one year or more have only experienced seizures during sleep, are unlikely to have attacks at other times of the day. In some girls seizures occur a few days before or shortly after their menstrual period.

A number of factors may precipitate not only a major attack but other epileptic manifestations as well:

1. Infection and fever: fever may induce a seizure not only in children suffering from febrile convulsions but also in patients who previously have had recurrent epileptic attacks unassociated with fever. In some children dehydration and ketosis accompanying an acute infectious illness may decrease seizure frequency.

2. Fatigue: in a few children excessive fatigue or lack of sleep appears to precede a seizure but probably does not represent an important precipitating factor. There is considerable clinical evidence to indicate that epileptic children have fewer seizures when actively engaged in strenuous physical activity. While fatigue seems to have little effect, sleep deprivation may activate the EEG of epileptics and precipitate seizures.[34]

Less commonly one may encounter a variety of tumors in the epileptogenic cortex. These include hamartomas, which occasionally may undergo malignant transformation, small gliomatous nodules, hemangiomas, and lesions suggestive of tuberous sclerosis.[43,44]

Typical psychomotor seizures are rarely seen prior to 10 years of age. Rather, children who later on develop psychomotor attacks may have an antecedent history of other seizure forms, a variety of behavior disorders, enuresis, nightmares, and sleep walking.[45,46]

Seizure manifestations in older children are presented in Table 11–4. A typical attack can be divided into four parts. The aura may consist of a variety of subjective phenomena. In children Glaser and Dixon have found an aura of intense anxiety usually associated with visceral sensations to be the most common antecedent to psychomotor seizures.[47] Olfactory hallucinations ("uncinate fits") are usually described as unpleasant but unidentifiable odors. Their association with tumors of the temporal lobe has been well-documented. In Daly's series almost 40% of 55 patients who experienced this aura were found to have neoplasms.[48]

Hallucinatory experiences, most commonly a feeling of déjà vu, an adventitious sense of familiarity, and visual hallucinations have been reported by children with psychomotor seizures.[49] According to Mullan and Penfield they are more common when the focus is in the nondominant temporal lobe.[50]

Paroxysmal emotional states, particularly fear, are not rare in children and are commonly reported by parents. Rage reactions

TABLE 11-4.
CLINICAL MANIFESTATIONS OF PSYCHOMOTOR SEIZURES IN CHILDHOOD

Seizure Manifestations	Number of Patients With Manifestations (Total 25)		
	Age 1–6	Age 7–16	Total
Aura	6	10	16
Altered consciousness	12	13	25
Change in position of body or limbs	10	11	21
Integrated but confused activity	8	11	19
Staring or dazed expression	10	8	18
Epigastric sensation, nausea, vomiting	9	5	14
Oral movements, drooling	8	5	13
Muttering, mumbling, hissing	5	5	10
Walking, wandering	4	6	10
Pallor or flushing	5	4	9
Rubbing or fumbling	4	5	9
Speech (usually irrelevant or incoherent)	3	5	8
Affective disturbance (fear, anger)	5	3	8
Stiffening of body or limbs	5	3	8
Falling	4	3	7
Aggressive activity	4	3	7
Dreamy state	2	3	5
Forced thinking or ideational blocking	1	4	5
Searching or orienting movements	1	3	4
Abdominal pain	3	1	4
Incontinence (urinary)	2	1	3
Perceptual disturbance (visual, auditory)	0	3	3

* After Glaser and Dixon.[47]

or temper tantrums are rarely auras of a psychomotor seizure, nor are purposeful aggressive acts common in the course of seizure. Nevertheless, the possibility of a temporal lobe seizure is often raised in a child with behavior problems who has an abnormal electroencephalogram. Aird and Yamamoto have examined this question and have found that about one-half of children with behavior problems have an abnormal EEG. In 27% of all patients there was EEG foci primarily involving the temporal lobe.[46]

Following the aura, the patient briefly stops all activity. He may stand still, stare, or turn pale. Shortly thereafter minor motor acts are initiated. Commonly these involve chewing and smacking movements, purposeless fumbling or patting of the hands, and picking at clothes. The final part of the seizure generally involves more complex motor acts. The child may move about the room, may begin to undress himself, and occasionally utter stereotyped or nonsensical phrases. These automatisms usually do not last longer than 5–10 minutes, although reliable observers have recorded prolonged psychomotor seizures and an occasional case of psychomotor status has been recorded. Psychomotor status is extremely rare, and to our knowledge it has never initiated psychomotor epilepsy.[51] It manifests itself as periods of amnesia and has to be differentiated from hysterical amnesia. Lennox stresses that the circumstances surrounding the onset of an attack are important in deciding on the diagnosis.[52]

Following his seizure the patient experiences postictal drowsiness or clouding of consciousness. When fully recovered he has complete amnesia for the entire attack.

As with major motor seizures, the frequency of psychomotor attacks varies, but unlike petit mal attacks, it is uncommon to see multiple attacks within a day.[47]

Focal Seizures. Focal seizures are characterized by the development of localized motor or sensory symptoms. In a large proportion of children these spread to other parts of the body, ultimately becoming generalized with loss of consciousness. On rare occasions there is an orderly sequential progression, a phenomenon known as the Jacksonian seizure or march.

Perhaps the most common focal attack observed in children is the adversive seizure.[53] This consists of turning of the eyes, or eyes and head away from the side of the focus. In some patients the upper extremity on the side toward which the head turns is abducted and extended, and the fingers are clenched. Thus the child "appears to look at his closed fist."

The patient may be aware of this movement or may lose consciousness simultaneously with it. According to Penfield and Jasper, the cortical areas of discharge responsible for this form of seizure are anterior to the rolandic gyrus and localized to the frontal lobes.[35] They attribute the early loss of consciousness in this type of seizure to a rapid spread of excitation from the anterior frontal areas to the brain stem centrencephalic system. Even though direct electric stimulation of the frontal lobes reproduces this seizure, interictal foci implicating the frontal lobes are only seen in about one-third of instances.[53,54]

Another common form of focal attack is the Sylvian seizure. Attacks commence with a somatosensory aura, usually referred to the tongue, cheek, or gums, less often to the abdomen. As a result of motor interference speech is arrested, the child salivates, and tonic or tonic-clonic movements involve the face. Attacks are common during sleep, and a good history is, therefore, difficult to obtain. The EEG will show mid-temporal spikes, probably a reflection of discharges arising from the rolandic cortex.[55]

Focal motor seizures are particularly common in hemiplegic children. The epileptic movements are usually clonic and begin in the hemiplegic hand, often heralded by localized sensory symptoms. The clonic movements spread over the entire affected side ultimately becoming generalized in many cases. Postictal weakness (Todd's paralysis) commonly follows this type of seizure and may last for several hours or up to a day or more.

In adults there is a high positive correlation between Todd's paralysis and a structural cortical lesion; this is not so in children and it is not unusual to see attacks of alternating left- and right-sided focal seizures with postic-tal paralyses as the initial events in a child with apparently idiopathic epilepsy.

Minor Motor Seizures. Three types of minor motor seizures can be distinguished: these are akinetic seizures, myoclonic seizures, and atypical petit mal.

Akinetic seizures are characterized by a sudden, momentary loss of posture or muscle tone. In the infant, who is able to sit but not yet stand, akinetic spells consist of a sudden dropping forward of the head and neck, the "salaam seizure." In older children the loss of postural tone precipitates the child violently to the ground. Loss of consciousness is only momentary, but the force of the fall not uncommonly produces injuries of the face and head. Akinetic spells recur frequently during the course of a day and are particularly common during the morning hours and shortly after the child awakens.

The term myoclonic seizure includes a variety of convulsive episodes characterized by single or repetitive contractures of a muscle or a group of muscles. Myoclonic seizures may be isolated as in benign essen-tial myoclonus, or may occur in association with other seizure forms. Myoclonus is encountered normally in the course of falling asleep, or as a nonspecific symptom in many diseases of the nervous system. These include several forms of viral encephalitis, metabolic disturbances such as uremia, or progressive cerebral degenerative diseases such as Unverricht's myoclonus (see Chapter 1), or Ramsay Hunt dentatorubral degeneration (see Chapter 2).[56,57] The anatomic substrate of myoclonus is still unknown. Myoclonic seizures are often precipitated by sensory stimuli, most commonly light or tapping on the face or chest. Physiologically, this suggests an abnormal susceptibility of neurons in the contralateral motor area of the cortex, or in some instances at lower levels of the neuraxis, to a variety of afferent stimuli.[58]

Atypical petit mal is characterized by absences, which in the majority of instances (86% in Janz's experience[59]) are unaccompanied by movement. Unlike true petit mal, they have a tendency to occur in cycles and may disappear for periods of several days.

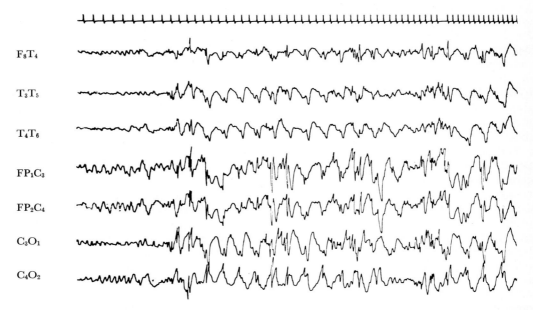

Fig. 11–3. Atypical polyspike and wave discharge. Photically (5/second) induced myoclonic seizure in a 14-year-old girl. The EEG shows 3/second multiple spike and wave discharges. (**Leads:** F_8T_4, right fronto-temporal; T_3T_5, left fronto-temporal; T_4T_6, right temporal; FP_1C_3, left frontopolar-central; FP_2C_4, right fronto-polar-central; C_3O_1, left central-occipital; C_4O_2, right central-occipital. Top lead is photo-stimulator.)

Minor motor seizures may occur by themselves or may be accompanied by grand mal, or psychomotor attacks.

Some 50% of patients with minor motor seizures have a history of perinatal cerebral injury, another 20% may have had an attack of encephalitis or meningitis, and 13% had major complications of gestation.[60]

These seizure forms correlate with an electroencephalogram, which was termed by Lennox and Davis as the petit mal variant (Fig. 11-3).[60] It is an asymmetric, sometimes lateralized, 2.0-2.5 per second polyspike and wave discharge (atypical spike-wave discharge), which in contrast to the 3 per second synchronous discharge of petit mal, is rarely provoked by hyperventilation. Gastaut has suggested that this type of electroencephalographic pattern indicates a secondary synchrony.[61]

Infantile Spasms. This form of seizure most commonly occurs between three and eight months of age, only 8% of cases being first encountered in infants over two years. It is twice as frequent in males as in females.[62] Attacks are characterized by a series of sudden muscular contractions by which the head is flexed, the arms extended, and the legs drawn up. A cry or giggling may precede or follow the seizure, and the infant may flush, turn pale or cyanotic.

Other clinical forms occur less commonly and include extensor spasms characterized by extension rather than flexion of arms, legs, and trunk, and head nodding. Rarely, the attacks are concluded by a brief clonic seizure.

Lightning attacks ("Blitzkrämpfe")[63] are a variant involving single, momentary, shock-like contraction of the entire body.[64]

Clusters of seizures recur frequently, particularly on waking, and some children have as many as 50-100 each day. In Jeavons and Bower's series of 112 children, mental development was normal up to the onset of seizures in 52% and was definitely or probably delayed in the remainder.[62] In 66% of patients the electroencephalogram has the characteristics of hypsarhythmia, namely diffuse dysrhythmia with high voltage slow waves and multiple spike and wave discharges (Fig. 11-4).[62]

Attacks are often associated with a discharge of multiple spike and wave or polyspikes. Sudden suppression of electric activity begins with an attack and persists for a brief time after its completion.

Gastaut and Roger[65] have proposed that infantile spasms indicate damage both to the cortex and to the diencephalon, with the discharging neurons located at the lower level. Immaturity of the cortex could provide an equally adequate explanation.

Infantile spasms are almost always associated with a variety of major underlying cerebral abnormalities. Cases are commonly classified as cryptogenic or symptomatic. The former represent a group of infants with normal birth and development until the onset of seizures, in whom no obvious etiology for the convulsions can be demonstrated. In the symptomatic group there may be a history of maternal infection, prematurity or birth injury, and development is retarded even prior to the appearance of seizures. Infantile spasms are also seen in tuberose sclerosis, neurofibromatosis, agenesis of the corpus callosum, and metabolic diseases such as phenylketonuria and maple syrup disease.[66] In a small group of infants spasms begin shortly after immunization, but it is not clear whether this relationship is other than coincidental.

As might be expected, a variety of neuropathologic findings have been reported. These include structural malformations of cortical gray matter,[67] and chronic edema and spongy degeneration of gray and white matter.[68] In most children the outlook for normal intellectual development is poor, even though in about 50% of children seizures will have ceased by three years of age or have been replaced by akinetic or major motor attacks.[69] According to Jeavons and Bower none of the patients whose development was already retarded by the time infantile spasms began had a subsequent normal intellectual development, while only 29% of infants believed to have developed normally up to the onset of seizures were found to be neurologically intact and intellectually in the normal or low normal range by the time their infantile spasms disappeared.[62] Treatment does not influence the developmental prognosis, although ACTH does have a beneficial effect

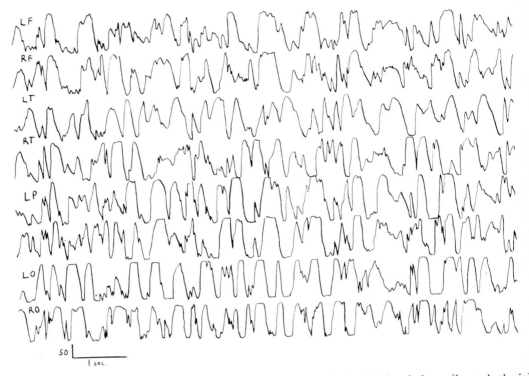

Fig. 11–4. Diffuse slowing, with independent sharp wave activity in both hemispheres (hypsarhythmia) in one-year-old infant with untreated phenylketonuria and infantile spasms. (**Marker** indicates 50 μV and 1 second.)

on seizures and the electroencephalogram in over half the cases.

Miscellaneous Seizure Forms. A number of seizure forms are seen too rarely to warrant more than a brief description. The following types deserve mention:

ABDOMINAL EPILEPSY. Paroxysmal attacks of abdominal pain may occur as an aura for a major motor attack or may be the only manifestation of a convulsive seizure. The abdominal pain is usually periumbilical, radiating to the epigastrium. In the majority of cases it lasts 5–10 minutes but can persist up to 24–36 hours. It is usually associated with disturbed awareness.[70,71]

Often the pediatrician sees a child who has recurrent bouts of paroxysmal abdominal pain, accompanied by vomiting, and in whom the usual gastrointestinal evaluation has been normal. Only a small proportion of these children have abdominal epilepsy. A more common cause for this complaint is childhood migraine. A history of pain and vomiting is common in small children who subsequently develop the usual clinical picture of migraine (see p. 452). The diagnosis of abdominal epilepsy rests upon the presence of other epileptic manifestations, an abnormal EEG pattern during or between attacks, and a favorable response to anticonvulsants, usually diphenylhydantoin (Dilantin).

EPILEPSIA PARTIALIS CONTINUA. This condition is characterized by clonic movements, usually localized to the face or upper extremities, which persist over long periods either continuously or with only brief interruptions. Consciousness is not impaired but postictal weakness is usually evident. We have seen several children with this condition who had an underlying chronic encephalitis of the type described by Rasmussen and McCann.[72] A variety of space-occupying lesions, including tumor, abscess, and cerebral cysticercosis may also be responsible.

PETIT MAL STATUS. This term has been used in different ways. Some authors employ it in referring to an exceedingly rare condition in which petit mal lapses occur in rapid succession. We, however, refer to a prolonged state of clouded mental activity usually accompanied by an electroencephalographic picture of atypical spike-wave complexes and multiple spike discharges. Petit mal status almost always occurs in children with preexisting organic cerebral lesions, a history of intellectual retardation, and a variety of other seizure forms (Fig. 11–5).[73]

Other seizure forms are summarized in Table 11–5.

Diagnosis

The diagnostic process in a child with epileptic seizures has two phases: 1) the ascertainment of the type of seizure that the child has experienced, and its focus, if any; and 2) an attempt to understand the cause for the attacks.

A thorough history taken not only from the parent but also from the child is the single most important prerequisite in arriving at a diagnosis. Usually the physician will not be able to witness an attack, and hospitalization of the child in the hope of recording a seizure is cumbersome and almost always fruitless.

The diagnosis of a grand mal seizure is usually made without much difficulty, although despite their current relative rarity, a hysteric convulsion should also be kept in mind. The best discussion of the differential diagnosis is Gowers' who emphasizes the following points:[84]

1. In the hysteric convulsion the aura is absent or consists of palpitation, malaise, or a choking sensation.

2. During a hysteric attack consciousness is impaired rather than lost.

3. The movements accompanying a hysteric seizure have a more or less coordinated character but lack the definite sequence of a true convulsion. Tonic spasms are long, severe, and often associated with opisthotonus or brief and irregular clonic movements.

4. Micturition and tongue biting are rarely seen in a hysteric attack.

5. The hysteric attack terminates suddenly and the patient often resumes his former activities.

To the above criteria, we can now add the absence of electroencephalographic abnormalities during a hysteric attack as a distinguishing feature.

Grand mal attacks should also be differentiated from syncope. The latter is rare in childhood, being more common in adolescence, particularly in girls. The attacks usually occur in the upright position and are preceded by fatigue or emotional stress. Syncopal attacks are occasionally terminated by a brief generalized convulsion, probably the result of cerebral anoxia. An electroencephalographic recording during a syncopic attack, if available, shows diffuse electric slowing rather than seizure activity.[85]

Another condition requiring differentiation from grand mal attacks is breath-holding. Breath-holding spells are limited to children younger than six years; they are precipitated by crying in response to emotional upsets. The attack is usually brief and accompanied by intense cyanosis or pallor. The child may be limp or opisthotonic. A short clonic convulsion induced by cerebral anoxia may terminate the spell.

The differentiation between a prolonged petit mal seizure with motor accompaniments and a brief psychomotor attack should take the following into account: 1) psychomotor attacks last longer and include a greater variety of movements; 2) petit mal attacks do not have an aura, occur far more frequently, and can often be elicited by hyperventilation; 3) the patient with a psychomotor seizure has partial clouding of consciousness for a brief period after the seizure has ended; and 4) the electroencephalographic abnormalities in petit mal epilepsy are often diagnostic.

Pavor nocturnus (night terror) should be distinguished from nocturnal psychomotor, or major motor seizures. Pavor nocturnus is a paroxysmal sleep disturbance occurring during arousal from slow wave (stage IV) sleep. The child appears agitated or may leave his bed crying and in apparent terror.

Laboratory studies are directed toward uncovering the cause of the seizures. The following diagnostic procedures are customary on patients presenting with seizures and lacking a history or neurologic findings that point to a diagnosis.

1. Blood chemistries: Serum glucose and calcium levels are obtained on all infants with convulsions and on older children whose history raises the possibility of a metabolic disturbance (see Chapter 9). In neonates an evaluation of renal function is also indicated. Serum electrolyte disturbances are rare in patients with recurrent seizures, and in the child with acute convulsions due to hypernatremia the history will usually be suggestive of a fluid imbalance.

2. Radiologic examination of the skull: This study is done in all children with seizures, except those presenting with uncomplicated petit mal attacks. Intracranial calcifications, asymmetry of skull development suggesting cerebral hemiatrophy, and increased intracranial pressure are points of particular importance.

3. Lumbar puncture: This procedure is not performed routinely in patients with seizure disorders. Because a significant proportion of infants with bacterial or tuberculous meningitis may have a febrile convulsion as their initial symptom (see Chapter 6) we believe a lumbar puncture is indicated in patients who have experienced their first febrile convulsion, when focal neurologic findings are uncovered by physical examination, and in all infants presenting with their first seizure.

Although the spinal fluid is normal in the majority of patients with idiopathic epilepsy, minor abnormalities were found by Lennox and Merritt.[87] In 4% of the patients there was a slight pleocytosis (4–10 cells per cu mm), and in 10% an increased protein content (45–85 mg%). Both abnormalities were believed to be related to the presence of small areas of cerebral contusion resulting from a fall attending the seizure and had disappeared when the spinal tap was repeated several weeks later.

4. Electroencephalography: The EEG may be useful in determining the type of seizure experienced by the patient, in particular to differentiate petit mal and psychomotor attacks, and between typical and atypical petit mal. Occasionally it may assist in establishing a diagnosis when the history is inadequate or not diagnostic.

The EEG must be interpreted in conjunction with the patient's history. A normal EEG does not exclude the diagnosis of epilepsy, nor does an abnormal one establish it.

Electric abnormalities may be seen during an overt attack and also between seizures. Generalized major convulsive seizures arising from subcortical excitation can be recorded on the EEG, but the abnormalities are usually obscured by movement artifacts. One exception is the major seizure with a focal cortical origin. In this condition random focal spiking seen during the interseizure period increases in frequency and in amplitude, and spreads both contiguously and via subcortical centers. Generalization may occur within a fraction of a second after the onset of the focal seizure or, less commonly, may develop slowly over as long as 20 seconds. Following the seizure electric activity is extinguished. Recovery starts with slow waves—normal cortical activity first appearing contralateral to the epileptic focus, then ipsilateral, and finally over the focus itself.

The electroencephalogram during a petit mal attack shows bilateral high voltage synchronous alternating spike and wave complexes, most commonly three per second (Fig. 11–1). As the discharge continues the spike and wave complexes tend to become less frequent.

In most patients with psychomotor seizures the EEG patterns accompanying the seizure are slow, rhythmic, usually bilaterally synchronous 1–4 cycles per second discharges, most prominent in the frontal and temporal areas, but becoming generalized as the seizure progresses. At the conclusion of the attack the EEG is featureless and recovery of normal activity is delayed for many minutes.

The interseizure record in patients with major motor attacks may be normal or may demonstrate a number of nonspecific abnormalities, including disorganization, spike discharges, loss of alpha rhythm, or loss of the highest frequency activity expected for the child's age and, occasionally, focal slowing. The latter finding should always raise the possibility of an underlying tumor or other structural lesion.

In the patient with petit mal epilepsy, the interseizure EEG record is almost always abnormal, with isolated or grouped symmetric three per second spike wave discharges, often most prominent in the frontal leads. The discharge frequency can be increased by hyperventilation.

In psychomotor epilepsy the interseizure tracing may be normal, or show nonspecific abnormalities or spike foci, usually arising from the anterior portions of the temporal lobes (Fig. 11–6). Often the seizure focus is only apparent during the transition between wake and sleep, and a combined wake and sleep tracing should always be obtained from children suspected of psychomotor epilepsy. In a number of patients secondary spike foci can be recorded from the opposite tem-poral lobe. It is rare to find focal temporal spike discharges in children under eight years of age, even in those with a classic clinical picture of psychomotor epilepsy.

The presence of atypical spike and wave discharges, that is to say spike and wave discharges at a frequency other than three cycles per second, and polyspike and wave discharges is common in children with minor motor seizures and indicates poor prognosis in terms of likelihood of seizure control and normal intellectual function. The high positive correlation between hypsarhythmia and infantile spasms has already been mentioned.

With time the EEG in patients with convulsive disorders may undergo significant changes. With maturation focal spike activity tends to migrate from the occipital to the midtemporal and ultimately to the anterior temporal leads.[88] In patients with three per second generalized spike and wave discharges, an improvement in clinical status may be associ-

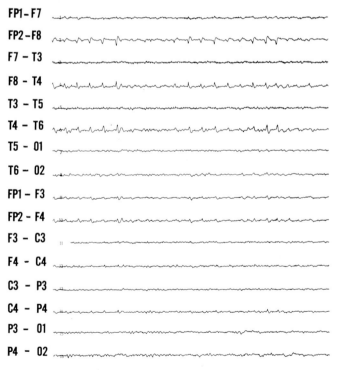

FP1–F7

FP2–F8

F7 – T3

F8 – T4

T3 – T5

T4 – T6

T5 – O1

T6 – O2

FP1 – F3

FP2 – F4

F3 – C3

F4 – C4

C3 – P3

C4 – P4

P3 – O1

P4 – O2

Fig. 11–6. Right anterior temporal spike discharge in patient with psychomotor seizures. (**Leads:** FP$_1$F$_7$, left frontopolar-frontal; FP$_2$F$_8$, right frontopolar-frontal; F$_7$T$_3$, left fronto-temporal; F$_8$T$_4$, right fronto-temporal; T$_3$T$_5$, left temporal; T$_4$T$_6$, right temporal; T$_5$O$_1$, left temporal-occipital; T$_6$O$_2$, right temporal-occipital. (Courtesy of Dr. Gregory Walsh, Department of Neurology, UCLA, Los Angeles.)

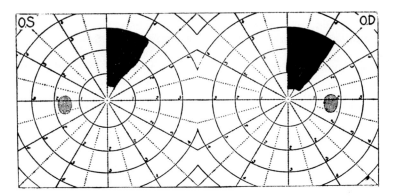

Fig. 11–7. Visual field defect in child with psychomotor seizures and temporal lobe tumor. There is a superior quadrantic hemianopia with sparing of the macula. (Courtesy of Dr. R. Hepler, Department of Ophthalmology, UCLA, Los Angeles.)

ated with disappearance of the abnormal EEG pattern, which often is replaced by a wandering spike focus.[89] In patients with focal epileptic discharges mirror spike activity may appear. In some this second focus may be suppressed by anticonvulsant medication, while in others it may become the only active focus.[89]

For further reading on the clinical aspects of electroencephalography the reader is referred to a number of excellent texts.[90,91]

5. Isotope brain scanning and echoencephalography are not routinely done on patients with epilepsy but are indicated when the EEG indicates a persistent discharge or slow wave focus, or when a focal abnormality is found on neurologic examination.

6. Contrast studies, such as pneumoencephalography or cerebral angiography, are major procedures and require hospitalization of the patient. We believe these studies to be indicated when there is reason to suspect a progressive neurologic disturbance, when neurologic examination shows focal abnormalities such as a mild hemiparesis or a visual field defect (Fig. 11–7), or when either the skull films or lumbar puncture is abnormal.

When focal EEG abnormalities are the only localizing finding, we hesitate to do contrast studies, preferring to do an isotope scan which, if normal, usually precludes a more extensive workup.

A small fraction of children with long-standing seizure disorder unaccompanied by neurologic abnormalities are subsequently found to harbor a cerebral glioma. In most of them neither the type of seizure nor the initial EEG suggests a focal disorder, and contrast studies performed at the initial evaluation may be normal. Page and associates[92] have compiled the clinical features which they consider indicative of a cerebral tumor (Table 11–7).

7. A considerable proportion of children with seizures and bilateral bursts of spike and wave activity have an underlying focal cortical lesion which may be amenable to surgical removal. In order to distinguish such a patient from one with multiple, bilateral epileptogenic foci, Lombroso and Erba have suggested evaluating the effect of intravenous thiopental (Pentothal) on the EEG.[24] Generally, 0.5 mg/kg are injected intravenously. If no appreciable fast (beta) activity is seen on the EEG, a second injection of 1 mg/kg is made. Fast activity normally appears bilaterally. In children with focal cerebral disease there is a regional depression or absence of beta activity, and focal epileptic discharges may be evoked in the area where beta rhythms are depressed. Such patients are potentially good candidates for excision of a cortical epileptogenic focus. When there is a diffuse cortical abnormality, beta rhythms are poorly evoked throughout, and the spike and wave discharges present initially may become enhanced by the injection of thiopental.

TABLE 11-7.
WARNING SIGNS OF CEREBRAL NEOPLASMS IN 23 CHILDREN WITH
LONG-STANDING SEIZURE DISORDER AND BRAIN TUMOR*

Parameter	Time Before Diagnosis of Tumor	
	6–24 Months	Less Than 6 Months
Deterioration of behavior and school performance	9	3
Slow wave focus on EEG	8	11
Seizure pattern changed or increased in frequency	8	5
Abnormalities on plain skull film	3	9
Specific neurologic signs	1	13
Signs reflecting increased intracranial pressure	0	12

* After Page et al.[92]

These patients tend to respond poorly to surgery. Children in whom beta activity is well-induced bilaterally and whose spike and wave discharges are depressed by thiopental usually have uncomplicated petit mal epilepsy and do well on anticonvulsant medication.

More recently methohexital (Brevital) has been used to activate focal epileptiform discharges from the temporal lobes, or generalized spike and wave discharges in patients suspected of petit mal epilepsy.[93] To activate a temporal lobe focus, the cumulative effect of intravenous methohexital is usually required, with the average most effective cumulative dose being 1.9 mg/kg.[94] By this means high amplitude spike discharges are produced in one or both temporal lobes in some three-quarters of patients with psychomotor seizures.

At our institution activation of the electroencephalogram by means of metrazol is no longer carried out.

8. Chromatographic screening of amino acids, keto-acids and organic acids is performed when a family history of seizures can be elicited.

Treatment

The objective in the treatment of the epileptic patient is complete control of seizures, or at least a reduction in their frequency to the point where they no longer interfere with physical and social well-being. Two aspects of therapy will be covered in this section: the questions of whom to treat and how to treat.

While there is unanimous agreement that all patients with recurrent seizures should be treated as soon as the diagnosis is established, there is considerable controversy regarding the optimum method of dealing with certain groups of patients.

1. Febrile convulsions: The treatment of febrile convulsions will be discussed in a subsequent section.

2. The child with an isolated major motor seizure: We believe that treatment of this type of a patient is optional and to a large measure is dependent on social factors. While phenobarbital, the drug of choice in this instance, has few side effects, it must be stressed that sudden withdrawal of the drug by the parents, unconvinced of its necessity, may precipitate status epilepticus.

3. Breath-holding spells: We have found antiepileptic drugs to be of no value in preventing recurrence of attacks. Our experience is shared by Livingston[95] and others.

4. Syncopal attacks: Here too, anticonvulsant therapy is of little use either in prevention of the attacks, or of the clonic seizure that may terminate it.

15

TABLE 11-8.
SOME DRUGS USED IN THE CONTROL OF CONVULSIVE DISORDERS*

Major Motor	Petit Mal	Psychomotor	Minor Motor	Focal Seizures	Infantile Spasms
Phenobarbital	Ethosuximide (Zarontin)	Diphenylhydantoin (Dilantin)	Clonazepam	Diphenylhydantoin (Dilantin)	Nitrazepam (Mogadon)
Diphenylhydantoin (Dilantin)	Clonazepam	Carbamazepine (Tegretol)	Diazepam (Valium)	Primidone (Mysoline)	ACTH and Corticosteroids
Primidone (Mysoline)	Trimethadione (Tridione)	Primidone (Mysoline)	Primidone (Mysoline)	Phenobarbital	
Carbamazepine (Tegretol)	Paramethadione (Paradione)	Phenobarbital	Ketogenic diet		
Mephenytoin (Mesantoin)	Methsuximide (Celontin)	Mephobarbital (Mebaral)			
Mephobarbital (Mebaral)	Quinacrine (Atebrine)	Phenacemide (Phenurone)			
Bromides					

* In this table drugs are arranged in order of preference. A number of other anticonvulsants which, in our hands have usually been less effective, have not been listed

440

5. The child with one or more episodes whose epileptic nature cannot be established with certainty: In this instance we either defer therapy until the clinical picture becomes clear, or if there is considerable likelihood that the patient did experience a seizure equivalent, we use an anticonvulsant in a therapeutic trial. Generally diphenylhydantoin (Dilantin), which is relatively more effective in seizure equivalents, is the drug of choice.

Drug Therapy. Once treatment has been decided upon, several therapeutic principles should be kept in mind:

1. The selection of the drug of first choice is based on the type of seizure and on the potential toxicity of the drug.

2. Treatment should be begun with one drug, its dosage being increased until seizures are controlled or the child develops toxicity. If the drug appears to be effective but not sufficiently so to control seizures completely, it is continued at its maximum tolerated dose, and a second drug is added, again slowly increasing its dosage.

3. Alterations in drug dosage should be made slowly, usually not more frequently than once every five to seven days.

4. The number of truly effective anticonvulsant drugs is small, and there is little likelihood of controlling a patient with a lesser-known drug when the usual medications have failed. However, the chances of inducing toxic side reactions with a new or rarely utilized drug are great.

5. Once seizures are controlled the medication should be continued for a prolonged period of time.

6. Medication should be given daily. In the case of phenobarbital and diphenylhydantoin (Dilantin), blood levels are maintained adequately by administering the drug no more frequently than twice daily.[96,97]

7. Determinations of anticonvulsant blood levels are helpful in patients whose seizures are not responding to therapy or who develop evidence of drug intoxication. While there is good correlation between blood levels and signs of intoxication, the relationship between drug dosage and blood levels is variable, particularly in the case of diphenylhydantoin and mephobarbital (Mebaral).

8. Anticonvulsant medication should be withdrawn gradually. Sudden withdrawal of medication, particularly barbiturates, is the most common cause of status epilepticus.

The selection of the drug for the treatment of a patient with a convulsive disorder depends on the type of seizure. Drugs of choice are presented in Table 11–8.

Phenobarbital is an effective anticonvulsant in the treatment of major motor and focal seizures. At anesthetic levels, barbiturates decrease the membrane potential of neurons and block generation of action potentials. At lower levels they depress the repetitive electric activity seen in grand mal convulsions, the activation of motor neurons in the spinal cord, and of secondary neurons in the medulla and thalamic nuclei.[98]

The effective dosage of phenobarbital varies from patient to patient; we, therefore, prefer to start at about 5 mg/kg/day, given in two divided doses. The drug is absorbed slowly from the gastrointestinal tract, and under clinical conditions (4 mg/kg body weight) 95% of the maximum serum level is reached in only two to three weeks.[99] Svensmark and Buchthal have shown that in most patients with grand mal seizures controlled by phenobarbital the drug did so at serum levels of 10–15 μg/ml. These were achieved by an oral dosage of 2–3 mg/kg in children weighing 10–20 kg and about 2 mg/kg in larger children (Table 11–9).[100] The maximum variation in serum concentration with one daily dose of phenobarbital is between 7%–14%. Therefore, in most cases two daily doses of the anticonvulsant suffice for seizure control.

Toxic levels of phenobarbital vary from one individual to another, but as a rule no permanent sedation is seen with levels below 35 μg/ml. Thirty percent of ingested phenobarbital is excreted unchanged in the urine, the rest is oxidized in the liver by *p*-hydroxylation to form *p*-hydroxyphenobarbital. Even though metabolism of phenobarbital is preserved in most patients with hepatic disease, a reduction in the usual dosage is indicated under these circumstances.[101] The principal side reactions experienced with phenobarbital are drowsiness and hyperkinetic behavior.

Mephobarbital (Mebaral) is commonly

TABLE 11-9.
RELATION BETWEEN SERUM LEVELS OF DIPHENYLHYDANTOIN AND PHENOBARBITAL, BODY WEIGHT IN KILOGRAMS, AND DAILY DOSE IN MILLIGRAMS*

Body Weight Kg (Pounds)	Serum Levels in μg/Milliliter			
	Diphenylhydantoin		Phenobarbital	
	10	15	10	15
	Daily Dose in Milligrams			
10 (22)	100		22	30
15 (33)	150	200	30	45
20 (44)	150	200	45	60
25 (56)	150	200	45	75
30 (67)	200	250	45	75
35 (78)	200	250	50	75
40 (89)	200	300	60	90
45 (100)	250	300	60	90
50 (111)	250	300	75	100

* After Svensmark and Buchthal.[100]

used in the place of phenobarbital, as it is believed to have less side effects. Since it is demethylated to phenobarbital in the liver, it would appear to have no real advantages.

Primidone (Mysoline) is an effective anticonvulsant for major motor and focal seizures due to organic disease of the brain. It is somewhat less effective against psychomotor attacks.

In children primidone (Mysoline) is started at low levels, generally 50 mg/day, given in two divided doses. The daily dose is gradually increased until the average effective dose (150–500 mg/day) is reached. This procedure is intended to circumvent marked sedation which often occurs when the drug is started at the latter levels. Toxic symptoms are due to primidone itself and appear at a time when only primidone is detectable in serum. As a rule, prior exposure to phenobarbital makes the subject less likely to develop primidone toxicity.[101a]

Diphenylhydantoin (Dilantin) is a very effective drug for major motor seizures and in combination with primidone (Mysoline) is often the best therapeutic regimen in patients with psychomotor attacks. Its effectiveness as an anticonvulsant is based on the ability to suppress spread of epileptic discharges to local and to distant, synaptically related neurons.[102] This is probably accomplished through a stabilizing action on excitable membranes[103] by limiting the increase in sodium permeability which occurs during stimulation of nerves.[104]

Depending on the size of the child the average effective dose of diphenylhydantoin in children is 5 mg–10 mg/kg/day (Table 11–9). The drug is slowly absorbed from the gastrointestinal tract and at a dose of 4–6 mg/kg/day equilibrium levels in the blood are established between 7 and 10 days after initiation of therapy.[96] The daily fluctuations in serum concentrations in children under 30 kg are sufficiently large to require the drug to be administered at approximately eight-hour intervals.[97,100] Diphenylhydantoin is metabolized in the liver, mainly by hydroxylation at the para-position.[103] The concurrent administration of phenobarbital has very little effect on diphenylhydantoin blood levels, and what little alterations do occur are unpredictable.[105] Diphenylhydantoin produces a number of untoward reactions, but in most instances these are related to overdosage and can be relieved by reducing the drug intake.

Clinically effective diphenylhydantoin levels range from 10 to 20 μg/ml. Nystagmus at lateral gaze appears at blood levels of 15–30 μg/ml, ataxia above 30 μg/ml, and lethargy or aggravation of seizures at levels of 40 μg/ml or higher.[106] Irreversible degeneration of the cerebellar Purkınje cells may occur after chronic intoxication or severe acute intoxication[107] and cerebellar atrophy may be demonstrable by pneumoencephalography.[107a] Since seizure control can be achieved at an average blood level of 18 μg/ml, reduction of dosage in patients with toxic levels usually has no adverse effects on the frequency of convulsions.[96]

A few patients have a defect in the para-hydroxylation of diphenylhydantoin and will develop toxic symptoms with the usual daily doses.[108] Low diphenylhydantoin tolerance is also seen with liver disease and in patients receiving chemotherapeutic drugs against tuberculosis. Small infants only eliminate 1%–20% of the drug in a 24-hour period and often develop toxic effects.[97]

About two to five percent of patients receiving diphenylhydantoin develop fever, a morbilliform rash, and lymphadenopathy within two weeks of the start of therapy. Blood levels at the time of the reaction are in the therapeutic range.[108a] After discontinuation of the medication the symptoms clear, and Schmidt and Wilder[13] state that diphenylhydantoin then can be restarted without recurrence. We have been hesitant to do so because the drug is known to precipitate lupus erythematosus on rare occasions in patients with a positive family history of the condition.[109] The incidence of malignant lymphomas in patients receiving long-term hydantoin therapy is 10 times greater than expected, a finding suggesting that lymphadenopathy is not necessarily benign.[110]

In a significant proportion of patients diphenylhydantoin causes gum hyperplasia and 75% of patients develop hirsutism. Neither complication has prompted us to discontinue the drug. Gingival hyperplasia, which usually appears two to three months after initiation of the drug, is seen at therapeutic blood levels of the drug. According to Kapus et al.,[110a] 93% of patients with diphenylhydantoin levels between 10 and 20 μg/ml display gum changes. These can be reduced by strict oral hygiene, daily massage of gums, and repeated excision of hyperplastic tissue.

Patients on prolonged diphenylhydantoin therapy develop megaloblastic anemia and lowered serum folate concentrations which respond to folic acid therapy.[111] The mechanism by which anemia develops in patients receiving not only diphenylhydantoin but also phenobarbital or primidone (Mysoline) is still unknown. Absorptive defects and interference in folate metabolism have been excluded. Although prolonged folate deficiency may induce an organic brain syndrome in the absence of subacute combined degeneration of the cord folate therapy has no effect on the behavior or mental deterioration of chronic epileptic patients.[112a]

A disturbed vitamin D metabolism resulting in hypocalcemic rickets, decreased serum calcium and phosphorus, and increased alkaline phosphatase is seen in some patients after long-term therapy with diphenylhydantoin, primidone, or phenobarbital.[113] The cause of these abnormalities is still unclear, but plasma levels of 25-hydroxycholecalciferol are lower than normal in patients receiving diphenylhydantoin and phenobarbital,[114] and it is possible that degradation of vitamin D_3 to inactive metabolites is accelerated. A low vitamin D intake and decreased exposure to sunshine may be contributory.

Peripheral neuropathy may also result from prolonged anticonvulsant therapy. Deep tendon reflexes are lost in about one-half of patients receiving diphenylhydantoin for longer than 15 years.[115]

Mephenytoin (Mesantoin), chemically related to diphenylhydantoin, is effective against major motor attacks. A starting dose for children of six years or over is 100 mg t.i.d. It is demethylated in the liver to 5,5-ethylphenylhydantoin (Nirvanol), which is probably responsible for the toxic effects of leukopenia, pancytopenia, and aplastic anemia seen in about five percent of patients receiving the drug. The hematologic abnormalities are usually reversible once the drug has been discontinued, but fatalities have been reported. Less common is a syndrome of fever, skin rash, and lymphadenopathy.

When abnormalities of the peripheral blood develop, they usually become apparent within six months after initial administration

of chronic idiopathic epilepsy. In Hunter's series, 23% of patients who were in status died.[132] This relatively high mortality justifies the use of vigorous methods for the termination of status. Hunter has analyzed the causes for status. In 23% of his patients status was preceded by changes in medication, and in 30% by intercurrent infections. All patients in the latter group were receiving anticonvulsant medication at the time of their status.

We believe that sodium phenobarbital is the drug of choice for the treatment of status epilepticus. The initial dose of 10 mg/kg is administered subcutaneously. If seizures do not subside within 20–30 minutes of administration of the barbiturate, we then give paraldehyde by muscular injection in a dosage of 1 cc per year of age, not exceeding 5 cc or in a dosage of 0.25 mg/kg. Should seizures continue for 20 to 30 more minutes, a second dose of sodium phenobarbital (10 mg/kg) is given subcutaneously. If these measures are ineffectual we ask the assistance of an anesthetist in the administration of ether by mask and open drop. If specialized help is not available the physician will have to proceed on his own, keeping in mind that an airway has to be secured before the ether is given. Work by Plum and his associates supports the concept that maintenance of an airway and abolition of muscular movements with succinylcholine or other curarelike drugs can prevent brain damage due to cerebral anoxia.[18]

A number of authorities have proposed diazepam (Valium) for the treatment of status epilepticus.[95,134,135,136] Carter and Gold suggest a dosage of 0.3 mg/kg up to a maximum dose of 10 mg, diluted with sterile water and given intravenously over a period no shorter than one minute. A repeat dosage of the same amount can be given 30 minutes later if necessary.[134] The use of diazepam is complicated by serious side reactions: cardiac arrest and severe respiratory depression. These are particularly common when diazepam is used as an adjunct to sodium phenobarbital.[136]

Intravenous diphenylhydantoin (Dilantin) has also been advocated in the treatment of status and is probably most desirable in patients whose seizures follow a head injury, and

in whom preservation of consciousness is important.[137] Intramuscular diphenylhydantoin is absorbed too slowly to produce effective anticonvulsant serum levels, and should not be used in the treatment of status epilepticus.[137a]

Following termination of status the patient is continued on intramuscular anticonvulsant therapy, usually sodium phenobarbital, until he has regained consciousness. Oral medication is then resumed.

Prognosis

The results of medical therapy depend on the type of seizure being treated and on its natural course.[138] Wilkins found spontaneous remissions for two or more years in 19% of epileptic children.[139] The incidence of remissions was 41% in patients whose attacks occurred less often than once a month, but only 16% in patients having attacks monthly or more often. Most of the remissions were experienced by patients who had attacks for periods between two and four years. The incidence of remissions was almost 60% in those children who had suffered only a few generalized convulsions, usually spaced at long intervals. Long or permanent remissions are unlikely in patients whose seizures start prior to four years of age.[138]

The chances for spontaneous remission are affected by the type of seizure. Remissions occurred in 37.1% of neurologically intact children with grand mal epilepsy,[139] and in 80% of children with pure petit mal epilepsy. Patients who have both petit mal and grand mal epilepsy become free of seizures in only 33% of instances. About one-third of patients with temporal lobe epilepsy experience complete seizure control for periods of one year or longer.[140] Complete remission is least likely in children with minor motor attacks.[35] It is not clear whether drug therapy influences the chances for a spontaneous remission. However severe the seizures may be, spontaneous improvement can still be looked for.

There has been considerable controversy as to whether or not and when medication should be discontinued after prolonged seizure control. We believe that reduction of medication can be considered after about two years of seizure control. In a recently published study anticonvulsant medication was discontinued after four years of seizure control. A relapse rate of 28% was encountered.[141] As a rule patients whose seizures started between four and eight years of age had a lower relapse rate than those whose seizures started in later childhood or in infancy. The relapse rate was highest in patients with Jacksonian seizures (53%), and those with multiple seizure types (40%). It was lowest in grand mal (8%) and in petit mal epilepsy (12%). Holowach and her co-workers found no relationship between the rate of relapse and the time of drug withdrawal, or the presence of electroencephalographic abnormalities at the time the medication was withdrawn.[141] Livingston, however, believes that when the time for planned withdrawal coincides with puberty, all medications should be continued throughout adolescence, particularly in girls.[5] In general, medication is withdrawn in the course of one to two years, the period for withdrawal being longer in children who have been receiving high doses of anticonvulsants.

Patients whose epileptic attacks are uncontrolled may suffer mental and emotional deterioration. Patients whose seizures are secondary to cerebral injury or malformations are far more likely to deteriorate than those with idiopathic epilepsy.[142] In Lennox's series of 2000 epileptic patients, 26% of the former and 10% of the latter group underwent intellectual deterioration.[142] Adverse factors in both groups included an early onset of seizures, and in the symptomatic group the duration of the epileptic disorder.

Deterioration was seen in 23% of patients whose seizures first appeared before one year of age, but in only 7% of children with idiopathic epilepsy with onset between two and nine years of age. Psychomotor and grand mal seizures were more likely to be associated with intellectual deterioration than petit mal attacks. "True" petit mal seizures, when not preceded by other seizure types, are perhaps never associated with mental deterioration.[143]

Behavior disturbances are common in epileptic children. In part they stem from the deleterious effects of a chronic illness, but children with psychomotor seizures appear particularly prone to disordered behavior. Abnormal behavior or psychoses may also be part of the ictal phenomenon—as in some patients with petit mal status—or may follow a seizure.[144,145] Occasionally they are induced by drug therapy and disappear spontaneously once the anticonvulsant is withdrawn.

Febrile Convulsions

The term febrile convulsion is used to designate seizures associated with fever, but excluding those due to infections of the central nervous system. It is one of the most common neurologic disorders of childhood. Patrick and Levy in 1924 found an incidence of 4.2% of febrile convulsions in an unselected group of children attending Well Baby Clinics,[146] a figure supported by most subsequent studies. Bridge found that febrile convulsions accounted for 35% of children attending the Johns Hopkins Seizure Clinic,[147] a value which is undoubtedly too low since most children with febrile convulsions may not be followed on a regular basis. The episodes are more common in males, and most series show boys to be affected nearly twice as frequently as girls.

The cause for febrile convulsions is still uncertain. In most patients the height of the body temperature appears to be an important factor in triggering the seizure, and Millichap has postulated a convulsive threshold beyond which the seizure is precipitated.[3,148] While the rate at which body temperature rises has been frequently cited as a contributing factor in the development of seizures, more recent EEG data obtained on children with artificially induced fever indicate that this is not the case.[149] Aside from roseola (exanthem subitum), which produces seizures in about one-quarter of cases and which is responsible for some 13% of febrile convulsions,[150] epidemic diseases are a relatively infrequent cause of febrile convulsions. More commonly, a convulsion accompanies an upper respiratory infection or severe gastroenteritis, particularly when due to *Shigella*.[151] In none of the infectious illnesses has there been evidence for direct involvement of the brain by the organisms. Rather, one is forced to conclude that as a result of genetic predisposition the immature neuronal membrane is particularly susceptible to temperature elevations and responds by breaking down.

The first febrile seizure usually occurs between six months and three years of age in 93% of children.[3,152] It is generally believed that patients with febrile convulsions consist of two distinct groups: 1) the majority (96.9%) who suffer with an entity designated by Livingston[5,95] as a simple febrile convulsion; and 2) 3.1% who are basically predisposed to idiopathic epilepsy and whose initial attack was triggered by fever.[150]

Patients in the latter group have, at the time of their initial seizure, either one of two findings:[5,95,152,153]

1. A generalized or focal convulsion of greater than 20 minutes duration.

2. Focal or generalized paroxysmal electroencephalographic abnormalities persisting for two weeks or more after the convulsion. In both groups the spinal fluid is normal, although a mild pleocytosis may occur in patients whose febrile convulsions are due to roseola.

Factors of lesser prognostic significance include a family history of seizures, abnormal birth history, and mental retardation. About 28% of the patients with simple febrile convulsions have a recurrence of seizures with subsequent infections and fever up to between 6 and 15 years of age.[154] In two-thirds of patients in the second group spontaneous seizures, usually major motor, will occur within one year of the onset of febrile convulsions (Table 11–11).

The treatment of the febrile convulsion consists of controlling the convulsion by means of sodium phenobarbital or diazepam (Valium) in dosages analogous to those recommended for the treatment of status epilepticus, reduction of body temperature by conductive or evaporative cooling of the patient, and treatment of the acute infection responsible for the fever.

There is considerable controversy as to whether a child who has experienced his first febrile convulsion should receive continuous prophylactic anticonvulsant therapy. The reader is referred to Hammill and Carter,[156]

TABLE 11-11.
TIME OF APPEARANCE OF SPONTANEOUS NONFEBRILE SEIZURES IN RELATION TO ONSET OF FEBRILE SEIZURES IN 313 PATIENTS WITH BOTH TYPES OF SEIZURES*

Time of Appearance of Nonfebrile Seizures	Patients With Febrile Seizures	
	Number	Percent
Prior to febrile seizures	20	6.4
Close to febrile seizures	21	6.7
Years after febrile seizures		
1/12 to 1	147	46.9
1 to 4	54	17.3
5 to 9	47	15.1
10 to 14	14	4.5
15 to 35	10	3.1

* After Lennox.[155]

proponents of continuous therapy, and Millichap[3] who advises against it. Controlled prospective studies suggest that the incidence of recurrent febrile convulsions is not significantly less in patients who have been placed on daily doses of phenobarbital or diphenylhydantoin than those on intermittent anticonvulsants administered only at the time of a febrile episode or on no therapy at all.[3,157] Faero and co-workers suggest that failure of phenobarbital prophylaxis is due to inadequate barbiturate blood levels, and believe that serum levels higher than 1.5 mg% are required to prevent febrile convulsions.[157a] In reconciling these viewpoints we suggest that patients who have a single simple febrile convulsion not be treated with continuous prophylactic anticonvulsants until a second seizure has occurred, and that the dosage of barbiturate be monitored with blood levels.

Neonatal Convulsions

As convulsions occur with relatively high frequency during the neonatal period and present special problems in terms of diagnosis and treatment, they will be considered separately.

The factors inducing seizures in the newborn infant, and their relative frequency as determined by autopsy are presented in Table 11–12.[158] The most common cause

TABLE 11-12.
MAJOR AUTOPSY FINDINGS IN INFANTS WITH NEONATAL SEIZURES*

Infections	29	
E. coli		9
Developmental anomalies of CNS	14	
Trauma	97	
Subdural hemorrhage		30
Intraventricular hemorrhage		23
Venous congestion, edema		16
Subarachnoid hemorrhage		14
Multiple hemorrhages		6
Sinus thrombosis		4
Other		4
Extracerebral hemorrhages, shock	9	
Kernicterus	4	
No abnormalities (? metabolic)	9	

* After Craig.[158]

is trauma, particularly subdural and intraventricular hemorrhage.[159] Developmental anomalies of the brain and metabolic disturbances are probably far more common than would appear from the autopsy studies of Craig, since a large proportion of those patients do not succumb to their illness. Convulsions due to subdural hemorrhage usually start in the second week of life, and it is rare to find such a lesion in infants presenting with seizures during the first week of life.

Only a small percentage of newborn infants present with classic tonic-clonic convulsions. More commonly one observes localized clonic movements, hypertonia of limbs and trunk, rhythmic eye movements, chewing or unusual rowing, swimming or pedalling movements of arms or legs.[160] These types of seizures reflect the immaturity of the nervous system of the newborn infant and its inability to propagate epileptic discharges.

Hypoglycemic and hypocalcemic convulsions are relatively common during the neonatal period; according to Keen they account for 6% and 34% of neonatal convulsions[161] (see Chapter 9). Therapy for convulsions, therefore, includes the administration of intravenous glucose and calcium, usually given on an emergency basis, even

before a cause for the convulsions has been clarified. Intramuscular pyridoxine (25–50 mg) should also be given as a therapeutic trial so as to exclude pyridoxine dependency as a cause for seizures.[162] As is shown in Table 11–13, inborn metabolic errors are only responsible for neonatal convulsions in exceptional instances.

Phenobarbital is the best anticonvulsant for use during the neonatal period. It is administered parenterally in doses up to 15 mg/kg/day. If necessary, paraldehyde, given intravenously, serves as an adjunct to phenobarbital. We have not had much success in the control of neonatal convulsions with diphenylhydantoin and have experienced a high incidence of toxic reactions, perhaps due to immaturity of the hepatic hydroxylating system responsible for diphenylhydantoin detoxification. Diazepam has also been suggested as an anticonvulsant in the newborn infant. We have found, however, that if seizures are not controlled by phenobarbital, they are usually poorly controlled by other drugs, including diazepam. The ultimate prognosis of such infants, most of whom have congenital cerebral malformations, is poor with respect to intellectual development.

The majority of infants having seizures as a result of cardiopulmonary disease die within a few months of birth, while those having convulsions due to birth injury or malformations of the central nervous system have a

TABLE 11-13.
SEIZURE ONSET REPORTED IN INBORN ERRORS OF METABOLISM

Phenylketonuria	1 to 18 months
Maple syrup disease	1 to 2 weeks
Argininosuccinic aciduria	7 days to 2½ years
Pyridoxine dependency	3 hours to 7 days
Hyperglycemia	First week
Citrullinemia	First week
Hypoglycemia	2½ hours or later
Galactosemia	First week
Congenital amaurotic idiocy	2 weeks
Hypocalcemia	
High phosphate intake	Third day or later
Other causes	First 48 hours
Hypomagnesemia	9 days to 6 weeks

headache, the possibility of an underlying space-occupying lesion should not be forgotten. We have seen two children in whom the appearance of a malignant posterior fossa tumor produced an aggravation of long-standing migraine.

Treatment

The treatment of migraine is symptomatic; the patient and his parents should be informed of his lifelong predisposition to headaches and of the essentially benign nature of the condition.

For most patients the drug of choice is ergotamine tartrate which induces strong arterial vasoconstriction. The medication is given orally at the beginning of an attack, usually in the form of Cafergot, a proprietary preparation containing ergotamine tartrate (1 mg) and caffeine (100 mg) per tablet. If necessary, it is followed by a second tablet at a 30-minute interval. Ergotamine is not indicated for patients who develop hemianopia or hemiparesis during the constrictive phase of an attack. Since children rarely inform their parents about the beginning of the headache, the usefulness of Cafergot is somewhat limited.

Sansert (methysergide maleate), a serotonin antagonist, has recently been advocated for the treatment of migraine. The medication is usually given as a 2 mg tablet after each meal. While headaches are prevented in about one-half of children, an occasional patient may develop thrombophlebitis as a result of therapy.[179]

The outlook for the patient with migraine headaches is excellent and in most instances the condition does not interfere with school work. In about two-thirds of the children the attacks persist throughout life, although many are intermittently free of them for prolonged periods or at least partly relieved by medication.[180]

SYNCOPE

Syncope or fainting is a condition characterized by transient loss of consciousness resulting from inadequate cerebral perfusion and anoxia. The most common cause for syncope is a sudden drop in blood pressure in a child who is in the upright posture. In about three-quarters of instances it is the result of some obvious emotional upset. Less commonly syncope is precipitated by hyperventilation, violent coughing, or hot baths. Adolescents subject to postural hypotension may faint when maintaining an upright posture for prolonged periods. Finally, children with cardiac asystole (Stokes-Adams syndrome), paroxysmal changes in cardiac rhythm, obstruction to left ventricular outflow, or anemia may be prone to syncope.

Syncope is rare in childhood but more common during adolescence, particularly in girls. Fainting spells consist of an initial period during which the patient experiences a number of premonitory symptoms including restlessness, pallor, sweating, and reduction in vision. These are followed by loss of consciousness. In two-thirds of the patients followed by Livingston for recurrent syncope, unconsciousness lasted less than 5 minutes; in the remainder it persisted for 5 to 30 minutes.[5] Rarely there are brief clonic convulsions, the result of cerebral anoxia.

The differentiation between syncope and epilepsy is difficult and has already been referred to. Generally, the longer the period of unconsciousness, the greater the likelihood of an epileptic equivalent. In the latter group anticonvulsant therapy is often beneficial in reducing the frequency of attacks. Finally, it should be emphasized that syncope may precipitate a convulsion in an epileptic individual.

BREATH-HOLDING SPELLS

It is common for a small child to hold its breath when crying. These episodes, termed breath-holding spells, are readily recognized and follow a distinct clinical pattern.

In a typical attack, the child who has been frightened or frustrated begins to cry and ceases breathing. Usually the breath is held in expiration,[181] and after a few seconds the infant becomes more or less cyanotic. Consciousness is lost, the infant becomes limp and may experience a few clonic convulsions of the extremities. It is a frequent experience that the longer the child cries, the less likely a spell is to follow. Lombroso and Lerman found breath-holding spells in 4.6% of infants; with the majority (76%) beginning between ages 6 and 18 months.[181] In a large number the first attack was observed during the neonatal period. The frequency of attacks varies considerably. About 10% of patients experience two or more attacks per day and another 20% an average of one spell a day.[5]

With increasing age spells become less common, finally disappearing by five to six years in almost all instances. Lombroso and Lerman[181] believe that these infants can be divided into two well-defined groups of about equal size; namely, one in whom breath-holding spells were conspicuously cyanotic, and another in whom spells were characterized by pallor. The latter group was particularly sensitive to vagus stimulation as elicited by ocular compression which induced a prolonged asystole and an occasional seizure. Gauk and co-workers have demonstrated a rapid fall in arterial oxygen saturation as measured by ear oximetry, probably the result of oxygen utilization.[182]

As has already been indicated, breath-holding spells accompanied by seizures are differentiated from the epileptic convulsions in that an obvious precipitating factor, which has induced the child to cry, can always be elicited in the former. Cyanosis in an epileptic attack generally follows the onset of convulsions but precedes breath-holding spells.[182a] Finally, the interseizure electroencephalogram is invariably normal in patients with breath-holding spells. Apneic seizures, which represent true epileptic attacks probably arising from the limbic system, may occur both during the waking and sleeping state. Generally they are seen in neurologically damaged children, and are accompanied by EEG abnormalities. Hooshmand has suggested treatment with atropine.[182b]

Drug therapy for breath-holding spells is neither indicated nor effective, although atropine is said to be helpful in the pallid type of breath-holding spell. Basically the attacks are triggered by a disciplinary conflict between parent and child, with the latter using the attacks or the threat of an attack to assert himself and to express his anger. Proper family counseling and assuring parents that the attacks do not represent any danger to the child is often effective in stopping them.[182]

Although breath-holding spells disappear spontaneously in every case, many patients become prone to syncope and develop behavior disturbances particularly temper tantrums. The incidence of true epilepsy in children with breath-holding spells is, however, no greater than is found in the general population.

NARCOLEPSY

Narcolepsy is a condition characterized by paroxysmal attacks of irrepressible sleep. Occasionally somnolence is associated with transient loss of muscular tone or cataplexy.

Although narcolepsy was first described by Westphal in 1877,[183] the neurophysiologic basis for the disorder has been recently found to represent abnormal recurrent episodes of rapid eye movement (REM) sleep. Normal subjects always go into nonrapid eye movement (NREM) sleep first, changing to REM sleep after a variable period, averaging 140 minutes in children aged 19–45 months.[184] By contrast, narcoleptic subjects show an immediate appearance of REM sleep. The cataplectic attack often associated can be explained as being the result of the motor inhibitory process which is an essential part of normal REM periods. Although there is considerable evidence that the pontile reticular formation is involved in REM sleep, no specific neuroanatomic abnormalities have been found in narcoleptic subjects. A disorder in the neurochemical regulation of sleep appears to be likely.[185]

Clinical Manifestations

Narcolepsy first appears during adolescence[186] although spells may develop as early as three years of age. Attacks of sleep usually occur while the child is at rest; while the patient can resist them, he can only do so briefly. If not disturbed, sleep lasts from a few minutes to half an hour, following which the patient awakens and is completely alert. Narcoleptic sleep is usually shallow and the patient can easily be aroused. Narcolepsy is only rarely characterized by abnormally excessive amounts of sleep.

Cataplexy is associated with narcolepsy in about 75% of children. Generally, the history indicates that during an emotional reaction, particularly laughter, anger, or surprise, the child loses all muscular tone, falls to the ground, but retains consciousness. The attack is short and rarely lasts more than a minute.

Some children experience both types of attacks on separate occasions, while others will experience somnolence as a result of excitement, and if sleep occurs undergo a cataplectic attack.

The condition persists throughout adult life, the frequency of attacks varying over the years, without showing a definite trend toward improvement or worsening.

A narcoleptic attack is distinguished from a true seizure in that the patient is easily aroused and once awake does not show postictal confusion which is a common sequel to an epileptic attack. This condition is unrelated to the Kleine-Levin syndrome of recurrent somnolence and morbid hunger which is occasionally encountered in adolescence,[187] and the excessive somnolence of the patient with obesity and carbon dioxide retention (Pickwickian syndrome).[188] The EEG during an attack shows the usual patterns of drowsy sleep with an occasional burst of 2–4 cps "saw-tooth" waves.[189] If EMG records are taken concurrently, the suppression of all EMG activity is diagnostic for REM sleep distinguishing this stage from NREM sleep.

Treatment

Methylphenidate (Ritalin), dextroamphetamine (Dexedrine), and phenelzine (Nardil), a monoamine inhibitor, have been used to reduce the tendency to fall asleep. Monoamine inhibitors suppress REM sleep for extended periods. Their adverse effects, including insomnia, hypotension, and alterations in personality, limit their usefulness.[190] Even though a child with narcolepsy tolerates large doses of these drugs (40 mg–60 mg methylphenidate per day), they rarely give complete relief although 50% of patients report a reduction in frequency and severity of attacks.

FAMILIAL PAROXYSMAL CHOREO-ATHETOSIS

This rare disorder, first described by Mount and Reback in 1940,[191] is characterized by sudden attacks of choreiform, athetoid, and dystonic movements of a few seconds to several minutes duration, which are associated with loss of consciousness. Attacks are regularly precipitated by movement, especially after immobility. The nature of the disorder is unknown. It is probably transmitted by an autosomal dominant gene with a low penetrance, or by an autosomal recessive gene. Stevens[192] has postulated that it represents a convulsive disorder. It, therefore, would be classified with the reflex epilepsies such as startle epilepsy previously described by Alajouanine and Gastaut.[193] The fact that hyperventilation may occasionally trigger an attack can be cited in support of this theory, but the absence of EEG abnormalities during an attack in at least some of the patients suggests that paroxysmal choreo-athetosis may have different underlying triggering mechanisms.[194]

Between attacks the patient is usually in excellent health, although we have detected mild choreiform movements in one child, and Pryles and associates have reported a patient in whom choreo-athetosis was associated with a seizure disorder in two other family members.[195]

A number of drugs have been suggested to eliminate attacks. Pryles and co-workers[195] and Stevens[192] have found diphenylhydantoin and phenobarbital to be effective. We have had a favorable response with methylphenidate (Ritalin) in one patient, with no effect on another. Perez-Borja and associates suggest the use of chlordiazepoxide (Librium) in patients whose EEG is normal during an attack, and anticonvulsants for those showing EEG abnormalities.[194]

REFERENCES

1. Tempkin, O.: *The Falling Sickness*, Baltimore: Johns Hopkins Press, 1945.
2. Jackson, H.: On convulsive seizures, Brit. Med. J. 1:703, 1890.
3. Millichap, J. G.: *Febrile Convulsions*, New York: The Macmillan Co., 1968.
4. Kurland, L. T.: The incidence and prevalence of convulsive disorders in a small urban community, Epilepsia (Amst.) 1:143, 1959.
5. Livingston, S.: *The Diagnosis and Treatment of Convulsive Disorders in Children*, Springfield: Charles C Thomas Publisher, 1954.

6. Gibbs, F. A., Gibbs, E. L., and Lennox, W. G.: Electroencephalographic classification of epileptic patients and control subjects, AMA Arch. Neurol. Psychiat. 50:111, 1943.

7. Jasper, H. H. and Kershman, J.: Classification of the EEG in epilepsy, Electroenceph. Clin. Neurophysiol. Suppl. 2:123, 1949.

8. Gibbs, E. L., Fleming, M. M., and Gibbs, F. A.: Diagnosis and prognosis of hypsarrhythmia and infantile spasms, Pediatrics 13:66, 1954.

9. Metrakos, K. and Metrakos, J. D.: Genetics of convulsive disorders. II. Genetic and electroencephalographic studies in centrencephalic epilepsy, Neurology (Minneap.) 11:474, 1961.

10. Bray, P. F. and Wiser, W. C.: The relation of focal to diffuse epileptiform EEG discharges in genetic epilepsy, Arch. Neurol. 13:223, 1965.

11. Metrakos, J. D. and Metrakos, K.: Childhood epilepsy of subcortical "centrencephalic" origin, Clin. Pediat. (Phila.) 5:536, 1966.

12. Ward, A. A., Jr. and Schmidt, R. P.: Some properties of single epileptic neurons, Arch. Neurol. 5:308, 1961.

13. Schmidt, R. P. and Wilder, B. J.: *Epilepsy*, Philadelphia: F. A. Davis Co., 1968.

14. Weichert, P. and Göllnitz, G.: Stoffwechseluntersuchungen des Cerebralen Anfallsgeschehens, J. Neurochem. 16:689, 1969.

15. Roberts, E. and Hammerschlag, R.: "Amino Acid Transmitters," in Albers, R. W., Siegel, G. J., Katzman, R., and Agranoff, B. W. (eds.): *Basic Neurochemistry*, Boston: Little, Brown & Co., 1972, pp. 131–165.

16. Tower, D. B.: *Neurochemistry of Epilepsy*, Springfield: Charles C Thomas Publisher, 1960.

16a. Meldrum, B. S. and Horton, R. W.: Physiology of status epilepticus in primates, Arch. Neurol. 28:1, 1973.

16b. Meldrum, B. S. and Brierley, J. B.: Prolonged epileptic seizures in primates, Arch. Neurol. 28:10, 1973.

17. Beresford, H. R., Posner, J. B., and Plum, F.: Changes in brain lactate during induced cerebral seizures, Arch. Neurol. 20:243, 1969.

18. Plum, F., Posner, J. B., and Troy, B.: Cerebral metabolic and circulatory responses to induced convulsions in animals, Arch. Neurol. 18:1, 1968.

19. Hughes, J. R.: Bilateral EEG abnormalities on corresponding areas, Epilepsia (Amst.) 7:44, 1966.

20. Efron, R.: Post-epileptic paralysis: Theoretical critique and report of a case, Brain 84:381, 1961.

21. Jasper, H. H., Ajmone-Marsan, C., and Stoll, J.: Corticofugal projections to the brain stem, Arch. Neurol. Psychiat. 67:155, 1952.

22. Moruzzi, G. and Magoun, H. W.: Brain stem reticular formation and activation of the EEG, Electroenceph. Clin. Neurophysiol. 1:455, 1949.

23. Penfield, W.: Epileptic automatism and the centrencephalic integrating system, A. Res. Nerv. Ment. Dis. 30:513, 1952.

24. Lombroso, C. T. and Erba, G.: Primary and secondary bilateral synchrony in epilepsy, Arch. Neurol. 22:321, 1970.

25. Niedermeyer, E., Laws, E. R., Jr., and Walker, A. E.: Depth EEG findings in epileptics with generalized spike-wave complexes, Arch. Neurol. 21:51, 1969.

26. Goldring, S.: The role of prefrontal cortex in grand mal convulsion, Arch. Neurol. 26:109, 1972.

27. Rossi, G. F., Walter, R. D., and Crandall, P. H.: Generalized spike and wave discharges and nonspecific thalamic nuclei, Arch. Neurol. 19:174, 1968.

28. Stewart, L. F. and Dreifuss, F. E.: "Centrencephalic" seizure discharges in focal hemispheral lesions, Arch. Neurol. 17:60, 1967.

29. Falconer, M. A., Serafetinides, E. A., and Corsellis, J. A. N.: Etiology and pathogenesis of temporal lobe epilepsy, Arch. Neurol. 10:233, 1964.

30. Earle, K. M., Baldwin, M., and Penfield, W.: Incisural sclerosis and temporal lobe seizures produced by hippocampal herniation at birth, AMA Arch. Neurol. Psychiat. 69:27, 1953.

31. Corsellis, J. A. and Falconer, M. A.: "Cryptic tubers" as a cause of focal epilepsy, J. Neurol. Neurosurg. Psychiat. 34:104, 1971.

32. Pollen, D. A. and Trachtenberg, M. C.: Neuroglia: Gliosis and focal epilepsy, Science 167:1252, 1970.

33. Van Buren, J. M.: The abdominal aura. A study of abdominal sensations occurring in epilepsy and produced by depth stimulation, Electroenceph. Clin. Neurophysiol. 15:1, 1963.

34. Mattson, R. H., Pratt, K. L., and Calverley, J. R.: Electroencephalograms of epileptics following sleep deprivation, Arch. Neurol. 13:310, 1965.

35. Penfield, W. and Jasper, H.: *Epilepsy and the Functional Anatomy of the Human Brain*. Boston: Little, Brown & Co., 1954.

36. Madsen, J. A. and Bray, P. F.: The coincidence of diffuse electroencephalographic spike-wave paroxysms and brain tumors, Neurology (Minneap.) 16:546, 1966.

37. Stevens, J. R.: Focal abnormality in petit mal epilepsy, Neurology (Minneap.) 20:1069, 1970.

38. Daly, D. D.: Reflections on the concept of petit mal, Epilepsia (Amst.) 9:175, 1968.

39. Dalby, M. A.: Epilepsy and 3 per second spike and wave rhythms, Acta Neurol. Scand. Suppl. 40, Vol. 45, 1969.

40. Lennox, W. G.: The petit mal epilepsies: Their treatment with Tridione, JAMA 129:1069, 1945.

41. Geier, S.: Minor seizures and behavior, Electroenceph. Clin. Neurophysiol. 31:499, 1971.

43. Cavanagh, J. B.: On certain small tumors encountered in the temporal lobe, Brain 81:389, 1958.

44. Malamud, N.: The epileptogenic focus in temporal lobe epilepsy from a pathological standpoint, Arch. Neurol. 14:190, 1966.

116a. Livingston, S., et al.: Use of carbamazepine in epilepsy: Results in 87 patients, JAMA 200:116, 1967.

117. Kirboe, E., et al.: Zarontin (ethosuximide) in the treatment of petit mal and related disorders, Epilepsia (Amst.) 5:83, 1964.

118. Gastaut, H., et al.: Treatment of status epilepticus with diazepam (Valium), Epilepsia (Amst.) 6:167, 1965.

119. Markham, C. H.: The treatment of myoclonic seizures of infancy and childhood with LA–1, Pediatrics 34:511, 1964.

120. Carson, M. J.: Treatment of minor motor seizures with nitrazepam, Develop. Med. Child Neurol. 10:772, 1968.

121. Hansen, R. A. and Menkes, J. H.: A new anticonvulsant in the management of minor motor seizures, Develop. Med. Child Neurol. 14:3, 1972.

122. Livingston, S.: "Seizure Disorders," in Gellis, S. and Kagan, B. (eds.): Pediatric Therapy, 5th ed., Philadelphia: W. B. Saunders Co., 1972, pp. 82–92.

123. Wilder, R. M.: The effect of ketonuria on the course of epilepsy, Mayo Clin. Proc. 2:307, 1921.

124. Millichap, J. G., Jones, J. D., and Rudis, B. P.: Mechanism of anticonvulsant action of ketogenic diet, Amer. J. Dis. Child. 107:593, 1964.

125. Huttenlocher, P. R., Wilbourn, A. J., and Signore, J. M.: Medium-chain triglycerides as a therapy for intractable childhood epilepsy, Neurology (Minneap.) 21:1097, 1971.

126. Hanson, R. A. and Menkes, J. H.: Iatrogenic perpetuation of epilepsy, Trans. Amer. Neurol. Ass. 97:290, 1972.

126a. Crandall, P. H.: "Developments in Direct Recordings from Epileptogenic Regions in the Surgical Treatment of Partial Epilepsies," in Brazier, M. A. B. (ed.): Epilepsy: Its Phenomena in Man. New York: Academic Press, 1973.

127. Bengzon, A. R. A., et al.: Prognostic factors in the surgical treatment of temporal lobe epileptics, Neurology (Minneap.) 18:717, 1968.

128. Griffith, H. B.: Cerebral hemispherectomy for infantile hemiplegia in the light of the late results, Ann. Roy. Coll. Surg. Eng. 41:183, 1967.

129. Falconer, M. A. and Wilson, P. J. E.: Complications related to delayed hemorrhage after hemispherectomy, J. Neurosurg. 30:413, 1969.

130. Bogen, J. E. and Vogel, P. J.: Treatment of generalized seizures by central commissurotomy, Surg. Forum 14:431, 1963.

131. Gazzaniga, M. S., Bogen, J. E., and Sperry, R. W.: Observations on visual perception after disconnexion of the cerebral hemisphere in man, Brain 88:221, 1965.

132. Hunter, R. A.: Status epilepticus. History, incidence and problems, Epilepsia (Amst.) 1:162, 1959.

133. Thurston, J. H., et al.: New enzymatic method for measurement of paraldehyde: Correlation of effects with serum and CSF levels, J. Lab. Clin. Med. 72:699, 1968.

134. Carter, S. and Gold, A. P.: The critically ill child: Management of status epilepticus, Pediatrics 44:732, 1969.

135. Lombroso, C. T.: Treatment of status epilepticus with diazepam, Neurology (Minneap.) 16:629, 1966.

136. Bell, D. S.: Dangers of treatment of status epilepticus with diazepam, Brit. Med. J. 1:159, 1969.

137. Wallis, W., Kutt, H., and McDowell, F.: Intravenous diphenylhydantoin in treatment of acute repetitive seizures, Neurology (Minneap.) 18:513, 1968.

137a. Wilensky, A. J. and Lowden, J. A. Inadequate serum levels after intramuscular administration of diphenylhydantoin, Neurology (Minneap.) 23:318, 1973.

138. Rodin, E. A.: The Prognosis of Patients With Epilepsy, Springfield: Charles C Thomas Publisher, 1968.

139. Wilkins, L.: Epilepsy in childhood, J. Pediat. 10:317, 1937.

140. Currie, S., et al.: Clinical course and prognosis of temporal lobe epilepsy, Brain 94:173, 1971.

141. Holowach, J., Thurston, D. L., and O'Leary, J.: Prognosis in childhood epilepsy: Follow-up study of 148 cases in which therapy has been suspended after prolonged anticonvulsant control, New Eng. J. Med. 286:169, 1972.

142. Lennox, W. G.: Brain injury, drugs, and environment as cause of mental decay in epilepsy, Amer. J. Psychiat. 99:174, 1942.

143. Currier, R. D., Kooi, K. A., and Saidman, L. J.: Prognosis of "pure" petit mal, Neurology (Minneap.) 13:959, 1963.

144. Yahr, M. D., et al.: Evaluation of standard anticonvulsant therapy in 319 patients, JAMA 150:663, 1952.

145. Goldensohn, E. S. and Gold, A. P.: Prolonged behavioral disturbances as ictal phenomenon, Neurology (Minneap.) 10:1, 1960.

146. Patrick, H. T. and Levy, D. M.: Early convulsions in epileptics and in others, JAMA 82:375, 1924.

147. Bridge, E. M.: Epilepsy and Convulsive Disorders in Children, New York: McGraw-Hill Book Co., 1949.

148. Millichap, J. G.: Studies in febrile seizures. I. Height of body temperature as a measure of the febrile-seizure threshold, Pediatrics 23:76, 1959.

149. Baird, H. W. III and Garfunkel, J. M.: Electroencephalographic changes in children with artificially induced hyperthermia, J. Pediat. 48:28, 1956.

150. VandenBerg, B. J. and Yerushalmy, J.: Studies on convulsive disorders in young children. I. Incidence of febrile and nonfebrile convulsions by age and other factors, Pediat. Res. 3:298, 1969.

151. Fischler, E.: Convulsions as a complication of shigellosis in children, Helv. Paediat. Acta 17:389, 1962.

152. Millichap, J. G., Madsen, J. A., and Aledort,

L. M.: Studies in febrile seizures. V. Clinical and electroencephalographic study in unselected patients, Neurology (Minneap.) 10:643, 1960.

153. Lennox, M. A.: Febrile convulsions in childhood: Their relationship to adult epilepsy, J. Pediat. 35:427, 1949.

154. Dodge, P. R.: Febrile convulsions, J. Pediat. 78:1083, 1971.

155. Lennox, W. G.: Significance of febrile convulsions, Pediatrics 11:341, 1953.

156. Hammill, J. F. and Carter, S.: Febrile convulsions, New Eng. J. Med. 274:563, 1966.

157. Frantzen, E., Nygaard, A., and Wulff, H.: Febrile kramper has born. Prognostiske studies og forsog pa vurdering af effekten af profylaktisk antiepileptisk langtidsbehandling, Ugeskrift for laeger 126:207, 1964.

157a. Faero, O., et al.: Successful prophylaxis of febrile convulsions with phenobarbital, Epilepsia (Amst.) 13:279, 1972.

158. Craig, W. S.: Convulsive movements occurring in first 10 days of life, Arch. Dis. Child. 35:336, 1960.

159. Hopkins, I. J.: Seizures in the first week of life. A study of aetiological factors, Med. J. Aust. 2:647, 1972.

160. Dreyfus-Brisac, C. and Monod, N.: "Electroclinical Studies of Status Epilepticus and Convulsion in the Newborn," in Kellaway, P. and Petersen, I. (eds.): Neurological and Electroencephalographic Correlative Studies in Infancy, New York: Grune & Stratton, Inc., 1964.

161. Keen, J. H.: Significance of hypocalcemia in neonatal convulsions, Arch. Dis. Child. 44:356, 1969.

162. Waldinger, C. and Berg, R. B.: Signs of pyridoxine dependency manifest at birth in siblings, Pediatrics 32:161, 1963.

163. Schwartz, J. F.: Neonatal convulsions—pathogenesis, diagnostic evaluation, treatment and prognosis, Clin. Pediat. (Phila.) 4:595, 1965.

164. Prichard, J. S.: "The Character and Significance of Epileptic Seizures in Infancy," in Kellaway, P. and Petersen, I. (eds.): Neurological and Electroencephalographic Correlative Studies in Infancy, New York: Grune & Stratton, Inc., 1964.

165. Wolff, H. G.: Headache and Other Head Pain, 2nd ed., New York: Oxford University Press, 1963.

166. Kimball, R. W. and Goodman, M. A.: Effects of reserpine on amino acid excretion in patients with migraine, J. Neurol. Neurosurg. Psychiat. 29:190, 1966.

167. Whitehouse, D., et al.: Electroencephalographic changes in children with migraine, New Eng. J. Med. 276:23, 1967.

168. Dalessio, D. J.: On migraine headache: Serotonin and serotonin antagonism, JAMA 181:318, 1962.

169. Chapman, L. F., et al.: A humoral agent implicated in vascular headache of the migraine type, Arch. Neurol. 3:223, 1960.

170. Sandler, M.: Migraine: A pulmonary disease, Lancet 1:618, 1972.

171. Menkes, M. M.: A study of family dynamics in children with migraine, Pediatrics (in press) (1974).

172. Holguin, J. and Fenichel, G.: Migraine, J. Pediat. 70:290, 1967.

173. Burke, E. C. and Peters, G. A.: Migraine in childhood, Amer. J. Dis. Child., 92:330, 1956.

173a. Hachinski, V. C., Porchawka, J., and Steele, J. C.: Visual symptoms in the migraine syndrome, Neurology (Minneap.) 23:570, 1973.

174. Verret, S. and Steele, J. C.: Alternating hemiplegia in childhood: A report of eight patients with complicated migraine beginning in infancy, Pediatrics 47:675, 1971.

175. Whitty, C. W. M.: Familial hemiplegic migraine, J. Neurol. Neurosurg. Psychiat. 16:172, 1953.

176. Vahlquist, B., and Hackzell, G.: Migraine of early onset: A study of 31 cases in which the disease first appeared between 1 and 4 years of age, Acta Paediat. 38:622, 1949.

177. Vahlquist, B.: Uber die Beziehungen zwischen acetonamischen Erbrechen und Migrane, Ann. Paediat. (Basel) 173:272, 1949.

178. Walsh, J. P. and O'Doherty, D. S. A.: Possible explanation of the mechanism of ophthalmoplegic migraine, Neurology (Minneap.) 10:1079, 1960.

179. Fenichel, G. M. and Battiata, S.: Thrombophlebitis secondary to methysergide maleate therapy, J. Pediat. 68:632, 1966.

180. Hinrichs, W. L. and Keith, H. M.: Migraine in childhood: A follow-up report, Mayo Clin. Proc. 40:593, 1965.

181. Lombroso, C. T. and Lerman, P.: Breathholding spells (cyanotic and pallid infantile syncope), Pediatrics 39:563, 1967.

182. Gauk, E. W., Kidd, L., and Prichard, J. S.: Mechanism of seizures associated with breathholding spells, New Eng. J. Med. 268:1436, 1963.

182a. Livingston, S.: Breathholding spells in children: Differentiation from epileptic attacks, JAMA 212: 2231, 1970.

182b. Hooshmand, H.: Apneic spells treated with atropine, Neurology (Minneap.) 22:1217, 1972.

183. Westphal, C.: Zwei Krankheitsfalle. II. Eigenthumliche mit Einschlafen verbundene Anfalle, Arch. Psychiat. Nervenkr. 7:631, 1877.

184. Ornitz, E. M., et al.: The EEG and rapid eye movements during REM sleep in normal and autistic children, Electroenceph. Clin. Neurophysiol. 26:167, 1969.

185. Dement, W., Rechtschaffen, A., and Gulevich, G.: The nature of the narcoleptic sleep attack, Neurology (Minneap.) 16:18, 1966.

186. Yoss, R. E. and Daly, D. D.: Narcolepsy in children, Pediatrics 25:1025, 1960.

187. Gilbert, G. J.: Periodic hypersomnia and bulimia—the Kleine-Levin syndrome, Neurology (Minneap.) 14:844, 1964.

188. Ward, W. A., Jr. and Kelsey, W. M.: The Pickwickian syndrome: A review of the literature and report of a case, J. Pediat. 61:745, 1962.

or are being phagocytized by satellite cells. Motoneurons in the brain stem, notably in the hypoglossal nucleus, are also affected. A number of authors have described supra-segmental lesions, including loss of Betz cells from the motor cortex. These findings must be interpreted, however, in the light of the severe agonal anoxia which is commonly encountered. An unusual finding, which may reflect the basic defect in this disease, is the prominent glial proliferation at the proximal portion of the anterior spinal roots. These changes may start during fetal life, and it is possible that the degeneration of neurons in the anterior horns represents a secondary process.[11]

Clinical Manifestations

The clinical picture is marked by reduction of muscle power and spontaneous movement.[12,13] Muscle weakness is symmetric and is more extensive in the proximal part of the limbs, and what little movement is left to the child is found in the small muscles of the hands and feet. At the same time the affected muscles undergo atrophy, though this is concealed by subcutaneous fat normally seen at this age. Muscles of the trunk, neck, and thorax are equally affected, although the diaphragm may be spared (Fig. 12–1). Cardiac and smooth muscles are usually spared as well. With progression of the disease, involvement of bulbar musculature becomes more prominent, and atrophy and fasciculation of the tongue are noted. Deep tendon reflexes are nearly always

TABLE 12–1.
AGE OF FIRST CLINICAL MANIFESTATIONS IN INFANTILE MUSCULAR ATROPHY*

Age	Percent of Cases
Newborn	37
0 to 1 month	10
1 to 3 months	12
3 to 6 months	6
6 to 9 months	12
9 to 12 months	9
More than 1 year	8

* Modified from Brandt.[12]

markedly reduced or absent. There is no sensory loss, no intellectual retardation, and no sphincter disturbance.

The age at which the first clinical manifestations become apparent is presented in Table 12–1.

In most cases the disease progresses rapidly. Children who already are severely hypotonic at birth rarely survive the first year of life, while in those whose weakness appears postnatally the disease may have a slower progression.[14,15] A few patients present with a clinical picture of a congenital nonprogressive myopathy.[15] Serum creatine phosphokinase levels are elevated in about half of these patients, and hypertrophy of the calves is not unusual.[15a] The benign form of infantile spinal muscular atrophy probably does not represent a distinct clinical entity, as this form and the rapidly progressive type of spinal muscular atrophy may coexist in the same family.[16] It is likely that many, bio-

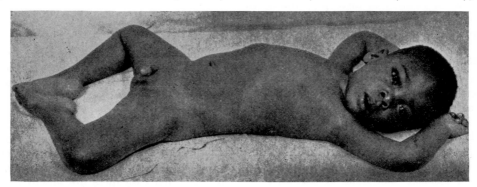

Fig. 12–1. Child with Werdnig-Hoffmann's disease, showing typical frog-legged posture. (From Ford, F. R.: *Diseases of the Nervous System in Infancy and Childhood and Adolescence*, 5th ed., 1966, courtesy of Charles C Thomas, Publisher, Springfield.)

chemically distinct types of spinal muscular atrophy will ultimately become clearly defined.[16a] Parents occasionally note a transient improvement in the child's motor faculties. In part this is due to a true stationary period in the course of the disease, such as that noted by Hoffmann in one of his earliest patients. Maturation of partially paralyzed muscles may also give an impression of transient improvement.

In most instances the disease is either fatal or leaves the child in a completely helpless condition and susceptible to infection.

A milder form of the disease consistent with survival into adult life was first described by Wohlfart et al.[16b] and by Kugelberg and Welander.[17] While in some instances this condition may not represent a clinical entity distinct from infantile muscular atrophy, in other families the disease is transmitted in an autosomal dominant manner distinct from the recessively transmitted infantile muscular atrophy.[18]

Diagnosis

Biochemical Studies. The study of serum enzymes is important in the differential diagnosis of motoneuron disease. Serum creatine phosphokinase is usually normal in the rapidly progressive, classic form of Werdnig-Hoffmann disease. The excretion of amino acids and of creatine is generally normal during the earlier stages of the illness.

Neurophysiologic Studies. Electromyographic findings help confirm the clinical diagnosis of motoneuron disease. The denervated muscles spontaneously contract, involving single muscle fibers (fibrillation) or entire motor units (fasciculation).[18a] The contractions exceed in strength and frequency the minimal fibrillations occasionally found in the distal musculature of young infants. Residual motor unit potentials are polyphasic and are increased in amplitude and duration. Conduction velocity in the motor nerves is somewhat decreased. This is due to the preferential involvement of the most myelinated and fastest conducting axons.

Histologic Studies

In evaluating a child with neuromuscular disease, a muscle biopsy is frequently used as a diagnostic procedure. The muscle selected for biopsy should be one that is clinically affected but not to such an advanced degree that all muscle tissue has degenerated beyond recognition. Care should be taken that the muscle had not been previously subjected to electromyography. The specimen is removed with the help of special tissue clamps which prevent crushing. For histochemical and most histologic studies, the tissue is frozen in liquid nitrogen and then stored at $-70°$ C. For histologic examination a portion of the specimen can be fixed in 10% buffered formalin and embedded in paraffin. Histochemical studies have shown that muscle fibers in human skeletal muscle can be differentiated into two types: type I fibers which are rich in oxidative enzymes but poor in ATPase and phosphorylase, and type II fibers for which the reverse is true. Normal muscle presents a mosaic of both types, but in infantile muscular atrophy fibers of a given type are grouped together. A fuller discussion of histochemical techniques, the histochemistry of developing muscles, and the histologic changes in neurogenic muscular atrophies is presented by Dubowitz[19] and Engel.[20,20a]

In Werdnig-Hoffmann disease a biopsy will show the classic features of denervation atrophy (Fig. 12–2). There are large patches of small, atrophic fibers, with residual muscle fibers of normal or somewhat enlarged diameter. Electron microscopy adds very little specific diagnostic information. The myo-

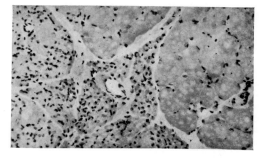

Fig. 12–2. Transverse section of muscle from patient with Werdnig-Hoffmann's disease. Note the relative preservation of muscle fibers in the right hand side of the field, and atrophied fibers on the left. (Hematoxylin and eosin $\times$ 20.) (Courtesy of Dr. P. Cancilla, Department of Pathology, UCLA, Los Angeles.)

filaments are loosened and mitochondria are diminished in number and show atrophic cristae. A similar picture is seen in a number of other conditions featuring neurogenic atrophy.

Differential Diagnosis

The infant with Werdnig-Hoffmann disease usually presents with poor muscle tone and a marked delay in motor development. Since a variety of well-defined diseases present the picture of the "floppy infant," differential diagnosis may be difficult in any one specific instance. The various conditions responsible for this syndrome are shown in Table 12–2. One common cause for diminished muscle tone in a small infant is "atonic cerebral palsy." In this syndrome hypotonia is the result of major abnormalities of the cerebrum and cerebellum. Invariably these infants have considerable intellectual retardation. Spontaneous movements are present, and the deep tendon reflexes are easily elicited. When the infant is lifted by his trunk, his legs will promptly become rigid, and there is a striking accentuation of the extensor thrust reflex. While some of these children will remain hypotonic, others will within one to three years develop extrapyramidal movements or a clear-cut hypertonicity (see Chapter 5).

Amyotonia congenita, a clinical syndrome reported briefly in a single case by Oppenheim in 1900,[22] represents a number of unrelated disease processes. It is important to differentiate these entities, now collectively termed

TABLE 12–2.
DIAGNOSIS IN 107 CASES OF "FLOPPY INFANTS"*

Diagnosis	Number of Cases
Infantile muscular atrophy	67
Congenital muscular dystrophy	3
Polymyositis	1
Myasthenia gravis	1
Scurvy	2
Cerebral disease (atonic cerebral palsy)	14
Benign congenital hypotonia	17
Complete recovery	8

* After Walton.[21]

"benign congenital hypotonias," from the usually fatal infantile muscular atrophy. Benign congenital hypotonia is used to describe "floppy" infants with a marked delay in motor development. Some of these children recover completely, while others can be considered to have a stationary or, at worst, a slowly progressive muscular disorder. In these infants the muscles are soft and flabby and a remarkable range of passive movement is possible. Tendon reflexes are elicitable, and spontaneous movements are more prominent than in infantile muscular atrophy. There is little involvement of respiratory muscles and intellectual development is normal. As will be noted later in this chapter, histochemical and electron microscopic studies of muscle biopsies have delineated a number of distinct entities.

Rarer causes for infantile hypotonia include myasthenia gravis, which can be diagnosed by the striking improvement in muscle strength following administration of an anticholinesterase drug. For this purpose a slowly metabolized drug, such as Prostigmin, is more suitable for infants than Tensilon, the effectiveness of which is often too fleeting to allow correct sequential assessment of muscle strength. Muscular dystrophy is only rarely seen in a small infant, but in no other condition is it common to see such a striking elevation in serum enzymes, particularly creatine phosphokinase. In the absence of a family history of a dystrophic process, the diagnosis will depend mainly on these biochemical alterations and a muscle biopsy.

Finally, mongolism, transsection of the spinal cord, intra-uterine poliomyelitis, congenital polyneuritis, and muscular hypotonia due to Marfan's disease, various chronic illnesses, or malnutrition must also be considered in the differential diagnosis of the hypotonic child.

Pathogenesis

The etiology of infantile spinal muscular atrophy is unknown.

Treatment

Treatment is purely symptomatic and is of no value in altering the course of the disease.

Active and passive exercise may help to delay the appearance of contractures.

ARTHROGRYPOSIS

At least three distinct clinical and pathologic syndromes have been grouped under the term arthrogryposis. Descriptively this entity refers to multiple congenital contractures of the limbs which are fixed in flexion or, less commonly, in extension accompanied by diminution and wasting of skeletal muscle. Other congenital malformations, particularly clubfoot and cerebral maldevelopment, are often part of the syndrome.[23] In the most common form anterior horn cells are markedly reduced, the muscle fibers are small and often hyalinized, and the EMG abnormalities are consistent with denervation.[24] In other instances there are changes compatible with congenital muscular dystrophy,[25] fibrosis of the anterior spinal roots, or evidence of embryonic denervation and maturation arrest of muscle.[25a] An increase in collagen synthesis, as measured by the rate of amino acid incorporation, has been reported but probably does not represent the basic chemical defect.[26] An early and vigorous orthopedic program has been advocated.[27]

DISEASES OF THE AXON

Disorders at this level of the motor unit are the result of traumatic, infectious, postinfectious, or toxic processes, and are therefore best discussed under their respective headings (see Chapters 7, 8, and 9). In the differential diagnosis of muscular weakness, a polyneuritic process must often be considered, and it is therefore appropriate at this point to enumerate some of its features.[28] One would suppose that the presence of sensory loss in the affected areas would easily distinguish polyneuritis from other disorders of the motor unit. However, an isolated motor neuropathy is far from rare. More commonly, motor weakness may overshadow sensory disturbances, the latter being particularly difficult to demonstrate in infants. In general the polyneuritides have a rapid onset, a feature they share only with the inflammatory muscular disorders, polymyositis, and dermatomyositis. The site of

muscular involvement is often a clue to the cause of the weakness. Werdnig-Hoffmann disease and the muscular dystrophies involve the proximal musculature preferentially, while the polyneuritides usually affect the distal musculature. Ascending paralysis such as was originally described by Landry (see Chapter 7) is not common in infants. As a result of the predilection for the distal musculature, ankle reflexes are lost early in the illness in contrast to their retention in the muscular dystrophies. The distinction between polyneuritis and Charcot-Marie-Tooth disease rests on the frequent association of the latter condition with cerebellar involvement and the presence of a similar condition in other members of the immediate family. In about two-thirds of children with polyneuritis the spinal fluid is abnormal. A classic picture of albuminocytologic dissociation, namely an elevated protein level in the absence of a cellular response, is common during the first two to eight weeks of the illness. Motor nerve conduction times are usually slowed, although they may be normal during the initial phases of the disease. While slowed motor conduction time, when present, is characteristic for polyneuritis, it may also be seen with severe atrophy in anterior horn cell disease (poliomyelitis and Werdnig-Hoffmann disease). The histologic changes in affected muscle are rarely significant during the acute phase of the illness, while in chronic polyneuritis the main abnormality is a widespread muscular atrophy.

DISEASES OF THE NEUROMUSCULAR JUNCTION

The principal disorder to be considered in this section is myasthenia gravis. The toxins of *Clostridium tetani* and *Clostridium botulinum* and the venom of cobras and of arachnoideae, such as the black widow spider, also affect the neuromuscular junction, but these are considered under their respective headings in Chapter 9.

MYASTHENIA GRAVIS

Myasthenia gravis is a chronic disease, first described by Willis in 1672,[29] and characterized by unusual fatigability of voluntary muscles.

Pathologic Anatomy

The microscopic changes may be minute even in severely affected muscles. Focal collections of small lymphocytes have been repeatedly found around necrotic muscle fibers, and less often in perivascular spaces of interstitial tissue. Engel and Warmolts have found that in more than one-half of the cases there is denervation atrophy similar to that seen in anterior horn cell disease.[29a] Special supravital staining techniques frequently show the neuromuscular junction to be abnormal. The region containing cholinesterase is reduced in size, and the terminal axon expansions are smaller than normal. On electron microscopy the nerve terminal area is decreased and there are growing axon tips, immature-appearing end plates, and postsynaptic regions denuded of their nerve terminals.[29b] In 70%–80% of patients there are pathologic changes in the thymus. In most instances, these consist of lymphoid hyperplasia. Although thymomas occur in about 10% of all patients with myasthenia, they are extremely rare in childhood. Myocardial abnormalities have been found in about one-half of autopsied patients.

Clinical Manifestations

In the child, myasthenia gravis may take one of three clinical forms.[30,31] "Neonatal" myasthenia is a transient disease seen on the average of one in seven infants born to mothers with myasthenia gravis. Symptoms usually appear during the first 24 hours or, at the latest, by the third day of life. In all instances there is a paresis of the lower bulbar muscles causing a weak cry and difficulty in sucking or swallowing. Generalized hypotonia is found in about one-half of the infants. The symptoms respond promptly to anticholinesterase medication and, even if untreated, the duration of the illness is usually less than five weeks.

"Congenital" myasthenia gravis is the term used to designate children with myasthenia born to mothers without the disease.[32] More than one sibling may be affected.[33] In many instances fetal move-

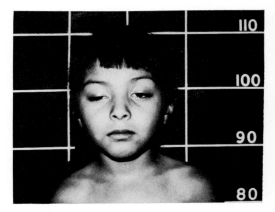

Fig. 12–3. Girl with myasthenia gravis. There is bilateral ptosis, more marked on the right, and the typical myasthenic facies. (Courtesy of Dr. Christian Herrmann, Jr., Department of Neurology, UCLA, Los Angeles.)

ments are reduced, and during the neonatal period, one may note feeding difficulties and a weak cry. The initial symptoms in congenital myasthenia gravis are not as severe as in the neonatal variety, and the diagnosis is therefore more difficult to establish. A few patients with congenital myasthenia have spontaneous remissions, but usually the course of the disease is protracted with mild symptoms which are somewhat refractory to therapy.

Myasthenia may also have its onset during childhood (juvenile myasthenia). In this form girls are affected two to six times as frequently as boys. The incidence of the condition increases progressively from age two to a peak at the end of the second decade. The onset of juvenile myasthenia may be insidious, or at times rapid, and often as a sequel to an acute febrile illness. As a rule muscles innervated by the cranial nerves are affected first, and ptosis is the commonest presenting sign (Table 12–3) (Fig. 12–3). The clinical course is highly variable. In some instances weakness may spread to the respiratory muscles and death may occur within a few months despite all therapy. About one-half of the patients experience one or more remissions. These usually occur during the early years of the illness. In others symptoms progress to a certain point and then they remain stationary. In about five

TABLE 12-3.
SYMPTOMS AND SIGNS IN 35 PATIENTS WITH
MYASTHENIA GRAVIS OF THE JUVENILE TYPE

Symptom and Sign	Number of Patients
Ptosis	32
Diplopia	30
Facial weakness	29
Dysphonia	29
Weakness of arms	29
Weakness of legs	29
Chewing weakness	22
External ophthalmoplegia	18
Respiratory difficulties	12

* After Millichap and Dodge.[31]

percent of cases myasthenia is restricted to the extraocular musculature.

The characteristic feature of all forms is the variability in muscular strength, with increasing weakness of the affected muscles upon repeated contractions (Fig. 12–4). The child is usually at his best in the morning, becomes progressively weaker during the day but experiences partial or complete recovery following a nap. In about 10%–20% of cases weakness becomes irreversible, and muscular wasting, particularly of the shoulder girdle and the extraocular muscles, becomes apparent. Despite hypotonia, the tendon jerks are normal or even exaggerated, but they may disappear after repeated elicitation.

The most common disease associated with juvenile myasthenia gravis is thyrotoxicosis, which occurs in about 10% of children.[34]

Disseminated lupus erythematosus and other collagen vascular diseases may also occur with greater than chance frequency.

Diagnosis

A distinction must be made between myasthenic syndromes secondary to a variety of more or less well-defined pathogenetic processes, and myasthenia gravis, the etiology of which is unknown.[35] All forms of myasthenia share the property of abnormal muscular fatigability and a prompt response to anticholinesterases. It is generally held that a clear-cut drug response indicates myasthenia gravis. The diagnosis is supported by a history of remissions and exacerbations and by the absence of any concurrent illness that might contribute to the muscular weakness. In some muscle diseases, notably dermatomyositis and polymyositis, slight but definite improvement has been observed with drug therapy. However, the distinction between myasthenia gravis and myositis is not absolute. Some patients with polymyositis show response of muscular weakness to anticholinesterase drugs and have a myasthenic distribution of affected muscles, while some patients with myasthenia gravis have round cell infiltration of muscle that resembles polymyositis.

An occasional patient with muscular weakness due to a dystrophic process, or disease of the central or peripheral nervous system may show a slight and inconsistent pharmacologic response.

For diagnostic purposes, the most widely used drug is edrophonium chloride (Ten-

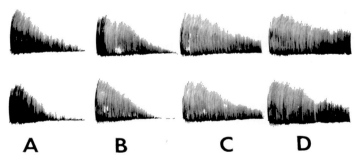

Fig. 12–4. Muscle ergograph in a patient with myasthenia gravis. (**A**) Resting state; (**B**) After i.v. atropine (0.4 mg); (**C**) After i.v. Tensilon (2.0 mg); (**D**) After i.v. Tensilon (8.0 mg). Note the progressive decrease in amplitude in **A** and **B**, partly or competely corrected by Tensilon. (Courtesy of Dr. C. Hermann, Jr., Department of Neurology, UCLA, Los Angeles.)

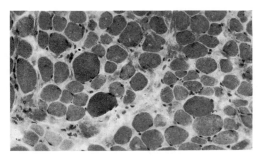

Fig. 12–5. Pseudohypertrophic muscular dystrophy. Transverse section from patient in early stages of the disease showing the variation in fiber size, the presence of occasional swollen fibers, and their homogenous appearance. The amount of connective tissue is increased. There is only a small amount of fat at this state of the illness. (Hematoxylin and eosin, × 30.) (Courtesy of Dr. P. Cancilla, Department of Pathology, UCLA, Los Angeles.)

When muscular dystrophy is associated with mental retardation, brain sections may disclose various developmental anomalies of the cortex, such as pachygyria and heterotopias and disorders of cortical architecture.[41]

Pathogenesis

Despite a wealth of investigative work in this field, the etiology of muscular dystrophy remains unknown. One currently held theory is that the dystrophies are the result of an abnormal muscular or sarcolemmal protein, which is either completely defective, or so altered as to be functionally inadequate. Although several abnormalities in the chemistry of muscle fibers have been described, their specific relationship to the dystrophic process has not been established.

A discussion of the biochemical processes underlying muscular contraction and relaxation are beyond the scope of this text. The reader is referred to reviews by Young,[42] and Katz and Epstein.[43] In essence, sarcolemmal depolarization induces the release of calcium ions from sarcoplasmic reticulum, which trigger myofibrillar contraction. Repolarization of the sarcolemma leads to the reaccumulation of calcium ions by the sarcoplasmic reticulum. In the presence of a minimal critical concentration of ATP, the accumulation of calcium, a process also termed the "relaxing factor," induces myofibrillar relaxation.

Samaha and Gergely have demonstrated that in muscle of dystrophic patients the initial rate and the total calcium uptake by fragmented sarcoplasmic reticulum is low, and that the actomyosin ATPase activity is reduced.[44] In addition, superprecipitation, a phenomenon reflecting the interaction of the contractile proteins of muscle, is delayed.[44a] Direct biochemical studies of diseased muscle have been of little value. Myosin from dystrophic human muscle is immunochemically and electrophoretically identical to normal myosin.[44b] However, as the profound anatomic changes occurring in atrophied muscle obscure any primary chemical alterations, these must be sought by biopsying unaffected muscle in children during the preclinical phase of the disease. Some of the other biochemical approaches to the problem of muscular dystrophy have been outlined by Peter.[44c]

For many years reduced blood creatine, and increased creatine excretion have been known to accompany muscular dystrophy. These findings, as well as the more recently substantiated aminoaciduria, reflect the diminution of muscle substance rather than a basic biochemical abnormality.

Of possibly greater significance is the low potassium and high intrafiber sodium concentrations seen in dystrophic muscle. These electrolyte changes may reflect ion leakage from dystrophic fibers, a process paralleling an enzyme leakage which induces an elevation in the serum levels of a variety of soluable enzymes.

Clinical Manifestations

Duchenne Muscular Dystrophy (Aran-Duchenne).[45] Transmitted in a sex-linked recessive manner, this disease has its clinical onset during early childhood. It is a relatively common condition, with prevalence of 1 per 25,000. The course is so gradual that initial symptoms are often overlooked. These may at first be confined to difficulty in climbing stairs, arising from the floor, or other activities which involve the pelvic musculature. An early indication of pelvic weakness is the manner by which patients arise from the floor by progressively climbing up their thighs (Gowers' sign). Lordosis commonly appears with progression of the disease, and the child "straddles as he stands and waddles as he walks." Muscular wasting and a progressive and early enfeeblement of deep tendon reflexes accompany the advance of the disease. Subsequent to the initial stages, muscular involvement is invariably symmetric. In contrast to the generalized atrophy there is striking pseudohypertrophy of the calves, less commonly of the deltoids and infraspinati (Fig. 12–6). Contractures are common and occur chiefly at the hamstrings.

Enlargement of the heart, persistent tachycardia, and myocardial failure are seen in 50%–80% of patients at some time during the disease, and are reflected in significant electrocardiographic abnormalities.

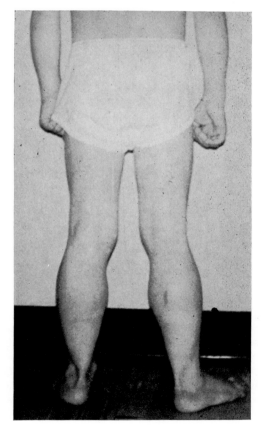

Fig. 12–6. Boy seven years old with pseudohypertrophic muscular dystrophy, showing hypertrophy of the calves which contrasts with the atrophic quadriceps muscles.

There are usually no symptoms of smooth muscle dysfunction. In a small number of patients a history of diarrhea, malabsorption, or megacolon can be elicited, and there may be a disturbance in motor function of the esophagus. These clinical findings correspond to pathologic changes in smooth muscle, most characteristically a fatty infiltration of the myofibers, necrosis of the muscle fibers, and degenerative changes in the nuclei.[45a]

A number of children with muscular dystrophy have defective intellectual development.[46] In the past this has been attributed to their physical handicap, but significant abnormalities in cortical architecture, suggestive of prenatal maldevelopment, have been found in recent pathologic studies.

The course of the illness is steadily downhill. Death usually occurs in adolescence and is due to secondary infections, or intractable congestive heart failure.

The female carrier for muscular dystrophy is usually asymptomatic but may occasionally demonstrate pseudohypertrophy and mild weakness of the pelvic musculature. All gradations from apparent complete normality to a marked dystrophy can be seen on biopsy.[47] The microscopic changes correlate well with the levels of serum creatine phosphokinase, which are abnormally high in about one-third of all female carriers. The findings of a population of dystrophic muscle fibers in some female carriers supports the view, postulated by the Lyon hypothesis, that in these cells the paternal X chromosome—on which the muscular dystrophy gene is located—is active.

In about 10% of children with X-linked muscular dystrophy the progression of the disease is slow. In these patients symptoms begin late, often after eight years of age, and the ability to walk is retained beyond 16 years of age. Pseudohypertrophy is less likely to be present than in the severe form of the disease, and the ankle reflexes are often lost. As a rule, mild and severe cases do not occur within the same family. Genetic studies suggest that the mild form of X-linked muscular dystrophy represents a mixture of entities, possibly alleles on the same locus.[47a]

The clinical form, termed Leyden-Möbius

muscular dystrophy, is probably identical with Duchenne muscular dystrophy. Like the latter it is transmitted in a sex-linked recessive manner, and is only distinguished from it by a less marked muscular hypertrophy.

Facioscapulohumeral Syndromes (Landouzy-Dejerine). As implied by its name, this form of dystrophy affects the muscles of the face, shoulder, and upper arm. It is usually transmitted as an autosomal dominant trait. Initial symptoms tend to appear at a somewhat later age than in the Duchenne form, and deterioration is not as rapid.

Pathologically, facioscapulohumeral dystrophy is a heterogenous group, with the clinical picture being caused by muscular dystrophy, neurogenic muscular atrophy, polymyositis, myasthenia gravis, myotubular myopathy or nemaline myopathy.[16a,48]

The initial symptoms are usually wasting of the shoulder girdle, prominent winging of the scapulae, and the development of myopathic facies. The lips cannot be pursed, and protrude in what has been termed a "tapir's mouth." The relative weakness of the zygomatic muscles results in an equally characteristic transverse smile. Muscular hypertrophy, contractures, and skeletal deformities are rare. Involvement tends to be symmetric, but asymmetric weakness is more common in this form than in any of the other dystrophies.

Although cardiac involvement has been encountered it occurs rarely, and the progression of this clinical entity is sufficiently slow, and interrupted by periods of seeming arrest, so as to allow a normal life span for a fairly large proportion of patients. Erb's muscular dystrophy is probably related to facioscapulohumeral dystrophy, differing only in that facial muscles retain their strength even up to an advanced stage of the disease.

Limb-Girdle Muscular Syndromes. This syndrome also comprises a number of distinct clinical conditions.[49] Transmission usually occurs in an autosomal recessive manner. Symptoms appear during the second or third decade, with muscles of either shoulder or pelvic girdle being affected initially. The rate of progression is highly variable, and the course is far more benign than that of Du-

chenne muscular dystrophy. About 30% of patients develop pseudohypertrophy, usually of the calves, less commonly of the lateral vasti and deltoids. Cardiac involvement is very rare, and intelligence is unaffected.

A variety of so-called restricted dystrophies have been reported. The most common of these conditions are those in which the process starts in and mainly involves the quadriceps[50] or the external ocular muscles.[51]

Diagnosis

A fully developed case of muscular dystrophy can readily be recognized by the distribution of the involved muscles, the presence of pseudohypertrophy, and the absence of the deep tendon reflexes. Occasionally, however, particularly in the early stages of the illness, the diagnosis is difficult, and auxiliary tests, such as measurement of serum enzyme levels, electromyography, or muscle biopsy will be required.

The early stages of the dystrophic process are accompanied by a marked outflow of muscle enzymes into the circulation. This may be the result of an abnormality in the muscle membrane permitting the passage of large molecules into the circulation. The serum level of many soluble enzymes, normally present in muscle tissue, is increased. These include glutamic-oxalacetic transaminase (SGOT), glutamic-pyruvic transaminase (SGPT), lactic dehydrogenase (LDH), aldolase, and creatine phosphokinase (CPK). Of these enzymes an elevation of creatine phosphokinase is the most specific for the presence of a dystrophic process.[5]

In the early stages of Duchenne muscular dystrophy, and even before clinical signs appear, serum creatine phosphokinase levels are strikingly increased. Neither liver disease nor hemolysis of blood samples change the serum activity of this enzyme, so that this abnormality is fairly specific for a dystrophic process. A large proportion of mothers transmitting Duchenne muscular dystrophy also have somewhat elevated serum creatine phosphokinase levels either at rest, or after standardized exercise. With progression of the disease, enzyme levels fall. Dystrophies other than the Duchenne form show only minor enzyme abnormalities, and clinically typical cases of limb-girdle dystrophy with normal serum enzymes are not rare.

The electromyogram may help distinguish myopathies from neuropathic muscular weakness. In myopathies, the EMG shows a shortened mean duration and lower amplitude of the motor unit action potentials. By contrast, neuropathic patterns are characterized by spontaneous activity at rest, and motor unit action potentials of increased duration and amplitude.

A muscle biopsy is valuable in differentiating primary muscle disease from other disorders. The alterations observed in the biopsy have already been described. When the appropriate muscle is selected for examination, pathologic findings are usually adequate for the diagnosis of a dystrophic process. Occasionally it is difficult to distinguish between muscular dystrophy and myositis by either clinical or histologic means. Generally, myositis has a more rapid onset and is accompanied by pain or tenderness of the affected musculature and, less commonly, by evidence of systemic involvement. Changes in one muscle section may be diagnostic of muscular dystrophy, while other areas have the appearance of myositis.

Treatment

At present there is no effective treatment for the muscular dystrophies. Courses of vitamin E, anabolic steroids, and combinations of amino acids have not withstood controlled trial. A significant proportion of patients with facioscapulohumeral dystrophy, when treated with corticosteroids, have experienced dramatic but often transient clinical improvement which is coupled with a striking fall in previously elevated serum creatine phosphokinase levels.[52]

A number of patients with apparent Duchenne muscular dystrophy have spontaneously recovered from their illness. In most cases these were children in whom the onset of symptoms was rapid, a feature strongly suggestive of myositis, from which recovery would not be unexpected.

Physiotherapy, when used routinely, may aid in preventing contractures which contribute to the immobilization of the patient. Orthopedic measures, particularly those followed by prolonged bed rest, seem to hasten the downhill process.

MYOTONIC DYSTROPHY
(Myotonic Atrophy)

Not at all a rare disease, myotonic dystrophy is transmitted as an autosomal dominant trait and is marked by the association of a dystrophic process, myotonia, and endocrine disturbances.

Pathologic Anatomy

On microscopic examination there is a nonspecific alteration in the appearance of the muscle fibers resembling that seen in muscular dystrophy. The fibers, most often those classified as type I on the basis of histochemical stains, are fragmented or atrophied, with small rows of pyknotic sarcolemmal nuclei. There is an increased amount of fibrous and adipose tissue, and usually no evidence for regeneration.

One of the histologic characteristics of the disease is a reorientation of the most peripheral myofibrils from a longitudinal disposition to one ringing the muscle fiber. The significance of this abnormality is uncertain, and it may be an artifact of the action of fixatives on the irritable myotonic muscle. None of the ultrastructural features of myotonic muscle are specific.[53]

Clinical Manifestations

Maas and Paterson and others have argued that myotonic dystrophy, myotonia congenita, and possibly paramyotonia represent expression of the same genetic disorder, with variability determined not by the pathologic gene but by an isoallele carried on the homologous chromosome.[54]

All these entities share the property of myotonia of voluntary muscles. Myotonia is characterized by a failure of voluntary muscle to relax after contraction ceases, and a slow, tonic response to mechanical and electric stimulation. This phenomenon is most readily observed in muscles of the hand, face, and tongue. Patients are unable to relax their grasp, and percussion of the thenar eminence can produce a dimple lasting several seconds. Repetitive movements lessen myotonia, while exposure to cold aggravates it.

some instances an accompanying cerebrospinal fluid pleocytosis indicates meningeal involvement. Pleurodynia is usually caused by a variety of group B coxsackie viruses.

BENIGN CONGENITAL HYPOTONIAS

For several years the term "benign congenital hypotonia" has referred to an infant with muscular weakness who, rather than getting progressively worse and finally dying of his condition, as is usually the case in Werdnig-Hoffmann's disease, may either improve with progressive muscular maturation or at least hold his own. Oppenheim's poorly described patients with amyotonia congenita would probably belong to this group,[22] as do a number of new and pathologically well-defined muscular disorders.

NEMALINE MYOPATHY

First described by Shy and co-workers,[68] this disorder is probably the most common entity in this group. The condition represents a group of disorders with transmission as either an autosomal dominant or autosomal recessive trait.[69] Affected individuals may show symptoms at birth or during the first year of life. There is moderate, slowly progressive or static weakness of the musculature of the pelvis, and of the muscles supplied by the cranial and upper cervical nerves. Deformities of the palate, spine, and feet have also been observed.

Aggregates of rods, staining red with modified trichrome stain, are present in most muscle fibers (Fig. 12–9). Chemical studies

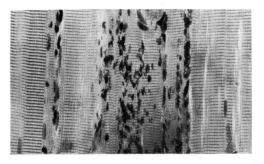

Fig. 12–9. Nemaline myopathy. Longitudinal section of muscle fibers showing rod-shaped structures occurring singly or in aggregates, the latter tending to a palisadelike arrangement. (Trichome stain × 300.) (Courtesy of Dr. P. Cancilla, Department of Pathology, UCLA, Los Angeles.)

on the rod material suggest that it is a protein, possibly tropomyosin B, originating from the Z band of muscle.[70] As similar rod-shaped particles have been produced in skeletal muscle fibers following tenotomy, there is some doubt as to the specificity of this pathologic finding.[71,71a]

CENTRAL CORE DISEASE

This disorder, probably transmitted by an autosomal dominant gene, is characterized by nonprogressive muscular weakness of early onset.[72,73] With the trichrome stain the central areas of affected muscle fibers stain blue while peripheral fibers appear red. When histochemical stains specific for the mitochondrial oxidative enzymes are used, the central area is found to stain less intensively than the periphery of the fiber. A central core, and the collection of rod-shaped structures characteristic for nemaline myopathy have been shown to coincide in some patients.[74]

MYOTUBULAR (CENTRONUCLEAR) MYOPATHY

Children affected with this disorder show a progressive weakness of the limb girdles and of the neck muscles with acute fluctuations coinciding with respiratory illnesses.[75] Ptosis and weakness of the extraocular muscles appear to be characteristic for this condition.[76] Pathological examination of the muscles reveals centrally positioned nuclei in all fibers, a picture similar to the myotubular stage of developing muscle. However, affected muscles do not contain fetal myoglobin, and it is uncertain whether this disease represents a developmental arrest of muscle.[77]

MYOPATHIES WITH ABNORMAL MITOCHONDRIA

Several childhood myopathies have been described in which mitochondrial abnormalities represent the earliest and most striking morphologic changes, and are therefore considered to be of major etiologic significance.[78] The clinical picture in these disorders is protean. Some patients demonstrate a slowly progressive or static myopathy, others have episodes of muscular weakness and salt craving, while in yet others the muscular disorder is overshadowed by a degeneration of the central nervous system highlighted by progressive ataxia and dementia.[78a]

The pathologic picture for all these disorders is similar. Muscle fibers have excessive amounts of red-staining material by the modified Gomori trichrome reaction ("ragged-red muscles"). On electron microscopy one observes an increased number of bizarre and often enlarged mitochondria accompanied by crystalline, and in some instances lipoid inclusions.[79] On biochemical examination of biopsy material, a variety of disorders in mitochondrial function have been noted.[80] The most common of these is a partial uncoupling of mitochondrial oxidative metabolism.[80] In other instances there may be complete uncoupling of oxidative phosphorylation.[81] In yet others the oxidation of glycerol-3-phosphate, NADH, or glutamate is impaired.[82,83,84]

At the present time the basic defect in these disorders is unclear. It is possible that they reflect disorders at the various stages of mitochondrial replication.

CONGENITAL DEFECTS OF MUSCLES

Unilateral or bilateral congenital absence of muscle is more frequently observed in the pectoral group than elsewhere. Absence of the abdominal musculature is commonly associated with defects of the urinary tract and hydronephrosis.[85]

MUSCULAR HYPERTROPHY

Congenital muscular hypertrophy can be associated with several different conditions. In 1934 De Lange reported three children with generalized muscular enlargement, severe mental retardation, and widespread porencephaly.[86] In some instances the hypertrophy diminished as the children matured, but all patients remained severely mentally defective.

Hypothyroidism (Debré-Sémélaigne syndrome)[87,88] and myotonic dystrophy are two other rare causes of congenital muscular hypertrophy. In muscular hypertrophy associated with hypothyroidism, there is an atrophy in Type I muscle fibers and abnormalities in oxidative enzyme activity, with a collection of glycogen in the subsarcolemmal areas.[89] Finally, muscular hypertrophy, including macroglossia, may be seen in infants as a completely unrelated condition.[90]

Biochemical Defects of Muscle

HYPOKALEMIC PERIODIC PARALYSIS

The clinical picture of acute transient paralysis of the musculature of the trunk and extremities with complete freedom from symptoms between attacks was first noted by Shakhnovitch in 1882[91] and by Westphal in 1885.[92]

Clinical Manifestations

This rare disorder is transmitted as an autosomal dominant with incomplete penetrance. For obscure reasons males are three times as frequently affected as females.[93] In 88% of cases, attacks first occur between the ages of 7 and 21. They may vary from slight transient weakness to almost complete paralysis.[94] Most attacks last 6–24 hours and primarily affect the lower limbs. Bulbar and respiratory muscles are the last to become paralyzed, and death during an attack occurs in only 10% of patients. The most consistent factors predisposing to an attack are prolonged rest after vigorous exercise, a heavy carbohydrate meal, and exposure to cold. Administration of ACTH and of a number of mineralocorticoid compounds, notably 2-methyl-9-alpha-fluorohydrocortisone, will also induce paralysis.

During an attack the child has a flaccid paralysis, most complete in the proximal musculature, a loss of deep-tendon reflexes, and absent electric and mechanical excitability. Between attacks, patients are free of symptoms; however, permanent wasting and proximal muscle weakness may develop, even in patients who experience only rare attacks.

Pathogenesis

In some sporadic cases, which are perhaps transmitted as a sex-linked dominant, thyrotoxicosis has been reported to be a major predisposing factor. As expected from a sex-linked recessive disorder, the syndrome of thyrotoxicosis and familial periodic paralysis is limited to males.[95,96] The importance of potassium and sodium metabolism in the etiology of the disease is well-documented. Severe attacks are generally preceded by sodium retention. During an attack the plasma potassium falls as weakness develops. Symptoms usually become evident at a serum potassium concentration of 3.0 mEq/liter, and are marked between 2.5 and 2.0 mEq/liter. Since normal subjects do not develop significant muscular weakness when, as a result of electrolyte imbalance, their serum potassium drops to 2.5 mEq/liter, this finding by itself makes it unlikely that weakness results directly from a potassium deficiency. More likely the converse actually takes place for weakened muscle has a higher potassium concentration than the same muscle sampled between attacks. Muscle sodium content is considerably elevated between attacks, and remains unchanged with the development of paralysis. These findings suggest that along with the onset of paralysis potassium shifts into the muscle. Increased water retention within the muscle may also be important in the development of symptoms.

When a muscle is biopsied during a paralytic attack, marked vacuolization of the sarcoplasm is found. This abnormality is due to an enormous dilatation of the endoplasmic reticulum and disappears once normal muscle function is regained. Vacuolation may not be the primary lesion, it may be secondary to myofibillary degeneration.[96a] Since the membrane potential remains essentially normal during an attack, the basic biochemical lesion has been postulated as a defect in carbohydrate metabolism, resulting in the accumulation of indiffusible metabolites with the consequent shift of potassium and water into the muscle cell. Another etiologic possibility is the intermittent hypersecretion of an aldosteronelike steroid.

Therapy

Paralytic attacks are best treated by the administration of potassium. Prophylactically, a low carbohydrate diet and administration of supplemental potassium at bed time is advisable. A low sodium intake and administration of diuretics, notably acetazolamide (Diamox), have also been very effective in preventing attacks or at least in reducing their frequency. Spironolactone, an aldosterone antagonist given in dosages of 100 mg–200 mg per day, appears to be also of benefit. None of these drugs, however, will prevent the development of progressive muscular atrophy.

HYPERKALEMIC PERIODIC PARALYSIS

For several years prior to Gamstorp's classic description of this condition, atypical cases of periodic paralysis had been recognized.[97] In these individuals attacks started in early childhood, did not respond to potassium, and were unaccompanied by an electrolyte imbalance.

Clinical Manifestations

Attacks often begin in infancy, and in 90% of cases the disease has become established by 10 years of age. The condition affects both sexes equally and is transmitted by an autosomal dominant gene. Attacks occur about once per week and are precipitated by rest following physical exertion. Weakness first affects the pelvic musculature but at times may become generalized. Average attacks last about one hour. During this time the plasma potassium levels are usually higher than normal. Between attacks muscle strength returns to normal, although a myopathy may develop in some families. Percussion myotonia is occasionally noted, and in some families potassium-induced paralysis and myotonia is jointly transmitted as a dominant disorder.[98]

Since hyperkalemia is not invariable, the diagnosis of hyperkalemic periodic paralysis is best established by inducing an attack through the oral administration of potassium.

Pathogenesis

By means of intracellular electromyography a normal resting muscle membrane potential averaging 72 mV is usually found. During an attack, the potential falls to about 45 mV. Depolarization of the muscle membrane may be due to an increased membrane permeability to sodium, or a failure in the sodium "pump" mechanism.[99]

Therapy

The administration of acetazolamide (Diamox) (125 mg/day for an eight-year-old child) has been successful in preventing attacks or reducing their severity.[100] Periodic attacks of severe weakness, commencing in early childhood and lasting up to several weeks, are the characteristic features of a third type of periodic paralysis, termed normokalemic paralysis, also transmitted as an autosomal dominant. Large amounts of sodium (460 mEq/24 hours for the average adult) may relieve the weakness in this condition, and attacks may also be prevented by the prolonged administration of acetazolamide.

Differential Diagnosis of Periodic Paralysis

When a child experiences recurrent attacks of muscular weakness, a number of conditions must be considered.

Hypokalemic periodic paralysis is diagnosed by the family history, a clinical response to potassium, and the concurrent hypokalemia. Hyperkalemic periodic paralysis is distinguished by the early onset of brief but frequent attacks, and their induction through the administration of potassium. In the rare form of normokalemic periodic paralysis, the attacks are more severe, of longer duration, but are also induced by potassium.

In myasthenia gravis weakness almost always affects the bulbar as well as the skeletal musculature, and deep tendon reflexes may be preserved during an attack. A clear-cut improvement in muscle strength following the administration of anticholinesterases will confirm the diagnosis. Periodic attacks of muscular weakness are seen in primary hyperaldosteronism. The striking alkalosis, hypernatremia, and hypokalemia which accompany the attacks aid diagnosis. Recurrent muscular weakness is also seen in myopathies associated with abnormal mitochondria, in polyneuropathies, particularly those accompanying intermittent acute porphyria, and is a prominent feature of paroxysmal myoglobinuria, McArdle's disease, and massive ingestion of licorice extract.

MUSCLE PHOSPHORYLASE DEFICIENCY
(McArdle's Disease, Glycogen Storage Disease, Cori Type 5)

This condition, first described by McArdle 1951,[101] is one of the inheritable myopathies for which the enzymatic abnormality, an absence of muscle phosphorylase activity, has been recognized. Clinical onset is in childhood, with muscle cramps following exertion and episodes of myoglobulinuria. In a typical case, when the forearm muscle is exercised with its arterial circulation occluded, the flexor muscles contract within a minute and remain in this state for an hour or longer after circulation is restored.[102]

Muscle biopsy shows an increased concentration of glycogen, and enzymatic studies reveal the specific defect in muscle phosphorylase activity. Erythrocyte and liver phosphorylase, enzymes which are chemically different, are present in normal amounts.

The sequence of biochemical events leading to contractures and myoglobinuria is still unclear. The uptake of calcium by sarcolemmal reticulum is normal, but it is likely that the amount of available ATP is reduced.[103] Since glycogenolysis is interrupted, energy for ordinary muscular effort must be derived from the oxidation of glucose or fatty acids.

CONGENITAL DEFECT OF PHOSPHOFRUCTOKINASE

Other disorders of muscle carbohydrate metabolism are even more rare. They include patients with a defect in phosphofructokinase who show a clinical picture similar to that of McArdle's disease.[104] Phosphofructokinase is absent from muscle in these patients. In erythrocytes, enzyme activity is reduced by some 50%, but is normal in leukocytes. Four isozymes of phosphofructokinase have been recognized with the muscle type subunit being absent in this disease.[105] Since in these individuals the enzymatic defect precludes glucose utilization, energy for muscular contraction must be derived from fatty acid oxidation or conceivably by enhancement of the usually unimportant hexose monophosphate shunt.

MYOGLOBINURIA

Myoglobinuria is a rare syndrome due to a variety of causes.[106] The hereditary form of myoglobinuria may be due to a deficiency in muscle phosphorylase or to other as yet unknown metabolic disorders. In sporadic myoglobinuria, patients character-istically suffer a sudden episode of severe muscle pain and weakness, accompanied by the passage of brown urine, following severe exertion, a febrile episode, convulsive seizures, or exposure to various toxins.

Serum enzymes, such as the transaminases and aldolase, are strikingly increased, and occasionally an acute renal tubular necrosis may accompany the attack.

Identification of the urinary pigment is made by the presence of a guaiac positive pigment in the erythrocyte-free urine. Spectroscopic analysis as described by Rowland et al.[106] will confirm the presence of myoglobin.

In one rare muscle disorder, associated with intermittent muscle cramps and myoglobinuria, but without weakness, attacks are induced not only by excercise but also by fasting, or by a high-fat, low-carbohydrate diet. Lipid droplets are seen in type I muscle fibers, and a defect in the utilization of long chain fatty acids by liver and muscle has been postulated.[107]

REFERENCES

1. Richardson, A. T. and Barwick, D. D.: "Clinical Electromyography," in Walton, J. N.: *Disorders of Voluntary Muscles*, London: Churchill, 1969, p. 813.
2. Richardson, A. T.: Clinical electrodiagnosis, Proc. Roy. Soc. Med. 55:897, 1962.
3. Lambert, E. H.: Neurophysiological techniques useful in the study of neuromuscular disorders, Res. Pub. Ass. Res. Nerv. Ment. Dis. 38:247, 1958.
4. Dunn, H. G., et al.: Conduction velocity of motor nerves in infants and children, Pediatrics 34:708, 1964.
5. Pearce, J. M. S., Pennington, R. T., and Walton, J. N.: Serum enzyme studies in muscle disease: Part II. Serum creatine kinase activity in muscular dystrophy and in other myopathic and neuropathic disorders, J. Neurol. Neurosurg. Psychiat. 27:96, 1964.
6. Dubowitz, V.: "Histochemical Aspects of Muscle Disease," in Walton, J. N.: *Disorders of Voluntary Muscles*, London: Churchill, 1969, p. 239.
7. Price, H. M.: "Ultrastructure of the Skeletal Muscle Fibre," in Walton, J. N.: *Disorders of Voluntary Muscles*, London: Churchill, 1969, p. 29.
8. Refsum, S. and Skillicorn, S. A.: Amyotrophic familial spastic paraplegia, Neurology (Minneap.) 4:40, 1954.
9. Werdnig, G.: Zwei fruhinfantile hereditare Falle von progressiver Muskelatrophie unter dem Bilde der Dystrophie, aber auf neurotischer Grundlage, Arch. Psychiat. Nervenkr. 22:437, 1891.
10. Hoffmann, J.: Uber chronische spinale muskelatrophie im Kindesalter auf familiarer Basis, Deutsch. Z. Nervenheilk. 3:427, 1893.
11. Chou, S. M. and Fakadej, A. V.: Ultrastructure of chromatolytic motoneurons and anterior spinal roots in a case of Werdnig-Hoffmann disease, J. Neuropath. Exp. Neurol. 30:386, 1971.
12. Brandt, S.: *Werdnig-Hoffmann's Progressive Muscular Atrophy*, Copenhagen: Ejnar Munksgaard, 1950.
13. Gamstorp, I.: Progressive spinal muscular atrophy with onset in infancy or early childhood, Acta Paediat. Scand. 56:408, 1967.
14. Pearce, J. and Harriman, D. G. F.: Chronic spinal muscular atrophy, J. Neurol. Neurosurg. Psychiat. 29:509, 1966.
15. Dubowitz, V.: Infantile muscular atrophy: A prospective study with particular reference to a slowly progressive variety, Brain 87:707, 1964.
15a. Van Wijngaarden, G. K. and Bethlem, J.: Benign infantile spinal muscular atrophy, Brain 96:163, 1973.
16. Munsat, T. L., et al.: Neurogenic muscular atrophy of infancy with prolonged survival: The variable course of Werdnig-Hoffmann disease, Brain 92:9, 1969.
16a. Emery, A. E. H.: The nosology of the spinal muscular atrophies, J. Med. Genet. 8:481, 1971.
16b. Wohlfart, G., Fex, J., and Eliasson, S.: Hereditary proximal spinal muscular atrophy—a clinical entity simulating progressive muscular dystrophy, Acta Psychiat. Neurol. Scand. 30:395, 1955.
17. Kugelberg, E. and Welander, L.: Heredofamilial juvenile muscular atrophy simulating muscular dystrophy, Arch. Neurol. Psychiat. 75:500, 1956.
18. Tsukagoshi, H., et al.: Kugelberg-Welander syndrome with dominant inheritance, Arch. Neurol. 14:378, 1966.
18a. Denny-Brown, D. and Pennybacker, J. B.: Fibrillation and fasciculation in voluntary muscle, Brain 61:311, 1938.
19. Dubowitz, V.: Enzyme histochemistry of skeletal muscle: Part III. Neurogenic muscular atrophies, J. Neurol. Neurosurg. Psychiat. 29:23, 1966.
20. Engel, W. K.: Selective and nonselective susceptibility of muscle fiber types, Arch. Neurol. 22:97, 1970.
20a. Engel, W. K.: Focal myopathic changes produced by electromyographic and hypodermic needles: Needle myopathy, Arch. Neurol. 16:509, 1967.
21. Walton, J. H.: The limp child, J. Neurol. Neurosurg. Psychiat. 20:144, 1957.

22. Oppenheim, H.: Uber allgemeine und local-isierte Atonie der Muskulatur (Myatonia) im fruhen Kindsalter, Monatsschr. Psychiat. Neurol. 8:232, 1900.

23. Peña, C. E., et al.: Arthrogryposis multiplex congenita: Report of two cases of a radicular type with familial incidence, Neurology (Minneap.) 18:926, 1968.

24. Amick, L. D., Johnson, W. W., and Smith, H. L.: Electromyographic and histopathologic correlations in arthrogryposis, Brain 86:75, 1963.

25. Pearson, C. M. and Fowler, W. G., Jr.: Hereditary non-progressive muscular dystrophy inducing arthrogryposis syndrome, Brain 86:75, 1963.

25a. Hooshmand, H., Martinez, A. J., and Rosenblum, W. I.: Arthrogryposis multiplex congenita, Arch. Neurol. 24:561, 1971.

26. Ionasescu, V., et al: Increased collagen synthesis in arthrogryposis multiplex congenita, Arch. Neurol. 23:128, 1970.

27. Williams, P. F.: The early correction of deformities in arthrogryposis multiplex congenita, Aust. Ped. J. 2:194, 1966.

28. McFarland, H. R. and Heller, G. L.: Guillain-Barre disease complex, Arch. Neurol. 14:196, 1966.

29. Willis, T.: *De Anima Brutorum Quae Hominis Vitalis ac Sensitiva Est, Exercitationes Duae*, London: Typis E. F., impensis Ric. Davis, 1672, pp. 287–289.

29a. Engel, W. K. and Warmolts, J. R.: Myasthenia gravis: A new hypothesis of the pathogenesis and a new form of treatment, Ann NY Acad. Sci. 183:72, 1971.

29b. Santa, T., Engel, A. G., and Lambert, E. H.: Histometric study of neuromuscular junction ultrastructure, Neurology (Minneap.) 22:71, 1972.

30. Osserman, K. E.: *Myasthenia Gravis*, New York: Grune & Stratton, Inc. 1958.

31. Millichap, J. G. and Dodge, P. R.: Diagnosis and treatment of myasthenia gravis in infancy, childhood and adolescence, Neurology (Minneap.) 10:1007, 1960.

32. Greer, M. and Schotland, M.: Myasthenia gravis in the newborn, Pediatrics 26:101, 1960.

33. Herrmann, C., Jr.: The familial occurrence of myasthenia gravis, Ann. NY Acad. Sci. 183:334, 1971.

34. Schlezinger, N. S. and Corin, M. S.: Myasthenia gravis associated with hyperthyroidism in childhood, Neurology (Minneap.) 18:1217, 1968.

35. Rowland, L. P., Hoefer, P. F. A., and Aranow, H., Jr.: Myasthenic syndromes, Res. Pub. Ass. Res. Nerv. Ment. Dis. 38:548, 1958.

36. Nastuk, W. L., et al.: Immunological changes following thymectomy in myasthenia gravis, Arch. Neurol. 15:1, 1966.

36a. Goldstein, G. and Manganaro, A.: Thymin: A thymic polypeptide causing the neuromuscular block in myasthenia gravis, Ann. NY Acad. Sci. 183:230, 1971.

37. Williams, D.: The management of myasthenia, Mod. Trends Neurol. 4:269, 1967.

38. Seybold, M. E., et al.: Thymectomy in juvenile myasthenia gravis, Arch. Neurol. 25:385, 1971.

39. Fonkelsrud, E. W., Herrmann, C., and Mulder, D. G.: Thymectomy for myasthenia gravis in children, J. Pediat. Surg. 5:157, 1970.

39a. Jenkins, R. B. Treatment of myasthenia gravis with prednisone, Lancet 1:765, 1972.

40. Ross, M. H., Pappas, G. D., and Harman, P. J.: Alterations in muscle fine structure in hereditary muscular dystrophy of mice, Lab. Invest. 9:388, 1960.

41. Rosman, N. P.: The cerebral defect and myopathy in Duchenne muscular dystrophy, Neurology (Minneap.) 20:329, 1970.

42. Young, M.: The molecular basis of muscle contraction. Ann. Rev. Biochem. 38:913, 1969.

43. Katz, A. I. and Epstein, F. H.: Physiologic role of sodium-potassium-activated adenosine triphosphatase in the transport of cations across biologic membranes, New Eng. J. Med. 278:253, 1968.

44. Samaha, F. J. and Gergely, J.: Biochemical abnormalities of the sarcoplasmic reticulum in muscular dystrophy, New Eng. J. Med. 280:184, 1969.

44a. Furukawa, T. and Peter, J. B.: Superprecipitation and adenosine triphosphatase activity of myosin B in Duchenne muscular dystrophy, Neurology (Minneap.) 21:920, 1971.

44b. Penn, A. S., Cloak, R. A., and Rowland, L. P.: Myosin from normal and dystrophic human muscle, Arch. Neurol. 27:159, 1972.

44c. Peter, J. B.: Biochemical approaches to the study of muscle disease, Birth Defects Original Article Series 7:38, 1971.

45. Rowland, L. P.: Muscular dystrophies, polymyositis and other myopathies, J. Chronic Dis. 8:510, 1958.

45a. Huvos, A. G. and Prudzanski, W.: Smooth muscle involvement in primary muscle disease. II. Progressive muscular dystrophy, Arch. Path. 83:234, 1967.

46. Rosman, N. P. and Kakulas, B. A.: Mental deficiency associated with muscular dystrophy: A neuropathological study, Brain 89:769, 1966.

47. Pearce, G. W., Pearce, J. M. S., and Walton, J. N.: The Duchenne type muscular dystrophy: Histopathologic studies of the carrier state, Brain 89:109, 1966.

47a. Shaw, R. F. and Dreifuss, F. E.: Mild and severe forms of X-linked muscular dystrophy, Arch. Neurol. 20:451, 1969.

48. Rothstein, T. L., Carlson, C. B., and Sumi, S. M.: Polymyositis with fascioscapulohumeral distribution, Arch. Neurol. 25:313, 1971.

49. Munsat, T. L. and Pearson, C. M.: The differential diagnosis of neuromuscular weakness in infancy and childhood: Part II. The dystrophic myopathies, Develop. Med. Child Neurol. 9:319, 1967.

50. Walton, J. N.: Two cases of myopathy limited to the quadriceps, J. Neurol. Neurosurg. Psychiat. 19:106, 1956.

51. Bray, G. M., Kaarsoo, M., and Ross, R. T.: Ocular myopathy with dysphagia, Neurology (Minneap.) 15:678, 1965.

52. Munsat, T. L., et al.: Inflammatory myopathy with fascioscapulohumeral distribution, Neurology (Minneap.) 22:335, 1972.

53. Schotland, D. L.: An electron microscopic investigation of myotonic dystrophy, J. Neuropath. Exp. Neurol. 29:241, 1970.

54. Maas, O. and Paterson, A. S.: Myotonia congenita, dystrophia myotonica, and paramyotonia, Brain 73:318, 1950.

55. Becker, P. E.: Neues zur Genetik und Klassifikation der Muskeldystrophien, Humangenetik 17:1, 1972.

56. Drager, G. A., Hammill, J. F., and Shy, G. M.: Paramyotonia congenita, Arch. Neurol. Psychiat. 80:1, 1958.

57. Calderon, R.: Myotonic dystrophy: A neglected cause for mental retardation, J. Pediat. 68:423, 1966.

58. Pruzanski, W.: Variants of myotonic dystrophy in preadolescent life, Brain 89:563, 1966.

58a.Dyken, P. R. and Harper, P. S.: Congenital dystrophica myotonica, Neurology (Minneap.) 24:465, 1973.

59. Dodge, P. R., et al.: Myotonic dystrophy in infancy and childhood, Pediatrics 35:3, 1965.

59a.Renwick, J. H., et al.: Confirmation of linkage of the loci for myotonic dystrophy and ABH secretion, J. Med. Genet. 8:407, 1971.

60. Norris, F. H., Jr.: Unstable membrane potential in human myotonic muscle, Electroenceph. Clin. Neurophysiol. 14:197, 1962.

60a.Lipicky, R. J., Bryant, S. H., and Salmon, J. H.: Cable parameters, sodium, potassium, chloride and water content, and potassium efflux in isolated external intercostal muscle of normal volunteers and patients with myotonia congenita, J. Clin. Invest. 50:2091, 1971.

61. Samaha, F. J. and Gergely, J.: Biochemistry of normal and myotonic human myosin, Arch. Neurol. 21:200, 1969.

61a.Peter, J. B. and Fiehn, W.: Distinctive lipid abnormalities in sarcolemma from patients with myotonic dystrophy, Clin. Res. 20:192, 1972.

61b.Walsh, J. C., et al.: Abnormalities of insulin secretion in dystrophia myotonica, Brain 93:731, 1970.

62. Wochner, R. D., et al.: Accelerated breakdown of immunoglobulin G (IgG) in myotonic dystrophy: A hereditary error of immunoglobulin catabolism, J. Clin. Invest. 45:321, 1966.

63. Sjaastad, O.: N-acetylhistaminuria in dystrophia myotonica, Europ. Neurol. 1:112, 1968.

63a.Swift, M. R. and Finegold, M. J.: Myotonic muscular dystrophy: Abnormalities in fibroblast culture, Science 165:294, 1969.

64. Banker, B. Q. and Victor, M.: Dermatomyositis (systemic angiopathy) of childhood, Medicine (Balt.) 45:261, 1966.

65. Wedgewood, R. J. P., Cook, C., and Cohen, J.: Dermatomyositis: Report of 26 cases in children with a discussion of endocrine therapy in 13, Pediatrics 12:447, 1953.

65a.Sullivan, D. B., et al.: Prognosis in childhood dermatomyositis, J. Pediat. 80:555, 1972.

65b.Currie, S. and Walton, J. N.: Immunosuppressive therapy in polymyositis, J. Neurol. Neurosurg. Psychiat. 34:447, 1971.

66. Eaton, L. M.: The perspective of neurology in regard to polymyositis, Neurology (Minneap.) 4:245, 1954.

67. Pearson, C. M.: Polymyositis, Ann. Rev. Med. 17:63, 1966.

68. Shy, G. M., et al.: Nemaline myopathy: A new congenital myopathy, Brain 86:793, 1963.

69. Peterson, D. I. and Munsat, T.: The clinical presentation of nemaline myopathy, Bull. Los Angeles Neurol. Soc. 34:39, 1969.

70. Nienhuis, A. W., et al.: Nemaline myopathy: A histopathologic and histochemical study, Amer. J. Clin. Path. 48:1, 1967.

71. Resnick, J. S., Engel, W. K., and Nelson, P. G.: Changes in the Z disk of skeletal muscle induced by tenotomy, Neurology (Minneap.) 18:737, 1968.

71a.Meltzer, H. Y., McBride, E., and Poppei, R. W.: Rod (nemaline) bodies in the skeletal muscle of an acute schizophrenic patient, Neurology (Minneap.) 23:769, 1973.

72. Shy, G. M. and Magee, K. R.: A new congenital non-progressive myopathy, Brain 79:610, 1956.

73. Armstrong, R. M., et al.: Central core disease with congenital hip dislocation: Study of two families, Neurology (Minneap.) 21:369, 1971.

74. Shy, G. M.: "Central Core Diseases and Nemaline Myopathy," in Stanbury, T. B., Wyngaarden, J. B., and Fredrickson, D. S. (eds.): The Metabolic Basis of Inherited Disease, 2nd ed., New York: McGraw-Hill Book Co., 1966, pp. 952–962.

75. Spiro, A. J., Shy, G. M., and Gonatas, N. K.: Myotubular myopathy, Arch. Neurol. 14:1, 1966.

76. Campbell, M. J., Rebeiz, J. J., and Walton, J. N.: Myotubular, centronuclear or pericentronuclear myopathy, J. Neurol. Sci. 8:425, 1969.

77. Munsat, T. L., Thompson, L. R., and Coleman, R. F.: Centronuclear ("myotubular") myopathy, Arch. Neurol. 20:120, 1969.

78. Shy, G. M., Gonatas, N. K., and Perez, M.: Two childhood myopathies with abnormal mitochondria, Brain 89:133, 1966.

78a.Drachman, D. A.: Ophthalmoplegia plus, Arch. Neurol. 18:654, 1968.

79. Price, H. M., et al.: Myopathy with atypical mitochondria in type I skeletal muscle fibers, J. Neuropath. Exp. Neurol. 26:475, 1967.

80. Kark, R. A. P., et al.: "Oxidative Metabolism in Small Samples of Normal and Diseased Human Muscle," in Kakulas, B. (ed.): Proceedings of the Second International Congress on Muscle Diseases, Perth, Australia, 1971.

81. Luft, R., et al.: A case of severe hypermetabolism of nonthyroid origin with a defect in the maintenance of mitochondrial respiratory control, J. Clin. Invest. 41:1776, 1962.

82. DiMauro, S., Schotland, D. L., and Rowland, L. P.: Ocular myopathy, glycogen storage and abnormal mitochondria, Neurology (Minneap.) 21:412, 1971.

83. Spiro, A. J., et al.: A cytochrome-related inherited disorder of the nervous system and muscle, Arch. Neurol. 23:103, 1970.

84. Spiro, A. J., Prineas, J. W., and Moore, C. L.: A new mitochondrial myopathy in a patient with salt craving, Arch. Neurol. 22:259, 1970.

85. Dodge, P. R.: Congenital neuromuscular disorders, Res. Pub. Ass. Res. Nerv. Ment. Dis. 38:479, 1958.

86. DeLange, C.: Congenital hypertrophy of the muscles, extrapyramidal motor disturbances and mental deficiency, Amer. J. Dis. Child. 48:243, 1934.

87. Debré, R. and Sémélaigne, G.: Syndrome of diffuse muscular hypertrophy in infants causing athletic appearance, Amer. J. Dis. Child. 50:1351, 1935.

88. Wilson, J. and Walton, J. N.: Some muscular manifestations of hypothyroidism, J. Neurol. Neurosurg. Psychiat. 22:320, 1959.

89. Spiro, A. J., et al.: Cretinism with muscular hypertrophy (Kocher-Debré-Sémélaigne syndrome), Arch. Neurol. 23:340, 1970.

90. Silver, H. K. and Schroeder, F. A.: Congenital muscular hypertrophy, Amer. J. Dis. Child. 108:406, 1964.

91. Shakhnovitch: On a case of intermittent paraplegia (abst.), London Med. Rec. 12:130, 1884.

92. Westphal, C.: Ueber einen merkwurdigen Fall von periodischer Lahmumg, Berl. Klin. Wchnschr. 22:489, 1885.

93. Pearson, C. M. and Kalyanaraman, K.: "Periodic Paralysis," in Stanbury, J. B., Wyngaarden, J. B., and Fredrickson, D. S. (eds.): The Metabolic Basis of Inherited Disease, 3rd ed., McGraw-Hill Book Co., New York, 1972, pp. 1180–1203.

94. Dyken, M., Zeman, W., and Rusche, T.: Hypokalemic periodic paralysis: Children with permanent myopathic weakness, Neurology (Minneap.) 19:691, 1969.

95. Brody, I. A. and Dudley, A. W., Jr.: Thyrotoxic hypokalemic periodic paralysis: Muscle morphology and functional assay of sarcoplasmic reticulum, Arch. Neurol. 21:1, 1969.

96. Creutzfeldt, O. D., et al.: Muscle membrane potentials in episodic adynamia, Electroenceph. Clin. Neurophysiol. 15:508, 1963.

96a.Macdonald, R. D., Rewcastle, N. B., and Humphrey, J. G.: Myopathy of hypokalemic periodic paralysis, Arch. Neurol. 20:565, 1969.

97. Gamstorp, I.: Adynamia episodica hereditaria, Acta Paediat. Scand. Suppl. 108:1, 1956.

98. Gamstorp, I.: Adynamia episodica hereditaria, and myotonia, Acta Neurol. Scand. 39:41, 1963.

99. Brooks, J. E.: Hyperkalemic periodic paralysis, Arch. Neurol. 20:13, 1969.

100. McArdle, B.: Adynamia episodica hereditaria and its treatment, Brain 85:121, 1962.

101. McArdle, B.: Myopathy due to a defect in muscle glycogen breakdown, Clin. Sci. 10:13, 1951.

102. Rowland, L. P., et al.: The clinical diagnosis of McArdle's disease, Neurology (Minneap.) 16:93, 1966.

103. Brody, I. A., Gerber, C. J., and Sidbury, J. B.: Relaxing factor in McArdle's syndrome: Calcium uptake by sarcoplasmic reticulum, Neurology (Minneap.) 20:555, 1970.

104. Layzer, R. B., Rowland, L. P., and Ranney, H. M.: Muscle phosphofructokinase deficiency, Arch. Neurol. 17:512, 1967.

105. Layzer, R. B. and Conway, M. M.: Multiple isoenzymes of human phosphofructokinase, Biochem. Biophys. Res. Commun. 40:1259, 1970.

106. Rowland, L. P., et al.: Myoglobinuria, Arch. Neurol. 10:537, 1964.

107. Engel, W. K., et al.: A skeletal muscle disorder associated with intermittent symptoms and a possible defect of lipid metabolism, New Eng. J. Med. 282:697, 1970.

Disorders of Mental Development

CHAPTER 13

Marcel Kinsbourne

Introduction

The most distinctive aspect of neurologic maturation in humans is the gradual acquisition of an extensive repertoire of cognitive skills. The newborn is considered as devoid of cerebrally controlled behavior patterns. Indeed, in the first six weeks after birth it is hard to distinguish a normal from an anencephalic baby. Subsequently, and particularly during the first three years, while the rate of cerebral maturation is at a maximum, a variety of mental processes becomes available for the child's use.

The rates of development of the components of intellect, as well as the level at which it reaches asymptote in adolescence, may be uniformly decreased by a variety of adverse influences, resulting in mental retardation proportionate to the severity of the decrease. In other cases, the decreased rate of development has uneven impact on different components of intelligence, resulting in a striking degree of "scatter" among some mental processes, which seem relatively well-developed for the child's age, and others that are pathologically delayed in their evolution. These instances of selective cognitive deficit may involve any subset of the spectrum of mental abilities, but the ones that most commonly come to clinical attention are those which are socially most prejudicial to the child, namely delayed language develop-

ment and the learning disabilities; these delays leave a child unready to acquire one or more academic skills by customary methods at the customary age. In yet other instances, although the development of mental abilities proceeds normally, the child has defective control over his distribution of attention in space and time; he therefore has difficulty in deploying his mental abilities in order to learn and to relate to others.

We will first consider general mental retardation, then attentional deficits, and then selective cognitive deficits. The discussion will be in the context of a model which postulates that impaired mental development results from neurodevelopmental lag.

As the normal brain matures, different areas of brain take control over specific aspects of behavior in a predictable sequence and timing.[1] When one area is damaged subsequent to the acquisition of the skill, then its control over that skill is impaired, and an acquired deficit results. When the damage is early and affects an area which has not yet begun to function, the child's behavior does not change at the time of the insult. Later, however, the impairment manifests as a delay in the evolution of the mental process from the damaged area. Whereas those forms of behavior which are supported by unimpaired brain evolve in normal sequence and with normal timing, the affected process appears later and thus out of sequence and evolves more slowly than expected once it has appeared. Thus, with respect to only one process, the child functions like a younger normal child.

The view that defective mental development is based on neurodevelopmental lag has practical consequences. It suggests that there exists for each variant of mental deficit a model at a particular stage of normal development. It becomes relevant to regard the deficits as "immaturities" and to relate their characteristics to normal development rather than to think of them as "disease" states with unique characteristics. Further, a model of management becomes available which is based upon the customary management of the younger normal child.

Neurodevelopmental lag may affect the nervous system at any level or any combination of levels. Thus the immaturities may become apparent in the conventional neurologic examination, in the form of so-called "soft signs." These are manifestations of modes of sensorimotor functioning which normally are transiently present during development, but are recognized as abnormal when their presence is observed at an age at which the progress of neural maturation should have caused them to be superseded. The overall trend of sensory development is toward a finer, more exact differentiation of various stimuli from each other.[2] The trend of motor development is toward increasingly precise control over an ever widening repertoire of movement combinations. The newborn is equipped with a limited number of synergisms, which in infancy become apparent both as "mass" responses to reflex stimulation, and in the context of the child's own voluntary movement, as "associated movements." Undue persistence of these primitive synergisms constitutes a "soft sign" of neurologic abnormality, for example, an elicitable obligatory tonic neck response, or the association of gripping with one hand with involuntary clenching of the other hand in an older child. The child is clumsy, without necessarily showing long tract signs[3] and has great difficulty in keeping still, a situation that has been termed the "choreiform syndrome."[4] These manifestations of sensorimotor im-

maturity are the lower level analogies of the mental immaturities already discussed. Sensorimotor immaturities and cognitive immaturities have sometimes been classified together under the heading of "minimal brain dysfunction." However, they do not necessarily coincide, and no conclusion about mental development or the nature of a cognitive deficit can be derived from the mere observation of neurologic "soft signs." Nor is there evidence that the antecedents of minimal brain dysfunction differ from those of major congenital nervous system disorders such as cerebral palsy or mental retardation. Whether minimal brain dysfunction or some other deficit occurs seems to depend on the distribution and severity of the insult rather than its pathogenesis.

Disorders of mental development could theoretically be classified on an etiologic basis. But while a wide range of noxious influences acting early in life have been incriminated, there is no evidence that highly specific relationships exist either between particular items in the patient's history and particular lesions, or between particular types of lesions and particular behavioral outcomes. Therefore, it is preferable to avoid inferences such as "cerebral dysfunction," "organicity," or "brain damage," and instead to focus attention on the characteristics of the disordered behavior. Is the child handicapped in reasoning, using language, remembering visual or auditory information, remembering spatial relationships, paying attention?

Differential Diagnosis of Mental Deficit

Children are brought for consultation either with a complaint of less than expected accomplishment or of deviant behavior, or both. With regard to his intellectual accomplishments, the basic decision to make is whether the child is in fact achieving up to what turns out to be a generally or selectively limited potential, or whether he is falling short of his potential. If he is achieving at the level of his potential, the main implication is for an adjustment of parental expectations and teaching techniques to that level. If he is truly underachieving, it is necessary to look for the causes of the underachievement in the child's social setting or his own emotional adjustment. Only in occasional cases—e.g. organic hyperactivity—is it possible to raise potential by physical measures.

Children who are mentally retarded usually are observed to be developing unduly slowly from the start. Motor and language milestones are reached with uniform delay. Of a variety of associated findings, microcephaly and hypotonia are the commonest but are often absent, and only in a minority of cases can a specific syndrome such as mongolism or phenylketonuria be identified. The diagnosis of mental retardation relies primarily upon the validation of a clinical impression of mental dullness by standard psychometric procedures.

The older the child, the more reliable is the prognostic value of mental testing. "Developmental" diagnosis during infancy[5,6] succeeds in pointing out only the more flagrant instances of mental deficiency. This is because the repertoire of cognitive function that is available at that age is so limited even in the normal case that it is possible only to evaluate accurately the infant's sensorimotor functions; these functions loosely correlate with but do not represent a child's cognitive skills, the lack of which constitutes mental retardation in later years. Many children are severely mentally defective in spite of normal sensorimotor development.

Since language ability is crucial in the socially relevant cognitive functions, the rate of language development is an important guide to the rate of overall mental development (although gross dissociations between the rate of language and of nonverbal mental development do occur and are discussed below). Mental testing becomes prognostically far more useful at an age at which some language competence is expected. As the child increases his language comprehension, he widens the range of test situations that can be used to evaluate the components of his intellect. Furthermore, when a child can speak he is far more accessible to specific test instruction than before that time. In preschoolers, the Stanford-Binet scale or the Wechsler Preschool and Primary Scale of Intelligence are used, and for school-age children the Wechsler Intelligence Scale for Children (WISC) becomes available. These are well-standardized test batteries that yield information about the child's actual as compared to expected (for his age) competence on a number of tasks. A normal outcome on such testing eliminates mental retardation as the reason for substandard preschool or school achievement. It does not eliminate the possibility that specific cognitive deficits handicap the acquisition of specific skills, since each subtest involves a variety of not always well-defined mental processes. Therefore, without one-by-one testing of each process involved, for example in the Block Design subtest of the WISC, the specific ability limiting the child's performance would remain unknown. A child might receive a below-normal score on one subtest, but one would not yet have identified which basic process is preventing him from learning to read.

"Scatter" between subtests on an intelligence scale may reflect a disparity in the level of development of different intellectual skills. Thus, the Wechsler tests are divided into verbal and performance subscales. Educable mentally subnormal children tend toward somewhat lower scores on the verbal than the performance scale.[7] A much lower verbal than performance intelligence quotient accompanies selective language delay; the opposite discrepancy is often found in association with developmental difficulties in spatial orientation and visuomotor control.

In many instances, however, the IQ scores, taken literally, underestimate the child's mental potential. The child's motivation to perform cannot be taken for granted, particularly when he comes from a subculture that has little understanding of and sympathy for the evaluator and his concerns. Anxiety may block the child's reasoning processes, alienation and withdrawal may make them unavailable for the task in hand, thought disorders may intrude, or impulsivity may degrade the thoroughness of the performance. Lapses of attention due to subclinical minor seizures may interrupt concentration, and the pathologically limited attention span of the hyperkinetic syndrome may impair performance on tasks that demand maintained attention. Finally, in young children, even the presence of gross sensory deficit such as deafness may go unnoticed, and the child's imperfect response to verbal questioning be attributed to mental deficiency. The intelligence test results must be considered in the light of these practical sources of misinterpretation, and it cannot be assumed that the psychologist has ruled them out unless these contingencies are specifically considered in the report.

Behavioral Diagnosis

The prediction of subsequent development from observations early in infancy is a much studied but as yet precarious exercise. Major neurologic deficit can be predicted with some success as early as birth, using the Apgar scoring system.[8] Early excitability has been found to predict choreiform movements later in childhood.[9] Orienting responses to acoustic[10] or other novel stimuli[11] are said to habituate more slowly in infants with brain damage. Intelligence tests in infancy[12] yield a "developmental quotient" (DQ) which evaluates skills that are measurable in infancy, and thus is heavily loaded with factors relating to motor development. Within a normal population the DQ is a poor predictor of subsequent cognitive development, presumably because it cannot take account of subsequent "growth spurts."[5] but it has some success in distinguishing a normal from a retarded population.[13] Infant testing is a highly specialized exercise, but the clinician can avail himself of a simple screening test[14] which will enable him to decide which children to send for further testing. If the child's cooperation cannot be enlisted, the mother can be given some standard questions about her child's social development.[15] The situation is complicated when the child comes from a deprived environment. Such children show relatively lower intelligence quotients, and the discrepancy increases with increasing age.[16]

Psychosocial Deprivation

Developmental retardation due to major abnormalities in the social environment, subsumed under the term cultural deprivation[17] is at times indistinguishable from that characteristic of mental retardation. Infants deprived of maternal attention were found to become depressed and to decline in cognitive skills.[18,19] Children reared in the home were found to be better able to reason than adopted infants, who in turn excelled infants in institutions.[20] There is some evidence that even handling of newborn infants has some effect on behavior, although the long-term consequences are unclear. The disadvantage that characterizes deprived children if anything increases with the passing years.[21]

Hunt[22] has summarized a variety of effects of experience on development. While the effects are definite, the mechanism is debatable. A direct effect on brain development cannot be assumed as there are gross and obvious effects on socialization and motivation which would impair performance even if the child possessed a potentially normal intellect. Thus, even within a relatively homogeneous retarded population, such as children with Down's syndrome, a group kept in the home was found to be more effective than a matched institutionalized group on tests of language manipulation, activities likely to be more encouraged and rewarded in the home than in the institution.[23]

MENTAL RETARDATION

Mental retardation is defined by the World Health Organization as an "incomplete or insufficient general development of mental capacities." As there is a continuum of mental abilities from very high to negligible in the population, the quantitative definition of mental retardation and of its subdivisions based on the intelligence quotient is necessarily arbitrary. IQ below 75 defines a retardate. An individual within the range 50–75, a so-called moron, is a slow learner but regarded as essentially educable, whereas children with IQ below 50, whether imbecile (20–50) or idiots (less than 20), are thought capable only of being trained in certain simple skills. Thus defined, the prevalence of mental retardation in the United States is some three percent, of whom all but 0.3 percent are educable; 400,000 require constant care. However, variable diagnostic

2. Repetitive aimless motor activites—52%
3. Explosive reactions—8%
4. Obsessive behavior—29%
5. Stereotyped play—19%
6. Unusual seeking of sensory experience—29%

The electroencephalogram is often abnormal in children with psychiatric disease. Eighteen studies[46] reported incidences between 5 and 15% of EEG abnormalities in normal children contrasted with their reports ranging from 33%–92% of abnormality in psychiatric cases. Among the latter, EEG abnormalities are concentrated among children with conduct disorders, whereas neurotic children's EEG abnormalities are no more frequent than in the general population.[47]

The EEG abnormalities usually reflect cerebral immaturity rather than structural disease. Children with normal intelligence but selective conduct disorder may or may not have EEG abnormalities, but their absence does not rule out the possibility of selective immaturity of part of the brain which controls conduct. Furthermore, the presence and extent of EEG abnormalities bear no relation to the natural course of the psychiatric disease. However, because of the possibility of brain immaturity causing the child's conduct disorder, psychotherapeutic methods that rely heavily on the child's cooperation are often impracticable, and certainly methods that rely on intelligent cooperation may not be helpful for severely retarded children. In such cases, behavior modification techniques and use of drugs offer greater promise.

CHANGES IN PREVALENCE

The incidence of a disorder is the frequency with which it arises in a population during a stated period of time. The prevalence of the disorder is its amount within a population at a given time. The prevalence of a condition thus is the product of its incidence and its duration. Prevalence may therefore increase although incidence remains constant or even falls, if longevity increases. This has occurred with Down's syndrome. Its prevalence at the age of 10 years was 1/6000 in 1929 and 1/100 in 1960.[48]

Yet fewer such children are being born, perhaps because of an increasing reluctance on the part of older women to bear children. The main cause of death, respiratory infection, is now controllable by antibiotics and immunization. Death is mainly due to associated anomalies, but even these can now more often be surgically corrected. The prevalence in general of handicapped persons who have to be cared for by the community has risen, although the incidence of mental retardation syndromes other than Down's syndrome is also falling. This again attests to longer life for these children. Indeed, between 1950 and 1960, the peak incidence of death due to congenital anomalies shifted from below five to between five and fourteen years of age.[49]

Further decreases in prevalence could be effected if there were fewer conceptions among at risk populations, such as older women and carriers of unfavorable genes who have benefit of genetic counseling; and if chromosomal defects are diagnosed by amniocentesis and the pregnancies terminated, as can now be done with Down's syndrome[50] and some metabolic causes of retardation (see Chapter 1). Finally, the severely mentally retarded may be helped to achieve at the level of their limited potentials by suitable placement and education, and the more mildly retarded taught well enough to join the ranks of the dull normal. Already it is found that the prevalence of mild retardation decreases from the mid-twenties onward, as these people gradually leave institutions to assume adult responsibilities.[51]

MANAGEMENT

As far as is known, the central nervous system is not capable of significant regeneration and, for the vast majority of cases of mental retardation, specific methods for improving intelligence are not available. The necessary measures are to provide for appropriate placement which safeguards the child, and at the same time permits him to function at the level of his admittedly limited potential. Custodial care is usual when the IQ falls short of 50, but the child's temperament and socialization are important factors which can differ widely between individuals at a given IQ level. Taught at an appropriately slow rate, the educable retarded can often become vocationally self-dependent,[52] not only as manual laborers, but as domestic servants and in routine industrial tasks, such as assembly and production line operations. Best results are obtained in structured rather than flexible situations.[53] With lower grade defectives the need is for training in basic hygiene self-care and the control of self-mutilation. Operant conditioning techniques have had impressive success in these areas.[54]

A more extensive review of the subject of mental retardation can be found in the book by Masland and associates.[55]

INFANTILE AUTISM

An alternative to the diagnosis of mental retardation in the child who performs inadequately on measures of mental development is infantile autism. This syndrome was first described by Kanner in 1943.[56] He emphasized the characteristic features of a profound withdrawal from contact with people, an obsessive desire to preserve sameness, and a failure to use language for communication. While many parents of the initially described group of children were cold, isolated, or withdrawn individuals ("refrigerated"), other etiologic variables have been found, and it is now clear that infantile autism is a behavioral syndrome of multiple causation.

Clinical Manifestations

It is rare to find more than one autistic child within the same family. The incidence of pre- and perinatal complications is probably greater in the autistic group than in controls.[57] During the early years two courses of development may be followed: one group of autistic infants appears normal until 18–26 months of age, when they begin to regress, often in association with emotional or physical trauma;[58] the other type of child already appears to be unusual at an early age in that he has a reduced level of activity or diminished crying and seems content to be left alone. Solid foods are rejected, and toys elicit little interest, or are held onto with

unusual obstinacy. Motor development is normal, or even precocious. During the second year of life there is an unusual sensitivity to auditory, visual, tactile, and labyrinthine stimulation, and repetitive mannerisms or gestures begin to appear.

The typical older autistic child has a multitude of symptoms. These may be classified as disturbances of relating, language, motility, and perception.[59] Most often, disturbances in relating manifest themselves by poor or absent eye contact and a lack of interest in people who are used rather than related to. Toys are handled bizarrely or are dropped when given to the child.

Language disturbances may consist of a complete lack of speech, a failure to communicate by pointing, or echolalia—a repetition of words or phrases out of social context. When speech does develop it is atonal, pronouns are poorly used, and there is a lack of comprehension of humor.[60] Mechanical language skills, such as reading, are at times developed out of all proportion to spontaneous verbal expression and are obsessively indulged in.[61] Autistic speech differs qualitatively from speech of mentally subnormal children of the same mental age in that subnormal children, within the limit of their sparse vocabulary, use it normally in a linguistic sense, while autistic children fail to use sentences either to organize their speech or to organize their memories.[62]

Disturbed motility manifests itself by repetitive, stereotyped movements, such as hand flapping, ear flicking, or head banging.[63] Toe walking, whirling, or rocking are also common. These movements, often complex in nature, become increasingly prominent when the child is anxious or is confronted with a novel situation.

There is a heightened sensitivity to a variety of stimuli, notably self-induced sounds or spinning objects. This may alternate with periods of nonresponsiveness to speech, objects, or pain. Sounds are also ignored, so that many autistic children are screened for presumptive deafness.

While the above picture pertains to the typical child with severe autism, transient or milder degrees of autistic behavior are common and perhaps more frequent than

Stuttering cannot be a disorder of auditory feedback because speech, like any highly practiced and automatized process, is not under continual feedback control. But it does seem that stutterers are unable to disengage their attention from their own speech, which therefore cannot become automatic. Stuttering is relieved by use of a loud noise that masks speech sounds, and it is very rare among the deaf.[82]

The stutterer has difficulty in passing smoothly from phoneme to phoneme. He explosively reiterates a single sound or blocks completely. He has most difficulty at the beginning of sentences, and of words of more than five letters. The severity of the disorder is situationally determined. Moments of self-consciousness and embarrassment yield maximal impediment, whereas distraction may result temporarily in nearly normal speech. Singing is mysteriously spared. Remedial methods divide into those which provide disincentive for stuttering (behavior modification) and those which address themselves to the disordered speech either by teaching patients to modify it to a more intelligible though still abnormal form (such as so-called syllabic speech) and those which release normal speech by use of a variety of distractions.[83] Typically most remedial methods will be temporarily effective, but the condition usually relapses.

Stuttering does not appear secondarily to organic brain disease, and therefore neurologic investigation is not needed. There is no justification for trying to modify children's hand preference to control stuttering.

ONTOGENESIS OF CEREBRAL DOMINANCE FOR LANGUAGE

In contrast to those of nonhuman primates, the human cerebral hemispheres are laterally specialized for certain cognitive functions. Notably, lesion and stimulation effects on behavior show that in almost all right-handers the left hemisphere is primarily concerned with neural processes underlying language, as well as the decoding of sensory stimuli and the programming of motor sequences. Some deficits in tasks that are not overtly verbal have been reported in children with language delay, notably in discriminating time differentials between rapidly successive clicks.[84] In respect of other functions like orientation in space and the spatial organization of nonverbal patterns, there is a less striking but definite asymmetry in favor of the right hemisphere.[85] This hemispheric specialization evolves progressively during the first decade of life.

The newborn infant shows no hemispheric specialization; indeed, his cerebrum is barely functional. Yet even at this early stage most infants show a bias toward turning their heads and eyes to the right rather than left, a turning tendency which will subsequently come under left hemisphere control. Congenital left hemispheric maldevelopment, and destruction in the context of acute infantile hemiplegia in the first year leads to no gross language disorder or delay; the right hemisphere assumes language representation,[86] the patient's general intellectual potential rather than specifically his language facility is reduced. The older the child is when left hemisphere destruction occurs, the less is the effect on general intelligence and the more on language. Preschoolers show transitory language deficits, but only toward the end of the first decade does the language disorder assume the characteristic severity and persistence of adult aphasia. Not only is there contralateral compensation for early lateralized lesions, but even bilateral disease of the potential (peri-Sylvian) language areas can be compensated for to a remarkable extent if sustained early in life.[87]

The ontogeny of the non-language functions that are asymmetrically represented is not yet elucidated. Presumably the changes over time resemble those for language.

There is considerable variability in the evolution of cerebral dominance, not only subsequent to disease, but also within the ostensibly normal population. The differentiation of limb preference is a rough guide, in that earlier emergence of handedness may reflect earlier hemispheric specialization. Some children who are late to manifest consistent handedness also show transient cognitive immaturities that result in school problems, but the relationship is too inconstant to be clinically useful in individual diagnosis.

The process of lateralization of language

involves not only increase of left hemisphere control of language but also an inhibition of the potential language processes on the right. Massive left hemisphere lesions release this inhibition, while disconnection of the hemispheres by callosal section reveals that the right hemisphere has the capability of decoding at least simple speech messages. The same is observed while the left hemisphere is temporarily anesthetized by means of the intracarotid injection of amobarbital.[88] The patient remains responsive to verbal commands as indicated by his facial and left hand movements. This perhaps explains the rarity of permanent total receptive aphasia; right hemisphere compensation for language disorder[89] is more complete for language decoding than encoding functions.

In view of the fact that early lateralized hemisphere lesions do not result in aphasia, the origins of language delay have to be sought elsewhere. The natural history of language delay, particularly the striking male predominance, support a genetic origin for at least some instances of this condition.

LANGUAGE DEVELOPMENT

Precursors

Even in the first six weeks of life, infants vocalize in the context of certain reflexes, notably when they orient by head and gaze turning and hand pointing (tonic neck reflex) to a novel stimulus. Subsequently babbling begins and soon includes the production of all the phonemes in human languages. Babbling is both spontaneous and imitative of the speech of others. While some severely retarded children are late to begin babbling, the characteristics of babbling when it occurs do not predict the quality of the language that will follow. Nor is babbling causally involved in the origin of language. When a child is precluded from babbling by long-term tracheotomy, this does not retard the development of speech once the aperture is closed. Babbling is not initially supported by auditory feedback; even profoundly deaf children babble.[90] However, toward the end of the first year, the deaf child's babbling diminishes and he falls silent.

Early Language

At around age one year, children begin to utter single words, of which "mama" and "dada" are often but unreliably reported first by parents. By 18 months, the child will be able to utter half a dozen distinguishable words, and after age two, words begin to be strung together in phrases. The excellence of a child's language development can be determined by use of measures such as the Peabody Picture Vocabulary Test,[91] in terms of developmental norms. At all stages children can understand more words and phrases than they can utter, and substantial comprehension of spoken speech may develop in the absence of vocalization.[92]

CAUSES OF LANGUAGE RETARDATION

Secondary and General

Imperfect language development follows a variety of patterns that depend on its pathogenesis. In the context of general mental retardation, speech is impoverished with regard to vocabulary and syntax,[93] but articulation is less affected. Even in the absence of cerebral structural lesions, as in Down's syndrome, delayed language maturation produces relative ultimate abnormality, because in these children, as in normals, language development is virtually complete by age 14.[90] The twin who shares a secret language with his fellow twin sounds coherent though incomprehensible and rapidly transfers to normal language when the twins are separated. The congenitally deaf child is silent until specifically taught when—if the deafness is of the customary type in which high frequencies bear the brunt of the deficit—he adopts a harsh "deaf tone." At times, children abruptly become deaf, usually as a consequence of meningitis. The effect depends on the stage of language development.[94] Children less than five years old gradually lose their ability to control articulation and voice production and behave increasingly like the congenitally deaf. However, even only one year of language experience makes it substantially easier to train children in language skills than the congenitally deaf. However, children who become deaf before age two become indistinguishable from the congenitally deaf. The early provision of hearing aids and training for all deaf children clinically improves their language progress.[95] Three million American children have hearing deficits; 0.1% of the school population is deaf, and 1.5% hard of hearing. Sixty percent of these are congenital, and most of the rest result from meningitis (see p. 169). Although deafness often goes unnoticed even by intelligent parents when a bright child uses contextual cues to guide his behavior, it can be suspected as early as $4\frac{1}{2}$ to 6 months of age if a child fails to move his eyes in the direction of a sound source beyond his visual field. In young children, free field audiometry is used for definitive diagnosis, which should be as early as possible so that the child does not go without appropriate language training (after the fitting of hearing aids, if these are shown to help) and does not acquire the recalcitrant habit of ignoring auditory stimuli. Blind children of normal intelligence tend to learn to speak slowly and they lack imitative gesture. The emotionally disturbed child may withhold speech either permanently, or only outside the home (so-called elective mutism)[96] but often will comprehend well. In infantile autism, speech is not only limited but pervaded by echolalia, stereotypic utterances and avoidance of the personal pronoun "I."[71] The rare normal child totally deprived of language experience will not speak but will rapidly learn once the opportunity is offered (unless he is secondarily emotionally disturbed). "Culturally deprived" children's language reflects local speaking patterns which are better described as deviant than as impaired. On formal tests that rely on middle class norms such children score poorly. Extreme instances of children isolated from language such as "wolf children"[97] have been reported, but even six years of total deprivation can, it is said, be overcome.[98] The notion of a "critical period" for language development lacks proof.[94]

Primary

Selective language delay, described as early as 1825,[99] results in speech that is not only late in developing, and semantically and syntactically impoverished as is language in mental retardation, but also characterized by severe articulatory disorder. This differs from speech defects such as stuttering, cluttering, lisping, and cleft palate nasality not only in its greater severity and wider range of affected phonemes, but in the far greater difficulty these children have in making the transition from phoneme to phoneme than in pronouncing the phonemes individually. This results in grossly curtailed word formation. Also, short binding words ("function" rather than "content" words) are frequently omitted. In contrast to the relatively fixed deficits of speech disorder, delayed ("dysphasic") language is very sensitive to context, and sound combinations that can be uttered at one time are unavailable at another. Greater mental effort often results in worse rather than better performance. The disorder is not limited to the spoken language. It includes not only writing but also metalanguages such as lip reading, finger language, and braille. Language delay invariably involves expressive speech, and verbal memory is also impaired. Speech comprehension may be relatively spared though these children have difficulty in discriminating speech sounds. When comprehension is severely affected—the "congenital auditory imperception" of Worster-Drought[100]—it is often initially mistaken for peripheral deafness. However, the clinical impression of fluctuation—which leads parents to suspect a functional element—is born out by audiometry in which stable thresholds are hard to obtain, and repeated testing is apt to lead to radically different audiometric profiles. Recording psychogalvanic skin responses to sound may then be informative. These instabilities are due to inconstant focusing of attention on the auditory modality,[101] a function normally subserved by the relevant cortical areas, had they not been underdeveloped.

A rare form of acquired aphasia in children[102] begins between the ages of five and six years with one or more seizures followed by a gradual loss of comprehension of speech, and finally loss of speech expression also. The only investigative abnormality is the presence of bitemporal focal discharge on EEG.[102a]

The condition may be spontaneously reversible or may improve with the use of anticonvulsant medication.

INVESTIGATION

The basic investigating tool is the intelligence test, by virtue of which the selective nature of the disorder is verified. Audiometry will exclude cases secondary to simple deafness, or it may reveal the fluctuating impairments of "cortical deafness." The language behavior itself is evaluated by one of the standard language test batteries.[103] Physical examination will reveal the role of mechanical and motor deficit of the vocal apparatus. Where emotional blocks are in question, projective testing may amplify clinical insights into the roots of the causative emotional maladjustment. In rare instances in which receptive aphasia and deafness resist clinical differentiation, the elicitation of auditory evoked potentials confirms the integrity of the auditory projections to cortex.

Classic neurologic procedures in search of structural intracranial disease (skull radiography, electroencephalography, neuro-radiologic procedures) are often undertaken, but the yield of practically useful information is trivial. Very occasionally, subclinical seizures are detected by EEG and thought to disrupt cognitive processes.[102a] In such cases, effective anticonvulsant management or, less often, excision of circumscribed foci defined at electrocorticography materially improves cognition.

MANAGEMENT

Language delay on an organic basis resists remedial methods. The greatest use of speech therapy is in improving children's articulatory skills.[104] Certain amplification techniques[104] and reinforcement techniques[105] help teach children to attend to spoken speech. But the central problem of impoverished vocabulary and syntax, and the resulting difficulty in verbal thought, is resistant to management, and the so-called "enrichment" techniques are unrewarding. Under these circumstances, it becomes important to re-create parental expectations with the realities of what is often an enduring problem, and to

organize the child's education so as to give him the opportunity to learn optimally at an admittedly limited rate. Individual tuition is usually required, and family therapy and behavior modification is often needed on account of secondary emotional disorder which usually involves the whole family unit.

LEARNING DISABILITY

INTRODUCTION

Unexpected school failure increasingly occasions referral for neurologic assessment. Some children who have ostensibly normal intelligence and are willing to learn do not benefit to the usual extent from conventional methods of education. In these cases, the question of a cognitive limitation on certain forms of learning arises. Terms applied to this situation variously emphasize an assumed neurologic basis ("minimal cerebral dysfunction"), a supposed perceptual deficit ("word blindness"), or the seemingly isolated character of the disorder ("dyslexia"), which is also often termed selective or specific, and hypothesized to be "organic" or "developmental." Such terms are distracting. Preoccupation with the brain basis of the difficulty may lead to investigations the outcome of which do not help in planning the child's future. Assumptions about the mechanism of the cognitive deficit preclude a rational search for exactly what the child finds particularly difficult to understand or remember. The "diagnostic" term "dyslexia" merely restates the problem and breeds the assumption that these cases are relatively homogeneous and amenable to one particular form of management. In fact, however, they are quite heterogeneous and require individualized remedial programs. Terms that describe the problem are preferable. If reading and writing only are selectively at fault, there is a selective reading disability. Selective arithmetic and drawing disabilities similarly occur but are much less frequently brought to clinical attention (unless the drawing disability involves the misshaping of letters). This is both because social pressure is concentrated on reading, and because schools use written texts as vehicles for all forms of learning and do so increasingly as possibility of copying are minimized, achievement tests[131,132] are helpful. The degree of underachievement that warrants clinical attention is a matter of definition, but a lag of two years behind the norm is always accepted as significant, and a one-year lag usually is.

Given that the achievement failure is real, and general intellect adequate, it becomes important to determine the extent of the child's motivation to learn. A teacher's report on classroom behavior is insisted upon and may be supplemented by a telephone conversation. If motivation is inadequate, the reason may be primary: a behavior deviancy often involving the whole family unit, an impulsive or hurried approach to the task,[115] or cultural differences with alienation from middle-class educational aspirations. Or the lack of motivation may be secondary to cumulative failure based on a learning disability in the face of mounting school and parental pressure to achieve.

If the evidence favors learning disability, there is sometimes a family history of similar problems;[124] the child, who is usually male,[114] will in perhaps half the cases show "soft signs" on neurologic examination. These are more likely when there is a primary attentional component than when the disorder is purely cognitive. At times the learning difficulty occurs in the context of frank cerebral palsy. The presence of positive family history and neurologic abnormalities may be used as circumstantial evidence in deciding between a social or cultural and a developmental cause for the learning difficulty. But neither positive family history nor neurologic abnormality offers any help in locating the limitation on performance, whether cognitive or attentional, or in assigning prognosis. For these purposes, it is necessary to scrutinize the psychiatric data, to perform further tests, and to find out what kind of mistakes the child makes.

Even though the full-scale intelligence quotient is normal, there may be "scatter" among tests within the scale, and the pattern of scatter may suggest the nature of the cognitive limitation. Some children score substantially less well on the verbal than the performance subscale of the WISC; a less common pattern is a lower performance than verbal score, with particular deficit on the performance subtests of block design and object assembly, as well as on arithmetic.[116] The children with verbal deficit yield a history of delayed language development, and their mistakes in reading and spelling suggest that they find it difficult to allocate appropriate letter sounds to a given word. The children with performance deficit, in contrast, make mistakes of letter sequence rather than letter choice. Their difficulty in remembering sequence is further illustrated in arithmetic, where they make errors in manipulations (such as subtraction) which involve the relative position of digits. Failure on tests of "finger order sense"[133] is similarly accounted for by a difficulty in making use of information about relative position. Finally, although most normal children can distinguish between their right and their left by seven years of age,[134] performance deficit children are delayed in right-left discrimination.

Another pattern is that of the child, often left-handed, who has a normal psychometric profile but occasionally reads or writes from right to left. Although these mistakes attract much attention, they are transient and of little consequence. They perhaps reflect incomplete or lacking left-hemisphere lateralization of language. A much publicized form of error is the mirror-image reversal of letters, which occurs in normal children who are not yet ready to learn to read and in some older but selectively immature children who have difficulty in the initial stages of reading. These children are showing developmental lags which are often transient. Where an enduring reading disability presents, it does not take this form.

Where specialized facilities are unavailable, the pediatrician can use certain test instruments that do not require special training for administration or interpretation. These are listed in Table 13–2. Such measures will enable the clinician to determine whether disparities exist between the child's intelligence and achievement, and whether apparent underachievement could be accounted for on the basis of selective language or other cognitive deficit. Such

TABLE 13-2.
OFFICE TESTS USEFUL IN EVALUATION OF LEARNING DISORDERS

Modality	Test	Reference
Developmental diagnosis (younger children)	Denver Developmental Test	14
	Vineland Social Maturity Test	15
Developmental diagnosis (school-aged children)	Raven's Colored Progressive Matrices Test	135
	Wide Range Achievement Test	131
Language	Peabody Picture Vocabulary	91
	Tokens Test	136
Developmental Gerstmann syndrome (finger agnosia, right-left disorientation, dysgraphia, dyscalculia)	Finger Recognition Test	137
Visual-motor integration	Figure Copying Test	138
Visual memory	Benton Visual Retention Test	139
	Bender Gestalt Test	140
Right-left discrimination	Benton Right-Left Discrimination Test	141
Intersensory integration	Birch Auditory-Visual Integration Test	142

inferences may then be checked against the prevalent error type in reading and spelling.[143]

There are certain commonly instituted investigations of reading disability which rarely if ever yield useful information. These include the electroencephalogram, which is only useful in the rare educational difficulty which arises from undiagnosed minor epileptic states, which momentarily interrupt the child's attention with great frequency, so that he fails to follow trains of thought in class. Geier has found that on the average, generalized 3/sec. spike and wave discharges lasting $5\frac{1}{2}$ seconds or more will interfere with mental activity.[143a] (See Chapter 11.) It is necessary to rule out gross deficits of hearing and of vision as components in the problem. However, diminished visual acuity impairs reading only when vision is reduced by half or more.[144] Orthoptic investigation is unnecessary, because none of the forms of strabismus results in learning disorder,[145] and strabismus is no more common in slow readers than among normal children.[146]

An ideal that is far from being realized is the prediction of reading failure in preschool children who are not mentally retarded. Reading readiness tests[147] do have a measure of success but rely unduly on establishing whether the entering first grader can already read. Also, the outcome does not specify the failing child's area of weakness and thus is no guide to how he should be taught. One study[148] reported 10 tests which, when combined, identified 91% of kindergarten children who later failed at the end of second grade. The test selection was empirical and will be replaced by more rational procedures when the precursors of reading readiness have been defined. In the meantime it has to be recognized that selective learning disability, as opposed to learning failures that arise from adverse social and economic circumstances,[148a] cannot be predicted, and it follows that group readiness testing is best performed shortly before school entry but soon enough to enable decisions based on the outcome to be implemented before schools' openings for the coming year are filled.

MANAGEMENT

The clinician has to clarify the situation and to dispose of a host of incorrect or irrelevant notions that are current about learning failure. He seeks to reconcile the aspirations of the parents and teachers with the realities of the case and to counteract feelings of guilt. He defines and attempts to

65. Rutter, M.: The influence of organic and emotional factors on the origins, nature and outcome of childhood psychosis, Develop. Med. Child Neurol. 7:518, 1965.

66. Eisenberg, L.: The autistic child in adolescence, Amer. J. Psychiat. 112:607, 1956.

67. Rutter, M.: Concepts of autism: A review of research, J. Child Psychol. Psychiat. 9:1, 1968.

68. Bergman, P. and Escalona, S. K.: Unusual sensitivities in very young children, Psychoanal. Stud. Child 3/4:333, 1949.

69. Rimland, B.: *Infantile Autism*, New York: Appleton-Century-Crofts, 1964.

70. Mahler, M. S. and Gosliner, B. J.: On symbiotic child psychosis, Psychoanal. Stud. Child 10:195, 1955.

71. Bettelheim, B.: *The Empty Fortress; Infantile Autism and the Birth of the Self*, New York: Free Press, 1967.

72. Spitz, R. A.: The psychogenic disease in infancy, Psychoanal. Stud. Child 6:255, 1951.

73. Mahler, M. S.: On childhood psychosis and schizophrenia, autistic and symbiotic infantile psychoses, Psychoanal. Stud. Child 7:286, 1952.

74. Stone, A. A.: Consciousness: Altered levels in blind retarded children, Psychosom. Med. 26:14, 1964.

75. Hollis, J. H.: Differential responses of profoundly retarded children to social stimulation, Psychol. Rep. 16:977, 1965.

75a.Tanguay, P. E.: A pediatrician's guide to the recognition and initial management of early infantile autism, Pediatrics 51:903, 1973.

76. ASHA Committee on the Mid-Century White House Conference: Speech disorders and speech correction, J. Speech Hearing Dis. 17:129, 1952.

77. Travis, L. E.: *Handbook of Speech Pathology and Audiology*, New York: Appleton-Century-Crofts, 1971.

78. Worster-Drought, C.: Congenital suprabulbar paresis, J. Laryng. 70: 453, 1956.

79. Bryngelson, B.: Sidedness as an etiological factor in stuttering, J. Genet. Psychol. 47:204, 1935.

80. Orton, S. T.: Some studies on the language function, Res. Pub. Ass. Nerv. Ment. Dis. 13:614, 1934.

81. Jones, R. K.: Observations on stammering after localized cerebral injury, J. Neurol. Neurosurg. Psychiat. 29:192, 1966.

82. Backus, O.: Incidence of stuttering among the deaf, Ann. Otol. 47:632, 1938.

83. Biggs, B. and Shehan, J.: Punishment or Distraction? Operant stuttering revisited, J. Abnorm. Psychol. 74:256, 1969.

84. Lowe, A. D. and Campbell, R. A.: Temporal discrimination in aphasoid and normal children, J. Speech Hearing Res. 8:313, 1965.

85. Kinsbourne, M.: "Lateralization of Human Cerebral Function," in Goldensohn, E. S. and Appel, S. H.: *Shy's The Cellular and Molecular Basis of Neurologic Disease*, Philadelphia: Lea & Febiger, in press.

86. Basser, L. S.: Hemiplegia of early onset and the faculty of speech with special reference to the effects of hemispherectomy, Brain 85:427, 1962.

87. Landau, W. M., Goldstein, R., and Kleffner, F. R:: Congenital aphasia; a clinicopathologic study, Neurology (Minneap.) 10:915, 1960.

88. Wada, J. and Rasmussen, T.: Intracarotid injection of sodium amytal for the lateralization of cerebral speech dominance: Experimental and clinical observations, J. Neurosurg. 17:266, 1960.

89. Kinsbourne, M.: The minor cerebral hemisphere as a source of aphasic speech, Arch. Neurol. 25:302, 1971.

90. Lenneberg, E. H.: Understanding language without ability to speak: A case report, J. Abnorm. Soc. Psychol. 65:419, 1962.

91. Dunn, L. M.: *Peabody Picture Vocabulary Test*, Minneapolis: American Guidance Service, 1959.

92. Lenneberg, E. H., Rebelsky, F. G., and Nichols, I. A.: The vocalization of infants born to deaf and to hearing parents, Vita Hum. 8:23, 1965.

93. O'Connor, N. and Hermelin, B.: *Speech and Thought in Severe Sub-normality*, Oxford: Pergamon Press, 1963.

94. Lenneberg, E. H.: *Biological Foundations of Language*, New York: John Wiley and Sons, Inc., 1967.

95. Fry, D. B.: "The Development of the Phonological System in the Normal and Deaf Child," in Smith, F. and Miller, G. A.: *The Genesis of Language: A Psycholinguistic Approach*, Cambridge: M.I.T. Press, 1966.

96. Reed, G. F.: Elective mutism in children: A reappraisal, J. Child Psychol. Psychiat. 4:99, 1963.

97. Singh, J. A. L. and Zingg, R. M.: *Wolf Children and Feral Man*, New York: Harper & Row Publishers, 1942.

98. Davis, K.: Final note on a case of extreme isolation, Amer. J. Sociol. 52:432, 1947.

99. Gall, F.: *On the Function of the Brain and Each of its Parts*, vols. 1–6, Phrenological Library, Boston: March, Capen and Lyon, 1825.

100. Worster-Drought, C. and Allen, I. M.: Congenital auditory imperception (congenital word deafness) with report of a case, J. Neurol. Psychopath. 9:193, 1929.

101. Myklebust, H. R.: *Auditory Disorders in Children: A Manual for Differential Diagnosis*, New York: Grune & Stratton, Inc., 1954.

102. Worster-Drought, C.: An unusual form of acquired aphasia in children, Folia Phoniat. (Basel) 16:223, 1964.

102a.Landau, W. M. and Kleffner, F. R.: Syndrome of acquired aphasia with convulsive disorder in children, Neurology (Minneap.) 7:523, 1957.

103. Spradlin, J. E.: "Procedures for Evaluating Processes Associated with Receptive and Expressive Language," Schiefelbusch, R. L., Copeland, R. H., and Smith, J. O. (eds.). *Language and Mental Retardation*, New York: Holt, Rinehart, & Winston, p. 118, 1967.

104. Van Riper, C. G.: *Speech Correction: Principles and Methods*, Englewood Cliffs: Prentice-Hall, Inc., 1963.
105. Sloane, H. N. and MacAulay, B. D. (eds.): *Operant Procedures in Remedial Speech and Language Training*, Boston: Houghton Mifflin, 1968.
106. Alwitt, L. F.: Decay of immediate memory for visually presented digits among non-readers and readers, J. Educ. Psychol. 54:144, 1963.
107. Birch, H. G. and Belmont, L.: Auditory-visual integration in normal and retarded readers, Amer. J. Orthopsychiat. 34:852, 1964.
108. Muehl, S. and Kremenak, S.: Ability to match information within and between auditory and visual sense modalities and subsequent reading achievement, J. Educ. Psychol. 57:230, 1966.
109. Belmont, L. and Birch, H. G.: Lateral dominance, lateral awareness and reading disability, Child Develop. 36:57, 1965.
110. Conners, C. K., Kramer, K. and Guerra, F.: Auditory synthesis and dichotic listening in children with learning disabilities, J. Spec. Educ. 3:163, 1969.
111. Bakker, D. J.: "Temporal Order Perception and Reading Retardation," in Bakker, D. J. and Satz, P. (eds.): *Specific Reading Disability*, Rotterdam: Rotterdam University Press, 1968.
112. Schenk, V. W. D.: Dyslexia and spatial disorientation, Psychiat. Neurol. Neurochir. 69: 337, 1967.
113. Rutter, M.: "The Concept of Dyslexia," in Wolff, D. H. and MacKeith, R. (eds.): *Planning for Better Learning Clinics for Developmental Medicine* 33, London: Heinemann Medical Books, Ltd., 1969, p. 129.
114. Critchley, M.: *Developmental Dysplexia*, London: Heinemann Medical Books, Ltd., 1964.
115. Kagan, J.: Reflection-impulsivity and reading ability in primary grade children, Child Develop. 36:609, 1965.
116. Kinsbourne, M. and Warrington, E. K.: Developmental factors in reading and writing backwardness, Brit. J. Psychol. 54:145, 1963.
117. Singer, H. and Ruddell, R. B.: *Theoretical Models and Processes of Reading*, Newark, Delaware: International Reading Association, 1970.
118. Chall, J.: *Learning to Read: The Great Debate*, New York: McGraw-Hill Book Co., 1967.
119. Satz, P., Rardin, D., and Ross, J.: An evaluation of a theory of specific developmental dyslexia, Child Develop. 42:2009, 1971.
120. Kinsbourne, M.: Minimal cerebral dysfunction as a neurodevelopmental lag, Ann. NY Acad. Sci. 205:268, 1972.
121. Orton, S. T.: *Reading, Writing and Speech Problems in Children*, London: Chapman and Hall, 1937.
122. Zangwill, O. L.: *Cerebral Dominance and its Relation to Psychological Function*, London: Oliver and Boyd, 1960.
123. Monroe, M.: *Children Who Cannot Read*, Chicago: The University of Chicago Press, 1932.
124. Hallgren, B.: Specific dyslexia: Cognitive word blindness, Acta Psychiat. Neurol. Suppl. 65, 1950.
125. Hermann, K.: *Reading Disability*, Springfield: Charles C Thomas Publisher, 1959.
126. Sabatino, D. A. and Becker, J. T.: Relationship between lateral preference and selected behavioral variables for children failing academically, Child Develop. 42:2055, 1971.
127. Hecaen, H. and de Ajuriaguerra, J.: *Left-Handedness*, New York: Grune & Stratton, Inc., 1964.
128. Annett, M.: "Handedness, Cerebral Dominance and the Growth of Intelligence," in Bakker, D. J. and Satz, P. (eds.): *Specific Reading Disability*, Rotterdam: Rotterdam University Press, 1970.
129. Zangwill, O. L.: "Dyslexia in Relation to Cerebral Dominance," in Money, J. (ed.): *Reading Disability: Progress and Research Needs in Dyslexia*, Baltimore: Johns Hopkins Press, 1962.
130. Otis, A. S.: *Otis Group Intelligence Scale*, Eng. ed., London, George G. Harrap & Co., Ltd., 1948.
131. Jastak, J. and Bijou, S.: *Wide Range Achievement Test*, rev. ed., New York: Psychological Corporation, 1965.
132. Gates, A.: *Gates Primary Reading Test*, New York: Bureau of Publication, Columbia University, 1958.
133. Kinsbourne, M.: Developmental Gerstmann syndrome: A disorder of sequencing, Pediat. Clin. N. Amer. 15:771, 1968.
134. Benton, A. L.: *Right-Left Discrimination and Finger Localization*, New York: Hoeber Medical Division, Harper & Row Publishers, 1959.
135. Raven's Colored Progressive Matrices. Psychological Corporation (H. K. Lewis & Co., Ltd), 1947–1963.
136. Tokens Test. Reported by de Renzi, E. and Vignolo, L. A., in Brain 85:665, 1962.
137. Kinsbourne, M. and Warrington, E. K.: The developmental Gerstmann syndrome, Arch. Neurol. 8:490, 1963.
138. Beery, K. E. and Butenica, K. A.: *Developmental Test of Visual-Motor Integration Test*, Chicago: Follett Educational Corporation.
139. *Benton Visual Retention Test*, Psychological Corporation, 1946–1955.
140. Bender, L.: *A Visual Motor Gestalt Test, and its Use*, New York, American Orthopsychiatric Association, 1938.
141. Benton, A. L.: Right-left discrimination, Pediat. Clin. N. Amer. 15:747, 1968.
142. Birch, H. G. and Belmont, L.: Auditory-visual integration in retarded readers, Amer. J. Orthopsychiat. 34:852, 1964.
143. Boder, E.: "Developmental Dyslexia: Prevailing Diagnostic Concepts and a New Diagnostic Approach through Patterns of Reading and Spelling," in Myklebust, H. R. (ed.): *Progress in Learning Disabilities*, vol. II, New York: Grune & Stratton, Inc., 1971.
143a. Geier, S.: Minor seizures and behavior, Electroenceph. Clin. Neurophysiol. 31:499, 1971.

Index

Page numbers in *italics* refer to illustrations; page numbers followed by t refer to tables and by n to footnotes.

Rash—(*Continued*)
   ethosuximide and, 444
   maculopapular, roseola and, 247
   measles encephalomyelitis and, 297
R. akari, rickettsialpox and, 269
   meningococcal meningitis and, 221
   mephenytoin and, 443
   methicillin and, 227
   morbilliform, diphenylhydantoin and, 443
   in Rocky Mountain spotted fever, 270
Rattlesnakes, neurologic symptoms from, 349t
Raven's Colored Progressive Matrices Test, 505t
Reaction. *See also* Reflex(es), Response *and specific*
      reactions
   labyrinthine accelerating, 190t
   "parachute," 192, *192*
   placing, 190t
Reading, ability, infantile autism and, 495
   associative complex for, 502
   auditory complex for, 502
   disability, selective, 501, 502
   readiness tests for, 505
   reflex seizure and, 434t
   remedial, learning disability and, 506
   visual complex for, 502
Reanastomosis, peripheral nerve injuries and, 334
Rebound phenomenon, cerebellar tumors and, 392
Reflex epilepsy(ies), 456
Reflex(es). *See also* Reaction, Response
   abdominal, spinal cord injuries and, 329
      abdominal, tuberculous meningitis and, 225
   in acute hemiparesis, 204
   ankle, in Duchenne muscular dystrophy, 473
   in ataxia-telangiectasia, 414
   biceps, in Erb-Duchenne paralysis, 208
   cardiovascular, 189
   crossed adductor, to quadriceps jerk, 190t
   crossed extensor, 190t
   coughing, 189
   extensor, spinal cord injuries and, 329
   extensor thrust, in "floppy infants," 466
   flexion, 189
   grasp, 190t, 208
      palmar, hemiplegia and, 197
   Landau, 191
   Moro, 190t, 191, 193
      in anencephaly, 131
      in Erb-Duchenne paralysis, 208
      in familial dysautonomia, 100
      in galactosemia, 26
      in kernicterus, 346
      Klumpke paralysis and, 208
   neck-righting, 190t
   in newborn, 189
   patellar, in Sydenham's chorea, 287
   plantar, barbiturate intoxication and, 344
   polymyxin B and, 228
   postural, 190t
   pupillary accommodation, paralysis of, in botulism,
      347
   sneezing, 189
   stretch, 190t, 192
   sucking, 189
   swallowing, 189

Reflex(es)—(*Continued*)
   tendon, Achilles, peroneal nerve injury and, 333t
      deep, acute cerebellar ataxia and, 307
         acute infectious polyneuritis and, 302
         barbiturate intoxication and, 344
         in benign congenital hypotonias, 466
         brain abscess and, 230t
         brain stem tumor and, 396
         cerebellar tumors and, 392
         in dermatomyositis, 477
         in grand mal epilepsy, 425
         hemiplegia and, 197
         hypokalemic periodic paralysis and, 481
         in infantile muscular atrophy, 464
         Klumpke paralysis and, 208
         in muscular dystrophy, 471, 473, 474
         in myasthenia gravis, 483
         paralytic poliomyelitis and, 244, 245
         peripheral nerve injuries and, 332
         rabies and, 257
         spastic diplegia and, 196
         in spastic infant, 191
         spinal cord injury and, 206, 329
         spinal cord tumors and, 405
         in Sydenham's chorea, 287
         transverse myelitis and, 295
         tuberculous meningitis and, 225
   tonic neck, 190t, 193
      language development and, 499
      obligatory, extrapyramidal cerebral palsy and,
         198–199
      intelligence and, 199
   triceps, in Erb-Duchenne paralysis, 208
Reflex seizure, epileptic, 434t
Refsum's disease, *51*, 54–55, *55*, 93, 96, 303t
   chronic polyneuropathy in, 97
   diagnosis of, 68
      differential, 414
   progressive hereditary nerve deafness and, 99
REM (rapid eye movement) sleep, narcolepsy and,
   455
Renal disease, hypocalcemia and, 354t, 355
   hypomagnesemia and, 354t, 355
   neurologic complications of, 357–359
"Rennes" galactosemia, 25
Renuart screening test, for urinary MPS, 36–37
Reovirus, 241
   Reye's syndrome and, 271
Repetition, infantile autism and, 495
   mental retardation and, 494
Reptiles, neurologic symptoms from, 349t
Respiration, abnormalities of, neonatal, 190
   artificial, closed head injury and, 316
   difficulties with, in juvenile myasthenia gravis, 469t
      in neonatal meningitis, 223t
Response. *See also* Reflex(es), Reaction *and specific*
      responses
   Babinski, hemiplegia and, 197
   extensor plantar, acute infectious polyneuritis and,
      302
      brain abscess and, 230t
      brain stem tumor and, 396
      closed head injury and, 314
      in grand mal epilepsy, 424